Atlas of the Prostate

Third Edition

Editors

Peter T. Scardino, MD
Florence and Theodore Baumritter/ Enid Ancell Chair of Urologic Oncology
Department of Urology
Memorial Sloan-Kettering Cancer Center
New York, New York

Kevin M. Slawin, MD
Professor and Dan L. Duncan Family Chair in Prostate Disease
Scott Department of Urology
Director, Baylor Prostate Center
Baylor College of Medicine
Houston, Texas

With 42 contributors

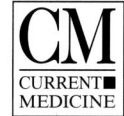

Developed by Current Medicine LLC
Philadelphia

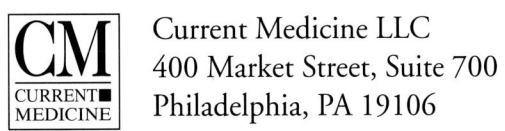 Current Medicine LLC
400 Market Street, Suite 700
Philadelphia, PA 19106

Director of Editorial, Design, Production	Wendy Vetter
Developmental Editor	Annmarie Piacentino
Editorial Assistant	Colleen Downing
Cover Design	William C. Whitman, Jr.
Design and Layout	William C. Whitman, Jr. and Christine Keller-Quirk
Illustrators	Wieslawa Langenfeld, Maureen Looney
Production Manager	Lori Holland
Assistant Production Manager	Margaret La Mare
Indexer	Holly Lukens

Library of Congress Cataloging-in-Publication Data

Atlas of the prostate.-- 3rd ed. / editors, Peter T. Scardino, Kevin M. Slawin ; with 42
contributors.
     p. ; cm.
  Includes bibliographical references and index.
  ISBN 1-57340-229-X (alk. paper)
 1. Prostate--Diseases--Atlases.
  [DNLM: 1. Prostatic Neoplasms--Atlases. 2. Prostatectomy--Atlases. 3. Prostatic
Hyperplasia--Atlases. 4. Prostatitis--Atlases. WJ 17 A88178 2006] I. Scardino, Peter T.
II. Slawin, Kevin M.
  RC899.A86 2006
  616.6'5--dc22

                       2005053786

ISBN 1-57340-229-X

For more information, please call 1 (800) 427-1796 or (215) 574-2266 or email us at inquiry@phl.cursci.com
www.current-science-group.com

10 9 8 7 6 5 4 3 2 1

Printed in Hong Kong by Paramount Printing Co, LTD

This book was printed on acid-free paper.

PREFACE

The medical and surgical management of prostatic diseases has undergone dramatic change in the past five years. Advances in medical imaging, laparoscopic and robot-assisted surgery, genetic research, new predictive tools, and new options for patients with advanced prostate cancer have transformed the way we work. Prospective randomized trials evaluating medical therapy for benign prostatic hyperplasia (BPH) have established that these drugs not only relieve symptoms, but also substantially reduce the risk of progression to acute urinary retention or the need for surgical intervention. Well-designed, randomized trials of herbal therapies for BPH have finally clarified many issues surrounding complimentary and alternative medicines for BPH therapy. Trials of common, therapeutic options for the treatment of chronic prostatitis have also changed long-standing views regarding this disease, so long an enigma to urologists and affected patients.

Evaluation of the patient with prostate cancer has also changed substantially. The focus is no longer on detection of metastases with bone or CT scan. With systematic biopsies and modum endorectal MRI with spectroscopy, we now expect to determine the size, location, and extent of the cancer in and around the prostate. With these studies, it is now feasible to tailor treatment to each patient and his particular cancer. Modern medical informatics has provided tools (nomograms) that allow for more accurate assessment, prediction of pathologic stage, and prognosis for the individual patient. With more accurate characterization of tumors, these nomograms will continually be improved. Available online, nomograms offer a rapid method for physicians and their patients to use in assessing the seriousness of their cancer.

Simultaneously, surgery for prostate cancer has undergone its own revolution. Laparoscopic surgery, whether free-hand or robotically-assisted, has caught the attention of the public as well as the medical profession. Regardless of the technique used, radical prostatectomy remains one of the most challenging operations in urology. The outcomes (cancer control and recovery of urinary and sexual function) are strongly related to the technical performance of the surgeon. The short-term benefits of laparoscopic surgery must be weighed against the difficulty of achieving surgical proficiency that produces the same long-term results in cancer control, continence, and potency as open surgery.

There have also been advances in radiation therapy. The development of intensity modulated radiotherapy (IMRT) followed the revolution achieved by 3-dimensional conformal techniques, and these approaches have enabled the delivery of higher dose radiation with markedly fewer complications than conventional therapy. The same technology is now being applied to brachytherapy, assuring optimum seed placement and minimizing complications. Finally, a host of new therapeutic options for patients with advanced prostate cancer are being proposed for FDA-approval, with the first effective chemotherapeutic agents for advanced, hormone-refractory prostate cancer already approved last year.

This third edition of the *Atlas of the Prostate* provides medical professionals with timely, straightforward, accessible, and well-illustrated descriptions of the very common diseases of the prostate and their management. We hope that this atlas, aimed at urologists in practice as well as those in training, will improve understanding of the rapidly changing environment of therapies for prostatitis, BPH, and prostate cancer.

Peter T. Scardino, MD
Kevin M. Slawin, MD

ACKNOWLEDGMENTS

The editors would like to thank the editorial staff at Memorial Sloan-Kettering Cancer Center - Barbara Kristaponis, Hope Lafferty, and Alixandra Gailunas - and Carolyn Schum at Baylor College of Medicine, for their patience, their tireless assistance, and their commitment to excellence that has been so important to achieving our goal of a thoroughly updated, scientifically sound, new edition of this atlas.

CONTRIBUTORS

Nelson E. Bennett, MD
Clinical Instructor
Department of Urology
Memorial Sloan-Kettering Cancer Center
Weill Medical College of Cornell University
New York, New York

Jeetesh Bhardwa, MBChB (UIC), MRCS (Eng)
Clinical Assistant in Urology
The London Clinic
London, England

Timothy B. Boone, MD, PhD
Professor and Chairman
Scott Department of Urology
Baylor College of Medicine;
Chief, Urology Service
The Methodist Hospital
Houston, Texas

Reginald C. Bruskewitz, MD
Professor of Surgery
Division of Urology
University of Wisconsin Medical School
Madison, Wisconsin

Mark K. Buyyounouski, MD
Associate Member
Attending Physician
Department of Radiation Oncology
Fox Chase Cancer Center
Philadelphia, Pennsylvania

Brett S. Carver, MD
Fellow
Department of Urology
Memorial Sloan-Kettering Cancer Center
New York, New York

Bob Djavan, MD
Vice Chairman
Department of Urology
University of Vienna Medical School
Vienna, Austria

James A. Eastham, MD
Associate Professor
Department of Urology
Memorial Sloan-Kettering Cancer Center
New York, New York

Ricardo R. Gonzalez, MD
Instructor
Department of Urology
Weill Medical College of Cornell University;
Assistant Attending Physician
New York Presbyterian Hospital
New York, New York

Bertrand D. Guillonneau, MD
Professor
Department of Urology
Weill Medical College of Cornell University;
Head of Minimally Invasive Surgery
Memorial Sloan-Kettering Cancer Center
New York, New York

Brian T. Helfand, MD, PhD
Resident
Department of Urology
Northwestern University Feinberg School
  of Medicine
Chicago, Illinois

William I. Jaffe, MD
Fellow
Department of Urology
Columbia University College of Physicians
  and Surgeons;
Clinical Instructor
New York Presbyterian Hospital
New York, New York

David F. Jarrard, MD
Associate Professor
Department of Surgery
Division of Urology
University of Wisconsin Medical School
Madison, Wisconsin

Steven A. Kaplan, MD
Given Foundation Professor
Department of Urology
Columbia University College of Physicians
  and Surgeons;
Vice Chairman
New York Presbyterian Hospital
New York, New York

Michael W. Kattan, PhD
Chairman
Department of Biostatistics and
  Epidemiology
Cleveland Clinic Foundation
Cleveland, Ohio

Naveen Kella, MD
Department of Urology
Baylor College of Medicine
Houston, Texas;
Director of Robotic Surgery
Urology San Antonio
San Antonio, Texas

Christopher E. Kelly, MD
Assistant Professor
Department of Urology
New York University School of Medicine;
Assistant Professor
New York University Urology Associates
New York, New York

Roger S. Kirby, MD, FRCS (Urol), FEBU
Professor
Department of Urology
St. George's Hospital
London, England

John N. Krieger, MD
Professor
Department of Urology
University of Washington School
  of Medicine
Seattle, Washington

Richard K. Lee, MD, MBA
Resident
Department of Urology
New York Presbyterian Hospital/Cornell
University Medical Center
New York, New York

Hans Lilja, MD, PhD
Professor
Department of Laboratory Medicine
University Hospital Malmö
Malmö, Sweden;
Attending Research Clinical Chemist
The Lilja Laboratory
Memorial Sloan-Kettering Cancer Center
New York, New York

Michael Marberger, MD
Professor
Department of Urology
University of Vienna Medical School
Vienna, Austria

John D. McConnell, MD
Professor and Chairman
Department of Urology
University of Texas Southwestern Medical
Center
Dallas, Texas

Kevin T. McVary, MD, FACS
Associate Professor
Department of Urology
Northwestern University Feinberg School
  of Medicine;
Attending Physician
Northwestern Memorial Hospital
Chicago, Illinois

Brian J. Miles, MD
Professor of Urology
Baylor College of Medicine;
Physician, Urology Institute at
  Methodist Hospital;
Chief, Urology Services
St. Luke's Episcopal Hospital;
Medical Director, St. Luke's Episcopal
  Hospital Cancer Program and the
  Texas Cancer Institute
Houston, Texas

Timothy D. Moon, MD, MBChB
Professor of Surgery
Division of Urology
University of Wisconsin Hospitals
  and Clinics
Madison, Wisconsin

John P. Mulhall, MD
Associate Professor
Department of Urology
Director, Sexual Health Programs
Weill Medical College of Cornell University;
New York Presbyterian Hospital
Memorial Sloan-Kettering Cancer Center
New York, New York

Rolf P. Muschter, MD, PhD
Associate Professor
Department of Urology
University of Munich School of Medicine
Munich, Germany;
Chairman of Urology
Diakoniekrankenhaus Academic
  Teaching Hospital
Rotenburg, Germany

Kenneth J. Pienta, MD
Professor
Departments of Internal Medicine
  and Urology
University of Michigan Medical Center
Ann Arbor, Michigan

Alan Pollock, MD, PhD
Senior Member and Chairman
Department of Radiation Oncology
Fox Chase Cancer Center
Philadelphia, Pennsylvania

Jaspreet S. Sandhu, MD
Clinical Instructor
Department of Urology
Wake Forest University School of Medicine
Winston-Salem, North Carolina;
Staff Physician
New York Presbyterian Hospital/Cornell
  University Medical Center
New York, New York

Peter T. Scardino, MD
Florence and Theodore Baumritter/
  Enid Ancell
Chair of Urologic Oncology
Department of Urology
Memorial Sloan-Kettering Cancer Center
New York, New York

Kevin M. Slawin, MD
Professor and Dan L. Duncan Family Chair
  in Prostate Disease
Scott Department of Urology
Director, Baylor Prostate Center
Baylor College of Medicine
Houston, Texas

Andrew J. Stephenson, MD
Fellow
A.F.U.D. Research Scholar
Department of Urology
Memorial Sloan-Kettering Cancer Center
New York, New York

Thomas Steuber, MD
Department of Urology
University of Hamburg School of Medicine;
Staff Physician
University Hospital Hamburg-Eppendorf
Hamburg, Germany

Maryrose P. Sullivan, PhD
Instructor
Department of Surgery
Harvard Medical School;
Biomedical Engineer
West Roxbury Veterans Affairs
  Medical Center
Boston, Massachusetts

Alexis E. Te, MD
Associate Professor
Department of Urology
Weill Medical College of Cornell University;
Director, Brady Prostate Center
Cornell Medical Center
New York, New York

Karim Touijer, MD
Department of Urology
Memorial Sloan-Kettering Cancer Center
New York, New York

Matthias Waldert, MD
Resident
Department of Urology
University of Vienna Medical School
Vienna, Austria

Subbarao V. Yalla, MD
Professor of Surgery
Department of Surgery
Harvard Medical School
Brigham and Women's Hospital;
Chief of Urology
West Roxbury Veterans Affairs Medical
Center
West Roxbury, Massachusetts

Michael J. Zelefsky, MD
Professor
Department of Radiation Oncology;
Chief, Brachytherapy Service
Memorial Sloan-Kettering Cancer Center
New York, New York

Philippe E. Zimmern, MD
Professor
Department of Urology
University of Texas Southwestern
  Medical School
Dallas, Texas

CONTENTS

Epidemiology and Pathophysiology of Benign Prostatic Hyperplasia

1

William I. Jaffe,
Steven A. Kaplan,
& John D. McConnell

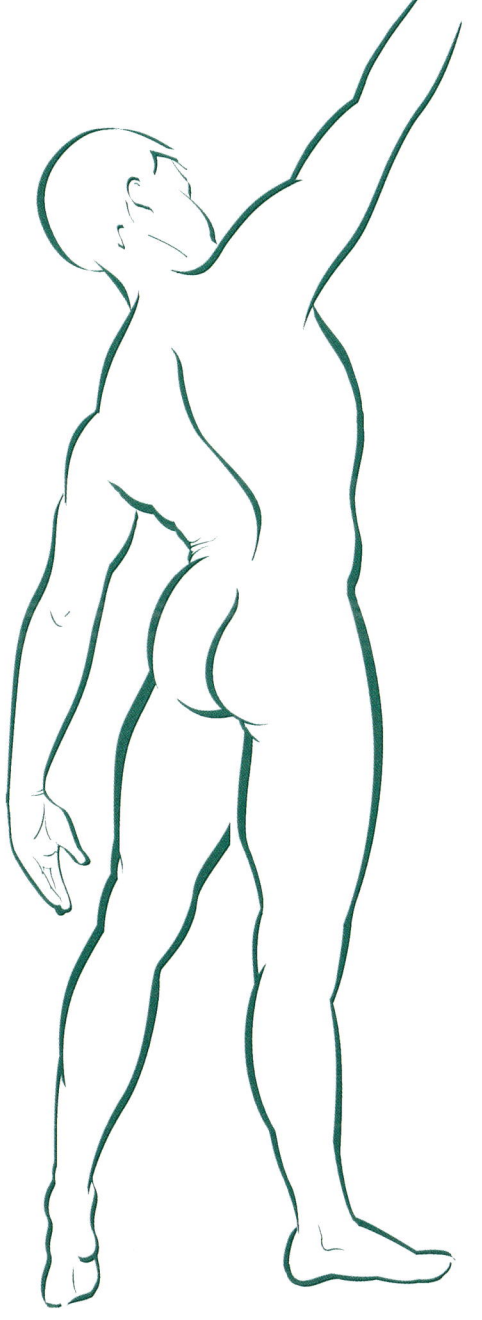

Prostatic growth is nearly ubiquitous in the adult male and is the focus of considerable research efforts. A comprehensive understanding of the pathophysiology of benign prostatic hyperplasia (BPH) remains elusive. As medical therapies, minimally invasive treatments, and other surgical procedures become more and more sophisticated, we are still unable to answer certain basic questions like why some older men have abnormal prostatic growth and others do not. Why do some men with enlarged prostates become symptomatic whereas others do not?

Population-based studies have revealed epidemiologic factors, such as erectile dysfunction, which co-exist with BPH. Investigation into common pathophysiologic pathways may yield new insights into the molecular biology of BPH. In the last decade there has been a refinement of the terminology of BPH which better reflects our current knowledge of the relationship between male lower urinary tract symptoms (LUTS), bladder outlet obstruction, prostatic hyperplasia, and bladder pathophysiology. A more complete understanding of these interrelationships will improve our ability to treat men with enlarged prostates and urinary symptoms.

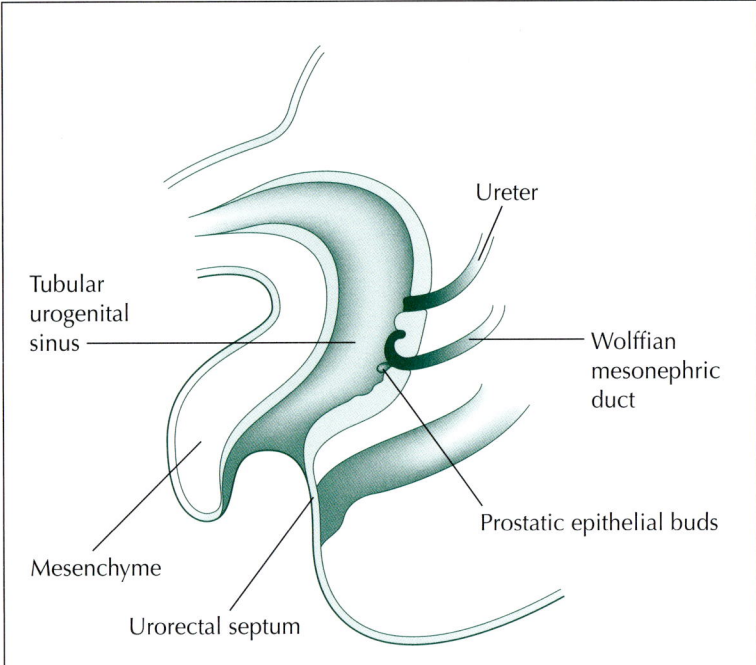

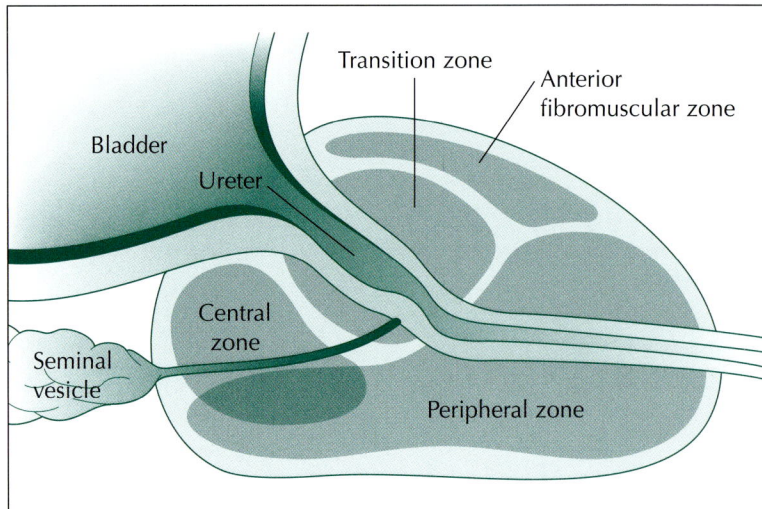

▶ **FIGURE 1-1.** Embryology. By the 6th week of gestation, the urorectal septum has divided the cloaca into the anterior urogenital sinus (UGS) and the posterior anorectal canal. The distal mesonephric ducts become incorporated into the urogenital sinus at this time and will give rise to the male sex accessory glands (except prostate) under the control of testosterone. In contrast, prostatic embryogenesis begins during the 12th week of gestation and is dependent on dihydrotestosterone. This process involves paired epithelial buds that arise from the UGS and penetrate the surrounding mesenchyme [1]. This interaction between the epithelium (glands) and mesenchyme (stroma) may be important in the pathogenesis of BPH [2]. (*Adapted from* www.endotext.org.)

▶ **FIGURE 1-2.** Anatomy of the male prostate. The zonal anatomy of the adult prostate is based on McNeal's seminal work [3]. The prostate is divided histologically into 4 discrete regions. BPH is limited to the preprostatic region that is comprised of the periurethral glands and the transition zone. The vascular supply to this area is from the urethral branches of the inferior vesical artery which course from the bladder neck to the verumontanum [4]. A critical anatomic structure to the pathophysiology of BPH is the capsule that causes BPH to compress the prostatic urethra. (*Adapted from* www.endotext.org.)

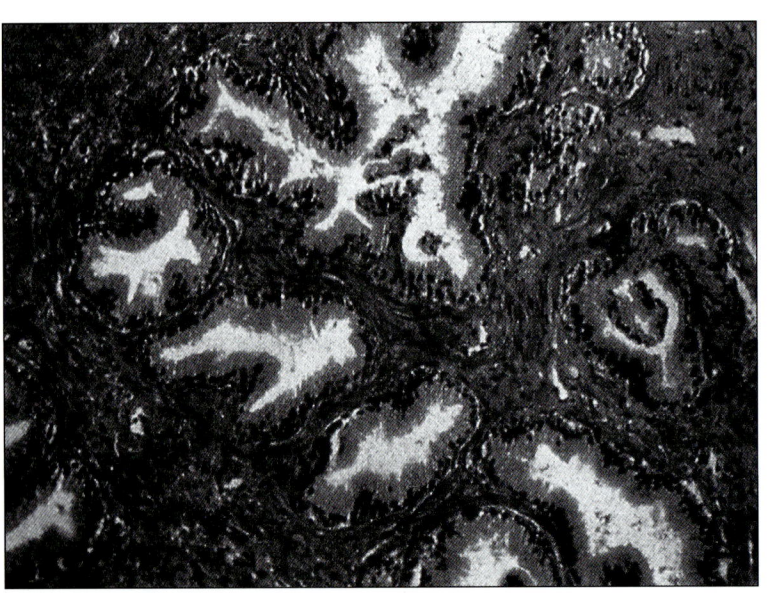

▶ **FIGURE 1-3.** Histology. The adult prostate is composed of branching acini and ducts embedded in a fibromuscular stroma. There is some controversy regarding the contributions of stromal and glandular elements to BPH. Although there tends to be significant heterogeneity between individuals, early BPH nodules tend to be predominately stromal; as the prostate grows larger glandular elements may predominate [5,6]. In either case, BPH is a truly hyperplastic process characterized by an increase in the total cell population.

Terminology for Benign Prostatic Hyperplasia

Benign Prostatic Hyperplasia (BPH)	**Benign Prostatic Enlargement (BPE)**	**Benign Prostatic Obstruction (BPO)**
Histologic diagnosis	Gross enlargement due to benign growth (can be without obstruction)	Urodynamically proven bladder outlet obstruction (BOO) (static/dynamic components)

▶ **FIGURE 1-4.** Terminology. Until recently, the nomenclature for BPH and male lower urinary tract symptoms (LUTS) was extremely nonspecific and led to a considerable amount of confusion. For investigative purposes, it is critical to have standardized terminology to allow study of similar groups of patients. Paul Abrams advanced the usage of more specific terminology that is becoming incorporated into the urologic lexicon [7]. Use of the term *benign prostatic hyperplasia* (BPH) should be limited to histologic changes of hyperplasia. *Benign prostatic enlargement* (BPE) refers to pathologic enlargement of the gland grossly, usually determined by digital rectal examination or transrectal ultrasound. *Benign prostatic obstruction* (BPO) is used to define urodynamically confirmed bladder outlet obstruction (BOO) attributed to the prostate. All of these "conditions" are not necessarily present in older men with LUTS.

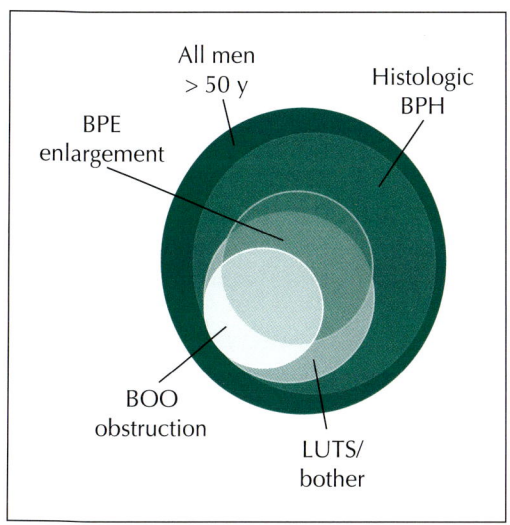

▶ **FIGURE 1-5.** Relationship of LUTS and BPH. LUTS can be caused by BPH, BPE, or BPO, or can exist independently. LUTS can be caused by outlet obstruction [8]. Conversely, although BPH is almost universal in the aged male, many of these patients have little in the way of symptoms or do not present for treatment [9]. The exact relationships between prostate enlargement, outlet obstruction, and urinary symptoms are the focus of considerable ongoing research. In defining patient populations for analysis or comparing studies, it is necessary to understand exactly which of these pathologic processes is being examined.

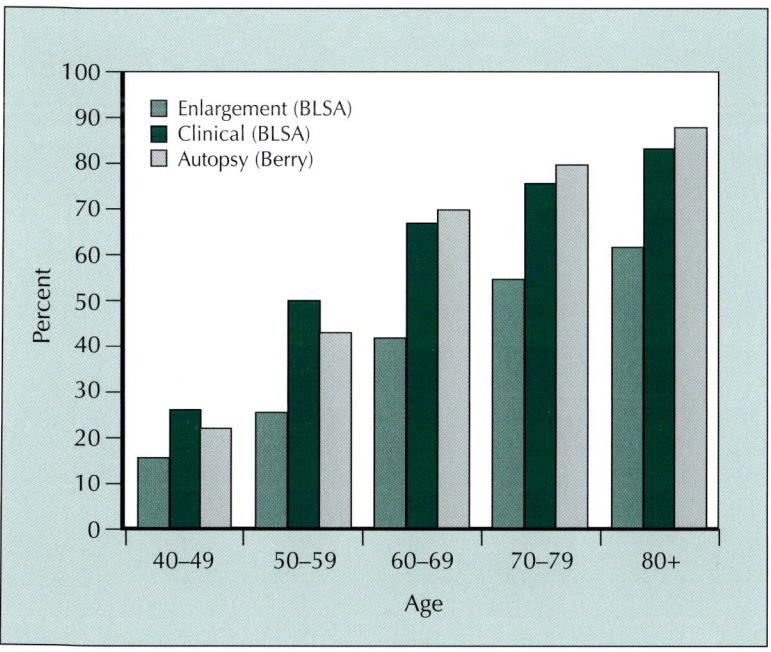

▶ **FIGURE 1-6.** Prevalence. Berry *et al.* published autopsy data from over 1000 prostate specimens from multiple studies and found histologic evidence of BPH in over 40% of men age 50 to 59 and almost 80% in the 70 to 79 age range [10]. Data from the Baltimore Longitudinal Study of Aging showed lower rates of BPE detected by digital rectal examination (DRE) but similar age-related increases [11]. The Triumph Project retrospectively reviewed the records of 80,774 Dutch men and found an overall prevalence of 10.3% for BPH/LUTS [12]. Reported prevalence is highly dependent on the diagnostic criteria and population studied, but in general, BPH or BPH/LUTS is a very common condition, and the prevalence tends to increase over time in a linear fashion. (*Adapted from* Berry *et al.* [10].)

Cost of Benign Prostatic Hyperplasia in the United States

Age groups, y	Incidence index*	Waiting only	Surgical only	Medical only	Mixed medical and surgical†	Mixed all‡
45–49	39	9619	14,007	23,366	30,899	22,960
50–59	488	6894	11,629	17,585	24,269	18,649
60–69	3180	4514	9703	12,099	18,708	15,046
70–79	4833	2821	9239	7874	14,875	12,846
80–85	1460	1140	9199	3328	11,687	10,551
All ages	10,000	3339	9516	9087	16,148	13,533

Implied rate per 10,000 BPH cases.
†*Assumes an unavoidable surgery rate of 27%.*
‡*Switch in therapy occurs at the terciles of the interval.*

▶ **FIGURE 1-7.** Cost of BPH. The total annual cost of BPH in the United States has estimated to be approximately $4 billion [13]. Chirikos and Sanford constructed a synthetic cohort of men with BPH and estimated the present value of watchful waiting, medical therapy, surgical therapy, or mixed (medical treatment progressing to surgical treatment). The overall cost of medical therapy and surgical therapy were almost equivalent over time when including all ages ($9087 vs $9516). Surgical therapy tends to be more cost-effective compared to medical treatment over time in younger patients, whereas the opposite is true in older patients [14]. Watchful waiting was by far the most cost-effective option ($3339). Indirect costs are, of course, more difficult to measure. Approximately 10% of working men with BPH will miss an average of 7.3 hours of work annually to inpatient or outpatient care [15]. (*Adapted from* Chirikos *et al.* [14].)

Symptoms and Bother for Patients with Benign Prostatic Hyperplasia (BPH) and Lower Urinary Tract Symptoms (LUTS)

Rank	Prevalence		Bothersomeness	
	Storage symptoms	Voiding symptoms	Storage symptoms	Voiding symptoms
1	-	Terminal dribble	-	Postmicturition dribble
2	-	Reduced stream	Urge incontinence	-
3	-	Intermittency	Nocturnal incontinence	-
4	-	Hesitancy	Miscellaneous incontinence	-
5	-	Incomplete emptying	Urgency	-
6	Urgency	-	-	Terminal dribble
7	Nocturia*	-	Frequency†‡	-
8	Repeated urination	-	-	Incomplete emptying
9	Frequency‡	-	Nocturia*‡	-

Urination at least 2 times a night.
†*Urination at least 9 times daily.*
‡*Includes all responders to bothersomeness question regardless of response to symptom occurrence question.*
§*Urination every 2 hours or more frequently.*

▶ **FIGURE 1-8.** Symptoms and bother for BPH/LUTS. The American Urologic Association Symptom Score (AUASSI) and the International Prostate Symptom Score (IPSS) are the two most commonly used questionnaires to assess the impact of BPH/LUTS on the patient. The ICS "BPH" study developed the ICS male questionnaire in which each question about symptom occurrence is followed by a question concerning bother from that symptom. The most prevalent symptoms tended to be voiding symptoms, whereas the most bothersome ones were typically storage symptoms [16]. Subgroup analysis from the Health Professionals Follow-up Study revealed that men with moderate to high LUTS (AUASSI 15 to 19) had deficits on SF-36 in two domains, one related to anxious, depressed mood and the other related to poor role functioning related to emotional problems from illness. Men with severe LUTS (AUASSI >19) had additional deficits in vitality/energy domain and the ability to work and carry out daily tasks [17]. (*Adapted from* Peters *et al.* [16].)

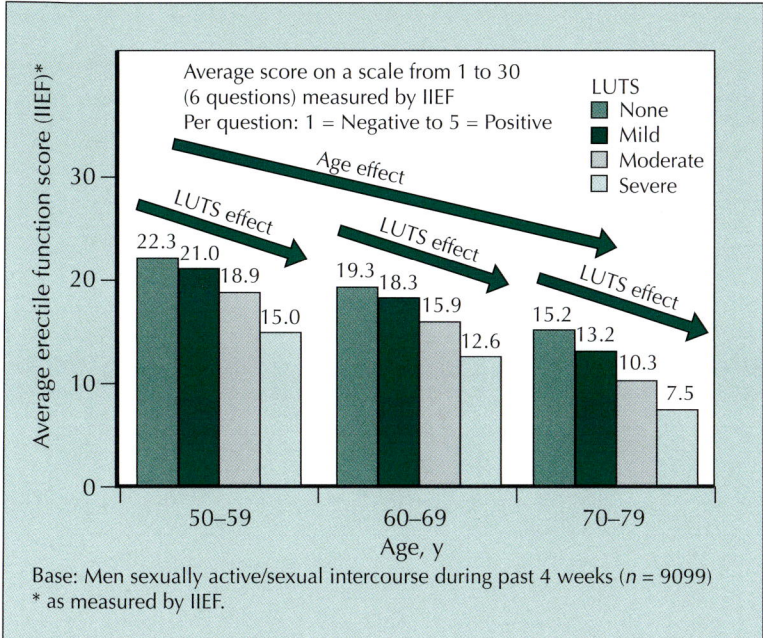

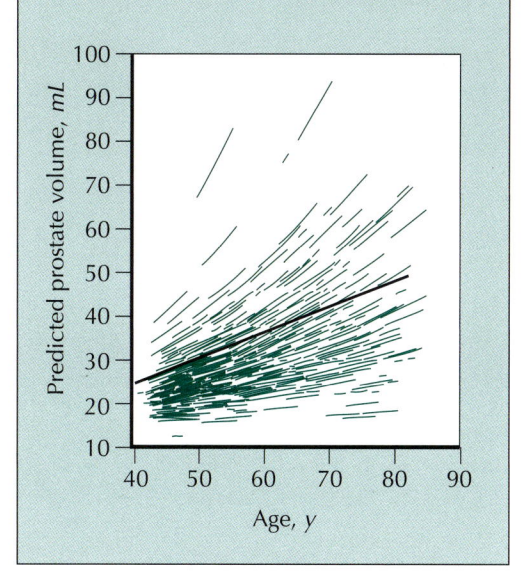

▶ **FIGURE 1-9.** Erectile dysfunction and BPH. BPH/LUTS and erectile dysfunction (ED) are both common conditions in the aging male and the prevalence of both increases with age. The causal relationship between these two entities has been the subject of emerging research over the last several years. The Multinational Survey of the Aging Male surveyed 14,000 men between the ages of 50 and 80 in the United States and Europe. Both erectile dysfunction and ejaculatory dysfunction increased significantly with age and severity of LUTS, independent of comorbidities [18]. Whereas the pathophysiologic link is still unclear, the evidence of an epidemiologic link is strengthening. The Cologne Male Survey and the UrEpik study both showed a significant correlation between LUTS and ED independent of age [19,20]. Subgroup data from Medical Therapy of Prostatic Symptoms (MTOPS) also showed a strong correlation between AUASS and sexual dysfunction and between decreased flow rates and sexual dysfunction [21]. (*Adapted from* Rosen *et al.* [18].)

▶ **FIGURE 1-10.** Natural history. Data from community-based cohorts yields fairly good insight into the natural history of BPH/LUTS. The Olmsted County Study (OCS) showed an annual prostate growth rate of 1.6% [22]. Men with larger prostates and clinical BPH (BPH/LUTS) tend to have higher growth rates than the general population (see figure). Data from Proscar Long-term Efficacy and Safety Study (PLESS) showed an overall growth rate of 14% at 4 years follow-up in the placebo arm. Mean baseline prostate volume in the placebo group was 55 mL [25]. In MTOPS, men in the placebo or doxazosin only group showed a mean growth of 29% over 4.5 years. Mean baseline prostate volume was 35 mL [23]. Almost all parameters relating to BPH/LUTS deteriorate with aging including decreases in flow rate, increases in symptom score, and risk of BPH-related surgery. How much of this change is related to progression of BPH and how much is related to age-related changes in detrusor function is unclear. It has been demonstrated, however, that altering the natural history of BPH with either medical or surgical therapy leads to fewer complications from BPH and a reduction in symptom severity [21,23]. In a selected cohort of 537 from the OCS, almost one in four men over the age of 70 received some form of treatment for BPH during the 6 years of follow-up. Risk factors for needing treatment included increasing age, worsening symptoms, decreasing flow rate, and prostate size [24]. (*Adapted from* Rhodes *et al.* [22].)

Complications of Benign Prostatic Hyperplasia (BPH)

	MTOPS data/rate per 100 person, y	
Surgery	AUR	0.6
Urinary retention	Symptom progression	3.6
Urinary tract infection	Renal insufficiency	0
Hematuria	Urinary tract infection	0.1
Bladder decompensation	Incontinence	0.3
Incontinence		
Bladder calculi		
Hydronephrosis		

▶ **FIGURE 1-11.** Complications of BPH. There are generally accepted sequelae of untreated, undertreated, or progressive BPH. The most commonly used endpoints in medical trials are symptom deterioration, BPH-related surgery, and acute urinary retention (AUR). Other complications of BPH include urinary tract infection, hematuria, bladder calculi, bladder decompensation, incontinence, and upper-tract deterioration. Acute urinary retention continues to be the most widely accepted and most scientific endpoint, although the exact pathophysiologic mechanism is not completely understood. The overall risk of AUR in the placebo arm of the MTOPS study was 0.6/100 person years and the risk increased with higher PSA levels [25]. Seven percent of the placebo arm in the PLESS trial suffered from AUR during 4 years of follow-up [26]. MTOPS also had very low rates of incontinence and urinary tract infection (0.3 and 0.1/100 person years). No cases of upper tract deterioration occurred during the study time. Historically, 7.6% to 13.6% of patients scheduled for TURP have upper tract deterioration [27]. The more modern data shows, however, that this is an extremely uncommon complication for patients with known BPH who are followed regularly. In reviewing 3 large finasteride trials, Kim concluded that PSA and baseline prostate volume are the strongest predictors of BPH progression [28].

Risk Factors for Benign Prostatic Hyperplasia	
Promote	**Protect**
Age	Smoking
Aspirin use	Alcohol
Heart disease	Asian ethnicity
Obesity	Exercise
Hypertension	

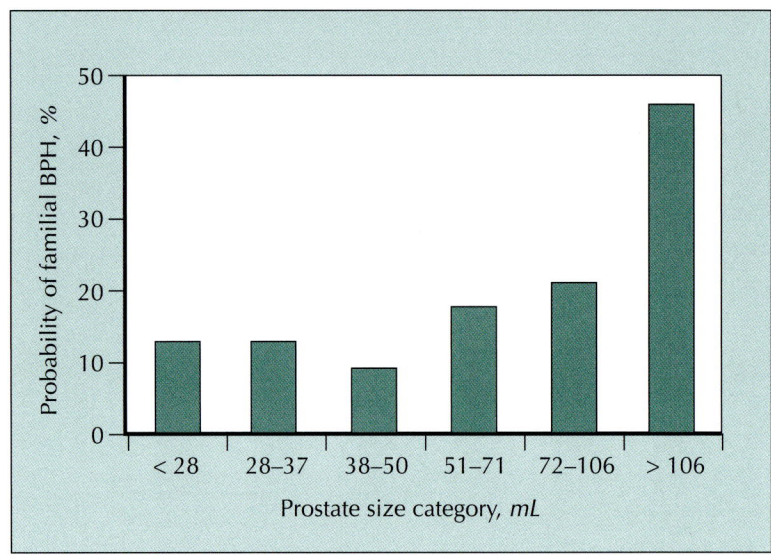

▶ **FIGURE 1-12.** Risk factors for the development of BPH. Although XY genotype and advancing age are undeniable risk factors for the development of BPH, evidence for comorbidity, environmental, dietary, or lifestyle-related risk factors is generally weak. In addition, the biochemical relationship between many of the postulated risk factors and development of BPH/LUTS is poorly understood. Kang *et al.* examined data from the National Cancer Institute sponsored Prostate, Lung, Colorectal and Ovarian Cancer Screening Trial and found statistically significant but mildly decreased rates for BPH and transurethral prostatectomy (TURP) among Asian men, current smokers, and alcohol consumers. There was no significant dose response relationship in the latter two groups. There was no difference between black and white males. Aspirin use was associated with a small increased risk for BPH and TURP [29]. The Massachusetts Male Aging Study found that cigarette smoking and increased physical activity were protective against BPH, whereas heart disease correlated positively with development of BPH. This study included a broad definition of BPH including men who reported frequent or difficult urination and were told by a health professional that they had an enlarged prostate [30]. There may also be a positive association between obesity and prostate volume and LUTS [31]. Systemic hypertension and symptomatic BPH are associated and may share a common pathophysiologic link due to either increased sympathetic tone or α-adrenoreceptor responsiveness [32].

▶ **FIGURE 1-13.** Hereditary BPH. There appears to be a clear hereditary component to the development of BPH, at least in some patients. The exact mechanisms remain unclear but there is a predisposition to younger age of onset and larger glands in patients with a family history of BPH. A case-control study by Sanda *et al.* showed a fourfold greater risk of prostatectomy in first-degree relatives of study subjects and that family history was positively associated with prostate volume [33]. Subgroup analysis of the U.S. Finasteride Trial identified 69 men with familial BPH (defined as 3 or more family members with BPH); these men were compared to 345 BPH control subjects. The familial BPH subjects had larger prostates compared to controls (82.7 vs 55.5 mL), but similar androgen levels and response to finasteride [34]. Most authors agree that there is an autosomal dominant or co-dominant Mendelian pattern of inheritance. Whereas investigation into specific genetic alterations in hereditary BPH certainly lags behind similar research for the urologic malignancies, discovery in this arena is ongoing and will likely lead to significant advances in diagnosis and treatment in the future. (*Adapted from* Sanda *et al.* [34].)

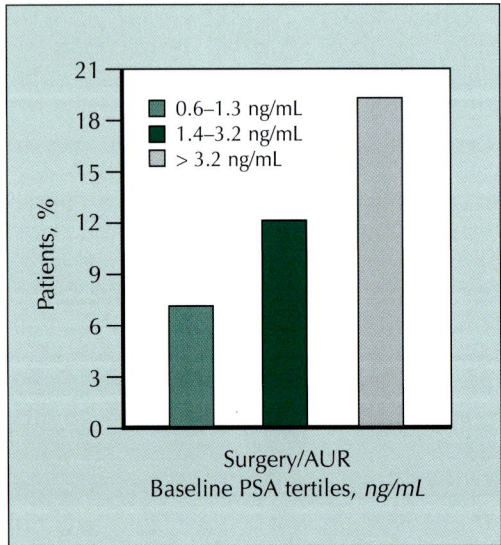

▶ **FIGURE 1-14.** Prostate size and BPH. There are two important questions relating to prostate size and BPH. First, does prostate size in and of itself cause problems unrelated to LUTS? This question has been answered more or less by the large finasteride studies. Reduction of prostate volume with finasteride reduces the risk of AUR and BPH surgery independent of other factors. In addition, men with larger prostate volumes or higher PSA levels (as a surrogate for prostate volume) are at higher risk for AUR [35]. Baseline prostate volume has been shown to be a strong predictor of BPH progression in most of the larger studies. Marberger *et al.* combined data from three prospective, randomized, placebo-finasteride trials and found prostate volume and PSA were risk factors for AUR. The second question is to what degree does prostate size influence symptoms. Generally, there has been a poor correlation between prostate size and symptoms [28]. Multiple other factors play a role in the development of male LUTS including age, medications, comorbid conditions, diet, and bladder physiology. Women have similar rates of LUTS compared to age-matched men in older populations. Prostate size has, however, been shown to be an independent factor in degree of obstruction. Eckhardt et al. studied 565 men with BPH/LUTS with pressure-flow urodynamics and found that 53% were obstructed. Prostate volume correlated positively with Schafer obstruction grade (except, interestingly, at grade 5–6 combined) [36]. Kaplan *et al.* developed the concept of transition zone index and showed that it correlated more strongly with symptoms, peak flow rates, and detrusor pressure at peak flow than total prostate volume [37]. (*Adapted from* Roehrborn *et al.* [35].)

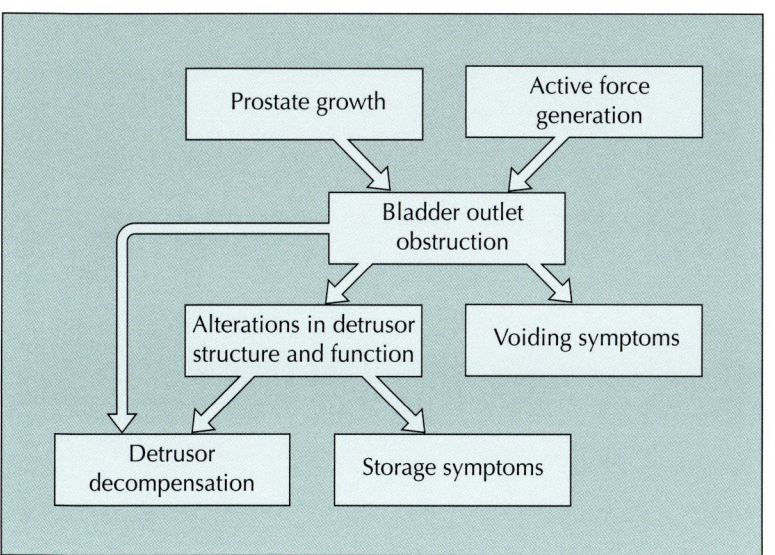

▶ **FIGURE 1-15.** Pathophysiologic framework for BPH. The commonly accepted paradigm for the development of BPH/LUTS begins with abnormal microscopic hyperplasia and macroscopic growth. This, along with the active force generation of prostatic and bladder neck smooth muscle, contributes to urine outflow obstruction and the classic voiding symptoms of decreased force of stream, intermittent stream, and hesitancy. The detrusor response to increased resistance is initially to generate higher pressures to overcome the outlet resistance. This leads to a variety of cellular and morphologic changes in the bladder. The common storage symptoms of frequency, urgency, and nocturia are likely the sequelae of these alterations in bladder physiology. Progression of the disease may eventually lead to bladder decompensation in which the bladder is no longer able to generate sufficient pressures to empty. This is analogous to the model of hypertensive cardiomyopathy in which increases in peripheral vascular resistance lead to cardiomyopathy and congestive heart failure.

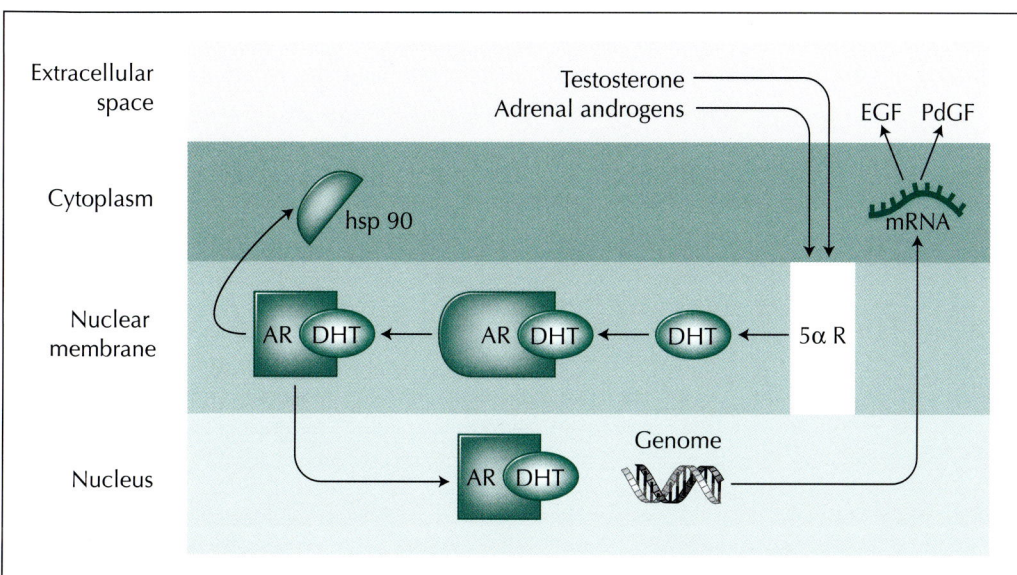

▶ **FIGURE 1-16.** Androgens. The role of both testosterone and dihydrotestosterone (DHT) is one of the most thoroughly studied areas in the development of BPH; the exact mechanism by which either of the steroid hormones promotes BPH is still unknown. It is clear, however, that DHT is required for

prostatic development. In patients with congenital deficiency of type 2 5 α-reductase, the prostate fails to develop, whereas the Wolffian duct structures develop normally under the influence of testosterone [38]. In men with BPH who are treated with androgen deprivation, there is a reduction in prostate volume of 35% after 24 weeks of treatment [39]. In prostatic stromal cells, testosterone is converted by 5 α-reductase to DHT that is the principal androgen in the prostate. DHT exerts its action through binding to the androgen receptor in stromal and epithelial cells. Whereas DHT is clearly a requirement for prostate growth and development of BPH, there is no convincing evidence that abnormalities in DHT concentration or metabolism have any further role in promoting BPH. Walsh *et al.* compared DHT concentrations in normal prostate and BPH tissue and found no difference in concentrations [40]. The overall effect seems to be that DHT plays a "permissive" role in the development of BPH. (*Adapted from* Griffiths *et al.* [61].)

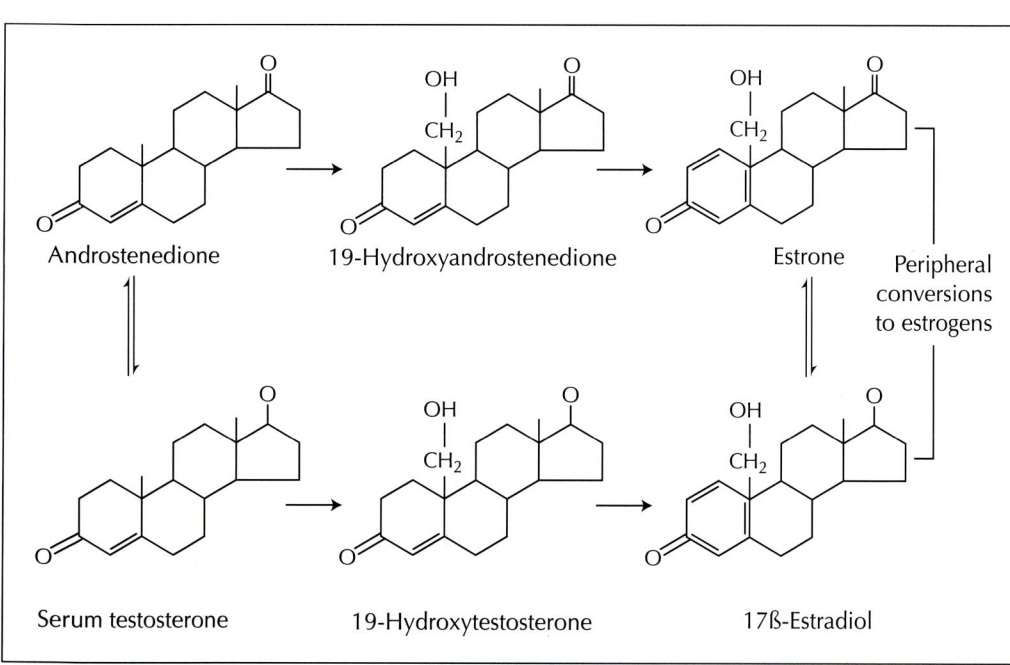

▶ **FIGURE 1-17.** Estrogens. The role of estrogens, specifically estradiol, is increasingly being recognized as a possible factor in the development of BPH. The vast majority of circulating estrogens in the male is produced by the peripheral conversion of testosterone and androstenedione to estrone and estradiol (*see* figure). In hyperplastic prostates, serum estradiol and estriol levels correlated positively with prostate size [41]. The estrogen receptor (ER) beta levels have been found to be lower in transition zone stromal cells than in normal tissue. Together with the knowledge that ER beta knockout mice develop prostatic hyperplasia, this suggests an inhibitory role in the development of BPH [42]. ER alpha levels (upregulated by estradiol) have been shown to correlate with concentrations of FGF-2 and FGF-7, both putative growth factors for BPH [43]. The exact importance of estrogen levels, estrogen receptors, and relative concentration to androgens remains unclear.

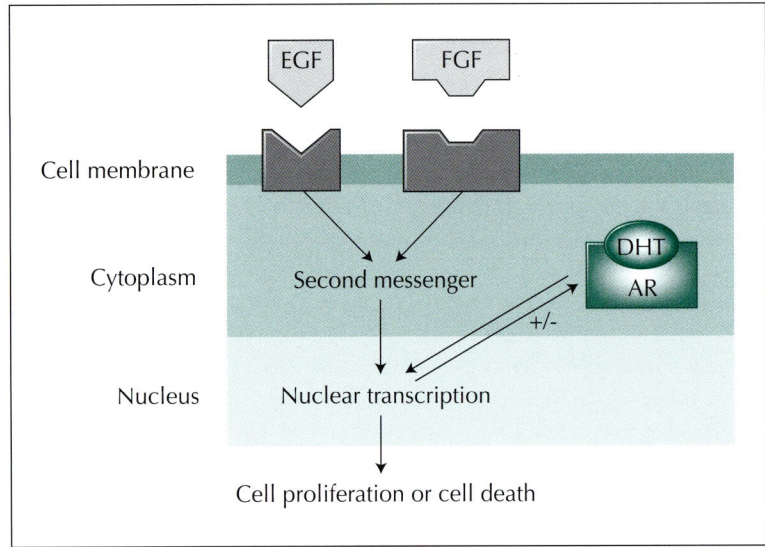

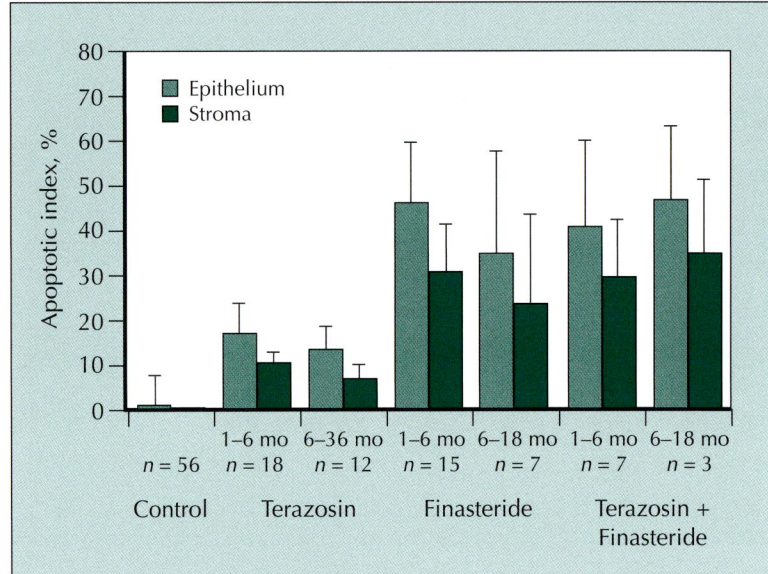

▶ **FIGURE 1-18.** Growth factors. Understanding the cellular signaling mechanisms that are altered in prostate hyperplasia may be key to developing new treatments including gene therapy applications. The fibroblast growth factor family (FGFs), transforming growth factor β (TGFβ), insulin-like growth factors (IGFs) and epidermal growth factors (EGFs) are among the many peptide molecules investigated in BPH tissue. FGF-2 and FGF-7 (also known as keratinocyte growth factor) have been implicated strongly in the development of BPH. These and other growth factors and hormones are involved in the paracrine communication between the stromal and epithelial compartments. There also seems to be a complex interaction between these growth factors and the hormonal milieu. The DHT-AR complex may exert influence on prostatic growth in part by regulating the expression of growth factors [44]. Local tissue hypoxia has been shown to be a possible herald event for the "embryonic reawakening" of stromal cells and their subsequent inductive influence on the epithelial cells [45].

▶ **FIGURE 1-19.** Apoptosis. Hyperplasia may be simply viewed as a disruption in the balance between normal cellular proliferation and programmed cell death (apoptosis). The effects of androgen deprivation on upregulating apoptosis have been well-studied in the animal and human prostate, however the precise roles of cellular proliferation and apoptosis in the pathophysiology of BPH have yet to be defined. Colombel *et al.* compared tissue from 10 normal prostate glands with 30 prostate adenomas and found significantly increased levels of glandular proliferation in the BPH tissue without compensatory increases in apoptosis [46]. Interestingly, they also found areas of rapid proliferation in BPH glands that were in contact with adjacent stroma. There is some evidence that in addition to anti-androgen therapies, α_1 blockers, specifically terazosin and doxazosin may contribute to apoptosis [47]. Both finasteride and combination treatment with α_1 blockers yield significant increases in the apoptopic index (see figure), likely mediated via increased TGF-β expression, a known inhibitor of cellular proliferation [48]. (*Adapted from* Glassman *et al.* [48].)

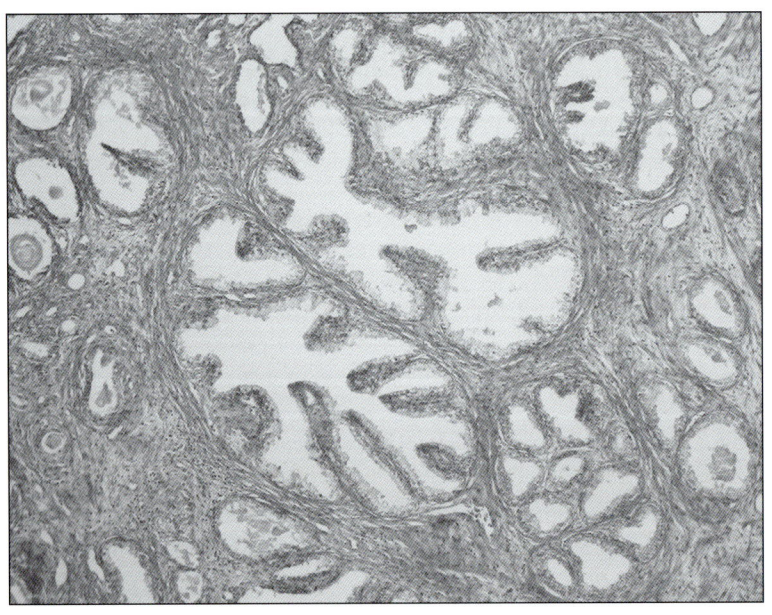

▶ **FIGURE 1-20.** Prostatic smooth muscle. The smooth muscle cells of the stromal compartment are a major contributor to urethral resistance and likely play a significant role in bladder outlet obstruction (BOO) related to BPH. By volume, smooth muscle cells may constitute 22% of the total prostate in BPH [49]. Smooth muscle of the prostate, prostatic capsule, and bladder neck is richly innervated with α_1 adrenoreceptors (AR) that are stimulated by the sympathetic nervous system and cause myosin-mediated contraction. The extent to which this process becomes pathologic in prostatic hyperplasia and BOO is not known. Endothelin, a potent vasoconstricting peptide that has known effects in the pulmonary, cardiac, renal, and nervous systems has been shown to have both a contraction effect and also mitogenic effect on prostatic smooth muscle [50].

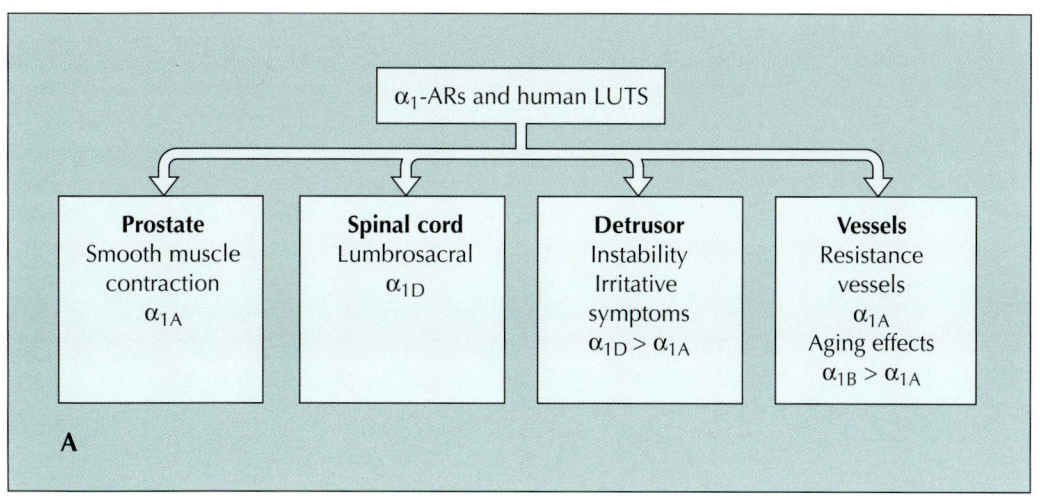

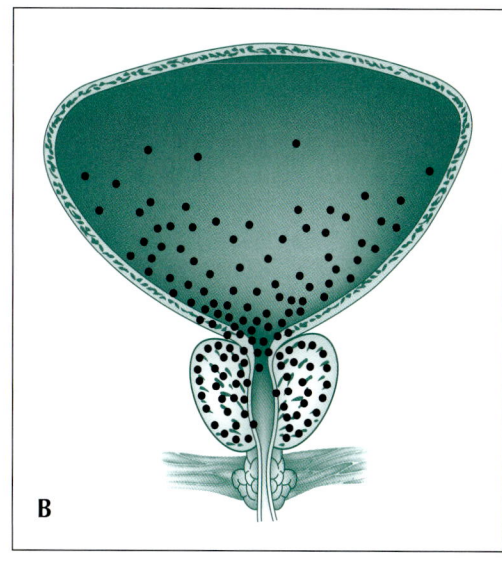

▶ **FIGURE 1-21.** α_1 adrenoreceptor distribution. **A,** Three distinct subtypes of α_1 ARs have been identified and their anatomic distribution has been described. The effects on lower urinary tract function seem to be mediated via receptors in prostatic smooth muscle, prostatic capsule, bladder neck/bladder, and the spinal cord. The most direct evidence for the role of α_1 ARs in bladder outlet obstruction is from a review of published urodynamic data which shows increases in flow rates and decreases in voiding pressures after treatment with α_1 AR antagonists [51]. **B,** The use of α_1 AR antagonists has been well accepted as a first line therapy for BPH/LUTS for over 25 years. (*Adapted from* Rudner *et al.* [62].)

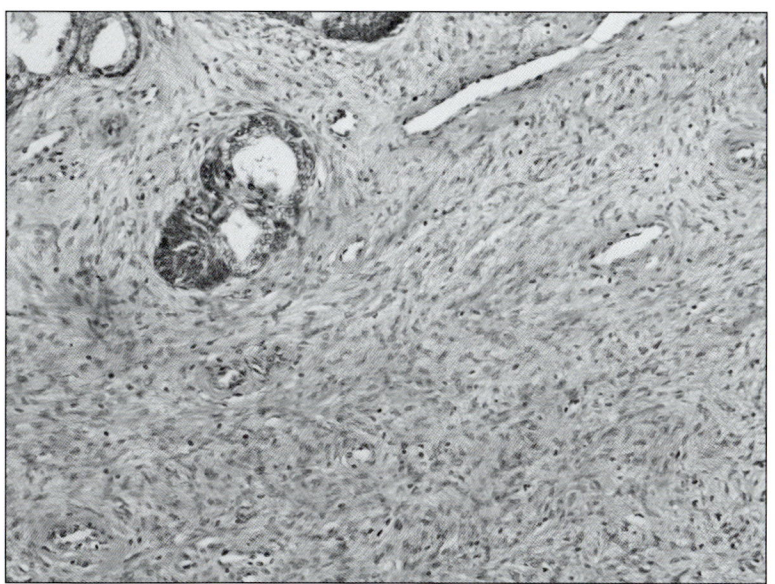

▶ **FIGURE 1-22.** Other stromal factors. BPH appears to be predominantly a stromal disease although this remains an area of controversy. Clearly there is both stromal and epithelial hyperplasia in BPH and both contribute to the total increase in prostate volume. There is wide heterogeneity in the stromal-epithelial ratio in BPH specimens which makes characterization difficult [52]. Besides the obvious contribution of smooth muscle content, other components of the stromal compartment have been shown to contribute to BOO. For instance, the ratio of chondroitin sulfate to dermatan sulfate is 4 times higher in BPH tissue compared to normal prostate. These glycosaminoglycans are known to alter the rate of epithelial cell proliferation in opposite directions such that this change in ratio favors proliferation [53].

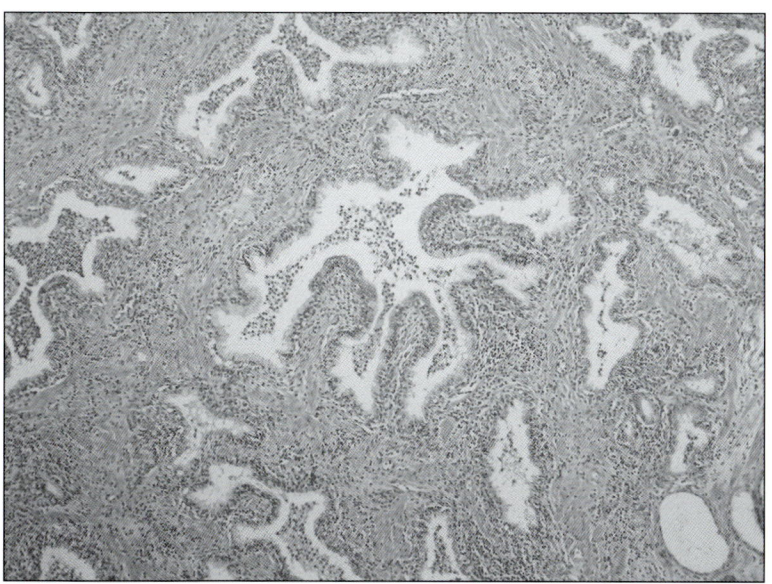

▶ **FIGURE 1-23.** Inflammation. Inflammatory infiltrates are a common finding in BPH tissues although the clinical significance is not known. Macrophage and T-cell infiltration may lead to destruction of glandular tissue and replacement by mesenchymal elements. Macrophage inhibitory cytokine-1, a member of the transforming growth factor-β superfamily, has been shown to be downregulated in symptomatic BPH patients compared to asymptomatic controls and nonBPH controls [54].

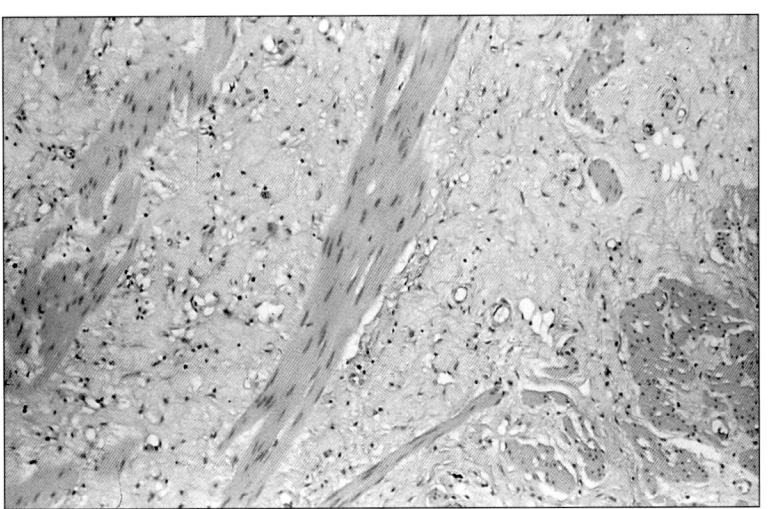

▶ **FIGURE 1-24.** *(See Color Plate)* Bladder dysfunction. It is now generally accepted that many of the symptoms previously attributed to "prostatism" are a consequence of both age-related changes in detrusor function and the bladder response to chronic outlet obstruction. Peak flow rates decrease with age with or without prostatic enlargement, indicative of specific age-related diminution of detrusor function [55]. The bladder is initially able to compensate for increases in outlet resistance by increasing work. Morphologically, there is smooth muscle hypertrophy and an overall increase in detrusor mass and deposition of interstitial collagen. In animal models of BOO, there is significant research into metabolic and structural derangements which are associated with the bladder dysfunction caused by BOO: detrusor overactivity and/or impaired contractility. One of the critical issues for preventing progression of BPH is understanding the mechanisms for bladder compensation and, ultimately, decompensation.

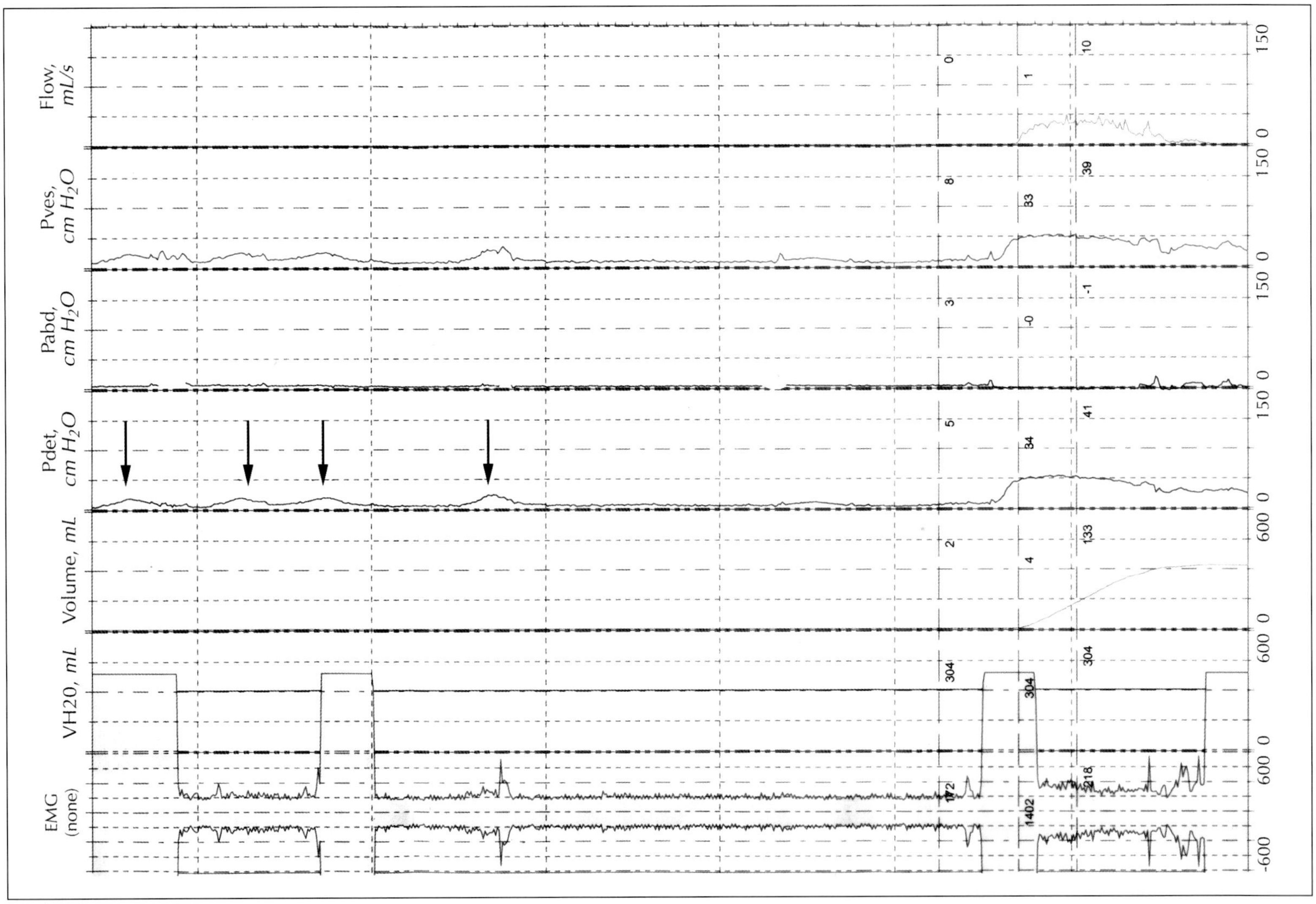

▶ **FIGURE 1-25.** Mechanisms for detrusor overactivity. Even after relief of obstruction, approximately 1/3 of patients will continue to have detrusor overactivity. The urodynamic tracing (*see* figure) shows a patient 9 months after TURP who continues to have storage symptoms. The study demonstrated detrusor overactivity (*large arrows*) and an unobstructed outlet. The cause of detrusor overactivity in patients with outlet obstruction is likely to due alterations in neurotransmission secondary to both ultrastructural and cellular changes. Obstructed bladders have been shown to have areas of denervation that is postulated to lead to autonomous activity of smooth muscle modules (denervation supersensitivity) [56]. There may be an increase in purinergic activity in overactive obstructed bladders that may explain why some patients do not respond to anticholinergic medication. O'Reilly *et al.* showed that the P2X1 was the predominant purinergic receptor subtype in the human bladder and that it was present in higher concentration in smooth muscle in the obstructed bladder compared to controls [57]. Other possible pathophysiologic links include alterations in muscarinic transmission and receptor subtypes, increased nerve growth factor production, and central nervous system changes.

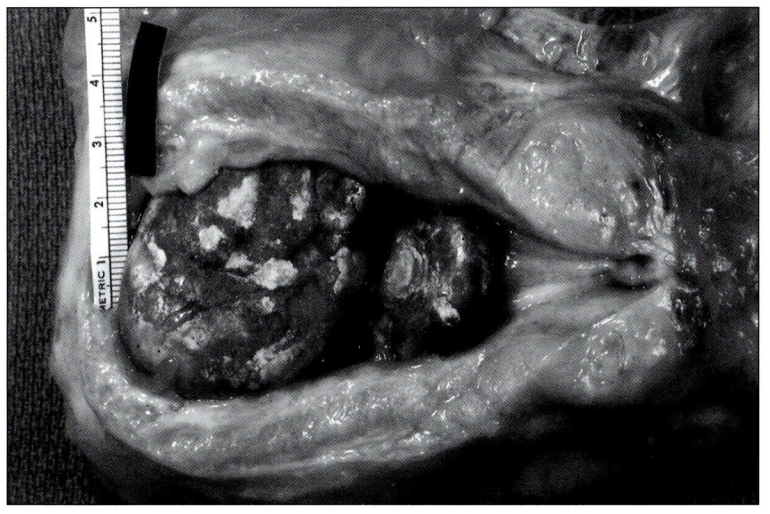

▶ **FIGURE 1-26.** *(See Color Plate)* Detrusor decompensation. The "end-stage" of progressive BPH is a decompensated bladder that is unable to empty even after the outlet obstruction is removed. In a partially obstructed rabbit bladder model, bladder decompensation can be judged according to at least five criteria described by Levin et al.: 1) increasing bladder mass; 2) decreasing compliance; 3) denervation; 4) decreased sarcoplasmic reticulum calcium-ATPase activity; and 5) mitochondrial dysfunction [58]. In terms of clinical usefulness, the first two criteria are the only ones that can be readily measured and potentially used as markers to guide treatment. Miyashita *et al.* have used ultrasound estimated bladder weights as potentially useful adjuncts to urodynamic evaluation of BOO. Patients with BPH/LUTS and a bladder mass >35g were over 13 times more likely to suffer from acute urinary retention than those with smaller bladders [59]. Loss of compliance may lead to renal deterioration, decreased functional capacity, and incontinence. Loss of compliance in BOO is thought to be mainly secondary to increasing connective tissue between muscle bundles that leads to a loss of bladder wall elasticity. Whereas abnormal histologic findings from bladder biopsies correlate well with loss of urodynamically measured compliance, they do not necessarily correlate with degree of BOO [60]. In both rabbit and rat animal models, relief of outlet obstruction can lead to improvements in both of these parameters. What causes these changes to become irreversible in some patients is a point of speculation. (*From* UAB Department of Pathology Digital Library www.peir.net, with permission.)

REFERENCES

1. Timms BG, Mohs TJ, Didio LJ: Ductal budding and branching patterns in the developing prostate. *J Urol* 1994, 151:1427–1432.

2. Eaton CL: Aetiology and pathogenesis of benign prostatic hyperplasia. *Curr Opin Urol* 2003, 13:7–10.

3. McNeal JE: The zonal anatomy of the prostate. *Prostate* 1981, 2:35–49.

4. Leventis AK, Shariat SF, Utsunomiya T, *et al.*: Characteristics of normal prostate vascular anatomy as displayed by power Doppler. *Prostate* 2001, 46:281–288.

5. Shapiro E, Berich MJ, Lepor H: The relative proportion of stromal and epithelial hyperplasia as related to the development of clinical BPH. *J Urol* 1992, 147:1293–1297.

6. McNeal J: Origin and evolution of benign prostatic enlargement. *Invest Urol* 1978, 15:340–345.

7. Abrams P: New words for old: lower urinary tract symptoms for "prostatism." *Brit Med J* 1994, 308:929–930.

8. Abrams P, Feneley RCL: The significance of the symptoms associated with bladder outflow obstruction. *Urol Int* 1978, 33:171–174.

9. Guess HA: Epidemiology and natural history of benign prostatic hyperplasia. *Urol Clin North Am* 1995, 22:247–261.

10. Berry SJ, Coffey DS, Walsh PC, *et al.*: The development of human benign prostatic hyperplasia with age. *J Urol* 1984, 132:474–479.

11. Arrighi HM, Metter EJ, Guess HA, *et al.*: Natural history of benign prostatic hyperplasia and risk of prostatectomy. The Baltimore Longitudinal Study of aging. *Urology* 1991, 38:4–8.

12. Verhamme KMC, Dieleman JP, Bleumink GS, *et al.*: Incidence and prevalence of lower urinary tract symptoms suggestive of benign prostatic hyperplasia in primary care-The triumph project. *Eur Urol* 2002, 42:323–328.

13. Tsang KK, Garraway WM: Prostatism and the burden of benign prostatic hyperplasia on elderly men. *Age Ageing* 1994, 23:360–364.

14. Chirikos TN, Sanford E: Cost consequences of surveillance, medical management or surgery for benign prostatic hyperplasia. *J Urol* 1996, 155:1311–1316.

15. Wei JT, Calhoun EA, Jacobsen SJ: *Benign Prostatic Hyperplasia*. Washington, DC: In *Urologic Diseases in America*. US Department of Health and Human Services, Public Health Service, National Institutes of Health, National Institute of Diabetes and Digestive and Kidney Diseases. US Government Publishing Office; 2004. [NIH publication no. 04-5512].

16. Peters TJ, Donovan JL, Kay HE, *et al.*: The International Continence Society "benign prostatic hyperplasia" study: the bothersomeness of urinary symptoms. *J Urol* 1997, 157:885–889.

17. Welch G, Weinger K, Barry MJ: Quality-of-life impact of lower urinary tract symptom severity: results from the health professionals' follow-up study. *Urology* 2002, 59:245–250.

18. Rosen R, Altwein J, Boyle P, *et al.*: Lower urinary tract symptoms and male sexual dysfunction: The multinational survey of the aging male (MSAM-7). *Eur Urol* 2003, 44:637–649.

19. Braun MH, Sommer F, Haupt G, *et al.*: Lower urinary tract symptoms and erectile dysfunction: co-morbidity or typical "ageing male" symptoms? Results of the "Cologne male survey." *Eur Urol* 2003, 44: 588–594.

20. Boyle P, Robertson C, Mazzetta C, *et al.*: The association between lower urinary tract symptoms and erectile dysfunction in four centers: the UrEpik study. *BJU Int* 2003, 92:719–725.

21. McVary KT, Foster H, Kusek J, *et al.*: Self-reported sexual function in men with symptoms of BPH- a MTOPS study. *Int J Impot Res* 2002, 14:ACP 1.32

22. Rhodes T, Girman CJ, Jacobsen SJ, *et al.*: Longitudinal prostate growth rates during 5 years in randomly selected community men 40 to 79 years old. *J Urol* 1999, 161:1174–1179.

23. Wasson JH, Reda DJ, Bruskewitz RC, *et al.*: A comparison of transurethral surgery with watchful waiting for moderate symptoms of benign prostatic hyperplasia. The Veterans Affairs cooperative study group on transurethral resection of the prostate. *N Engl J Med*, 1995, 332:75–79.

24. Jacobsen SJ, Jacobson DJ, Girman CJ, *et al.*: Treatment for benign prostatic hyperplasia among community dwelling men: The Olmstead County study of urinary symptoms and health status. *J Urol* 1999, 162:1301–1306.

25. McConnell JD, Roehrborn CG, Bautista OM, *et al.*: The long-term effect of doxazosin, finasteride and combination therapy on the clinical progression of benign prostatic hyperplasia. *N Engl J Med* 2003, 349:2387–2398.

26. McConnell JD, Bruskewitz R, Walsh P, *et al.*: The effect of finasteride on the risk of acute urinary retention and the need for surgical treatment among men with benign prostatic hyperplasia. *N Engl J Med* 1998, 338:557–563.

27. McConnell JD, Barry MJ, Bruskewitz RC, *et al.*: Benign prostatic hyperplasia: Diagnosis and treatment. Clinical Practice Guideline, No 8. Rockville, MD, AHCPR, Public Health Service, U.S. Department of Health and Human Services, 1994.

28. Kim ED: The use of baseline clinical measures to predict those at risk for progression of benign prostatic hyperplasia. *Curr Urol Rep* 2004, 5:267–273.

29. Kang D, Andriole GL, van de Vooren RC, *et al.*: Risk behaviours and benign prostatic hyperplasia. *BJU Int* 2004, 93:1241–1245.

30. Meigs JB, Mohr B, Barry MJ, *et al.*: Risk factors for clinical benign prostatic hyperplasia in a community-based population of healthy aging men. *J Clin Epidemiol* 2001, 54:935–944.

31. Roehrborn CG, McConnell JD: Etiology, pathophysiology, epidemiology, and natural history of benign prostatic hyperplasia. In *Campbell's Urology, edn 8.* Philadelphia: WB Saunders; 2002:1297–1336.

32. Michel MC, Heemann U, Schumacher H, *et al.*: Association of hypertension with symptoms of benign prostatic hyperplasia. *J Urol* 2004, 172:1390–1393.

33. Sanda MG, Beaty TH, Stutzman RE, *et al.*: Genetic susceptibility of benign prostatic hyperplasia. *J Urol* 1994, 152:115–119.

34. Sanda MG, Doehring CB, Binkowitz B, *et al.*: Clinical and biological characteristics of familial benign prostatic hyperplasia. *J Urol* 1997, 157:876–879.

35. Roehrborn CG, McConnell JD, Lieber M, *et al.*: Serum prostate-specific antigen concentration is a powerful predictor of acute urinary retention and need for surgery in men with clinical benign prostatic hyperplasia. PLESS Study Group. *Urology* 1999, 53:473–480.

36. Eckhardt MD, van Venrooij GEPM, Boon TA: Interactions between prostate volume, filling cystometric estimated parameters, and data from pressure-flow studies in 565 men with lower urinary tract symptoms suggestive of benign prostatic hyperplasia. *Neurourol Urodyn* 2001, 20:579–590.

37. Kaplan SA, Te AE, Pressler LB, *et al.*: Transition zone index as a method of assessing benign prostatic hyperplasia: correlation with symptoms, urine flow and detrusor pressure. *J Urol* 1995, 154:1764–1769.

38. McConnell JD: Prostate growth: new insights into hormonal regulation. *Br J Urol* 1995, 76:5–10.

39. Eri LM, Tveter KJ: A prospective, placebo-controlled study of the luteinizing hormone-releasing hormone agonist leuprolide as treatment for patients with benign prostatic hyperplasia. *J Urol* 1993, 150:359–364.

40. Walsh PC, Hutchins GM, Ewing LL: Tissue content of dihydrotestosterone in human prostatic hyperplasis is not supranormal. *J Clin Invest* 1983, 72:1772–1777.

41. Partin AW, Oesterling JE, Epstein JI, *et al.*: The influence of age and endocrine factors on the volume of benign prostatic hyperplasia. *J Urol* 1991, 145:405–409.

42. Tsurusaki T, Aoki D, Kanetake H, *et al.*: Zone-dependent expression of estrogen receptors alpha and beta in human benign prostatic hyperplasia. *J Clin Endocrinol Metab* 2003, 88:1333–1340.

43. Smith P, Rhodes NP, Ke Y, *et al.*: Relationship between upregulated oestrogen receptors and expression of growth factors in cultured, human, prostatic stromal cells exposed to estradiol or dihydrotestosterone. *Prostate Cancer Prostatic Dis* 2004, 7:57–62.

44. Niu Y, Xu Y, Zhang J, *et al.*: Proliferation and differentiation of prostatic stromal cells. *BJU Int* 2001, 87:386–393.

45. Berger AP, Kofler K, Bektic J, *et al.*: Increased growth factor production in a human prostatic stromal cell culture model caused by hypoxia. *Prostate* 2003, 57:57–65.

46. Colombel M, Vacherot F, Gil Diez S, *et al.*: Zonal variation of apoptosis and proliferation in the normal prostate and in benign prostatic hyperplasia. *Brit J Urol* 1998, 82:380–385.

47. Chon JK, Borkowski A, Partin AW, *et al.*: Alpha 1-adrenoceptor antagonists terazosin and doxazosin induce prostate apoptosis without affecting cell proliferation in patients with benign prostatic hyperplasia. *J Urol* 1999, 161:2002–2008.

48 Glassman DT, Chon JK, Borkowski A, *et al.*:Combined effect of terazosin and finasteride on apoptosis, cell proliferation and transforming growth factor-b expression in benign prostatic hyperplasia. *Prostate* 2001, 46:45–51.

49. Shapiro E, Hartanto V, Lepor H: Quantifying the smooth muscle content of the prostate using double-immunoenzymatic staining and color assisted image analysis. *J Urol* 1992, 147:1167–1170.

50. Saita Y, Yazawa H, Koizumi T, *et al.*: Mitogenic activity of endothelin on human cultured prostatic smooth muscle cells. *Eur J Pharmacol* 1998, 349:123–128.

51. Kortmann BBM, Floratos DL, Kiemeney LALM, *et al.*: Urodynamic effects of alpha-adrenoceptor blockers: a review of clinical trials. *Urology* 2003, 62:1–9.

52. Sherwood JB, McConnell JD, Vazquez DJ, *et al.*: Heterogeneity of 5 alpha-reductase gene expression in benign prostatic hyperplasia. *J Urol* 2003, 169:575–579.

53. Goulas A, Hatzichristou DG, Karakiulakis G, *et al.*: Benign hyperplasia of the human prostate is associated with tissue enrichment in chondroitin sulphate of wide size distribution. *Prostate* 2000, 44:104–110.

54. Taoka R, Tsukuda F, Ishikawa M, *et al.*: Association of prostatic inflammation with down-regulation of macrophage inhibitory cytokine-1 gene in symptomatic benign prostatic hyperplasia. *J Urol* 2004, 171:2330–2335.

55. Roberts RO, Jacobsen SJ, Jacobson DJ, *et al.*: Longitudinal changes in peak urinary flow rates in a community based cohort. *J Urol* 2000, 163:107–113.

56. Charlton RG, Morley AR, Chambers P, *et al.*: Focal changes in nerve, muscle and connective tissue in normal and unstable human bladder. *BJU Int* 1999, 84:953–960.

57. O'Reilly BA, Kosaka AH, Chang TK, *et al.*: A quantitative analysis of purinoceptor expression in the bladders of patients with symptomatic outlet obstruction. *BJU Int* 2001, 87:617–622.

58. Levin RM, Haugaard N, O'Connor L, *et al.*: Obstructive response of human bladder to bph vs. rabbit bladder response to partial outlet obstruction: A direct comparison. *Neurourol Urodyn* 2000, 19:609–629.

59. Miyashita H, Kojima M, Miki T: Ultrasonic measurement of bladder weight as a possible predictor of acute urinary retention in men with lower urinary tract symptoms suggestive of benign prostatic hyperplasia. *Ultrasound Med Biol* 2002, 28:9985–9990.

60. Horn T, Kortmann BB, Holm NR, *et al.*: Routine bladder biopsies in men with bladder outlet obstruction? *Urology* 2004, 63:451–456.

61. Griffiths K, Morton MS, Nicholson RI: Androgens, androgen receptors, antiandrogens and the treatment of prostate cancer. *Euro Urol* 1997, 32(suppl 3):24–40.

62. Rudner XL, Berkowitz DE, Booth JV, *et al.*: Subtype specific regulation of human vascular alpha(1)-adrenergic receptors by vessel bed and age. *Circulation* 1999, 100:2336–2343.

Clinical Evaluation of Lower Urinary Tract Symptoms Due to Benign Prostatic Hyperplasia including Urodynamics

2

Subbarao V. Yalla,
Maryrose P. Sullivan,
Timothy B. Boone,
Christopher E. Kelly,
& Philippe E. Zimmern

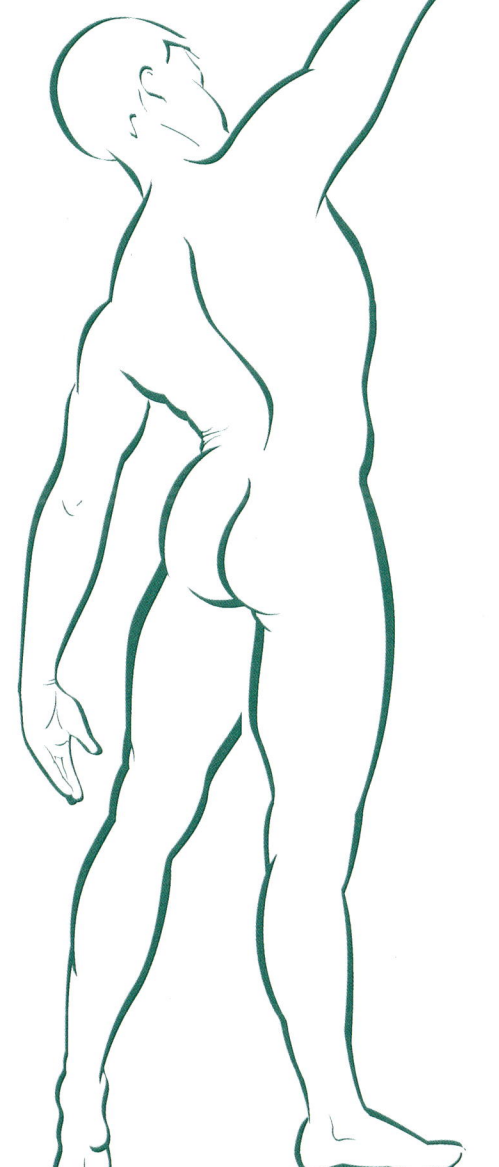

In 2000, lower urinary tract symptoms (LUTS) representing a "diagnosis of BPH" led to 4.5 million office visits in the United States [1]. The old term "prostatism" was replaced by LUTS in the mid 1990s to reflect the significant role that the bladder plays in both "irritative" and "obstructive" symptoms. Whereas it is well-established that LUTS can be precipitated by benign prostatic enlargement (BPE) and bladder outlet obstruction (BOO), LUTS can also occur secondary to aging, neurologic disease, and extravesical causes [2,3]. The term BPH is often misused. BPH implies a histologic diagnosis, which should be reserved for known prostatic tissue pathology. Therefore, the International Consultation on BPH (IC-BPH) recommended that the terms "BPE" and "BOO" be used, when appropriate, to increase accuracy of communication [4]. Dividing LUTS into "irritative" and "obstructive" components is imprecise and confusing as well, as a patient complaining of a weak force of stream (obstruction) may suffer from detrusor hypocontractility and not BOO. Furthermore, irritative symptoms associated with detrusor overactivity may or may not be attributable to BOO. BPE associated with BOO is the principal cause of LUTS; however, some patients with BPE, regardless of their degree of prostatic enlargement, may not have LUTS and may not have urodynamically defined BOO [5]. Furthermore, other patients with urodynamically confirmed BOO may not have LUTS [6]. Studies have shown that patients with BPE and no urodynamic evidence of BOO can have LUTS. It is not clear how BPH alone can induce LUTS.

Prostatic enlargement, LUTS, and BOO are all age-dependent. Based on this finding, it has been assumed that they are causally related. Two studies have shown clear data that it is an oversimplification to blame LUTS, in an aging male, on bladder outlet obstruction secondary to an enlarged prostate [7,8]. It has been proposed that altered sensory afferent input secondary to BPE may be responsible for the symptoms [9,10].

LUTS can also be secondary to pharmacologic agents that may directly or indirectly affect lower urinary tract function [11]. These agents include antihistamines, diuretics, calcium channel blockers, tricyclic compounds, sedatives, and cold remedies coupled with alpha-adrenergic agonists.

The 1994 Agency for Health Care Policy and Research (AHCPR) Clinical Practice Guidelines for the Diagnosis and Management of BPH were updated in 2000. The clinical evaluation of LUTS must take into account all participating factors, including BPH with or without BOO. The initial evaluation of LUTS starts with a detailed medical history, a genitourinary examination including a digital rectal examination (DRE), a urinalysis, and a prostate-specific antigen (PSA) test when the result would be used to make management decisions. Optional studies include a serum creatinine and a blood urea nitrogen (BUN) [12].

The medical history should search for any comorbid diseases and include a detailed pharmacologic history and a voiding diary. Also recommended is the use of patient symptom questionnaires. The most widely used and most intensively studied lower urinary tract symptom questionnaire is the International Prostate Symptom Score (IPSS), an adopted version of the American Urological Association Symptom Score [12,13]. Another popular symptom-measuring instrument is the ICS-BPH Study Questionnaire [14]. Measuring voiding symptoms allows the physician to ascertain symptom severity, may uncover symptoms not brought up during the interview, and helps monitor symptoms on therapy. It has been shown that questionnaires cannot establish the diagnosis of BPE, nor can they screen for BPE. In fact, some of the highest scores are generated by women with LUTS [15,16]. Although controversy continues as to which questionnaire measuring symptom severity is superior, more attention is now given to validated questionnaires measuring bothersomeness or quality of life indices.

The physical examination should evaluate the patient for a distended bladder, skin integrity, urethral discharge, and the presence of genital abnormalities like phimosis or meatal stenosis. A focused neurourologic examination is necessary to rule out a neurologic deficit. Assessment of the sacral cord, bulbocavernosus reflex, and anal sphincter tone are important to note, along with an assessment of motor and sensory functions of the lower extremities.

Digital rectal examination has traditionally been used to evaluate prostate size, consistency, shape, symmetry, tenderness, and induration suggestive of prostate cancer. However, the DRE is only moderately effective in estimating prostatic size when compared with transrectal ultrasound or MRI [17]. It should also be noted that in population-based studies, prostate size did not correlate with the severity of LUTS [18].

The laboratory investigation considered standard by most guidelines is the urinalysis to rule out urinary tract infection. Both serum creatinine and BUN levels to ascertain renal function are now optional [13]. Other tests like urinary cytology may be used to screen for carcinoma in situ of the bladder. The PSA measurement is recommended for the initial evaluation of LUTS when knowing the value would change potential management. For this reason, the clinician should take into account the patient's age, life expectancy, and intent to treat. For example, a life expectancy of more than 10 years and a plan to treat prostate cancer, if it is diagnosed, is required by some guideline panels, including the IC-BPH [18].

Endoscopic evaluation may be helpful in the clinical evaluation of LUTS. Some causes of LUTS, other than BPE, may be discovered using cystourethroscopy. These would include urethral stricture, bladder cancer, cystitis, and bladder stones. Bladder trabeculation has recently been shown to correlate significantly with urodynamically proven BOO and detrusor overactivity. However, 11% of patients with no trabeculations were found to be obstructed, whereas 8% with severe trabecula-

tions had no obstruction [20,21]. Because endoscopic identification of a large median lobe may influence some therapeutic decisions, cystoscopy is encouraged in patients with BOO who are seeking minimally invasive therapies.

Although now considered standard by the IC-BPH panel, urinary flowmetry can serve as a noninvasive screening test for selecting patients who should undergo more sophisticated urodynamic studies. This test, however, has several limitations. First, peak flow rates (Q_{max}) less than 15 mL/sec do not necessarily differentiate between obstruction and detrusor impairment. Additionally, the peak flow rate (Q_{max}) can be highly variable among individual sequential voids [22] and does not correlate with the degree of obstruction. Lastly, a normal flow rate does not exclude obstruction [4].

The predictive role of postvoid residual (PVR) measurement is poor. A large residual urine volume can be secondary to detrusor failure or as a direct result of BOO [23]. A high PVR, although unable to differentiate between obstruction and bladder decompensation, might predict a slightly higher failure rate with a "watchful waiting" strategy. Threshold values have been poorly defined. However, very high PVR values (>300 mL) may increase the risk of upper tract dilatation and renal failure [24].

Urodynamic evaluation with pressure flow testing is the gold standard for determining the true etiology of LUTS. A filling cystometrogram can detect the presence of detrusor overactivity, compliance changes, or a reduction in maximum bladder capacity. Also, combined voiding pressure with flow studies can help distinguish between obstruction and impaired detrusor contractility or hypocontractility. Although not required for all patients, multichannel urodynamic evaluation is recommended for the following patients:

• Those in whom a diagnosis is difficult to infer from history, physical examination, and simple tests.

• Those with a complex history of multiple prior surgeries.

• Those with documented or suspected neurologic disease (eg, multiple sclerosis, spinal stenosis, Parkinson's disease, diabetes, stroke, chronic alcoholism, and neuropathies).

• Those in whom empiric treatment such as pharmacotherapy and biofeedback fail.

• When irreversible or potentially morbid treatments are planned.

• When results from uroflowmetry or PVR are grossly abnormal.

• In young patients in whom underlying voiding dysfunction more so than BPE or BOO may be associated with LUTS [25].

Imaging of the lower urinary tract (videourodynamics or voiding cystourethrography) is sometimes helpful to diagnose the site of obstruction when BOO is suspected. For example, radiographic imaging may help establish the exact location of obstruction in a patient with a prior history of failed lower urinary tract surgery. Transrectal ultrasound of the prostate can accurately assess prostate volume and guide surgical decisions. Symptomatic patients with BPE in excess of 75 cm³ might be considered for an open procedure, whereas those with smaller glands may be offered more minimally invasive, outflow-relieving procedures. Imaging of the upper urinary tract is very selectively recommended in men with a history of urinary tract infection, urolithiasis, hematuria, or renal insufficiency [19].

In summary, the clinician must judiciously select appropriate methods of evaluation for successful management of elderly men with LUTS. Diagnosis before, rather than after, empiric treatment can avoid morbidity and is likely more cost effective in the long run.

THE RELATIONSHIPS AMONG LOWER URINARY TRACT SYMPTOMS, BENIGN PROSTATIC ENLARGEMENT, AND BLADDER OUTLET OBSTRUCTION

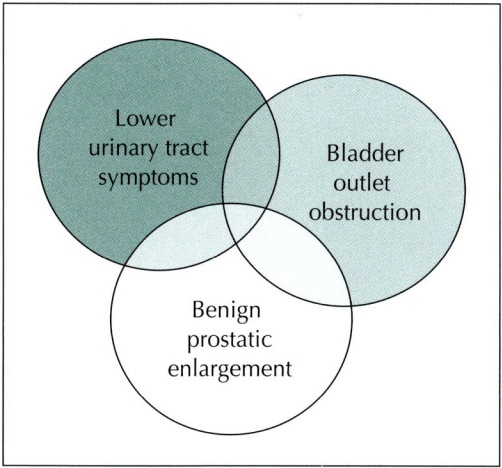

▶ **FIGURE 2-1.** The interrelationships among lower urinary tract symptoms (LUTS), benign prostatic enlargement (BPE), and bladder outlet obstruction (BOO). These interrelationships can be complex [26]. As this Venn diagram shows, patients with BPE can have symptoms with or without BOO [27]. Furthermore, some patients with LUTS do not have BOO [28]. Other prostatic diseases, such as prostatitis or prostatic carcinoma, can lead to LUTS. Conversely, varying degrees of BOO have been detected in asymptomatic elderly men [6].

Although BPE without detectable BOO could produce LUTS via increased or altered afferent neural input [9], no large-scale studies have supported this hypothesis. (*Courtesy of* Subbarao V. Yalla, MD and Maryrose P. Sullivan, PhD).

A. Causes of Urologic Lower Urinary Tract Symptoms

Ureter
  Acute distal ureteral irritation
    Secondary to calculi or stent
Bladder
  Increased postvoid residual urine
    From bladder outlet obstruction
    From detrusor hypo- or areflexia
  Involuntary detrusor contraction
    Detrusor instability
    Detrusor hyperreflexia
  Intrinsic bladder wall disorder
    Poor compliance
  Bacterial cystitis
  Interstitial cystitis
  Trigonitis
  Bladder aging
  Bladder neoplasm
Prostate
  Benign prostatic enlargement
  Prostate cancer
  Prostatitis
Urethra
  Urethritis
  Stricture

▶ **FIGURE 2-2.** Urologic (**A**) and nonurologic

(*Continued on next page*)

B. Nonurologic Causes of Lower Urinary Tract Symptoms

Excessive fluid intake
  Learned behavior
  Drug-induced polydipsia
    Anticholinergics
    Chlorpromazine
  Psychogenic polydipsia
  Hypothalamic disease
Inadequate tubular reabsorption of water
  Diabetes insipidus
    Central
    Nephrogenic
Altered renal absorption of solutes
  Glucose (diabetes mellitus)
  Mannitol
  Diuretics
Sleep disorders
Excess fluid mobilization when supine (eg, CHF)
Pelvic floor muscle spasm
CNS disorders
  Multiple sclerosis
  Parkinson's disease
  Cerebral vascular accident
  Trauma
PNS disorders
  Trauma
    Iatrogenic (eg, after abdominal perineal resection)
    Noniatrogenic
  Infection
    Herpes zoster
Drugs
  Inhibiting bladder contractility
    Antihistamines
    Antimuscarinics
    β-antagonists
    Psychotropic medications
  Increasing outlet resistance
    Adrenergic agonists
    Imipramine
  Increasing renal blood flow
    Caffeine

▶ **FIGURE 2-2.** (*Continued*) (**B**) causes of lower urinary tract symptoms (LUTS). LUTS can be produced by several factors that may or may not be primarily urologic in origin. CHF—congestive heart failure; CNS—central nervous system; PNS—peripheral nervous system.

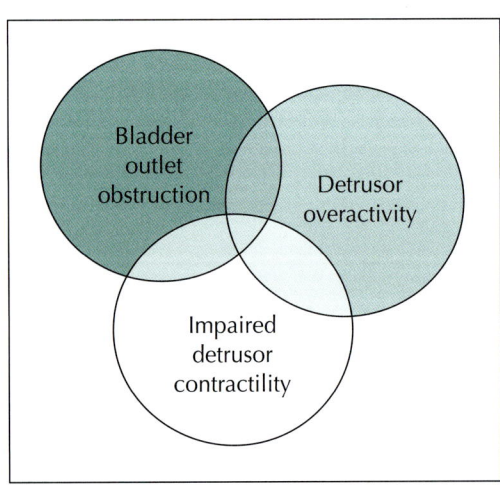

▶ **FIGURE 2-3.** Functional abnormalities associated with benign prostatic enlargement (BPE). These include bladder outlet obstruction (BOO), detrusor overactivity (DO), and impaired detrusor contractility (IC). A combination of BOO, DO, and IC may coexist. Conversely, prostatic enlargement presumed to be caused by benign prostatic hypertrophy can sometimes be asymptomatic and manifest no urodynamic abnormalities. (*Courtesy of* Subbarao V. Yalla, MD and Maryrose P. Sullivan, PhD).

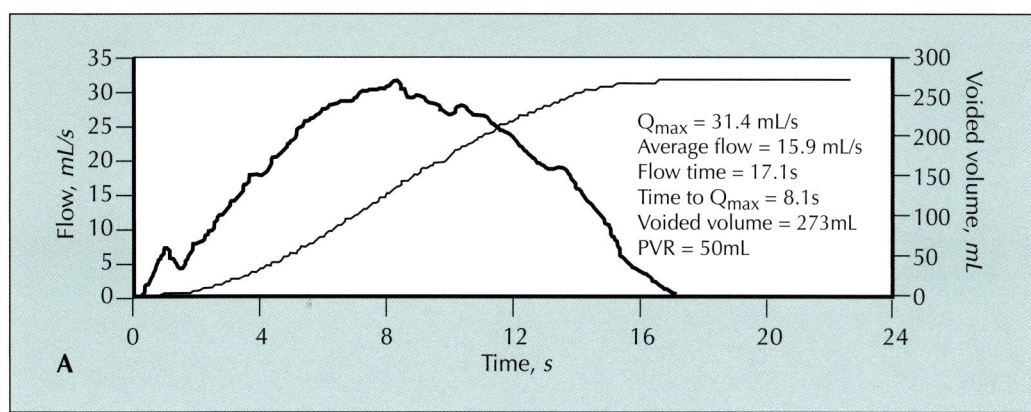

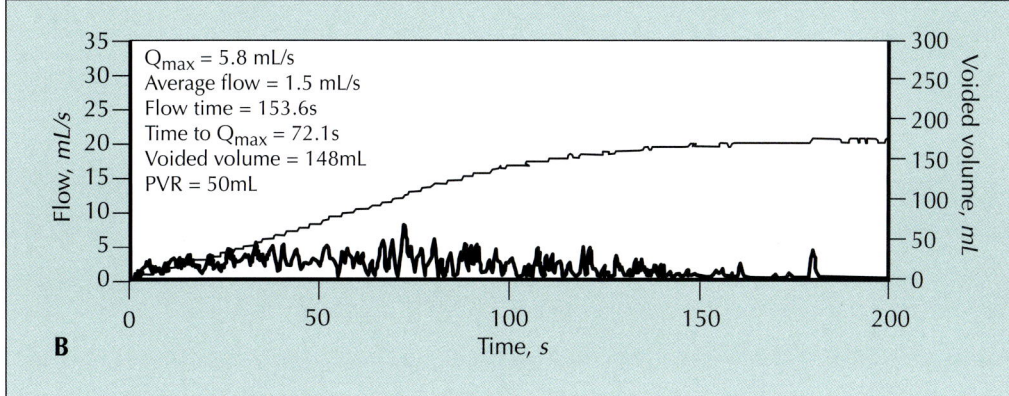

▶ **FIGURE 2-4.** Uroflowmetry. Uroflowmetry is a simple, noninvasive urodynamic test that can be an invaluable screening tool for identifying those patients who require more extensive urodynamic evaluation. Thus, a patient with a low urinary flow rate will need further testing to discriminate between poor detrusor contractility and bladder outlet obstruction [29]. Various types of abnormal voiding patterns can be recognized from uroflowmetry parameters, and from the flow curve. Note that many studies report the maximum urinary flow rate (Q_{max}) as a measure of response to treatment. However, the dependence of Q_{max} on age and bladder volume (>150 mL) should not be overlooked in the final analysis. **A,** A normal urinary flow pattern is characterized by a bell-shaped curve with high Q_{max}. Note the short micturition time and the volume voided. Voided volumes less than 150 mL make uroflowmetry interpretation difficult. **B**, Abnormal uroflowmetry is characterized by a low maximum flow rate and a prolonged duration. Several flow patterns have been described that typify "obstructive flow," detrusor impairment, Valsalva voiding, and superflow [30]. Uroflowmetry can alert the clinician when voiding is abnormal, thus prompting the recommendation for a pressure-flow study. PVR—postvoid residual. (*Courtesy of* Subbarao V. Yalla, MD and Maryrose P. Sullivan, PhD).

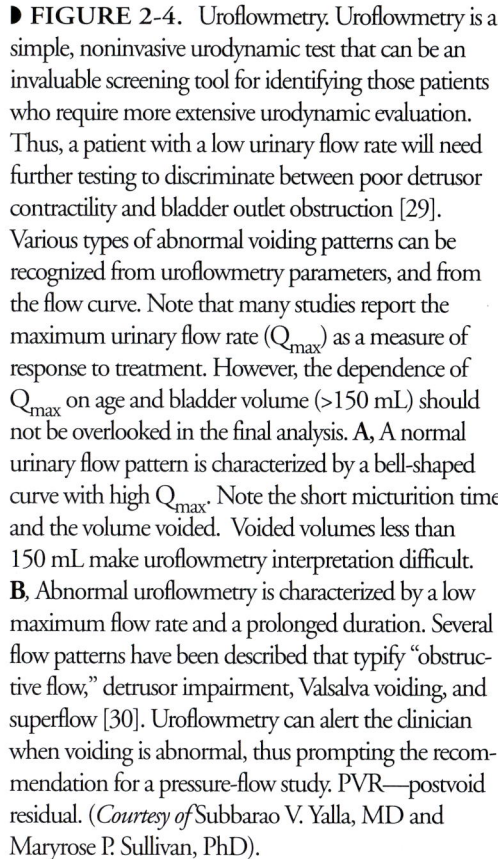

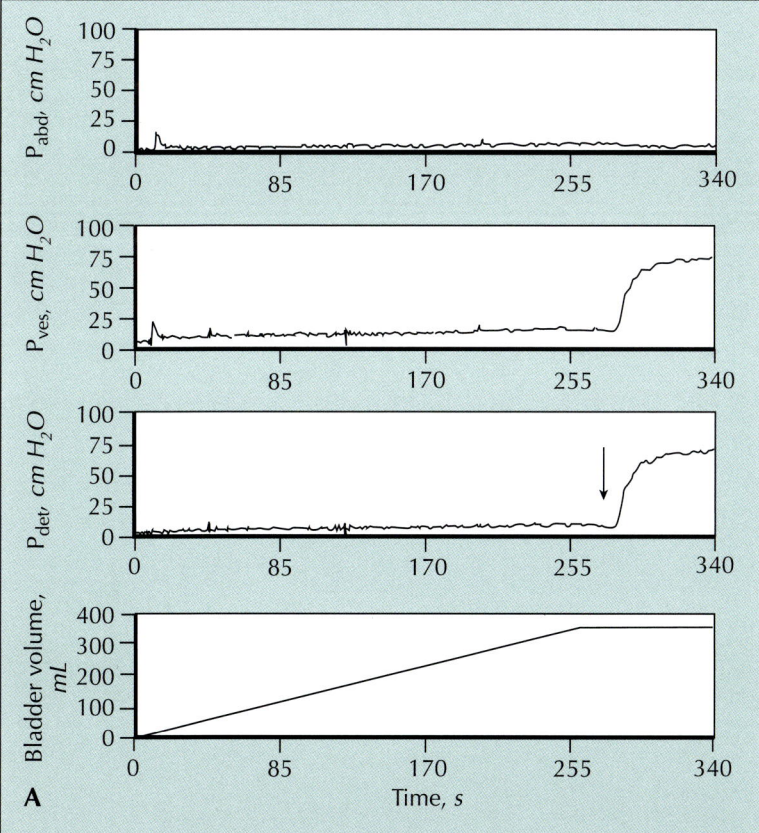

▶ **FIGURE 2-5.** Cystometry. The multichannel cystometrogram (CMG) uses simultaneous pressure transducer catheters in the bladder (P_{ves}) and in the rectum (P_{abd}). The true bladder pressure (P_{det}) ($P_{det} = P_{ves}-P_{abd}$) is a mathematical derivative obtained from subtracting the abdominal pressure from the total pressure measured within the bladder.

A filling CMG provides objective data on bladder filling, desire to void, detrusor capacity, and detrusor compliance. It is particularly helpful when the patient's symptoms are reproduced during the test. Therefore, it is imperative that the clinician be highly observant of the patient's experience during the study. Also, several points can help to avoid pitfalls in interpretation. Rapid filling can artifactually cause detrusor overactivity. Thus, an involuntary detrusor contraction corresponds to a symptomatic involuntary intravesical pressure rise, which the patient cannot actively inhibit. One should also remember that spontaneous rectal contractions can affect P_{abd} and result in a falsely reduced detrusor pressure. Lastly, detrusor compliance, measured by dividing the change in the bladder volume to the rise in detrusor pressure, is dependent on filling rate and volume [31].

A, A normal filling CMG in an adult man is characterized by a bladder capacity of 350 to 500 mL with low detrusor pressure and absence of involuntary contractions. In this 64-year-old asymptomatic man, bladder capacity was 360 mL with a bladder compliance of 60 mL/cm H_2O. The *arrow* indicates the onset of a voluntary bladder contraction.

(*Continued on next page*)

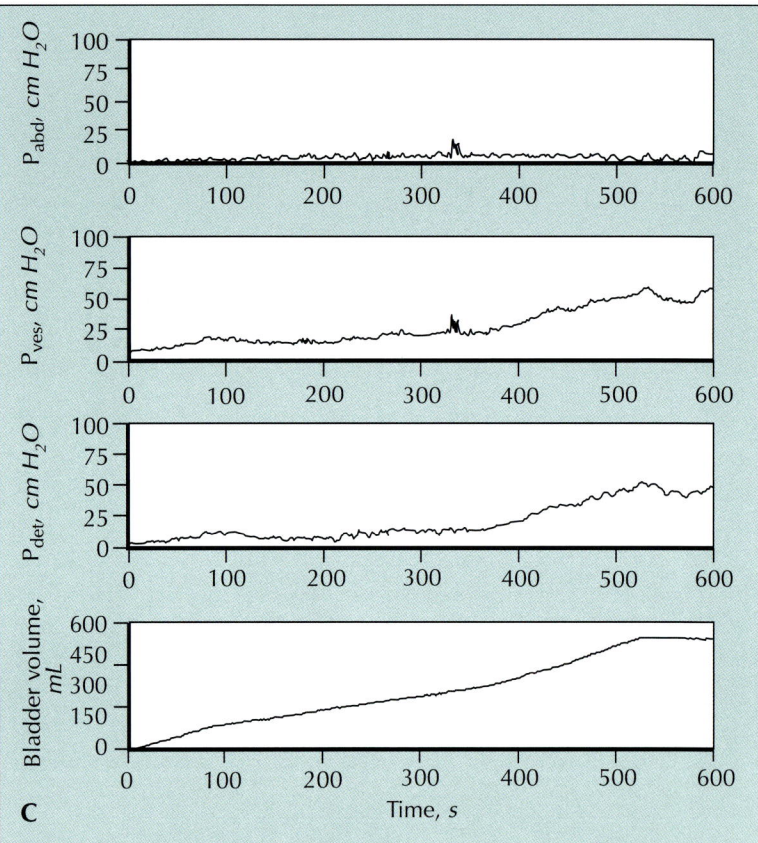

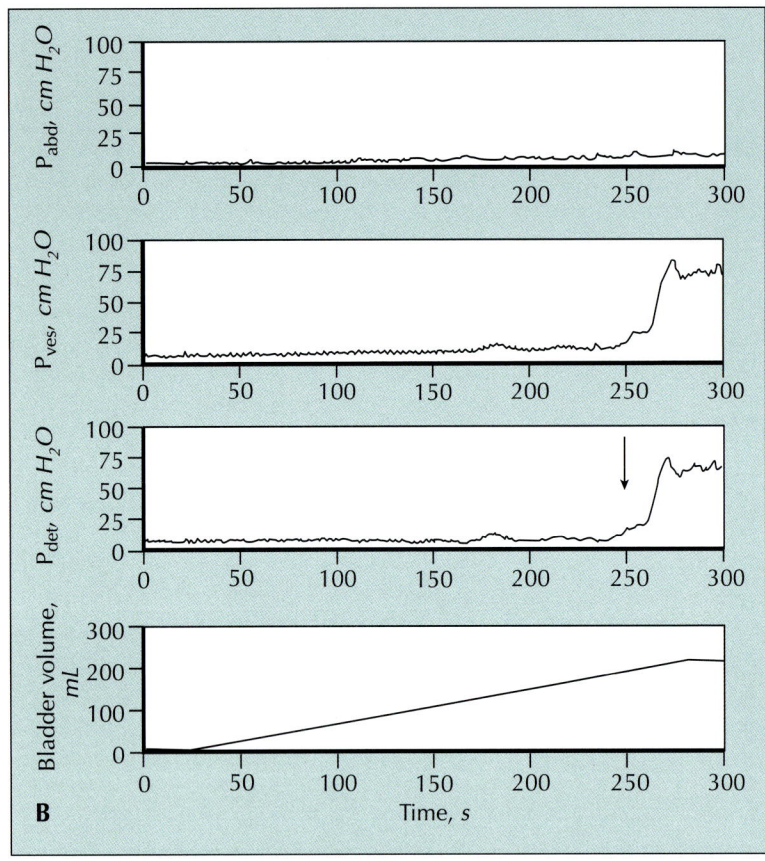

▶ **FIGURE 2-5.** (*Continued*) **B,** This CMG shows a strong uninhibited detrusor contraction at 190 mL. Stopping the flow of infusant may help distinguish detrusor overactivity from end-fill compliance changes. **C,** In the literature, diminished bladder compliance was arbitrarily defined by the International Continence Society as less than 20 mL/cm H_2O [32]. This filling CMG demonstrates an increased slope of detrusor pressure in a patient with bladder outlet obstruction as the bladder was filled beyond

400 mL. This increased slope occurred in the later phase of bladder filling and could be mistaken for the onset of a detrusor contraction. However, the sustained increase in bladder pressure after cessation of bladder filling indicates decreased compliance. In this patient, bladder compliance (10.9 mL/cm H_2O) was considered abnormal, because bladder pressure did not return to baseline after filling stopped. (*Courtesy of* Subbarao V. Yalla, MD and Maryrose P. Sullivan, PhD).

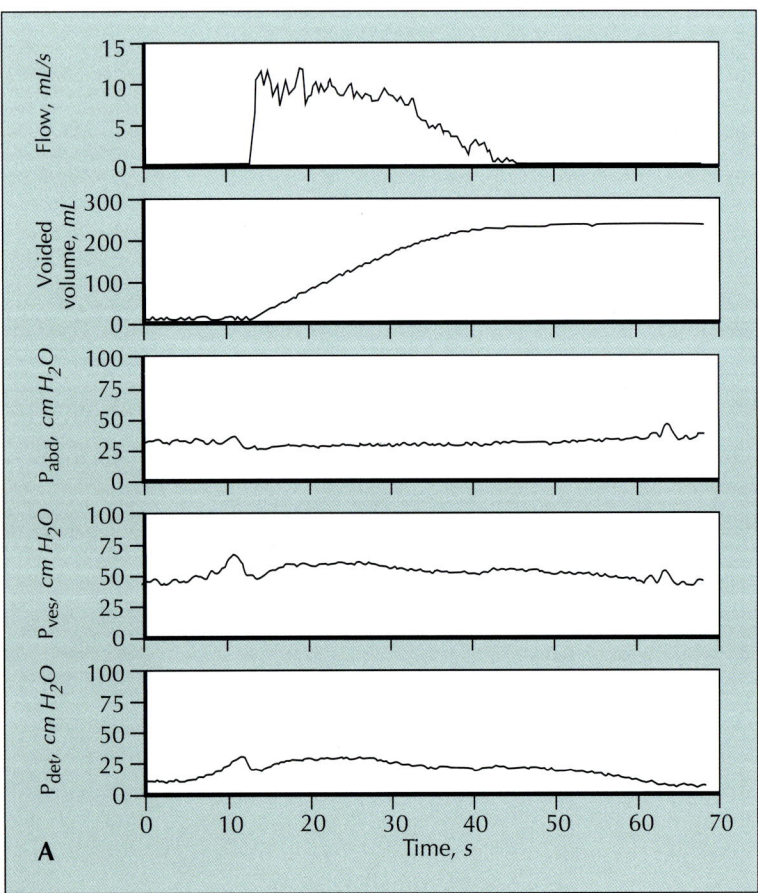

▶ **FIGURE 2-6.** The pressure-flow study is widely accepted as an important urodynamic step to assess bladder contractility and outlet resistance. Simultaneous intravesical pressure, intrarectal pressure, and urinary flow rate are recorded during voiding in either the sitting or standing positions. This study can be performed under fluoroscopic monitoring to detect bladder changes such as diverticuli and vesicoureteral reflux. The pressure and flow tracings obtained from a nonobstructed (**A**), a mildly obstructed

(*Continued on next page*)

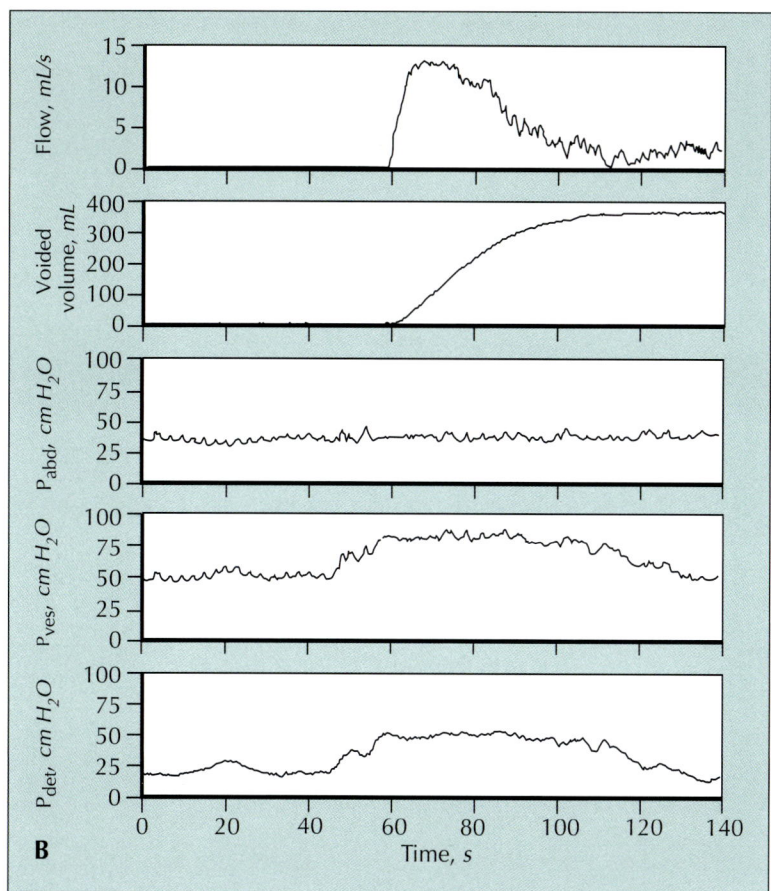

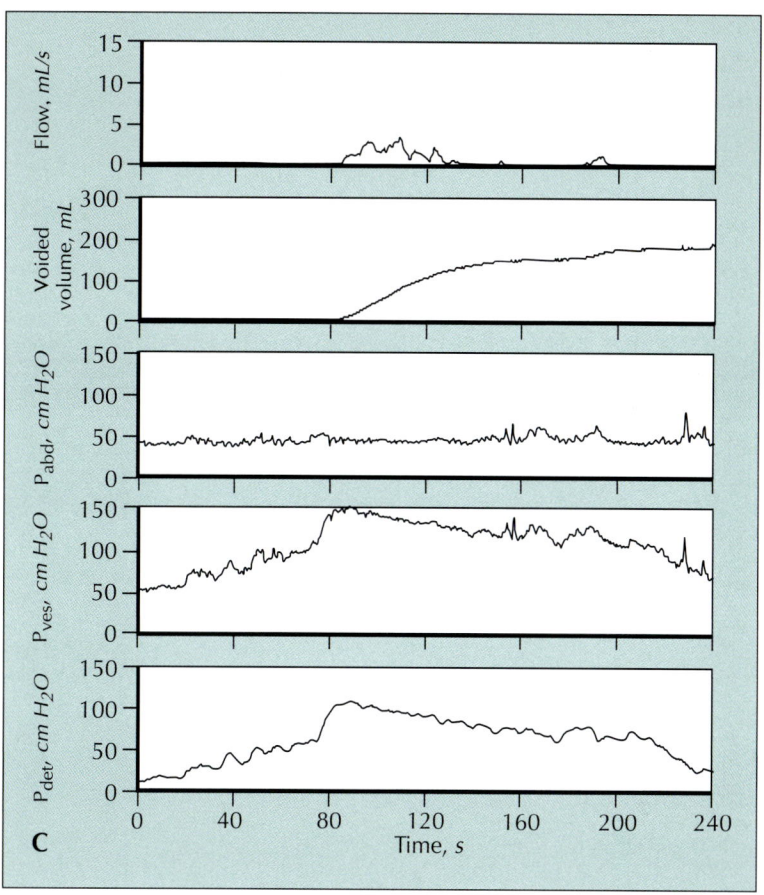

▶ **FIGURE 2-6.** (*Continued*) (**B**), and a severely obstructed (**C**) patient are shown. P_{abd}—abdominal pressure; P_{det}—detrusor pressure; P_{ves}—vesical pressure. (*Courtesy of* Subbarao V. Yalla, MD and Maryrose P. Sullivan, PhD).

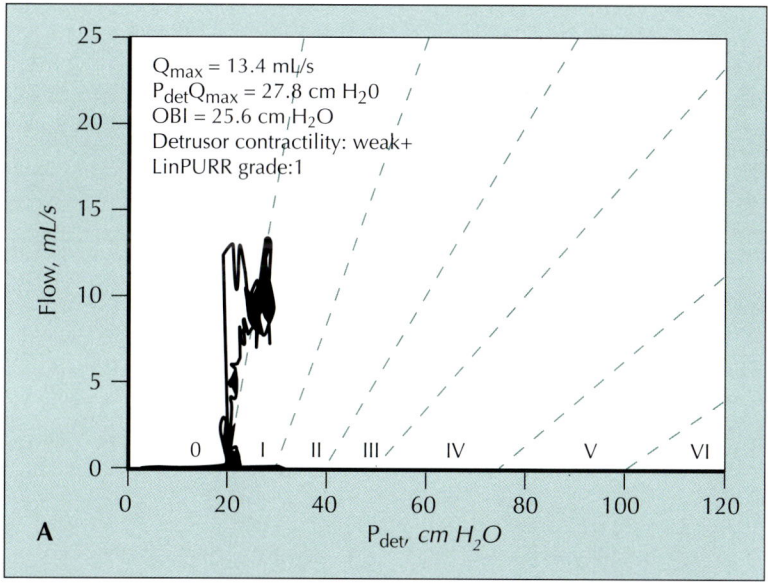

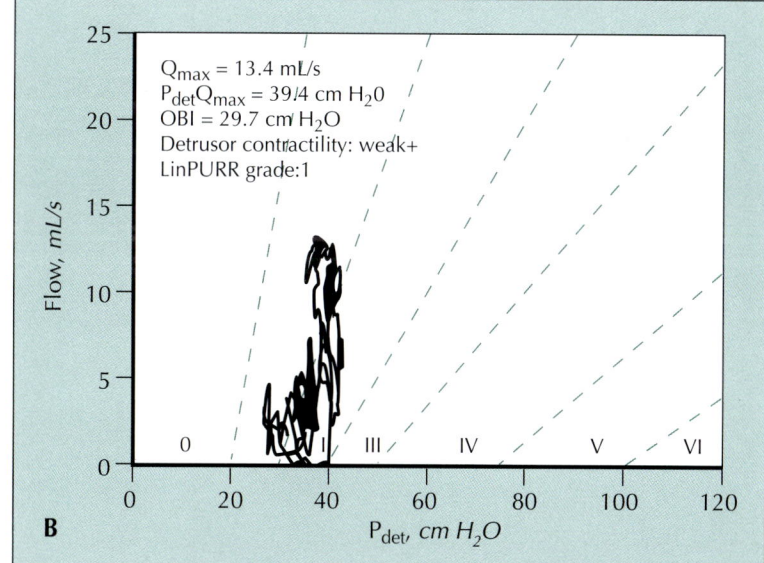

▶ **FIGURE 2-7.** Pressure-flow (P-Q) studies can be analyzed using a number of sophisticated methods that are based on similar concepts and thus produce fairly comparable results [23]. After eliminating artifacts and correcting the time lag between detrusor pressure and onset of flow, the urinary flow is plotted against the corresponding detrusor pressure during voiding. The nomogram proposed by Schafer for grading bladder outlet obstruction (BOO) is based on the concept of the passive urethral resistance relation (PURR) [33]. PURR represents the passive state of bladder outlet, which is presumed to be free from smooth muscle and striated sphincter influences during voiding. The resistance offered by the bladder outlet under these conditions is assumed to be entirely due to the mechanical properties of the posterior urethra, including the prostate gland. This analysis can be simplified by approximating the PURR with a straight line (LinPURR). LinPURR is graded into six categories (0 through 5), with grade 2 and higher representing BOO. Detrusor contractility is classified in the nomogram as very weak, weak, normal, and strong. The P-Q plots, generated from the same patients studied in Figure 2-6, are superimposed on Schafer's nomogram to determine the severity of BOO and detrusor strength. Data from Figures 2-6*A* and 2-6*B* fall into grade 1 on Schafer's nomogram (**A** and **B**), whereas data

(Continued on next page)

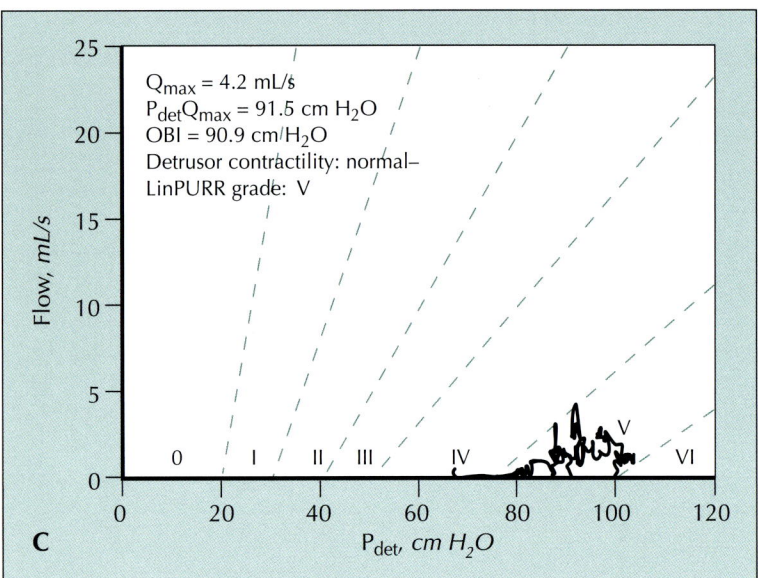

Q_max = 4.2 mL/s
$P_{det}Q_{max}$ = 91.5 cm H_2O
OBI = 90.9 cm/H_2O
Detrusor contractility: normal–
LinPURR grade: V

C

▶ **FIGURE 2-7.** (*Continued*) from Figure 2-6*C* fall into grade 5, indicating severe obstruction (**C**). $P_{det}Q_{max}$—detrusor pressure at maximum flow. (*Courtesy of* Subbarao V. Yalla, MD and Maryrose P. Sullivan, PhD).

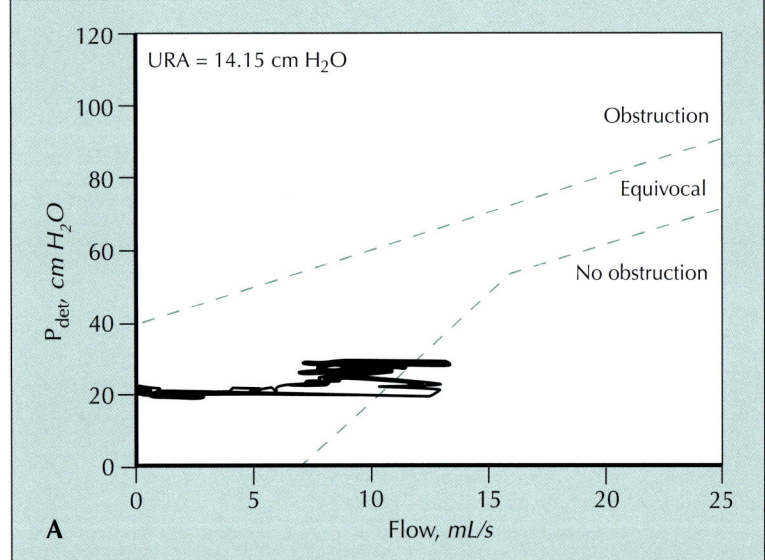

URA = 14.15 cm H_2O

Obstruction
Equivocal
No obstruction

A

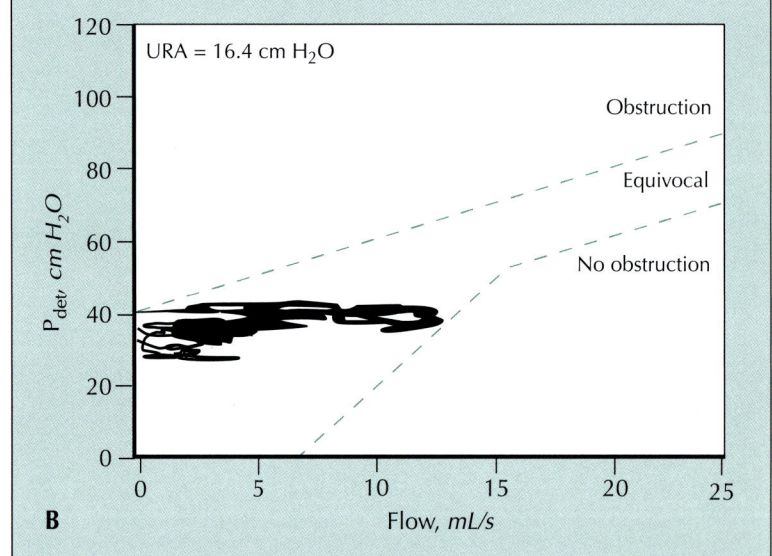

URA = 16.4 cm H_2O

Obstruction
Equivocal
No obstruction

B

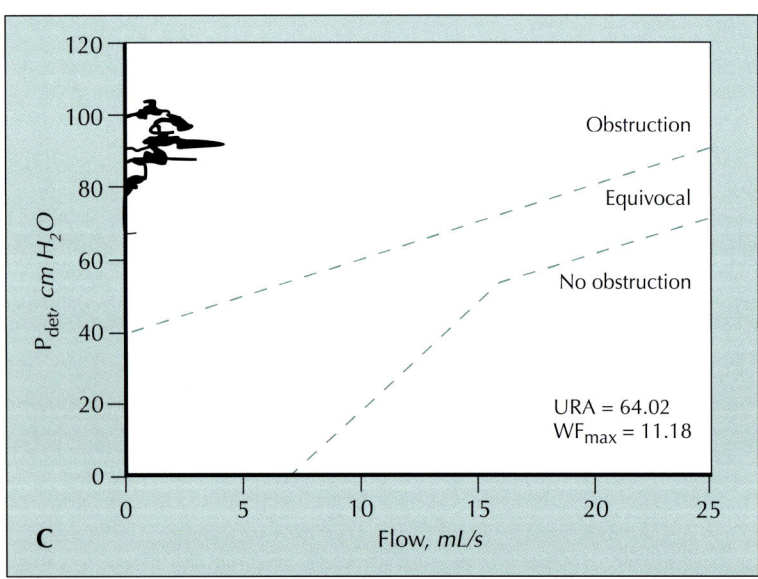

Obstruction
Equivocal
No obstruction
URA = 64.02
WF_max = 11.18

C

▶ **FIGURE 2-8.** The Abrams-Griffiths (A-G) nomogram also can be used to characterize the bladder outlet as obstructed, nonobstructed, and equivocal based on the location of the point determined by the detrusor pressure at maximum flow ($P_{det}Q_{max}$) and the maximum flow rate (Q_{max}) [23]. The line on the graph is a continuous plot of P_{det} versus flow. The provisional standard of the International Continence Society for pressure-flow (P-Q) analysis is a modified A-G nomogram in which the slope separating equivocal from unobstructed zones is constant [34]. The A-G number ($P_{det}Q_{max} - 2 \times Q_{max}$) is used to further distinguish equivocal values. Values greater than 40 are correlated with obstruction, whereas values less than 20 are associated with no obstruction. A-G numbers between 20 and 40 are deemed equivocal. The urethral resistance factor (URA), a prostate-specific parameter that approximates the passive urethral resistance relation also can be used to diagnose bladder outlet obstruction on a continuous scale [35]. The P-Q plots generated from the data in Figure 2-6 are superimposed on the A-G nomogram. This analysis results in a diagnosis of no obstruction (**A**), equivocal obstruction (**B**), and obstruction (**C**) for the patients shown in Figure 2-6*A* to *C*, respectively. Detrusor contractility can be assessed by calculating the maximum Watts factor (WF_max) [36] or by generating the maximum isovolumetric detrusor pressure (P_{iso}). The Watts factor has been shown to correlate well with P_{iso} [37]. (*Courtesy of* Subbarao V. Yalla, MD and Maryrose P. Sullivan, PhD).

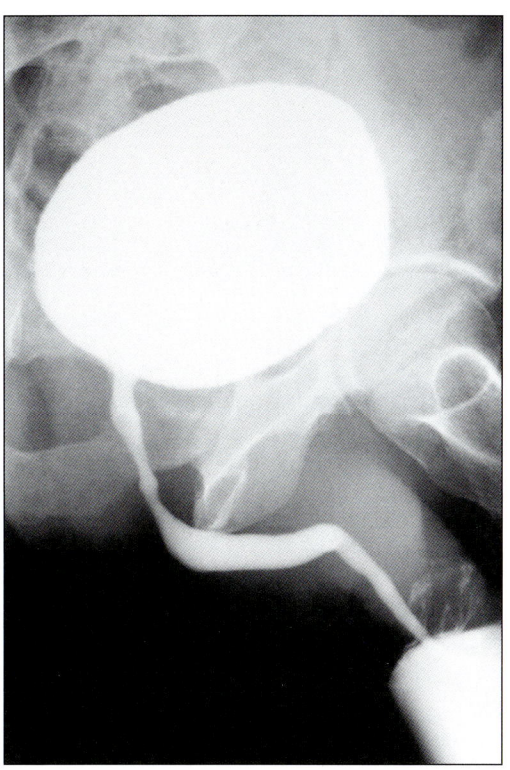

▶ **FIGURE 2-9.** Normal voiding cystourethrography (VCUG) result. Patients undergoing video-urodynamics have the benefit of radiologic imaging of the lower urinary tract to identify significant structural abnormalities that may be associated with voiding dysfunction. When fluoroscopic-assisted urodynamic evaluations are not available, VCUG can be performed as an important adjunct to the functional urodynamic evaluation. By observing the detrusor contour, the degree of bladder neck funneling, the degree of prostatic fossa and bulbous urethral filling, and any degrees of reflux can be determined. This normal VCUG of a 35-year-old asymptomatic volunteer with a normal urodynamic study is characterized by a smooth bladder contour, opened bladder neck and prostatic urethra, and well-distended bulbous urethra. The smooth filling defect in the middle of the prostatic urethra corresponds to the verumontanum. (*Courtesy of* Subbarao V. Yalla, MD and Maryrose P. Sullivan, PhD).

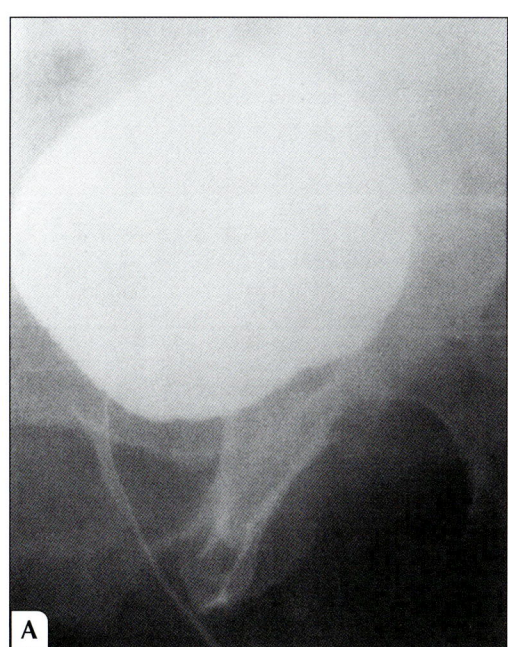

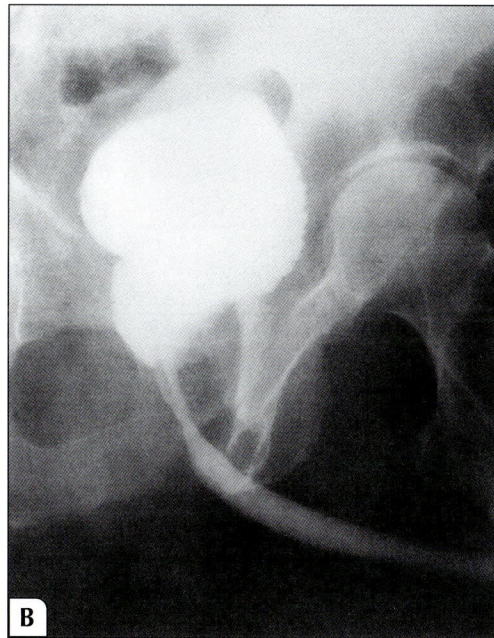

▶ **FIGURE 2-10.** Abnormal voiding cystourethrography (VCUG) results. **A,** VCUG of an elderly man with lower urinary tract symptoms and radiographic evidence of bladder outlet obstruction. The bladder neck and prostatic urethra appear narrow. **B,** VCUG of an elderly man after transurethral resection of the prostate. The prostatic fossa is wide and the bladder neck is open. There is no evidence of bladder neck contracture or filling defect, suggesting incomplete resection or prostatic regrowth.

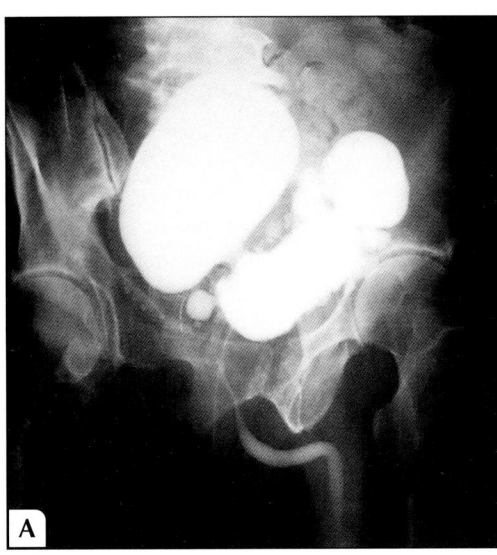 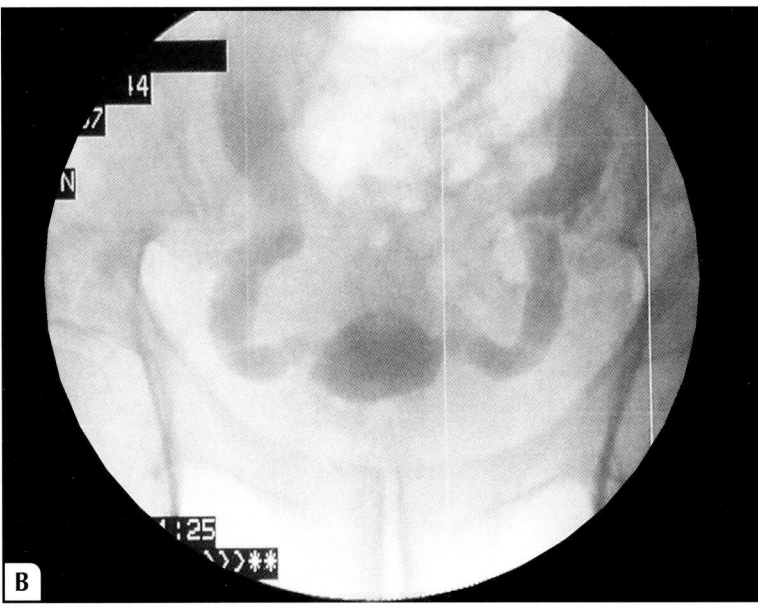

▶ **FIGURE 2-11.** Large bladder diverticula and high-grade vesi-coureteral reflux. These conditions can be the result of chronically elevated vesical pressures. It is important to recognize that both diverticula can confound the urodynamic evaluation by falsely lowering the true bladder capacity and voiding pressure. By providing a venting mechanism to elevated intravesical pressures, they narrow the margin between bladder outlet obstruction (BOO) and detrusor hypocontractility. **A,** Voiding cystourethrogram (VCUG) of an elderly man with lower urinary tract symptoms shows a large bladder diverticulum with a capacity greater than 50% of the total bladder capacity and multiple small diverticula. Bladder diverticula may be congenital but more commonly result from BOO.

Diverticula can be the source of recurrent urinary tract infections (persistent contrast in the diverticulum on the postvoid film) or incomplete bladder emptying. **B,** The VCUG of an 80-year-old man with severe lower urinary tract symptoms and a poorly compliant bladder showed high-grade bilateral ureteral reflux with most of the radiocontrast solution entering the renal pelvis and widely dilated ureters. Despite the marked redundancy in the upper urinary tract, the bladder pressures were elevated during filling. His renal function was impaired as demonstrated by elevated serum creatinine and blood urea nitrogen. (*Courtesy of* Subbarao V. Yalla, MD and Maryrose P. Sullivan, PhD).

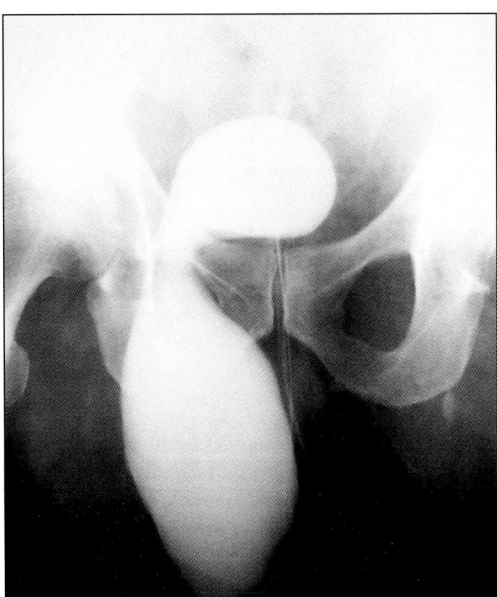

▶ **FIGURE 2-12.** In some cases, the structural abnormalities identified on voiding cystourethrogram (VCUG) can change the management strategy. This VCUG of a 65-year-old man with an American Urological Association Symptom Index score of 25 shows scrotal herniation of the urinary bladder. Urodynamic evidence of mild outlet obstruction with detrusor instability was noted. Cystoscopy and pressure-flow studies without radiologic assistance would have missed this important structural abnormality. In fact, this patient had been treated for several months with an α-adrenergic blocker (terazosin) without relief of symptoms. Following reduction of a wide-mouthed bladder diverticulum, the direct inguinal hernia was repaired. (*Courtesy of* Subbarao V. Yalla, MD and Maryrose P. Sullivan, PhD).

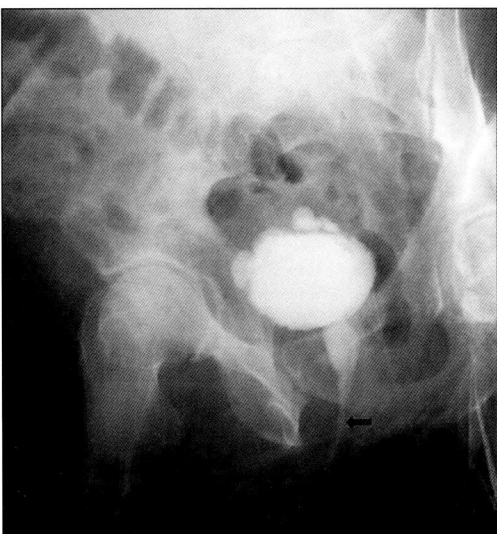

▶ **FIGURE 2-13.** In patients with bladder outlet obstruction, the site of obstruction cannot be determined by pressure-flow studies, although the prostate is the most likely location in elderly patients with nonneuro-pathic, nontraumatic lower urinary tract dysfunction. However, this voiding cystourethrogram in an elderly man with lower urinary tract symptoms reveals a narrow membranous urethra with proximal dilation of the prostatic urethra (*arrow*), suggesting obstruction in the region of the membranous urethra but not in the prostatic urethra. Note the small diverticula in the bladder dome. (*Courtesy of* Subbarao V. Yalla, MD and Maryrose P. Sullivan, PhD).

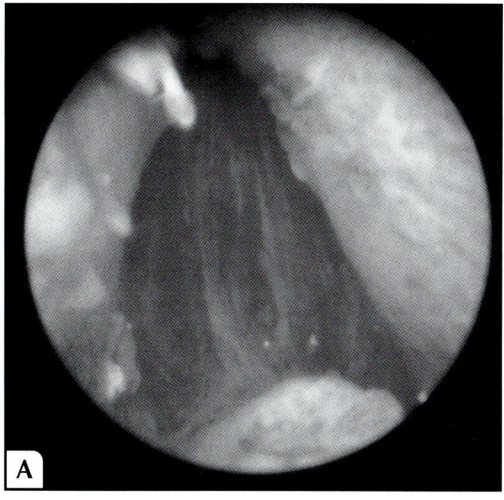

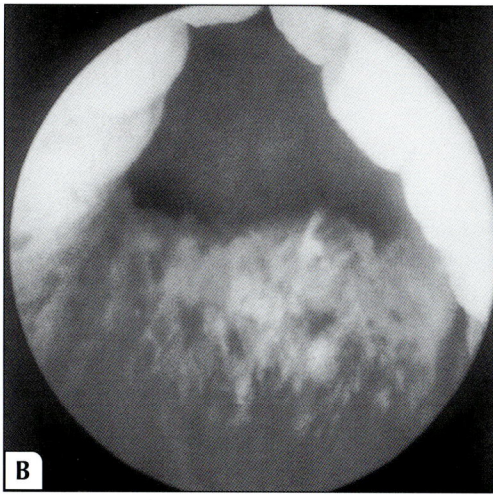

▶ **FIGURE 2-14.** Because cystoscopy is done in a retrograde fashion, endoscopic findings regarding the prostatic urethra cannot reliably determine bladder outlet obstruction [38]. **A,** Cystoscopy of the bladder neck and midprostatic urethra shows minimal prostatic lobes and a closed bladder neck. No obstruction was found urodynamically. **B,** Up to 25% of patients have median lobe enlargement, which may be responsible for obstruction and lower urinary tract symptoms. (**A** *Courtesy of* Subbarao V. Yalla, MD and Maryrose P. Sullivan, PhD).

CLINICAL APPROACH FOR THE ASSESSMENT OF LOWER URINARY TRACT SYMPTOMS

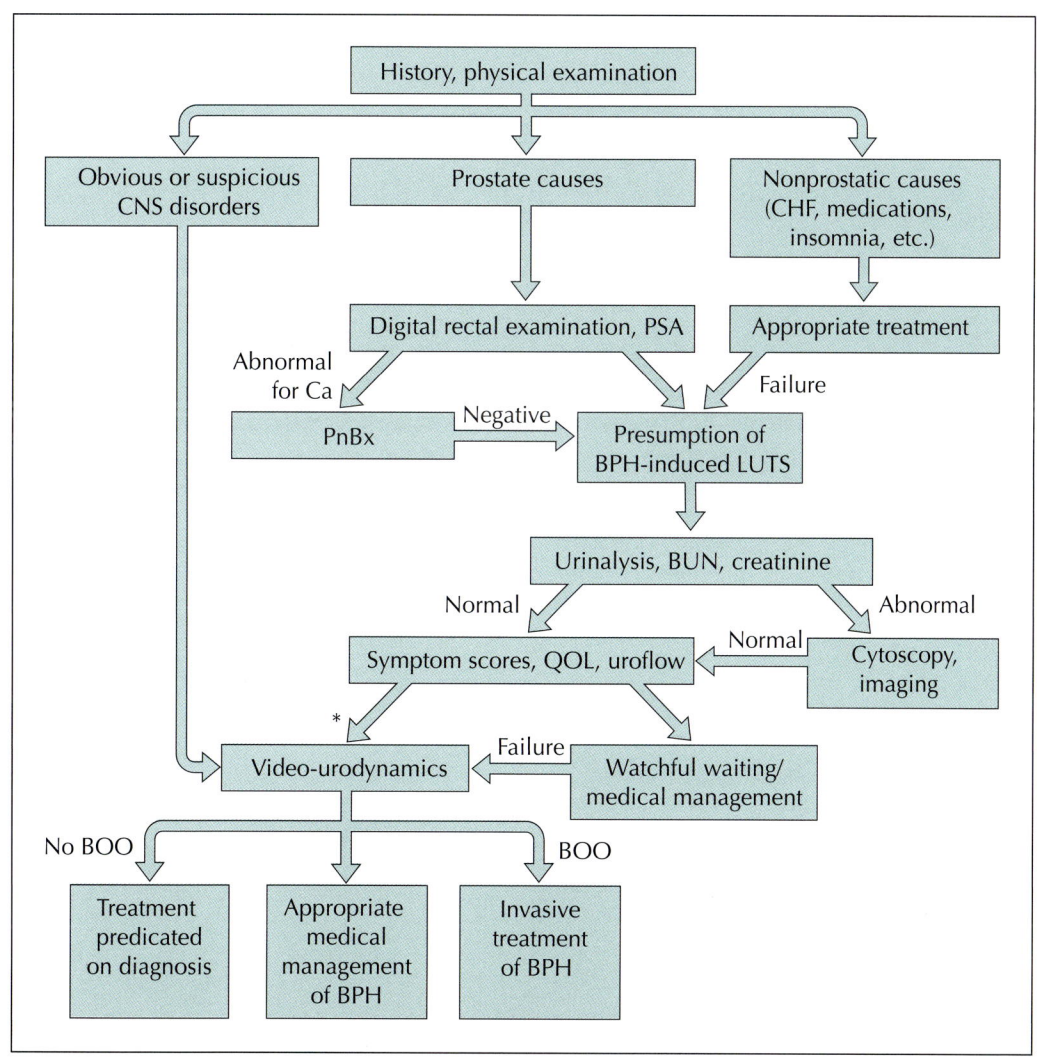

▶ **FIGURE 2-15.** Algorithm for evaluating adult and elderly men with lower urinary tract symptoms (LUTS). Prostatic causes are separated from other factors that can produce symptoms. After deciding whether benign prostatic hyperplasia (BPH) is presumed responsible for LUTS, the symptom scores decide the remaining part of the work-up of patients with LUTS. The decision to perform cystoscopy, intravenous pyelogram, ultrasonic imaging, or other ancillary tests is prompted by abnormal urinalysis, blood urea nitrogen (BUN), and creatinine, but not by symptom scores alone. The *asterisk* denotes that urodynamic studies are indicated in patients with obvious or suspicious central nervous system (CNS) disorders, in patients who may be candidates for invasive procedures, in younger patients in whom a more accurate diagnosis is required before pharmacologic or surgical intervention, and in frail, elderly patients who are prone to a higher morbidity. BOO—bladder outlet obstruction; CHF—congestive heart failure; PnBX—prostatic needle biopsy; PSA—prostate-specific antigen; QOL—quality of life. (*Courtesy of* Subbarao V. Yalla, MD and Maryrose P. Sullivan, PhD).

REFERENCES

1. Abrams P: In support of pressure flow studies for evaluating men with lower urinary tract symptoms. *Urology* 1994, 44:153–155.

2. Dyro FM, DuBeau CE, Sullivan MP, *et al.*: Covert comorbid neurologic abnormalities in patients presenting with symptoms of prostatism. *J Urol* 1992, 147:269A.

3. Resnick NM: Voiding dysfunction in the elderly. In *Neurourology and Urodynamics: Principles and Practice.* Edited by Yalla SV, McGuire EJ, Elbadawi A, Blaivas JG. New York: MacMillan; 1988:303–330.

4. Abrams P, Griffiths D, Hofner K, *et al.*: The urodynamic assessment of lower urinary tract symptoms. In *Benign Prostatic Hyperplasia.* Edited by Chatelain C, Denis L, Foo KT, *et al.*: Plymouth, UK: Plymbridge Distributors Ltd; 2001:229–281.

5. Hald T: Urodynamics in benign prostatic hyperplasia: a survey. *Prostate* 1989, 2 (suppl):69–77.

6. Resnick NM, Elbadawi A, Yalla SV: Age and the lower urinary tract: what is normal? *Neurourol Urodynam* 1995, 14:577–579.

7. Jacobsen SJ, Girman CJ, Lieber MM: Natural history of benign prostatic hyperplasia. *Urology* 2001, 58:5–16.

8. Barry MJ, Cockett ATK, Holtgrewe HL, *et al.*: Relationship of symptoms of prostatism to commonly used physiological and anatomical measures of the severity of benign prostatic hyperplasia. *J Urol* 1993, 150:351–358.

9. Chalfin SA, Bradley WE: The etiology of detrusor hyperreflexia in patients with intravesical obstruction. *J Urol* 1982, 127:938–942.

10. Nordling J, Artibani W, Hald T, *et al.*: Pathophysiology of the urinary bladder in obstruction and aging. In *Benign Prostatic Hyperplasia.* Edited by Chatelain C, Denis L, Foo KT, *et al.* Plymouth, UK: Plymbridge Distributors Ltd; 2001:107–166.

11. Resnick NM, Yalla SV: Geriatric incontinence and voiding dysfunction. In *Campbell's Urology.* Edited by Walsh PC, Retik AB, Vaughan ED, Wein AJ. Philadelphia: WB Saunders; 1997:1044–1058.

12. Resnick M, Ackermann R, Bosch J, *et al.*: Initial evaluation of LUTS. In *Benign Prostatic Hyperplasia.* Edited by Chatelain C, Denis L, Foo KT, *et al.* Plymouth, UK: Plymbridge Distributors Ltd; 2001:169–188.

13. AUA practice guidelines committee: AUA guidelines on management of benign prostatic hyperplasia (2003). Chapter 1: Diagnosis and treatment recommendations. *J Urol* 2003, 170:530–547.

14. Donovan JL, Abrams P, Peters TJ, *et al.*: The ICS-'BPH' study: The psychometric validity and reliability of the ICS male questionnaire. *Br J Urol* 1996, 77:554–562.

15. Lepor H, Machi G: Comparison of the AUA symptom index in unselected males and females between 55 and 79 years of age. *Urology* 1993, 42:36–41.

16. Chancellor MB, Rivas DA: American Urological Association Symptom Index for women with voiding symptoms: lack of index specificity for benign prostatic hyperplasia. *J Urol* 1993, 150:1706–1709.

17. Roehrborn CG, Girman CJ, Rhodes T: Correlation between prostate size estimated by digital rectal examination and measured by transrectal ultrasound. *Urology* 1997, 49:548–553.

18. Chute CG, Guess HA, Panser LA, *et al.*: The non-relationship of urinary symptoms, prostate volume and uroflow in a population based sample of men. *J Urol* 1993, 149:356A.

19. Roehrborn CG, Bartsch G, Kirby R, *et al.*: Guidelines for the diagnosis and treatment of benign prostatic hyperplasia: a comparative, international overview. *Urology* 2001, 58:642–650.

20. el Din KE, de Wildt MJ, Rosier PF, *et al.*: The correlation between urodynamic and cystoscopic findings in elderly men with voiding complaints. *J Urol* 1996, 155:1018–1122.

21. Chapple C, Turner-Warsick R: *Bladder Outflow Obstruction in the Male: Urodynamics. Principles, Practice and Application.* Edited by Mundy AR, Stephenson TP, Wein AJ. New York: Churchill Livingston; 1994:233–262.

22. Golomb J, Lindner A, Siegel Y, Korczak D: Variability and circadian changes in home uroflowmetry in patients with benign prostatic hyperplasia compared to normal controls. *J Urol* 1992, 147:1044–1047.

23. Abrams P, Griffiths DJ: The assessment of prostatic obstruction from urodynamic measurements and from residual urine. *Br J Urol* 1979, 51:129–134.

24. George NJ, O'Reilly PH, Barnard RJ, *et al.*: High pressure chronic retention. *BMJ* 1983, 286:1780–1783.

25. Nitti VW: Overactive bladder: strategies for effective evaluation and management. *Cont Urol* 2001 (suppl):14–21.

26. Barry MJ, Cockett ATK, Holtgrewe L, *et al.*: Relationship of symptoms of prostatism to commonly used physiologic and anatomic measures of the severity of benign prostatic hypertrophy. *J Urol* 1993, 150:351–358.

27. Sirls LT, Kirkemo AK, Jay J: Lack of correlation of the American Urological Association Symptom Index with urodynamic bladder outlet obstruction. *Neurourol Urodynam* 1996, 15:447–457.

28. el Din KE, Kiemeney LA, de Wildt MJ, *et al.*: The correlation between bladder outlet obstruction and lower urinary tract symptoms as measured by the international prostate symptom score. *J Urol* 1996, 156:1020–1025.

29. Chancellor MB, Blaivas JG, Kaplan SA, Axelrod S: Bladder outlet obstruction versus impaired detrusor contractility: the role of uroflow. *J Urol* 1991, 145:810–812.

30. Rivas DA, Chancellor M: Uroflowmetry. In *Atlas of Urodynamics.* Edited by Blaivas J, Chancellor M. Baltimore: Williams & Wilkins; 1996:48–59.

31. Kelly CE, Krane RJ: Current concepts and controversies in urodynamics. *Curr Urol Rep* 2000, 1:217–226.

32. Stohrer M, Goepel M, Kondo A, *et al.*: The standardization of terminology in neurogenic lower urinary tract dysfunction: with suggestions for diagnostic procedures. International Continence Society Standardization Committee. *Neurourol Urodynam* 1999, 18:139–158.

33. Schafer W: Principles and clinical application of advanced urodynamic analysis of voiding function. *Urol Clin North Am* 1990, 17:553–566.

34. Griffiths D, Hofner K, van Mastrigt R, *et al.*: Standardization of terminology of lower urinary tract function: pressure-flow studies of voiding, urethral resistance, and urethral obstruction. *Neurourol Urodynam* 1997, 16:1–18.

35. Griffiths DJ, VanMastrigt R, Bosch R: Quantification of urethral resistance and bladder function during voiding, with special reference to the effects of prostate size reduction on urethral obstruction due to benign prostatic hyperplasia. *Neurourol Urodynam* 1989, 8:17–27.

36. Griffiths DJ: Assessment of detrusor contraction strength or contractility. *Neurourol Urodynam* 1991, 10:1–18.

37. Sullivan MP, DuBeau CE, Resnick NM, *et al.*: Continuous occlusion test to determine detrusor contractile performance. *J Urol* 1995, 154:1834–1840.

38. Payne C: The breadth of neurology [editorial]. *J Urol* 1996, 155:1030–1031.

Medical Management of Benign Prostatic Hyperplasia

3

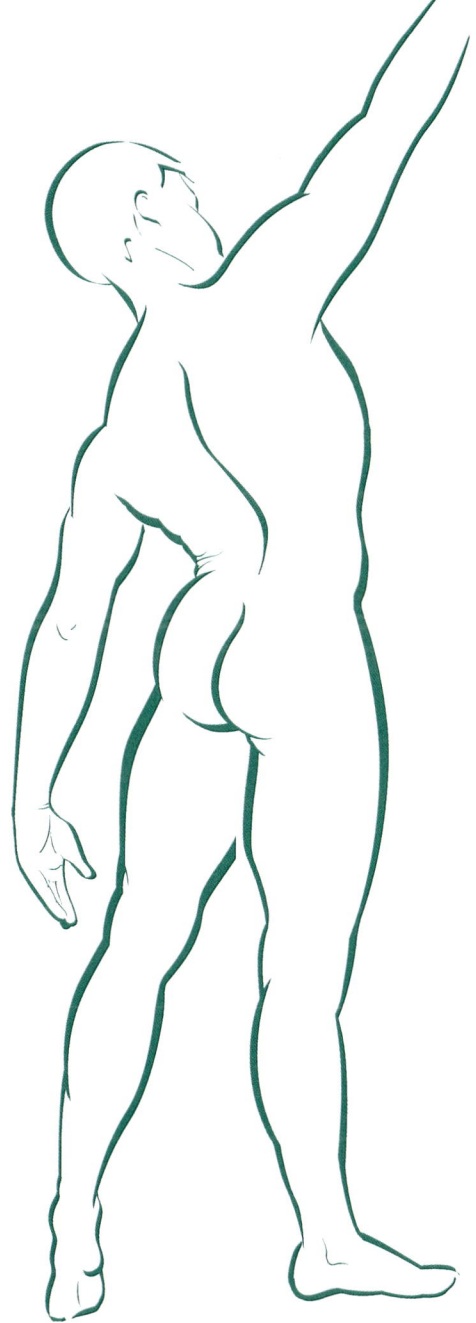

Brian T. Helfand, Timothy D. Moon, & Kevin T. McVary

Benign prostatic hyperplasia (BPH) remains a complicated issue for both the primary care physician and the urologist. The term *BPH* is a histologic definition related to the stromal and epithelial cell proliferative process that occurs in the transition zone of the prostate [1,2]. This process requires increasing age, the presence of androgens at critical points over time, and an intact autonomic nervous system [3,4]. Autopsy data estimate that the presence of histologic BPH may be as high as 70% in men by their seventh decade of life [5]; however, quantifying and defining the clinical incidence of the problematic voiding symptoms specifically caused by macroscopic BPH remain a challenge [6–8]. Although the exact number of men in the United States with lower urinary tract symptoms (LUTS) secondary to BPH is unknown, it is estimated that approximately 9 million men currently living in the United States seek some form of treatment for the voiding disturbances and quality-of-life changes attributed to BPH [9].

Clinical symptoms of BPH occur because of bladder outlet obstruction due to an enlarged prostate gland that physically impinges on the prostatic urethra (static component) and increased smooth muscle tone within the prostatic stroma (dynamic component). Symptomatic or clinical BPH largely refers to the presence of bothersome voiding disturbances known as LUTS. LUTS represent a complex of irritative voiding symptoms (nocturia, frequency, urgency) and obstructive voiding symptoms (hesitancy, weak stream, incomplete bladder emptying, and straining to void). Although these particular symptoms are not specific for the diagnosis of BPH, they are commonly present in older men with BPH-related bladder outlet obstruction and the resultant detrusor dysfunction caused by this process [1,10].

Treatment intervention for clinical BPH has mostly been directed toward the alleviation of bothersome LUTS; however, more recent attention has been focused on the prevention of BPH-related disease progression [11,12]. This attention is focused on the potential sequelae of BPH-related disease progression, which may include events such as acute urinary retention, renal insufficiency, detrusor dysfunction, development of bladder calculi, progressive worsening of LUTS, urinary incontinence, and recurrent urinary tract infection [12,13].

Treatment philosophy for clinical BPH has changed dramatically over the past 20 years, evolving from a paradigm that relied almost exclusively on surgery to one of medical treatment [14]. Recent US Medicare data show that the number of prostatectomies for BPH-related disease decreased from 250,000 in the mid-1980s to 88,000 in 1997 [15,16]. This decrease in the number of prostatectomies in lieu of the increasing number of men diagnosed with clinical BPH each year is likely multifactorial; however, the most apparent reason appears to be the development of safe, effective medical therapy. Other reasons for this decline in surgical intervention include the increased development of newer, minimally invasive therapies for BPH, and patient avoidance of the risks and complications associated with prostatectomies.

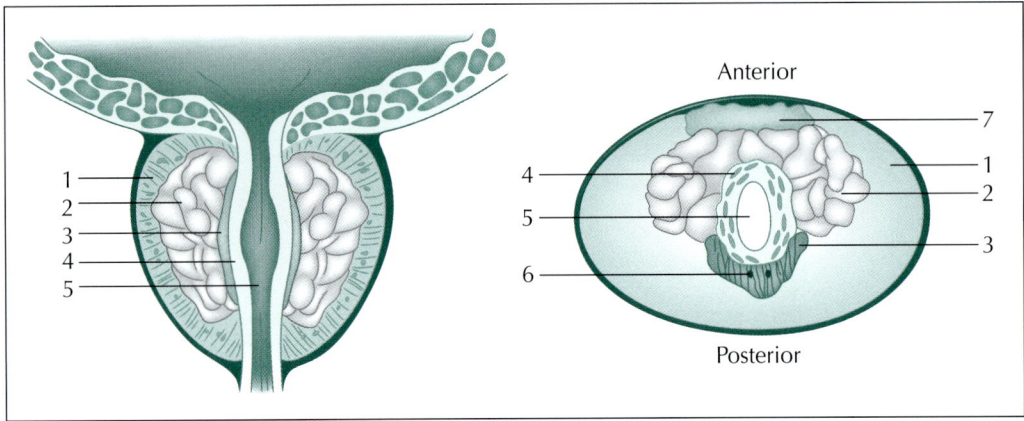

▶ **FIGURE 3-1.** Anatomy of benign prostatic hyperplasia (BPH). The prostate can be roughly divided into three different zones of tissue that include the 1) peripheral zone, 2) transition zone, and 3) central/periurethral zone. BPH has its origin within the transition zone [17]. Starting at around age 30, both the stromal (collagen and smooth muscle) and epithelial elements of the prostate begin to increase in cell number and form nodules within the prostate (seen schematically in the transition zone) [18]. Bladder neck obstruction occurs as the nodules enlarge in size, which may lead to clinical symptoms of BPH. In addition, bothersome lower urinary tract symptoms may occur because of the increased tone caused by the proliferation of smooth muscle cells. The contribution of the central nervous system (*ie*, innervation to the bladder and the bladder detrusor) to this process is currently being elucidated [4,19].

The type of proliferation that occurs within the prostate in BPH (*ie*, a predominance of smooth muscle vs a predominance of epithelial growth) may ultimately determine the responsiveness to different types of medical therapies. For example, a patient who has increased stromal proliferation may respond better to α-blocker therapy, whereas a patient with a relative increase in epithelial proliferation may theoretically respond better to 5α-reductase inhibitors [20].

The figures on the *left* and *right* represent coronal and transverse views of the prostate gland. 1—peripheral zone; 2—transition zone; 3—central zone; 4—urethral muscle; 5—urethra; 6—ejaculatory ducts; 7—anterior fibromuscular area.

Lower Urinary Tract Symptoms	
Irritative	Frequency
	Urgency
	Nocturia
Obstructive	Sensation of incomplete bladder emptying
	Decreased and/or intermittent flow of urinary stream
	Hesitancy
	Straining to void

▶ **FIGURE 3-2.** Lower urinary tract symptoms (LUTS): symptoms of benign prostatic hyperplasia (BPH). The majority of patients seeking treatment options for BPH do so because of bothersome symptoms that affect the quality of their lives [21,22]. Such symptoms are referred to as lower urinary tract symptoms (LUTS) and can roughly be divided into irritative and obstructive symptoms. Irritative symptoms include urinary frequency (increased number of times that a patient has to urinate), urgency (a sensation of having to urinate immediately), and nocturia (having to urinate during sleep hours). Obstructive symptoms include a sensation of incomplete bladder emptying, decreased or nonfluent flow of stream of urine, hesitancy (having difficulty starting stream of urine), and having to strain to void (having to use abdominal musculature to facilitate bladder emptying).

Although the symptomatology of BPH varies considerably among men, most diagnosed cases will have some degree of LUTS. However, it is important to note that LUTS are not necessarily indicative of BPH, as other conditions unrelated to the prostate may cause these symptoms [23]. Therefore, LUTS are sensitive but not specific for BPH.

Natural History of Benign Prostatic Hyperplasia

Histologic prevalence
  30% at age 50 y
  90% at age 80 y
AUA-IPSS scores >7
  12%–26% at age 40–49 y
  46% at age 70+ y
Likelihood of treatment
  3/1000 person-years at age 40–49 y
  30/1000 person-years at age 70+ y
Progression of disease over 5 y
  37%–42%
Risk of urinary retention over 1 yr
  0.3%–3.5%
Risk of urinary retention over 5 y
  3%–7%

▶ **FIGURE 3-3.** Natural history of benign prostatic hyperplasia (BPH). Part of the difficulty in studying the natural history of BPH comes from the variability in clinical presentation and the lack of a universally accepted case definition and diagnostic criteria [13,24]. Therefore, the definitive diagnosis of BPH has been made based on histologic examination of a tissue specimen obtained during biopsy, surgery, or autopsy procedure. However, obtaining tissue on every normal subject is impractical because the most frequent consequences of BPH are related to decreases in quality of life and are usually not medical emergencies. Therefore, autopsy studies have been the only source to provide data on the prevalence of histologically diagnosed BPH [18].

Autopsy studies from many different countries show the progressive development of BPH with age starting in some individuals as early as 25 to 30 years [18]. The clinical prevalence of BPH is much lower because it depends on the degree of bothersome symptoms and the patient's ability/desire to seek treatment. In addition, there appears to be substantial variation in prevalence estimates among different countries despite the use of community- or population-based study designs [25–27]. The likelihood of treatment for BPH has therefore been shown to relate to age and symptomatology.

Results from the Olmsted County Study (OCS) of Urinary Symptoms and Health Status Among Men suggest a measurable progression in symptom severity over 3.5 to 4 years, but also suggest that these lower urinary tract symptoms (LUTS) may "wax and wane" over time [28]. The likelihood of progression of LUTS also appears to depend on initial severity of symptoms. Sixty-seven percent of men with mild urinary symptoms at the beginning of observation experienced worsened symptoms over a 4-year period (50% progressed to moderate symptoms, 7% to severe symptoms, and 10% chose surgery). Forty-one percent of men with moderate symptoms at the beginning of observation progressed to severe symptoms, and 24% underwent surgery. Thirty-nine percent of patients with severe symptoms at the initial time of observation chose surgery over a 4-year period [29].

Benign prostatic hyperplasia may lead to complications such as acute urinary retention, serious or recurrent urinary tract infections, hydronephrosis, bladder calculi, and rarely, renal failure [12,13,28–30]. AUA-IPSS—American Urological Association–International Prostate Symptom Score (*see* Figure 3-4 for further explanation).

AUA-IPSS Questionnaire

Questions	Score
1. Over the past month, how often have you had a sensation of not emptying your bladder completely after you finished urinating?	0–5
2. Over the past month, how often have you had to urinate again less than 2 hours after you finished urinating?	0–5
3. Over the past month, how often have you found you stopped and started again several times when you urinated?	0–5
4. Over the past month, how often have you found it difficult to postpone urination?	0–5
5. Over the past month, how often have you had a weak urinary stream?	0–5
6. Over the past month, how often have you had to push or strain to begin urination?	0–5
7. Over the past month, how many times did you most typically get up to urinate from the time you went to bed until the time you got up in the morning?	Once = 1; 5 or more = 5

▶ **FIGURE 3-4.** American Urological Association–International Prostate Symptom Score (AUA-IPSS): evaluation of benign prostatic hyperplasia symptoms. This self-administered questionnaire assesses urinary symptomatology, both irritative (questions 2, 4, and 7) and obstructive (questions 1, 3, 5, and 6). Severity is scored on a scale of 0 to 5, with total scores of 0 to 35 possible. A score of 0 to 7 is considered mild, 8 to 19 moderate, and 20 to 35 severe.

Types of Medical Therapies for BPH

Hormonal therapy
5α-Reductase inhibitors
α-Adrenergic antagonists
Combination therapy
Phytotherapy

▶ **FIGURE 3-5.** Types of medical therapies for benign prostatic hyerplasia (BPH). BPH produces bladder outlet obstruction via two general mechanisms: 1) the static component (*ie*, the mechanical and physical compression exerted by the increased prostate size) and 2) the dynamic component (*ie*, increased prostatic smooth muscle tone caused by smooth muscle cell proliferation and increased neural input). A number of different medical therapies have been developed to treat both of these components. Discussion and efficacy of these treatments are discussed in the figures below.

The development and progression of benign prostatic hyperplasia (BPH) appears to be the result of a series of interactions between the different cell types in the prostate (*ie*, stromal and epithelial cells), endocrine, hereditary, neural influences, and environmental factors [31]. One of the most important factors for the development of BPH, aside from increasing age, appears to be the effect of testicular androgens on prostate cell growth. Therefore, the regulation of testicular hormone function is integral to the medical treatment of BPH.

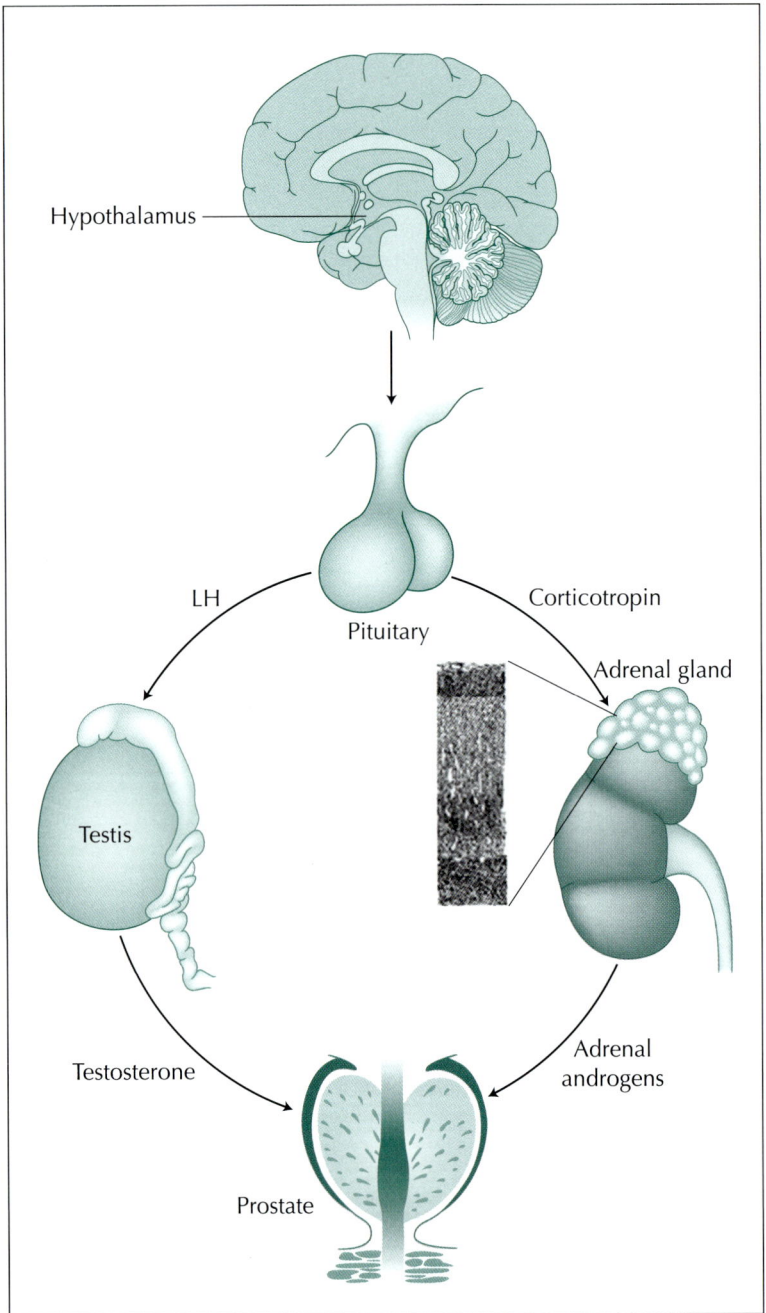

▶ **FIGURE 3-6.** Hypothalamic-gonadal axis in benign prostatic hyperplasia (BPH). Adequate levels of circulating testosterone are necessary for the prostate to develop and grow. This is essential during prostate development but appears to be the major driving factor for prostatic growth in BPH. Gonadotropin-releasing hormone (GnRH) is released in a pulsatile fashion by the hypothalamus of the brain into the portal-venous circulation, stimulating the anterior pituitary to secrete luteinizing hormone (LH). LH enters the systemic circulation and then stimulates the Leydig cells of the testes to release testosterone. In addition, androgens are also released from the adrenal gland. To this end, the hypothalamus releases corticotropin-releasing hormone, which acts on the anterior pituitary gland and causes the release of corticotropins. Corticotropins then act on the adrenal gland cells located within the zona fasciculata and zona reticulata, and induce the release of adrenal androgens such as dehydroepiandrosterone sulfate. Of circulating androgens, 95% are released from the testes and the remaining 5% are released from the adrenal glands. Approximately 98% of circulating androgens are bound to plasma proteins such as albumin and sex hormone–binding globulin [32]. Only free testosterone is biologically active and available to enter prostate cells by a process of simple diffusion.

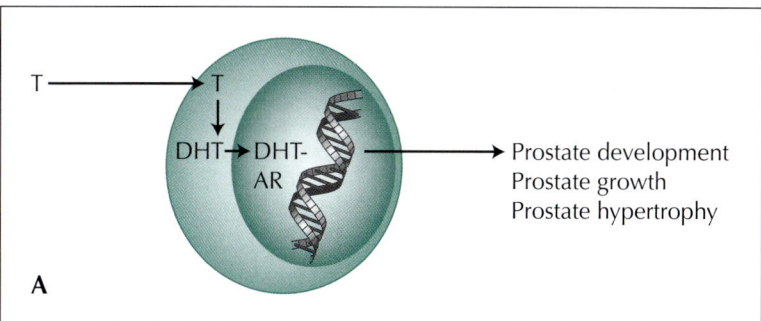

A

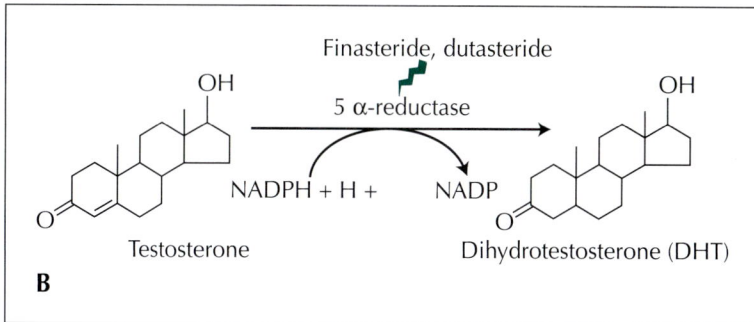

B

▶ **FIGURE 3-7.** The mechanism of action of 5α-reductase inhibitors. The development of benign prostatic hyperplasia (BPH) is clearly linked to the presence of functioning testes because eunuchs and men castrated before puberty have atrophic prostate glands and do not develop BPH. However, testosterone does not act alone. The mechanism by which testosterone exerts many of its physiologic effects on the prostate gland is through dihydrotestosterone (DHT). As mentioned in Figure 3-6, androgens, including testosterone, are produced by the Leydig cells of the testes and by the adrenal glands. **A,** The mechanisms by which testosterone subsequently influences prostate cellular growth. After production, testosterone is circulated by the bloodstream to the prostate gland and then freely diffuses into the cells by simple diffusion. Once intracytoplasmic, testosterone is converted to its active metabolite, DHT, by the enzyme 5α-reductase, type 2. DHT forms a complex with androgen receptors (AR)

that is then transported to the nucleus. Within the nucleus, this complex exerts its effects on the transcription of DNA. These effects are necessary for the normal development of the prostate gland (*see* Fig. 3-8) as well as the normal growth and hypertrophy of the prostate.

B, Drugs have been developed that target and inhibit the enzyme 5α-reductase, such as finasteride and dutasteride. These drugs virtually eliminate the production of DHT and thus inhibit normal prostate growth and hyperplasia (*see* Figs. 3-9 to 3-14). For example, finasteride administration results in an 80% decrease in the concentration of DHT within both the prostate and the general circulation [33,34]. Accompanying this response is a 56% increase in the local concentration of testosterone within the prostate, without a significant change in the total serum concentration of testosterone [35–37].

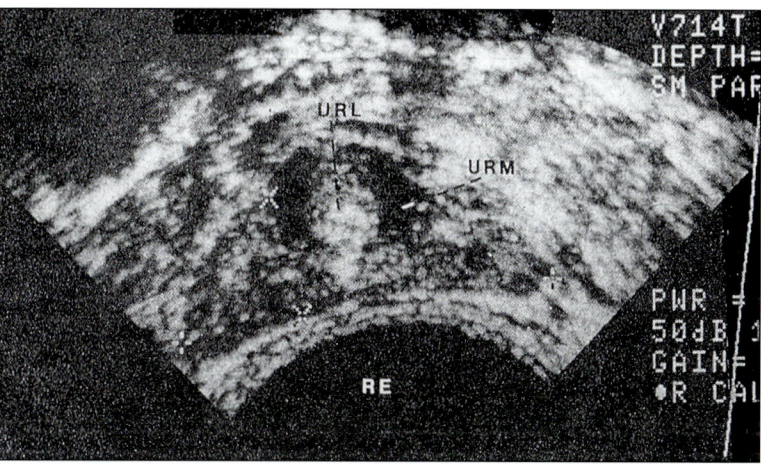

▶ **FIGURE 3-8.** Rationale for the suppression of dihydrotestosterone (DHT) as a treatment for benign prostatic hyperplasia (BPH). As mentioned in the previous figures, androgens are necessary for the development and normal growth of the prostate gland. BPH rarely occurs in men castrated prior to puberty [38]. Numerous clinical studies have documented the regression of BPH and improved voiding symptomatology in men with large prostates following bilateral orchiectomy [39–41]. As indicated by Figure 3-7, free testosterone is converted to its active form by the enzyme 5α-reductase. Male human pseudohermaphrodites resulting from congenital deficiency of the 5α-reductase enzyme have abnormal vestigial prostates, consisting only of a central zone, despite normal serum testosterone levels and normal-func-

tioning androgen receptors [42–44]. Administration of DHT in these individuals results in prostatic growth, indicating that DHT is the primary mediator of prostate growth and that testosterone cannot act alone to support the normal growth and development of the prostate gland [45]. The rationale for the hormonal treatment of BPH is based on these clinical findings. DHT is necessary for the embryonic development and maintenance of the normal prostate gland.

The image is a transrectal ultrasound of the rudimentary prostate (indicated by *cursors*) in a male pseudohermaphrodite with 5α-reductase deficiency. RE—rectal lumen; URL—urethral lumen; URM—urethromuscular wall. (*Courtesy of* the *Journal of Clinical Endocrinology*).

Short-Term Effects of a 5α-Reductase Inhibitor

Agent	Year	Dose, mg	Follow-up, y	↑Qmax, mL/s (% change)	↓Symptom Score (% change)	↓Prostate Volume, cm³ (% change)
Finasteride [46]	1992	5	1	1.6 (17*)	2.7 (26*)	11.1 (19*)
Placebo	1992	0	1	0.2 (2)	1.0 (1.0)	1.2 (2)

Statistically significant compared with placebo-based studies.

▶ **FIGURE 3-9.** Short-term effects of a 5α-reductase inhibitor: a randomized, double-blind, placebo-controlled phase III trial of finasteride. As mentioned above, finasteride is a 5α-reductase inhibitor that exerts its effects on the prostate gland by inhibiting the formation of dihydrotestosterone. The results of a 1-year clinical trial with finasteride were the first to demonstrate that finasteride has efficacy in the medical management of benign prostatic hyperplasia. Entry criteria for the initial multicenter, randomized, double-blind, placebo-controlled studies with finasteride included men with lower urinary tract symptoms, a maximum urinary flow rate of less than 15 mL/s and an enlarged prostate on digital rectal examination. The data obtained from the study demonstrated a mean decrease in circulating dihydrotestosterone levels by 80%. This level was sustained without escape during 12 months of treatment and without significant change in circulating serum testosterone levels (*ie*, there was no positive feedback on the level of testosterone [46]). Approximately 3% to 5% of patients in these studies experienced side effects of decreased libido, impotence, and ejaculatory disorder. All of these changes were statistically significant compared with findings of the placebo group [46]. Q$_{max}$—maximum urine flow rate.

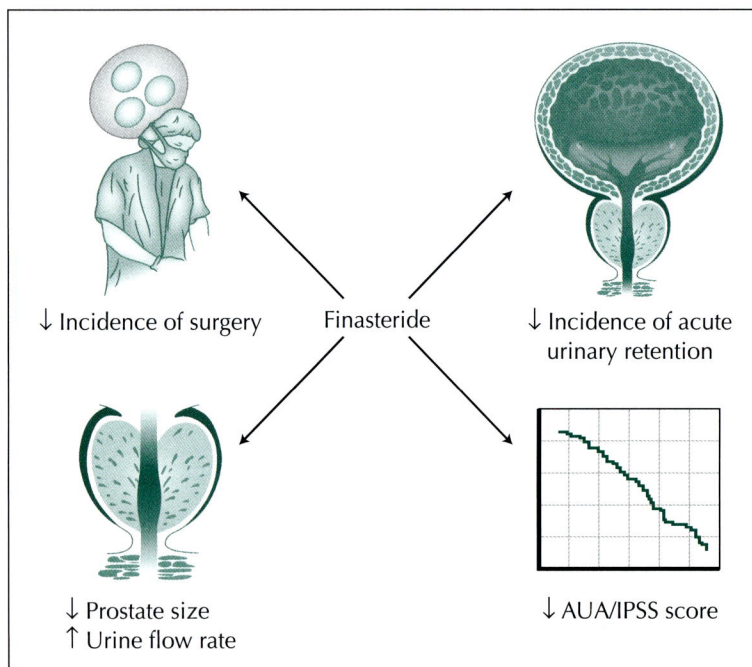

▶ **FIGURE 3-10.** Long-term effects of a 5α-reductase inhibitor: the Proscar Long-Term Efficacy and Safety Study (PLESS) [47]. The PLESS trial was the largest clinical study to investigate the effects of finasteride on the management of benign prostatic hyperplasia (BPH) [47]. In this multicenter, double-blind, placebo-controlled study conducted in the United States, more than 3000 men with moderate to severe urinary symptoms and an enlarged prostate on digital rectal examination were randomized to a finasteride group, 5 mg/day, or a placebo group. During the 4-year study period, 10% of the 1516 men in the placebo group and only 5% of the 1524 men in the finasteride group underwent surgery for BPH (a 55% reduction in risk with the use of finasteride). Acute urinary retention developed in approximately 7% of the men in the placebo group and approximately 3% of the men in the finasteride group (a 57% reduction in risk with the use of finasteride). There was a significant ($P < 0.001$) decrease in mean American Urological Association–International Prostate Score (AUA-IPSS), with a 3.3 reduction in the finasteride group and a 1.3 reduction in the placebo group (*see* Fig. 3-12). Treatment with finasteride improved urinary flow rates and significantly ($P < 0.001$) reduced prostate volume (*see* Fig. 3-11). This study suggested that long-term medical therapy can affect the natural history of BPH as manifested by acute urinary retention and surgery. A 5α-reductase inhibitor is now recommended as prevention for BPH because it may alter the natural history of BPH (*see* Fig. 3-35). In addition, this class of medications is recommended for patients with large prostates (> 30 g) with moderate to severe symptoms of BPH.

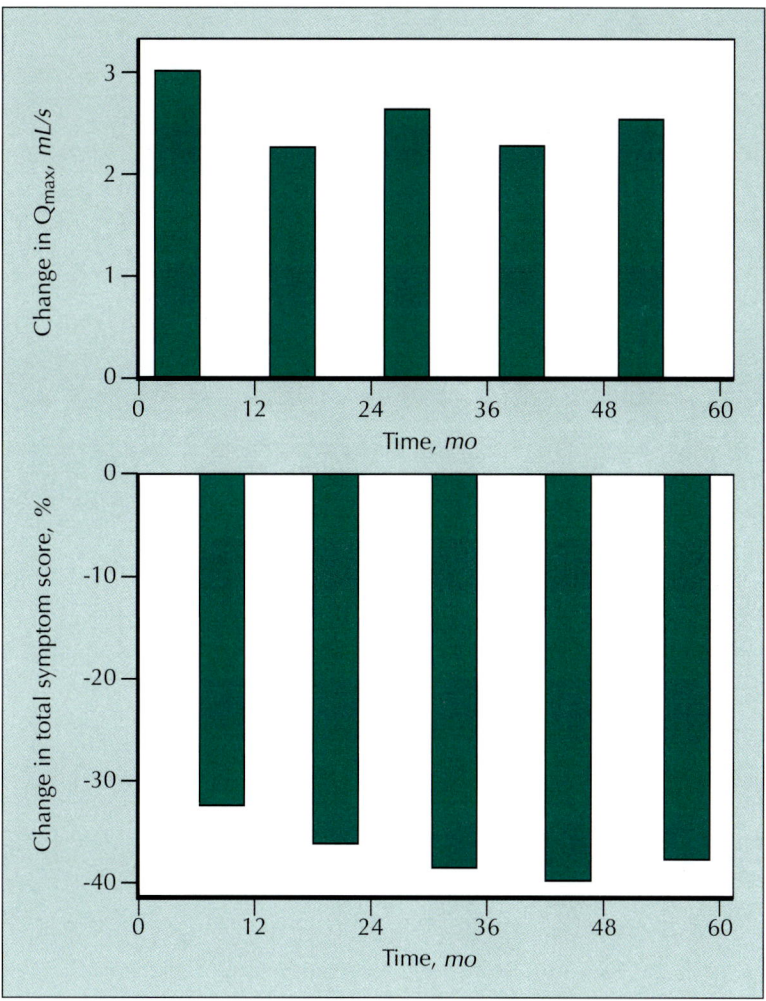

▶ **FIGURE 3-11.** A detailed analysis of the long-term effects of finasteride. Data obtained from the Proscar Long-Term Efficacy and Safety Study (PLESS) showed that men had statistically significant improvement in symptom scores and maximum urine flow rates [47]. Men with larger prostate glands and lower urinary flow rates at the beginning of the study appeared to benefit most from hormone treatment with finasteride [48]. The graph demonstrates the improvement in urinary symptom score and maximum urine flow rate over the 4-year treatment with finasteride. Q_{max}—maximum urine flow rate.

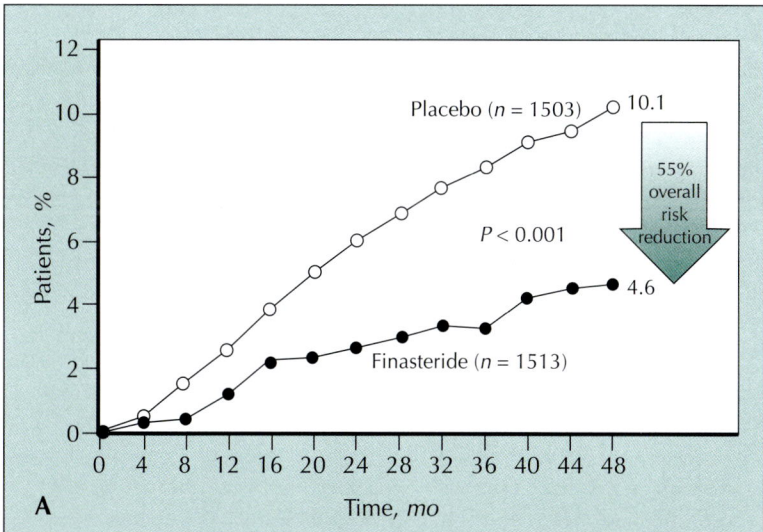

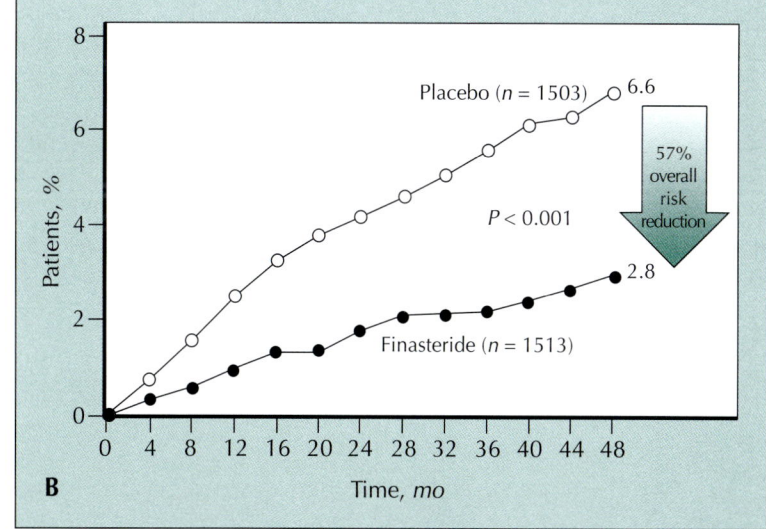

▶ **FIGURE 3-12.** Effect of finasteride on acute urinary retention (AUR) and the incidence of surgery related to benign prostatic hyperplasia (BPH). Several large-scale population-based longitudinal epidemiologic studies of aging reveal an increased risk of AUR and BPH-related surgery (*eg*, transurethral resection of the prostate) over time for men with lower urinary tract symptoms and enlarged prostates [28,30,49]. As mentioned in

Figure 3-11, finasteride reduced the risk of AUR by 57% and the need for BPH-related surgery by 55% compared with placebo during the 4-year study period [47]. The graphs demonstrate the significantly decreased risk of AUR (**A**) and BPH-related surgery (**B**) in patients assigned to the finasteride group compared with the placebo group over the 4-year study period. (*Adapted from* McConnell *et al.* [47].)

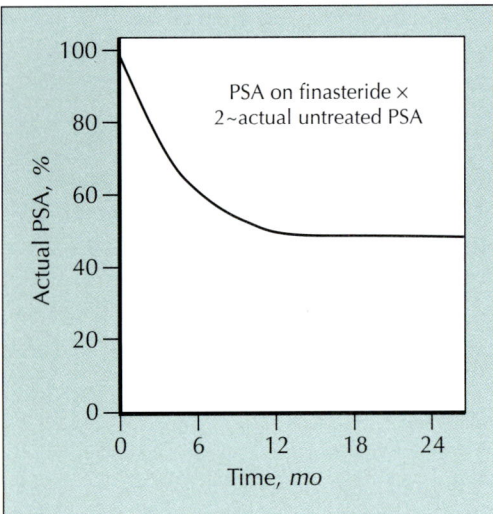

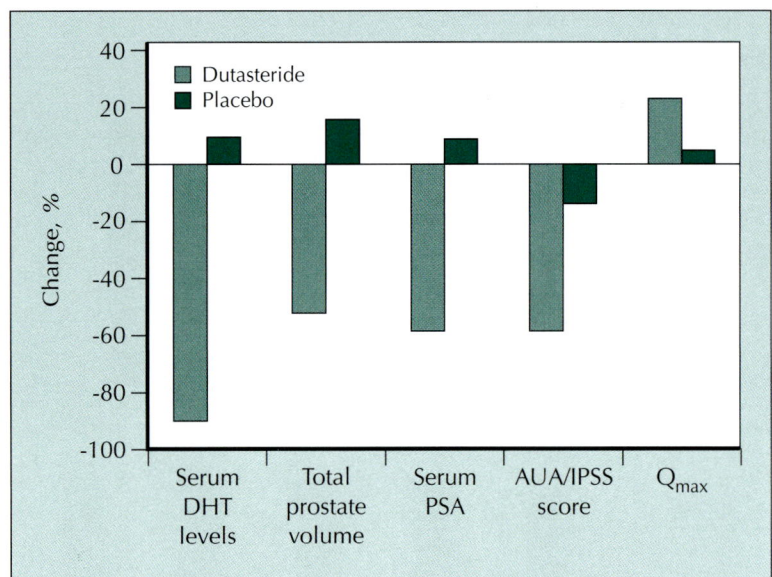

▶ **FIGURE 3-13.** Effect of finasteride treatment on prostate-specific antigen (PSA) levels over time. Prostate cancer is the most common cancer affecting men and the third most common cause of cancer death in American men. Early detection of prostate cancer has been enhanced since the introduction of the PSA screening assay [50]. PSA is an enzyme produced by the prostate gland and is usually only detectable at low levels in the blood. Most men with prostate cancer have elevated serum levels of PSA. Other variables that can increase PSA levels include other lower genitourinary conditions, such as prostatitis, prostate infarction, and recent ejaculation. In addition, PSA levels also rise as prostate volume increases secondary to benign prostatic hyperplasia (BPH) [51,52].

Treatment with finasteride decreases serum PSA levels by approximately 50% over a 4- to 6-month time period [53–55]. Because BPH and prostate cancer may coexist in the same patient, there has been some concern regarding the detection of prostate cancer in patients taking 5α-reductase inhibitors. Stoner [56] demonstrated that despite an approximately 60% decrease in intraprostatic concentrations of testosterone, there appears to be no increased risk of prostate cancer for patients taking finasteride. Doubling the serum PSA for patients taking finasteride and then interpreting the resulting PSA value as in untreated men has been recommended [55]. Oesterling *et al.* [57] suggested that doubling PSA levels in finasteride-treated patients allows for appropriate interpretation of PSA and does not mask the detection of prostate cancer. Any sustained increases in PSA levels during finasteride treatment should be carefully evaluated. To date, 5α-reductase inhibitors have been shown to play a role in the reduction in incidence of prostate cancer. However, it should be noted that a recent report demonstrated a significant increase in more aggressive prostate cancer types in patients who were diagnosed with prostate cancer after taking a 5α-reductase inhibitor [58].

▶ **FIGURE 3-14.** Dutasteride: a dual type 1 and type 2, 5α-reductase inhibitor. As mentioned above, the prostate gland depends on androgen stimulation in the form of dihydrotestosterone (DHT) for its normal development and growth. The enzyme 5α-reductase is responsible for the production of DHT (*see* Fig. 3-7). 5α-Reductase occurs as two different isozymes, referred to as type 1 and type 2. The prostate gland expresses predominantly the type 2 isozyme, whereas the skin and liver express an abundance of the type 1 isozyme [59–61]. The contribution of DHT is primarily derived from the type 2 isozyme found in the prostate stomal tissue. However, type 1 5α-reductase in the liver and skin and a small amount in the prostate may play a role in prostatic enlargement.

Dutasteride is a drug indicated for benign prostatic hyperplasia (BPH) that is a dual inhibitor of both the type 1 and type 2 5α-reductase isozymes [62]. Dutasteride has been evaluated in men with lower urinary tract symptoms (LUTS) and large prostate glands (> 30 cm³) and was shown to produce a near-complete suppression of DHT (> 90%). Dutasteride reduces the levels of DHT relatively rapidly, and most patients experience a significant reduction by 1 month [63,64].

As demonstrated above, dutasteride has been shown to significantly reduce the LUTS produced by BPH. In addition, it has been shown to significantly decrease prostate volume, increase urinary flow rate, decrease the risk of acute urinary retention, and decrease the risk of requiring BPH-related surgery compared with placebo [63]. By decreasing prostate size, dutasteride is also useful in the prevention of BPH progression [65]. The efficacy of dutasteride has been maintained in results of long-term phase IIIa multicenter, randomized placebo-controlled studies [64]. Dutasteride, like finasteride, has also been shown to halve the serum levels of prostate-specific antigen (PSA) without affecting the ratio of free PSA to total PSA. Thus, the serum PSA can still be used in the evaluation of prostate cancer in patients taking dutasteride [62]. AUA-IPSS—American Urological Association–International Prostate Symptom Score; Q_max—maximum urine flow.

Clinical Studies of GnRH Agonists and Nonsteroidal Antiandrogens for the Treatment of BPH

Clinical Study	Agent	Patients, n	Decrease in Prostate Volume, %	Q_{max}	Symptom Score
Gabrilove *et al.* [66]	GnRH agonist	15	46	↑	↓
Eri and Tveter [67]	GnRH agonist	50	35	↑	↓
Stone *et al.* [68]	Antiandrogen	84	41	↑	↓
Eri and Tveter [69]	Antiandrogen	30	26	↑	↓

▶ **FIGURE 3-15.** Clinical studies of gonadotropin-releasing hormone (GnRH) agonists and nonsteroidal antiandrogens for the treatment of benign prostatic hyperplasia (BPH). Inhibiting testosterone, and dihydrotestosterone production, prevents the formation of BPH. Castration can be achieved by chemical means. Androgen receptor antagonists such as flutamide, progestin-estrogen combination, and GnRH agonists have all been tested in patients with BPH. As the data demonstrate, these drugs are quite effective in reducing prostate size and improving symptoms. However, their cost and increased frequency of adverse effects (decreased libido, painful gynecomastia, and hot flashes) have excluded these drugs from clinical use. Q_{max}—maximum urine flow rate.

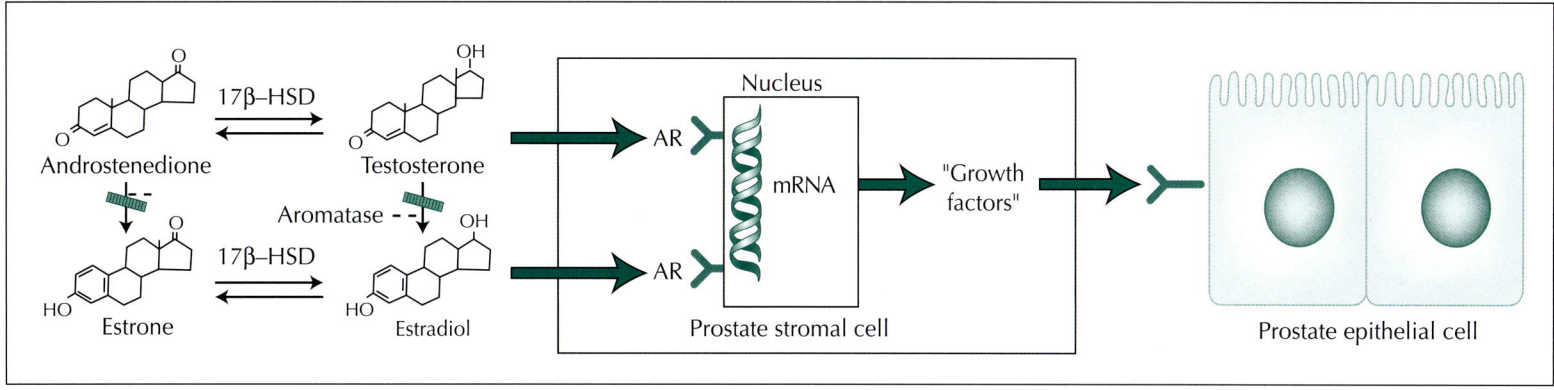

▶ **FIGURE 3-16.** Aromatase inhibitors as a potential treatment for benign prostatic hyperplasia (BPH). It has been demonstrated that estrogens exert effects on the pathophysiology of BPH. As men age, there is a direct correlation between prostate volume and increased serum levels of free testosterone, estradiol, and estriol [70]. In a canine model of BPH, experiments have shown that estrogens act synergistically with androgens to promote BPH. The hormones increase the expression of the androgen receptor (AR), which promotes increased prostatic concentrations of dihydrotestosterone and reduces the rate of prostate cell death [71–73]. BPH can be induced in castrated dogs via supplementation with aromatizable androgens, and this effect can be blocked by concomitant administration of aromatase inhibitors that prevent conversion of testosterone to estrogen [72,73]. However, clinical studies using aromatase inhibitors, such as atamestane or testolactone, as monotherapy for the treatment of BPH have failed to yield encouraging results [74–77]. Failure of aromatase inhibitors to improve BPH symptomatology may be related to a simultaneous rise in testosterone concentration that leads to glandular epithelial hyperplasia of the prostate [74–77]. 17β-HSD—17β-hydroxysteroid dehydrogenase.

Adverse Effects of Hormonal Therapy

Effect	5α-Reductase Inhibitor, Type 2 (Finasteride), %	5α-Reductase Inhibitor, Types 1 and 2 (Dutasteride), %	GnRH Agonists, %	Antiandrogens, %
Impotence	3–4	1–6	95–100	10–20
Loss of libido	4–5	4	95–100	10–20
Ejaculatory disorder	4–5	1–2	—	—
Hot flashes	—	—	95–100	—
Gynecomastia	—	1–2	0–5	50–100
Diarrhea	—	—	—	50

▶ **FIGURE 3-17.** Adverse effects of hormonal therapy. The most deleterious effects of agents that alter the hypothalamic-gonadal axis at different levels along the pathway are related to varying degrees of sexual dysfunction. Interventions that markedly lower serum testosterone levels are associated with greater degrees of sexual dysfunction (*eg*, loss of libido) than are agents that block the effect of testosterone on target organs [78].

MEDICAL THERAPIES FOR THE TREATMENT OF BENIGN PROSTATIC HYPERPLASIA: α-ADRENERGIC ANTAGONISTS

As mentioned above, benign prostatic hyperplasia (BPH) has two major components: static and dynamic. The dynamic component is associated with an increase in smooth muscle tone mediated by the autonomic nervous system. Prostatic smooth muscle cells contract under the influence of noradrenergic sympathetic nerves, and subsequently constrict the urethra and impair the flow of urine. In addition, there is recent evidence that adrenergic receptors mediate lower urinary tract symptoms via their activation within the central nervous system and bladder detrusor [79]. The prostate gland contains high levels of both α_1- and α_2-adrenergic receptors [80–83]. However, the majority (~98%) of the α_1-adrenoreceptors are associated with the stromal elements of the prostate and subsequently have the largest influence on urethral tone. Thus, blockade of the α_1-adrenergic receptor would relax prostatic smooth muscle, relieve bladder outlet obstruction, and enhance urine flow.

Promise for medical therapy using α-adrenergic receptor blockers first came from studying phenoxybenzamine. Phenoxybenzamine is a nonselective α_1/α_2-receptor blocker that was found to be effective in relieving the symptoms of BPH [84–87], although side effects such as dizziness, weakness, and palpitations limited the use of this drug for the treatment of BPH. However, it was noticed that although both α_1- and α_2-receptors are in the prostate, prostatic smooth muscle contraction is predominated by α_1-receptors. Therefore, it was presumed that many of the adverse effects associated with this drug are induced by α_2-receptor blockers. These findings led to the development of α_1-selective blockers for the successful medical treatment of BPH. These therapies are discussed below.

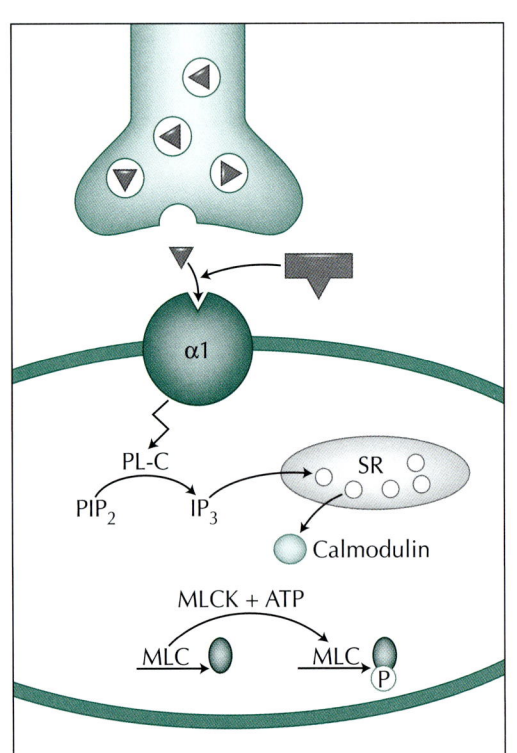

▶ **FIGURE 3-18.** Molecular mechanisms underlying adrenergic-induced smooth muscle contraction and blockade by α-adrenergic antagonists. An understanding of the molecular mechanisms regulating smooth muscle tone is integral to the understanding of benign prostatic hyperplasia. Smooth muscle tone within the prostate gland is dictated, at least in part, by input from α-adrenergic receptors (for review [88]). These receptors are normally activated by norepinephrine (depicted as *triangles*) released from the sympathetic nervous system. This induces a cascade of events that activate phospholipase C (PL-C), causing the formation of inositol triphosphate (IP_3) from phosphatidylinositol (PIP_2) [89]. The IP_3 then stimulates the sarcoplasmic reticulum (SR) to release its store of calcium (depicted as *circles*). Calcium then activates calmodulin, which activates myosin light chain kinase (MLCK), an enzyme that is capable of phosphorylating myosin light chains (MLCs) in the presence of ATP [90]. MLCs are regulatory subunits found on the myosin heads. MLC phosphorylation leads to cross-bridge formation between the myosin heads and actin filaments, and hence smooth muscle contraction.

α-Adrenergic receptor antagonists competitively inhibit the norepinephrine binding sites on the α-adrenergic receptor. When these sites are occupied by α-adrenergic antagonists, then PL-C is not activated and the chain of events that cause smooth muscle contraction do not occur. Therefore, α-adrenergic receptor blockers prevent smooth muscle contraction by preventing one of the main pathways that lead to smooth muscle contraction.

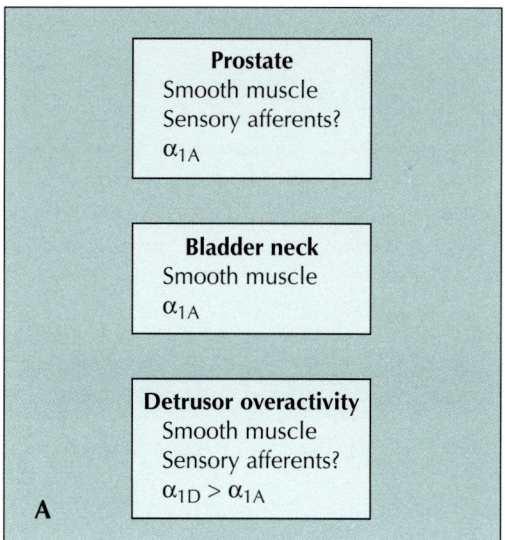

Prostate
Smooth muscle
Sensory afferents?
α_{1A}

Bladder neck
Smooth muscle
α_{1A}

Detrusor overactivity
Smooth muscle
Sensory afferents?
$\alpha_{1D} > \alpha_{1A}$

A

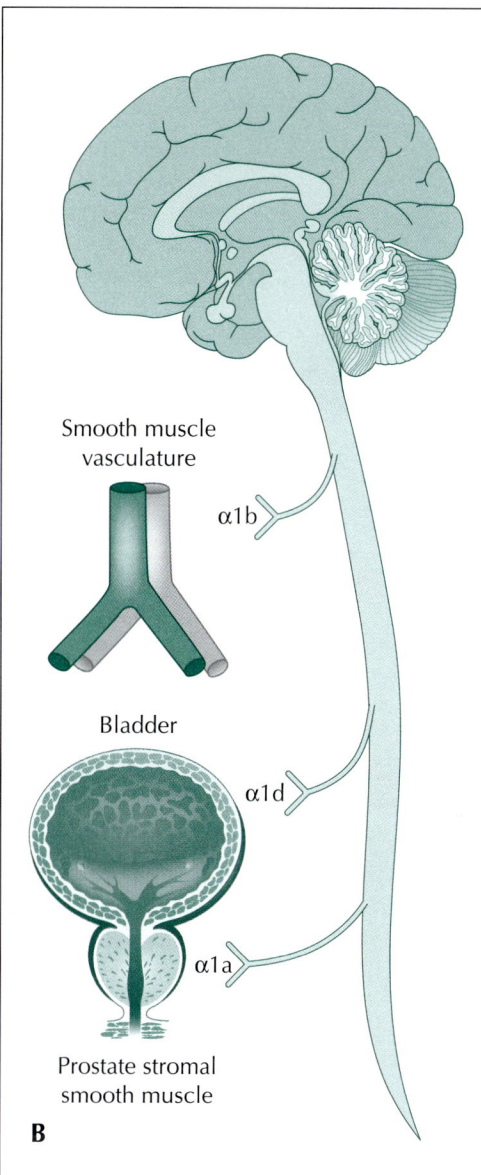

Smooth muscle
vasculature

$\alpha 1b$

Bladder

$\alpha 1d$

$\alpha 1a$

Prostate stromal
smooth muscle

B

▶ **FIGURE 3-19.** α_1-Adrenergic receptor subtypes and function within the lower genitourinary tract. **A** and **B**, α-Receptors are distributed ubiquitously throughout the human body. There are two basic subtypes of these receptors, α_1 and α_2. α_2-Receptors are located presynaptically and cause down-regulation of norepinephrine release via a negative feedback mechanism. α_1-Receptors are located postsynaptically and are the target of treatment in benign prostatic hyperplasia (BPH) [83]. Based on the molecular characterization, differential binding affinities, and cloning of unique DNA sequences, a number of subtypes of the α_1-adrenoreceptors have been identified [91]. These subtypes have been classified into three groups: α_{1A}, α_{1B}, and α_{1D} [92].

Although both α_{1A} and α_{1B} are present in the prostate, α_{1A} is the dominant adrenoreceptor expressed by smooth muscle cells in this location [83]. Therefore, blockade of the α_{1A}-adrenoreceptors reduces prostatic tone and improves the dynamic aspects of voiding [93]. The α_{1D}-adrenoreceptors are located mainly in the bladder body and dome. Detrusor instability appears to occur via stimulation of these receptors, and blockade of these receptors has been shown in animal models to reduce irritative voiding symptoms [19,94]. α_{1D}-Receptors are also located in the spinal cord, where they are presumed to play a role in the sympathetic modulation of parasympathetic activity [95]. The α_{1B}-receptors are located in the smooth muscle of arteries and veins, including the microvasculature contained within the prostate gland [92]. Blockade of these receptors in the cardiovascular system causes symptoms of dizziness and hypotension because of decreased total peripheral resistance via veno- and arterial dilatation. Taken together, it appears that combined α_{1A}- and α_{1D}-receptor antagonist action is one of the best options for the management of BPH.

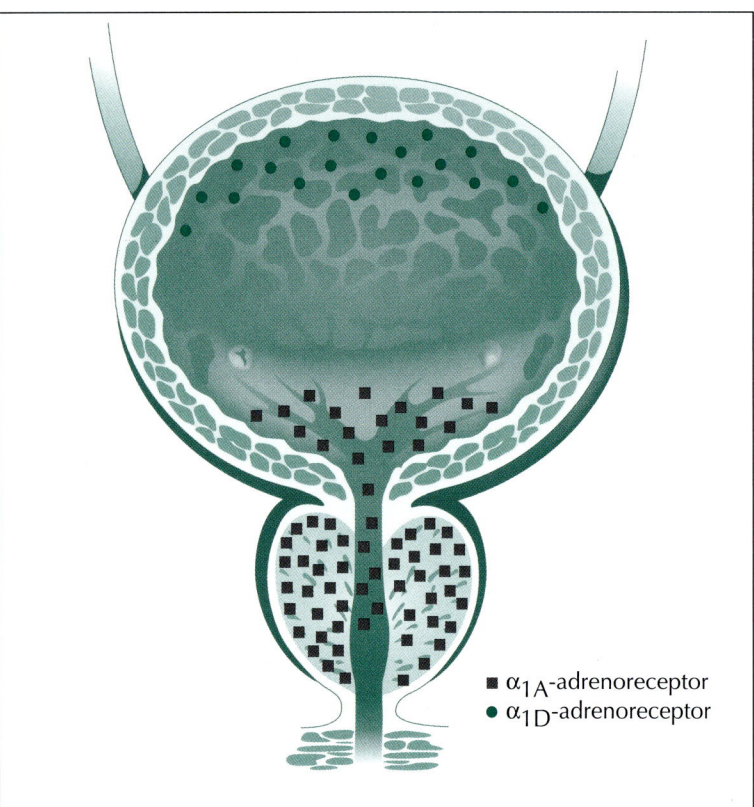

■ α_{1A}-adrenoreceptor
● α_{1D}-adrenoreceptor

◗ **FIGURE 3-20.** Distribution of α_1-adrenoreceptors in the bladder and prostate [96]. α_{1D}-Adrenoreceptors are located primarily within the dome of the bladder. α_{1A}-Receptors predominate in the prostatic epithelial tissue, bladder trigone, and urethra. α_{1A}-Receptors are also expressed within the prostatic vascular smooth muscle. However, with aging, the expression of α_{1B}-receptor in the vasculature is increased and ultimately predominates. This transition occurs at around age 50 years. Taken together, blockade of α_{1A}-receptors is believed to improve obstructive lower urinary tract symptoms by decreasing smooth muscle tone within the epithelial tissue of the prostate, bladder trigone, and urethra.

Types and Characteristics of Different α-Adrenergic Antagonists

Name	Rank Order of Receptor Selectivity*	α_{1A}/α_{1B} Selectivity Ratio†	$T_{1/2}$, hr	Metabolism
Prazosin	$\alpha_{1A} = \alpha_{1B} = \alpha_{1D}$	0.95	2–3	Hepatic
Doxazosin	$\alpha_{1A} = \alpha_{1B} = \alpha_{1D}$	0.43	9–22	Hepatic
Terazosin	$\alpha_{1B} = \alpha_{1D} > \alpha_{1A}$	0.38	9–14	Hepatic
Alfuzosin	$\alpha_{1A} = \alpha_{1B} = \alpha_{1D}$	0.33	5–61	Hepatic
Tamsulosin	$\alpha_{1A} = \alpha_{1D} > \alpha_{1B}$	20.0	0–15	Hepatic

*Selectivity defined as ≥ 1 order of magnitude's difference in affinity for individual α_1-adrenoreceptors.
†Ratio is determined from ratio of pKi values.
Adapted from Lyseng-Williamson et al. [97].

◗ **FIGURE 3-21.** Types and characteristics of different α-adrenergic antagonists [97]. Three generations of α-adrenergic antagonists have been used in the treatment of benign prostatic hyperplasia (BPH). First-generation agents (*eg*, phenoxybenzamine) were the first pharmaceuticals to be used in the treatment of BPH. They antagonize both prostatic and vascular α_1- and α_2-adrenoreceptors. As a result, first-generation agents cause many dose-related side effects, such as syncope, orthostatic hypotension, reflex tachycardia, cardiac arrhythmias, and retrograde ejaculation [84,86]. Because of these adverse effects, first-generation agents have been replaced by second- and third-generation agents. Second-generation agents (*eg*, prazosin, terazosin, doxazosin, alfuzosin) selectively antagonize α_1-adrenoreceptors and relatively leave α_2-receptors alone. Therefore, they improve urinary symptoms, with fewer vasodilatory related effects. Third-generation α_1-adrenergic antagonists (*eg*, tamsulosin) are thought to be more selective antagonists for prostatic α_{1A}-receptors [98,99]. Therefore, these agents theoretically affect adrenergic receptors located specifically within the prostate and urethra [100].

The different types of specific α_1-receptor antagonists are presented in the figure. The table shows the affinities that the different drugs have for each of the different subtypes of adrenoreceptors. Selectivity ratios between the affinity of the drug for α_{1A}- and α_{1B}-receptors have also been determined, and higher values indicate a greater pharmacologic selectivity for α_{1A}- and α_{1B}-adrenoreceptors. Interestingly, pharmacologic selectivity (determined from animal models) does not always correlate with clinical selectivity (determined from human subjects) [100].

The half-life ($T_{1/2}$) and route of metabolism are presented for each drug. Drug half-life has been shown to greatly affect the frequency of adverse effects. For example, prazosin has a short half-life, producing large differences between peak and trough serum prazosin levels after each dose. These differences have been implicated to an increased frequency of vasodilatory side effects (*see* Fig. 3-26). Longer-acting α_1-receptor antagonists allow once-daily dosing and have recently been favored over short-acting selective α_1-antagonists because of their lowered rate of side effects. All of the drugs are metabolized through the liver. Therefore, caution should be taken in patients with hepatic dysfunction. (*Adapted from* Lyseng-Williamson *et al.* [97].)

Clinical Trials of Terazosin

Study	Year	Patients, n	Dose, mg	Follow-up, wk	↑ Q_{max}, mL/s	↓ Symptom Score, %	% Significant Response	
							>25% Improvement in AUA-IPSS, %	>30% Increase in Q_{max}, %
Fabricius et al. [101]	1992	30	10	12	2.3	NR	NR	NR
Lepor et al. [102]	1992	285	2–10	12	0.7–1.3	23–44	51–69*	35–52
Lepor et al. [103]	1992	45	2–10	24	1.5	33	47†	NR
Di Silverio [104]	1992	137	2–10	8	1.2–2.9	58–69	NR	NR
Brawer et al. [105]	1993	160	1–20	24	1.4	31	14	NR
Debruyne et al. [106]	1996	186	5–10	24	0.6–3.2	25	85.2	NR
Elhilali et al. [107]	1996	164	1–10	24	2.0	31	57‡	36‡
Lepor et al. [108]	1996	610	1–10	52	2.7	38	NR	NR
Roehrborn et al. [109]	1996	2084	2–10	52	2.2	38	55§	40*

>30% improvement in Boyarsky score.
†Significant in urinary symptoms as determined by investigators.
‡>30% improvement in AUA-IPSS and >50% improvement in Q_{max}.
§>35% improvement in AUA-IPSS.

▶ **FIGURE 3-22.** Randomized, placebo-controlled, double-blind clinical trials of terazosin. The efficacy of terazosin, a long-acting α_1-selective antagonist that allows for once-a-day dosing, has been studied in many clinical trials. The largest of these clinical trials, the Hytrin Community Assessment Trial (HCAT), is representative of the results obtained from many clinical trials of patients treated with terazosin [109]. The HCAT study enrolled 2084 men 55 years of age or older with moderate to severe urinary symptoms who were randomized to receive treatment with terazosin or placebo. Terazosin was significantly superior to placebo in all measurements of efficacy; the American Urological Association–International Prostate Symptom Score (AUA-IPSS) improved from a baseline mean of 20.1 points by 37.8% in the terazosin group, compared with 18.4% in the placebo group. The mean change from baseline in peak urinary flow rate was 2.2 for terazosin compared with 0.8 for placebo. Treatment failure occurred in approximately 11% of the terazosin study group compared with approximately 25% in the placebo group. Withdrawal from the study because of adverse effects of treatment occurred in 20% of the terazosin group. In conclusion, terazosin given once daily in community-based settings is an effective medical treatment for reducing urinary symptoms, perception of bother, and impairment of quality of life due to urinary symptoms created by benign prostatic hyperplasia. NR—not reported; Q_{max}—maximum urine flow rate.

Clinical Trials of Doxazosin

Study	Year	Patients, n	Dose, mg	Follow-up, wk	↑ Q_{max}, mL/s	↓ Symptom Score, %	% Significant Response	
							>25% Improvement in AUA-IPSS, %	>30% Increase in Q_{max}, %
Holme et al. [110]	1991	100	4	29	1.7	NR	NR	NR
Gillenwater and Mobley [111]	1993	100	8	6	2.9	56	NR	NR
Janknegt and Chapple [112]	1993	456	1–16	4–29	1.2–3.9	NR	NR	NR
Chapple et al. [113]	1994	135	4	12	1.0	NR	33–60*	36†
Fawzy et al. [114]	1995	100	2–8	16	2.9	40	39–43*	39
Gillenwater et al. [115]	1995	216	2–12	16	2.3–3.6	NR	NR	37–39
Kirby [116]	1995	232	4	9–12	2.0–2.4	NR	NR	47.4
Roehrborn and Siegel [117]	1996	322	2–12	16	2.2	16.4	27	35

*Significant improvement in symptoms as determined by investigators.
†>50% increase in Q_{max}.

▶ **FIGURE 3-23.** Randomized, placebo-controlled, double-blind clinical trials of doxazosin. Doxazosin is another long-acting α_1-selective blocker that allows for once-daily dosing. Short-term clinical trials have shown that doxazosin can increase peak flow rates by about 1 to 4 mL/s and decrease symptom scores by up to 50% in men with symptomatic benign prostatic hyperplasia (BPH). The clinical response to α_1-receptor antagonists in terms of decreased symptomatology and increased urinary flow rates is dose dependent; however, the side effect profile is also dose dependent. Studies attempting to determine variables that are predictive of the clinical response to α_1-receptor blockers (eg, patient age, prostate size, total symptom score, and flow rate) have failed to delineate a significant association between baseline factors and treatment effect.

Doxazosin therapy for BPH is typically initiated at a dose of 1 mg administered once daily. This low starting dose is intended to minimize the frequency of side effects such as postural hypotension and syncope. Depending on the patient's response to therapy and urodynamics, the dosage may be increased to 8 mg/day. Overall, doxazosin is an effective therapy for symptomatic BPH. Like terazosin, it has been proven to relieve symptoms and improve urinary flow rates. AUA-IPSS—American Urological Association–International Prostate Symptom Score; NR—not reported; Q_{max}—maximum urinary flow rate.

Clinical Trials of Tamsulosin

Study	Year	Patients, n	Dose, mg	Follow-up, wk	↑ Qmax, mL/s	↓ Symptom Score, %	PVR, %	% Significant Response >25% Improvement in AUA-IPSS, %	% Significant Response >30% Increase in Qmax, %
Abrams *et al.* [118]	1995	296	0.4	12	1.4	36	21	67	29
Schulman *et al.* [119]	1996	244	0.4	60	1.6	34	NR	69	32
Chapple *et al.* [120]	1996	575	0.4	12	1.6	35	23	66	32
Lepor [121]	1998	1488	0.4	13	1.8	42	NR	78–81	31–36
Lepor [122]	1998	755	0.4–0.8	13	1.75–1.78	50	NR	59–78	39–40
Narayan and Tewari [123]	1998	239	0.4–0.8	13	1.52–1.79	55	NR	55–56	33
Narayan and Bruskewitz [124]	2000	248	0.4–0.8	13	1.52	30	NR	56	34

▶ **FIGURE 3-24.** Randomized, placebo-controlled, double-blind clinical trials of tamsulosin. As mentioned in Figure 3-23, tamsulosin is an α-blocker with specificity for the α_{1A}-adrenoreceptor in relation to the α_{1B}-adrenoreceptor. Theoretically, this drug would target the smooth muscle cells contained within the prostate gland, with minimal effects on the other α-adrenergic receptor subtypes that regulate blood pressure and vasodilation. Clinical trials suggest that tamsulosin provides a rapid onset of action, based on symptom improvement and peak urinary flow rate. The initial short-term clinical trials suggested that tamsulosin increases peak flow rates approximately 1.5 mL/s and decreased American Urological Association–International Prostate Symptom Scores (AUA-IPSS) by more than 35% [118]. Long-term studies (up to 60 weeks) examining the effects of tamsulosin demonstrated that the beneficial effects of tamsulosin are sustained over time, as measured by maximum urinary flow rates and total Boyarsky symptom score. Tamsulosin continued to be well-tolerated during the study period, with side effects occurring in approximately 21% of patients. The most common side effects experienced were dizziness and abnormal ejaculation, each of which occurred in approximately 5% of patients. Clinical studies have also demonstrated that tamsulosin can be coadministered with antihypertensive medications such as nifedipine, enalapril, and atenolol without any increase in risk of hypotensive or syncopal episodes [125]. Taken together, tamsulosin is a safe and efficacious drug for the treatment of benign prostatic hyperplasia, without major vascular side effects. NR—not reported; Q_{max}—maximum urinary flow rate; PVR—postvoid residual.

Clinical Trials of Alfuzosin

Study	Year	Patients, n	Dose, mg	Follow-up, wk	↑ Qmax, mL/s	↓ Symptom Score, %	% Significant Response >25% Improvement in AUA-IPSS, %	% Significant Response >30% Increase in Qmax, %
Jardin *et al.* [126]	1991	518	2.5 tid	26	1.4	42	50–61	NR
Buzelin *et al.* [127]	1993	48	2.5 tid	4	2.6	32	NR	NR
Hansen *et al.* [128]	1994	178	2.5 tid	12	2.0	29	NR	NR
Schulman *et al.* [129]	1994	50	2.5 qd	4	2.6	38	NR	NR
Buzelin *et al.* [130]	1997	382	5 SR bid	12	2.4	33	42*	38
Buzelin *et al.* [131]	1997	588	2.5 tid	4–12	2.3	NR	64	42
van Kerrebroeck *et al.* [132]	2000	297	10 XL qd	12	2.3	40	NR	NR
Roehrborn *et al.* [133]	2001	353	10–15 XL qd	12	0.9–1.7	19–20	39–56	40–41
Roehrborn *et al.* [134]	2003	473	10 XL qd	12	2.3	32	76	NR

*>25% improvement in Boyarsky score.

▶ **FIGURE 3-25.** Randomized, placebo-controlled, double-blind clinical trials of alfuzosin. Alfuzosin is a second-generation α_1-adrenoreceptor antagonist indicated for the management of moderate to severe benign prostatic hyperplasia. It has been shown to improve bothersome urinary symptoms and to increase urine flow rates while having minimal cardiovascular side effects. The immediate-release formulation requires administration two to three times per day. Alfuzosin is also available in extended-release (XL) and sustained-release (SR) formulations that necessitate once-daily administration. Interestingly, it has been reported that cardiovascular side effects occur more frequently with the immediate-release preparation compared with the extended-release preparation, which is probably the result of fluctuation in serum drug levels. Alfuzosin is similar to other second-generation α_1-adrenoreceptor antagonists with regard to clinical efficacy and adverse effects. AUA-IPSS—American Urological Association–International Prostate Symptom Score; bid—twice a day; NR—not recorded; qd—every day; Q_{max}—maximum urinary flow rate; tid—three times a day.

Adverse Effects of α-Adrenergic Antagonists

Effect	Phenoxybenzamine, %	Prazosin, %	Terazosin, %	Doxazosin, %	Tamsulosin, %	Alfuzosin, %
Hypotension	15–20	10–15	2–8	1–2	<1	<1
Dizziness	10–14	15–17	7–14	10–15	15	6–9
Headache	4–15	13–15	4–10	9–10	19	8–14
Sexual dysfunction	5–8	NR	2–7	NR	8	1–2
Fatigue	10–15	10	4–8	1–2	8	1–7
Syncope	NR	NR	<1	<1	<1	<1
Nasal congestion	8	NR	2	NR	13	5–6

▶ **FIGURE 3-26.** Adverse effects of α-adrenergic antagonists [117,133,135,136]. Dizziness is the most common side effect of α-adrenergic antagonists. It is possible that this side effect may be caused by effects on the central nervous system or by other unconventional drug mechanisms and may be unrelated to effects on the blood vessels themselves. The fact that some dizziness is seen with tamsulosin (a selective α$_{1A}$-adrenergic antagonist) suggests that a central effect may mediate this symptom. Hypotension decreases with longer-acting drugs and is least with α$_{1A}$-adrenergic selective agents. Tamsulosin has been safely administered concurrently with other hypotensive agents (*see* Fig. 3-24). Dizziness and hypotension are more common in those older than 65 years. Ejaculatory dysfunction may occur but when explained to the patient, does not generally cause a problem. Its effect may be mediated through drug interactions with the vas deferens itself. NR—not recorded.

MEDICAL THERAPIES FOR THE TREATMENT OF BENIGN PROSTATIC HYPERPLASIA: COMBINATION THERAPY

As mentioned above, both hormonal therapy and α-adrenergic therapy are effective treatments for benign prostatic hyperplasia (BPH). Hormonal therapy targets the static component whereas α-adrenergic therapy is concentrated on the dynamic component of BPH. However, it was of interest to determine the results of combination therapy that targets both of the major components of BPH simultaneously.

The first randomized, double-blind, placebo-controlled study investigating combination therapy using α-adrenergic antagonists and 5α-reductase inhibitors was a four-arm Veterans Administration Cooperative Trial comparing placebo, finasteride alone, terazosin alone, and combination therapy with finasteride and terazosin [108] (*see* Fig. 3-29). The conclusions derived from this study were that short-term combination therapy was no more effective than a single agent in the treatment of BPH. However,

this was a relatively short-term study that did not examine BPH progression or the long-term effects of combination therapy.

The Medical Treatment of Prostatic Symptoms (MTOPS) study asked a different question about the ability of combination therapy [137]. This study was designed to determine whether medical therapy could prevent or delay the clinical progression of BPH as defined by acute urinary retention, renal insufficiency caused by BPH, recurrent urinary tract infections, incontinence, and progression of American Urological Association–International Prostate Symptom Score (AUA-IPSS) [138]. The results suggested that in a large but select population of patients, combination therapy was the most effective treatment for BPH to reduce the risk of clinical progression, improve AUA-IPSS, and improve maximum urinary flow rate (*see* Figs. 3-29 to 3-33).

Combination Therapy for Benign Prostatic Hyperplasia

Agent	Patients, n	Q$_{max}$, mL/s	↓ Symptom Score, Units	Change in Prostate Volume, mL
Placebo	254	1.4	2.6	0.5
Terazosin	256	2.7	6.1	0.5
Finasteride	243	1.6	3.2	-6.1
Terazosin + Finasteride	254	3.2	6.2	-7.0

▶ **FIGURE 3-27.** Combination therapy for the treatment of benign prostatic hyperplasia (BPH): the Veterans Affairs Cooperative Study. As mentioned above, the Veterans Affairs Cooperative Study [108] was the first clinical trial to investigate the usefulness of combination therapy for the treatment of BPH. In this multicenter, double-blind trial, patients were randomly assigned to treatment with placebo, terazosin, finasteride, or a combination of terazosin and finasteride. After 1 year of treatment, the investigators concluded that terazosin alone produced superior results in terms of improvement of symptom score and peak urinary flow rates. Note that treatment with finasteride decreased prostate size the most significantly, but report of bothersome symptoms decreased the most with terazosin or combination therapy. The applicability of this study's conclusion to the general population of men with symptomatic BPH has been challenged because of the relatively small percentage of men with larger prostates included in this study. This study also failed to address whether combination therapy affected BPH progression or whether a longer duration of therapy affected the outcome. Q$_{max}$—maximum urinary flow rate.

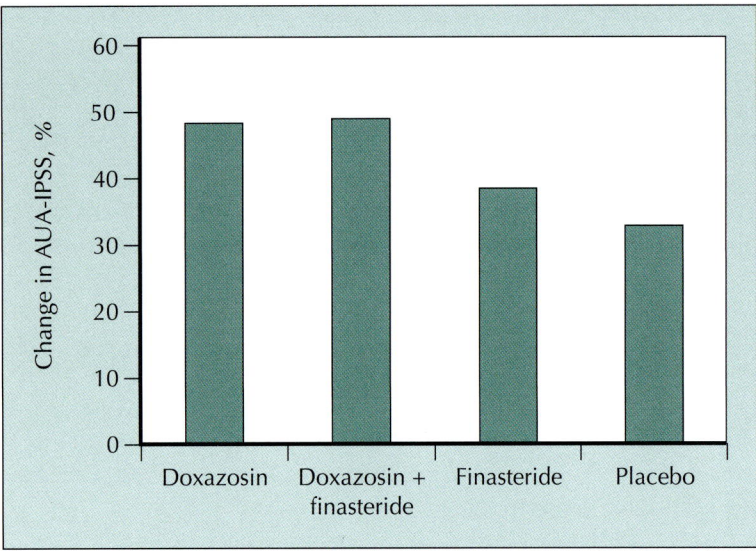

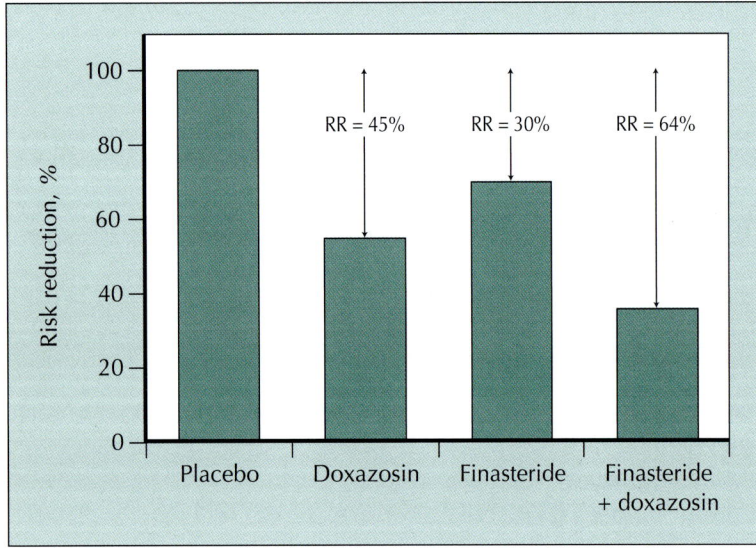

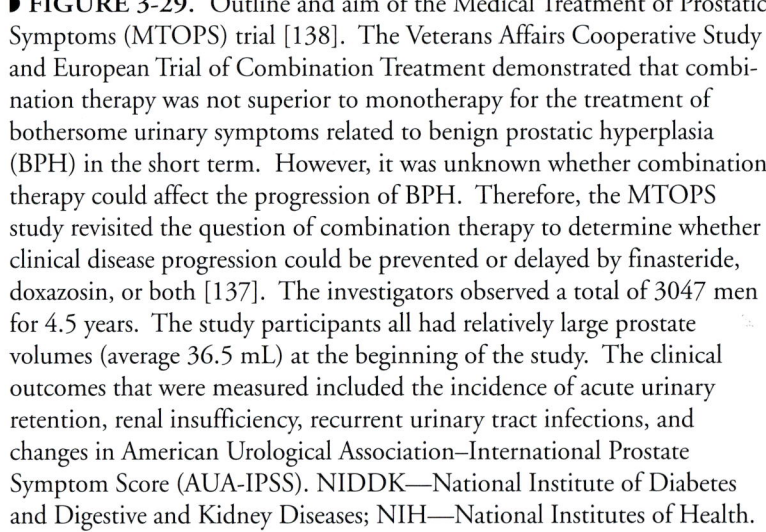

FIGURE 3-28. Combination therapy for the treatment of benign prostatic hyperplasia (BPH): the Prospective European Doxazosin and Combination Therapy (PREDICT) trial [139]. The PREDICT trial also examined whether combination therapy with α-adrenergic inhibitors and 5α-reductase inhibitors could be used for the symptomatic treatment of BPH. In this prospective, double-blind, placebo-controlled study, 1095 men were randomized to 1-year treatment with doxazosin, finasteride, the combination of doxazosin and finasteride, or placebo. The drug treatment groups all had decreases in American Urological Association–International Prostate Symptom Scores (AUA-IPSS). In addition, the maximum urinary flow rate increased by 3.6, 3.8, 1.8, and 1.4 mL/s in the doxazosin, doxazosin and finasteride combination, finasteride, and placebo groups, respectively. The conclusions of this study confirmed that doxazosin is a superior treatment for BPH compared with finasteride alone or placebo. Also, the addition of finasteride to doxazosin did not provide any additional benefit compared with doxazosin alone. Therefore, combination therapy is not recommended solely for the relief of bothersome urinary symptoms caused by BPH. However, as with the Veterans Affairs Cooperative Study, this study failed to address whether combination therapy played a role in the prevention of BPH progression or whether a longer duration of combination therapy affected the outcomes.

FIGURE 3-29. Outline and aim of the Medical Treatment of Prostatic Symptoms (MTOPS) trial [138]. The Veterans Affairs Cooperative Study and European Trial of Combination Treatment demonstrated that combination therapy was not superior to monotherapy for the treatment of bothersome urinary symptoms related to benign prostatic hyperplasia (BPH) in the short term. However, it was unknown whether combination therapy could affect the progression of BPH. Therefore, the MTOPS study revisited the question of combination therapy to determine whether clinical disease progression could be prevented or delayed by finasteride, doxazosin, or both [137]. The investigators observed a total of 3047 men for 4.5 years. The study participants all had relatively large prostate volumes (average 36.5 mL) at the beginning of the study. The clinical outcomes that were measured included the incidence of acute urinary retention, renal insufficiency, recurrent urinary tract infections, and changes in American Urological Association–International Prostate Symptom Score (AUA-IPSS). NIDDK—National Institute of Diabetes and Digestive and Kidney Diseases; NIH—National Institutes of Health.

FIGURE 3-30. Risk of increasing American Urological Association–International Prostate Symptom Score (AUA-IPSS) with benign prostatic hyperplasia (BPH): doxazosin versus finasteride versus combination therapy. Patients enrolled in the Medical Treatment of Prostatic Symptoms (MTOPS) trial completed AUA-IPSS questionnaires [137] (*see* Fig. 3-4, for example). An increase in the AUA-IPSS of more than four points above baseline values was the most common individual event in all groups at the end of the study. There was a 3.6 per 100 person-year risk of having this four-point increase in the placebo arm of the study. This value is represented as 100% in the graph (*see Placebo column*). In comparison, the risk of having a four-point increase in AUA-IPSS was reduced to 1.9 person-years (45% reduction in risk [RR]) in the doxazosin group. This value is represented as 55% in the graph (*see Doxazosin column*). Similarly, patients in the finasteride group had a 30% reduction in risk (*see Finasteride column*). Patients enrolled in the combination therapy arm experienced a 66% reduction in the risk of AUA-IPSS progression. In fact, this risk reduction was larger than that for any of the medical therapies used alone.

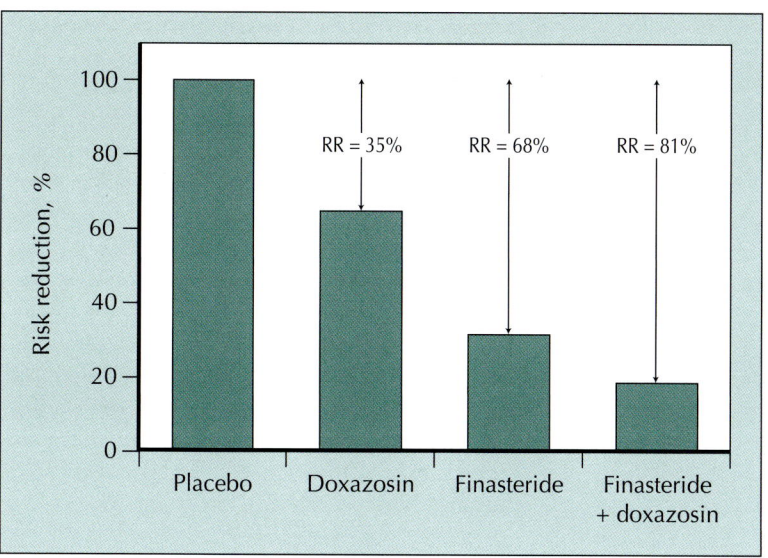

▶ **FIGURE 3-31.** Risk of urinary retention: doxazosin versus finasteride versus combination therapy. The Medical Treatment of Prostatic Symptoms (MTOPS) trial also analyzed the contribution of single and combination therapy to the incidence of acute urinary retention [137]. Doxazosin did not significantly reduce the rate of acute urinary retention compared with the placebo group (0.4 per 100 person-years). However, both the finasteride monotherapy (0.4 per 100 person-years) and combination therapy (0.1 per 100 person years) groups significantly lowered the rate of development of urinary retention compared with the placebo group (0.6 per 100 person-years). The graph demonstrates an insignificant decrease of 35% in the doxazosin group and a significant decrease of 68% and 81% in the finasteride monotherapy and combination therapy groups, respectively. RR—risk reduction.

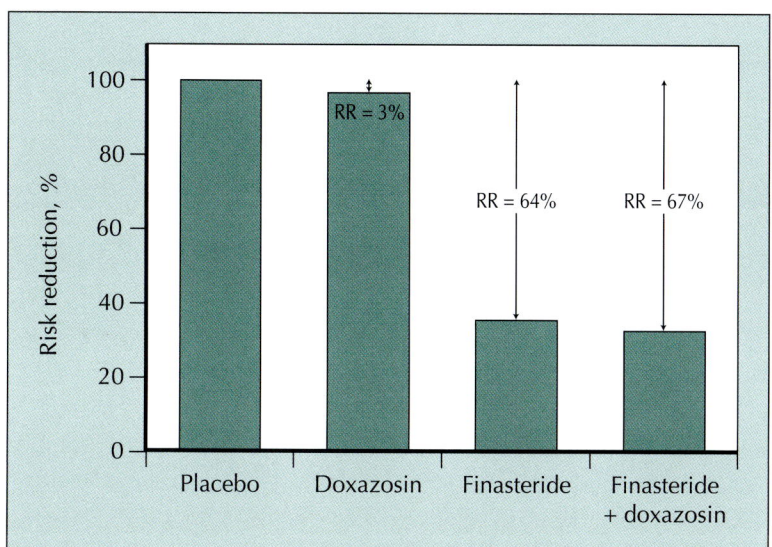

▶ **FIGURE 3-32.** Risk for surgery related to benign prostatic hyperplasia (BPH): doxazosin versus finasteride versus combination therapy. Analysis of the Medical Treatment of Prostatic Symptoms (MTOPS) trial demonstrates that there is a significant reduction in the rate of invasive therapy with surgery over a 5-year period when either finasteride monotherapy or combination therapy with finasteride and doxazosin is used [137]. Men enrolled in the placebo group had a 1.3 per 100 person-year risk of having invasive surgery for BPH, such as transurethral prostatectomy or transurethral microwave therapy. The risk of requiring these invasive therapies for progression of BPH was reduced by 64% and 67% in the finasteride and combination therapy groups, respectively. Doxazosin did not significantly reduce the incidence of invasive therapy. RR—risk reduction.

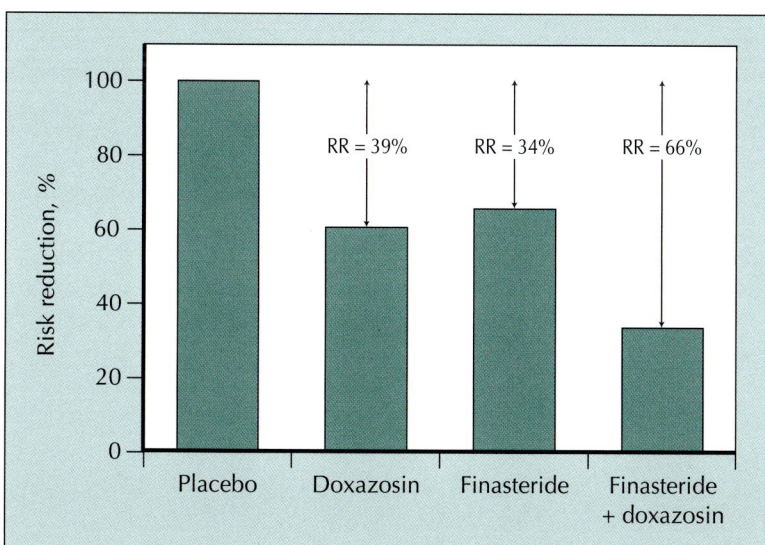

▶ **FIGURE 3-33.** Risk of clinical progression of benign prostatic hyperplasia (BPH): doxazosin versus finasteride versus combination therapy. Taken together (*see* Figs. 3-30 to 3-32), combination therapy significantly reduces the clinical progression of BPH [137]. The Medical Treatment of Prostatic Symptoms (MTOPS) trial served to analyze this rate and found that the rate of overall clinical progression among men in the placebo group was 4.5 per 100 person-years. In comparison, doxazosin reduced the risk of progression by 39%, to 2.7 person-years. Finasteride reduced the risk of progression by 34% (2.9 person-years). Combination therapy with both these drugs affected the rate of progression more than either drug alone and reduced the risk by 66%, to 1.5 per 100 person-years. Taken together, combination therapy reduces the risk of American Urological Association–International Prostate Symptom Score progression, urinary retention, and surgery because it significantly inhibits the natural progression of BPH. RR—risk reduction.

Adverse Reactions Reported in 100 Person-Years of Follow-Up				
Effect	Placebo	Doxazosin	Finasteride	Combination
Hypotension	2.29	4.03	2.56	4.33
Dizziness	2.29	4.41	2.33	5.35
Asthenia	2.06	4.08	1.56	4.20
Erectile dysfunction	3.32	3.56	4.53	5.11
Decreased libido	1.40	1.56	2.36	2.51
Abnormal ejaculation	0.83	1.10	1.78	3.05
Allergic reaction	0.46	0.85	0.58	0.73

Adapted from McConnell et al. [137]

▶ **FIGURE 3-34.** Adverse effects of combination therapy for benign prostatic hyperplasia. The Medical Treatment of Prostatic Symptoms (MTOPS) trial also evaluated the rate of side effects between single and combination therapy [137]. As mentioned above, patients assigned to the doxazosin group had an increased rate of dizziness, postural hypotension, and asthenia compared with the placebo group. Similarly, erectile dysfunction, decreased libido, and abnormal ejaculation were increased in frequency compared with placebo. The adverse events experienced by patients taking combination therapy were similar to those for each drug alone. However, the rates of abnormal ejaculation, peripheral edema, and dyspnea were increased in this group. (*Adapted from* McConnell *et al.* [137].)

ALGORITHM FOR THE MEDICAL MANAGEMENT OF BENIGN PROSTATIC HYPERPLASIA

Benign prostatic hyperplasia (BPH) will continue to be a major challenge for all health care providers because of the increasing aging population. Therefore, it is important for clinicians to be knowledgeable and up to date on the latest treatments for this disorder. The previous sections describe many different proven medical therapies for the treatment of BPH, including 5α-reduc-tase inhibitors and α-adrenergic antagonists. Knowing when to implement these therapies and how to cater them to the needs of each individual patient is critical to the successful relief and prevention of symptoms and complications related to BPH. The following section outlines the most current evidence-based practices for the medical treatment of BPH.

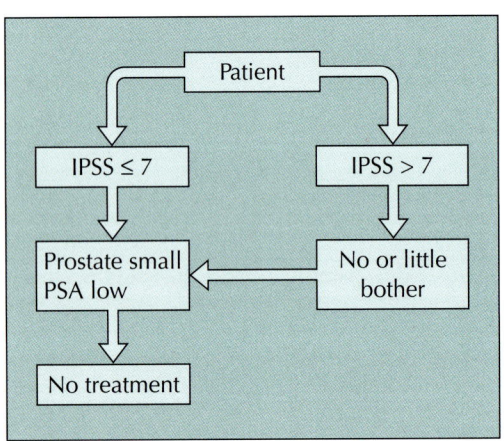

▶ **FIGURE 3-35.** Evaluation of patients who present with lower urinary tract symptoms (LUTS): role for watchful waiting. The decision to treat a patient for benign prostatic hyperplasia (BPH) is based on the degree of bothersome symptoms and assessment of the risk of BPH progression (*ie*, acute urinary retention, urinary tract infections, bladder stones). The initial evaluation of a patient who presents with complaints of LUTS is to use the American Urological Association–International Prostate Symptom Score (AUA-IPSS) to determine the degree of LUTS and their impact on the quality of the patient's lifestyle. Medical or surgical therapies

are generally not indicated for patients who experience mild or moderate symptoms (AUA-IPSS 0 to 18) and who are not significantly bothered by these symptoms. In addition, the initial clinical evaluation of all patients should include a digital rectal examination (DRE), serum prostate-specific antigen (PSA) level, and a prostatic volume estimate (transrectal ultrasound [TRUS], PSA, MRI, or DRE; see below for description) [140].

Diagnostic methods for estimating prostatic volume include DRE, TRUS, MRI, and PSA testing. Although TRUS and MRI are limited by their high cost and low availability, they are the most accurate methods of estimating prostate volume. In contrast, DRE is inexpensive but notoriously underestimates the prostatic volume. Serum PSA measurements can easily be obtained and have been shown to directly correlate with prostate volume [52,141]. In addition, determination of serum PSA levels has the additional benefit of screening for prostate cancer. Because of this, it is recommended that the diagnostic workup of every patient at minimum include a PSA measurement as an approximation of prostate volume.

Elevated serum PSA has been shown to correlate with progression of BPH [51,141]. PSA is produced almost exclusively by the epithelial cells of the prostate. Serum PSA is related to prostate volume [51,141]; therefore, increased levels of serum PSA are present in patients with increased prostate volume, such as that which occurs in BPH and prostate cancer. Elevated serum PSA in patients with BPH has been shown to be associated with a higher incidence of surgical treatments and acute urinary retention [52]. In addition, increased serum PSA levels at the initial evaluation for BPH have been associated with increased bothersome LUTS, faster symptom deterioration, reduced urinary flow rate, and impaired quality of life. Therefore, serum PSA values greater than 1.3 ng/mL are associated with increased BPH progression [52,142].

If it is determined that patients are not bothered by their LUTS, have a small prostate (< 30 g) by DRE or TRUS, and have a relatively low serum PSA (< 1.3 ng/mL), then it is reasonable to hold medical treatment modalities for BPH until a later time. Data from the Olmsted County Study suggest that approximately 40% to 60% of patients who present with mild to moderate symptoms will not progress over a 4-year period of time. Therefore, in this group, it is reasonable to employ a "watchful waiting" strategy and reassess these patients' symptoms on an annual basis [175].

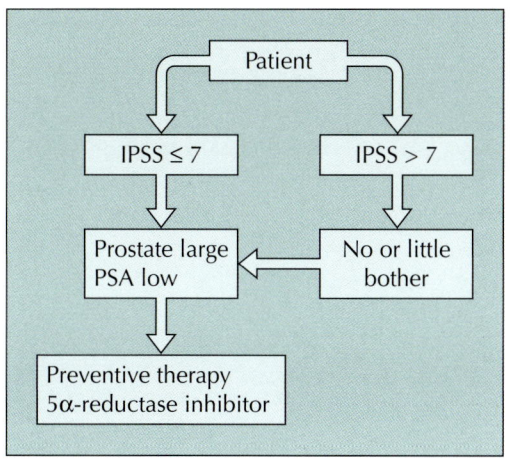

FIGURE 3-36. Evaluation of patients who present with lower urinary tract symptoms (LUTS): role for medical therapy as prevention. Multiple studies have demonstrated a strong association between baseline prostate volume and risk of benign prostatic hyperplasia (BPH) progression [52]. Men with large prostate glands compared with men with normal-sized or small prostate glands are 3.5 times more likely to have moderate symptoms, 2.5 times more likely to have decreased urinary flow rates, approximately three to four times more likely to suffer from acute urinary retention, and four times more likely to need medical or surgical treatments [30].

Given the fact that there is convincing evidence for disease progression [143–145] and that identification of patients at greatest risk of disease progression is possible using estimates of prostate volume and serum prostate-specific antigen (PSA) values, medical management strategies that are aimed at preventing BPH progression can be employed. At present, only 5α-reductase inhibitors have been shown to prevent BPH progression [47,137] (*see* Figs. 3-11 to 3-13). Long-term treatment with 5α-reductase inhibitors such as finasteride and dutasteride has been shown to significantly reduce prostate volume and improve bothersome LUTS derived from BPH (*see* Figs. 3-10 to 3-12). Thus, these drugs are efficacious in decreasing the progression of BPH, incidence of acute urinary retention, and surgical treatments for BPH. Therefore, it is possible that men with large prostate glands and few bothersome LUTS (mild to moderate American Urological Association–International Prostate Symptom Scores [AUA-IPSS]) could be prophylactically started on a 5α-reductase inhibitor for prevention of BPH progression.

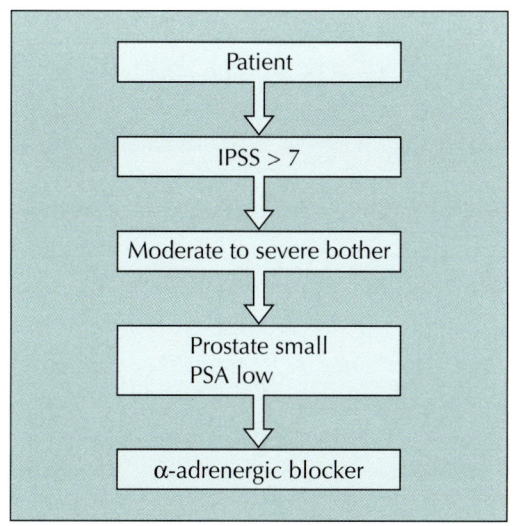

FIGURE 3-37. Evaluation of patients who present with lower urinary tract symptoms (LUTS) with a relatively small prostate volume: role for medical therapy as treatment. Patients with moderate to severe American Urological Association–International Prostate Symptom Scores (AUA-IPSS) should be evaluated with digital rectal examination, serum prostate-specific antigen (PSA) testing, and transrectal ultrasound. Patients who experience significant decreases in their quality of life because of LUTS and who have a small prostate gland (< 30 g) and a serum PSA less than 1.3 ng/dL should be started on therapy with an α-adrenergic blocker. Both short- and long-term studies with α-adrenergic blockers have shown significant efficacy in the treatment of BPH in that they reduce the mean AUA-IPSS by approximately 35% to 55%, depending on the dose and type of α-adrenergic blocker used (*see* Figs. 3-22 to 3-25 for more details).

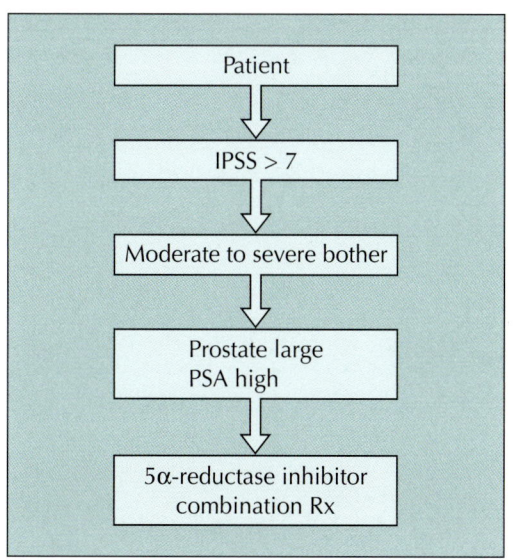

FIGURE 3-38. Evaluation of patients who present with lower urinary tract symptoms with a relatively large prostate volume: role for combination medical therapy as treatment. Patients who present with moderate to severe urinary symptoms that affect their lifestyle and who are found to have a large prostate volume or an elevated prostate-specific antigen (PSA) level need to be evaluated by transrectal ultrasound biopsy to rule out histologic evidence of prostate cancer. Once it is determined that these patients have benign prostatic hyperplasia (BPH), combination therapy with a 5α-reductase inhibitor and an α-adrenergic blocker should be initiated. The Medical Treatment of Prostatic Symptoms (MTOPS) trial demonstrated that combination therapy for BPH was the most effective means to reduce the risk of clinical progression, improve maximum urinary flow rate, improve American Urological Association–International Prostate Symptom Score (AUA-IPSS), and reduce the risk of urinary retention and invasive therapy (*see* Figs. 3-29 to 3-33 for more details).

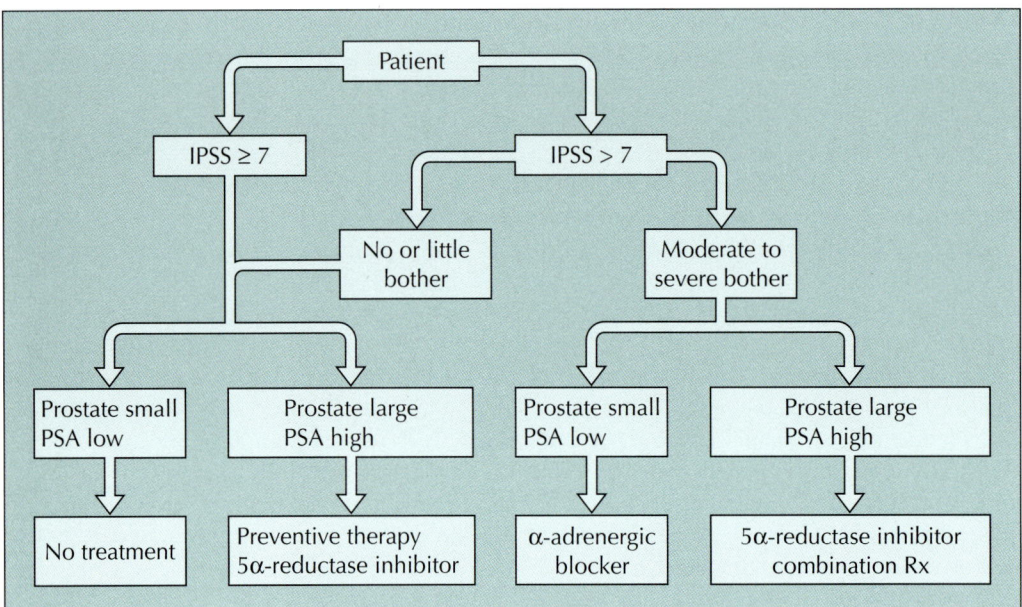

▶ **FIGURE 3-39.** Overview of the evaluation of patients with lower urinary tract symptoms: an algorithm for the clinical workup and medical management of benign prostatic hyperplasia. IPSS—International Prostate Symptom Score; PSA—prostate-specific antigen.

MEDICAL THERAPIES FOR THE TREATMENT OF BENIGN PROSTATIC HYPERPLASIA: PHYTOTHERAPY

Phytotherapy is defined as the use of plants or plant extracts for medical treatment. Plant extracts for the treatment of symptoms related to benign prostatic hyperplasia (BPH) have been used since ancient times. The current use and prevalence of phytotherapy for BPH therapy tends to be based on geographic location. Although their use is not as common in the United States, plants and plant extracts are widely used in Europe. For example, in Germany, up to 90% of all patients with BPH are treated with phytopharmaceutical agents, and it has been reported that approximately 50% of German urologists prefer plant-based therapies to chemically derived ones [146].

Although these agents have been used for centuries, little is known about the true mechanism of action that gives phytopharmaceuticals their therapeutic nature. Several problems have significantly affected the evaluation of the effectiveness of these drugs for use in treating BPH [147]. First, only a limited number

of double-blind trials have been conducted using these phytotherapies. In addition, most of these studies have been uncontrolled and have not been able to rule out the possibility of a placebo effect. Second, the active ingredient in most of these plant extracts is unknown because of the abundance of compounds contained within the extracts. Therefore, the dosage of an active drug in a specific preparation is unknown, which makes direct comparison between medications nearly impossible. Finally, most previously reported studies did not use standardized urinary symptoms scores (eg, American Urological Association–International Prostate Symptom Score) in their evaluation of efficacy, which makes quantitation and direct comparison extremely difficult.

Despite these problems, many phytotherapies are currently being used for the treatment of BPH. In fact, there are approximately 30 different phytotherapeutic compounds used for the treatment of BPH. Some of these treatments are discussed in detail below.

Phytotherapeutic Agents Used in the Treatment of Benign Prostatic Hyperplasia

Plant	Common Name	Trade Name	Proposed Active Agent(s)	Proposed Method of Action
Serenoa repens	Saw palmetto	Permixon	Fatty acids, sterols	Antiandrogen β-FGF, EGF
Pygeum africanum	African prune	Tadenan	β-Sitosterol	Cholesterol mechanism
			Fatty alcohols	Inhibits β-FGF
			Fatty acids	EGH
				Anti-inflammatory
Hypoxis rooperi	South African star grass	Harzol	β-Sitosterol	Anti-inflammatory
				Anticholesterol metabolism
Pinus picea	Pine flower spruce	Azurusat (combination)	β-Sitosterol	Anti-inflammatory
				Anticholesterol metabolism
Secale cereale	Rye grass pollen	Cernilton	β-Sterols	Antiandrogen
				Inhibitors of prostaglandins
				Leukotriene synthesis

▶ **FIGURE 3-40.** Some of the phytotherapeutic agents used in the treatment of benign prostatic hyperplasia. The true chemical nature of these plants and plant extracts is generally unclear. The listed "active" agent represents only one of the probably many active ingredients contained within the extract. In general, the components of plant extracts are phytosterols, phytoestrogens, and terpenoids [147,148]. Likewise, the postulated action is often broader than that shown in the figure [147]. Unfortunately, many of these studies evaluating the mechanisms of action have used supraphysiologic doses of extracts [147]. In addition, as mentioned above, many of these studies have failed to be double-blind and placebo-controlled. EGF—epidermal growth factor; EGH—equine growth hormone; β-FGF—β-fibroblast growth factor.

Results of Clinical Studies Using Saw Palmetto

Study	Year	Daily Dose, mg	Patients, n	Study Duration, mo	Urinary Symptoms	Change in Flow Rate, mL/s Treated	Placebo
Boccafoschi and Annoscia [149]	1983	320	22	2	Decreased	4.1*	1.9
Emili *et al.* [150]	1983	320	30	1	Decreased	3.4*	0.2
Champault *et al.* [151]	1984	320	110	1	Decreased	3.0*	0.3
Cukier *et al.* [152]	1985	320	146	2	Decreased	NR	NR
Tasca *et al.* [153]	1985	320	30	1–3	Decreased	3.3*	0.6
Reece-Smith *et al.* [154]	1986	320	70	3	Not decreased	2.5	2.5
Carbin *et al.* [155]	1990	480	53	3	Decreased	3.0*	0.6
Descotes *et al.* [156]	1995	320	215	1	Not decreased	3.5	1.1
Carraro *et al.* [157]	1996	320	1098	5–6	Not decreased	2.7	3.2
Braeckman *et al.* [158]	1997	320	238	3	Decreased	2.8	1.2
Willetts *et al.* [159]	2003	320	100	12	Not decreased	1.5	4.4*

▶ **FIGURE 3-41.** Results of placebo-controlled trials using saw palmetto (*Serenoa repens*). Extract from the saw palmetto plant is the most widely used phytotherapeutic agent for benign prostatic hyperplasia (BPH). Saw palmetto is a dwarf palm tree native to the West Indies and the Southeastern United States. It was initially used by the American Indians to increase testicular function and relieve genitourinary irritation [160]. The lipid-soluble components of the saw palmetto berries are believed to contain the active components for the treatment of BPH [160]. The purified lipid extract is used medicinally and consists of fatty acids and sterols, such as β-sitosterol. The active constituents are believed to be those compounds related to steroids. For example, sitosterols are chemically related to cholesterol. However, the exact mechanism by which these compounds exert their antiandrogen effects remains to be determined.

Double-blind clinical studies using saw palmetto berry extract for the treatment of BPH have been performed. Data supporting the efficacy of saw palmetto for BPH therapy have been produced, although it should be noted that many of these studies are inconclusive because of problems with inclusion/exclusion criteria, lack of a uniform symptom score analysis, lack of power, lack of a placebo run-in period, and short duration of therapy. The available data indicate that *S. repens* may improve urinary tract symptoms and urinary tract flow measures. Compared with placebo, *S. repens* may modestly improve urinary tract symptoms. A recent meta-analysis suggests that saw palmetto increases the maximum urinary flow rate by 1.0 mL/s compared with placebo and reduces the mean number of episodes of nocturia by 0.37 episodes per night compared with placebo [161]. However, the clinical significance of a reduction in episodes of nocturia is not known. Overall, saw palmetto may have some efficacy in the treatment of BPH. Future multicenter, randomized, placebo-controlled studies need to be performed to determine the effectiveness of saw palmetto in the treatment of BPH.

Comparison of the Effects of *Serenoa repens* With Those of Other Medical Therapies

Study	Year	Drug	Daily Dose, mg	Patients, n	Study Duration, d	Change in AUA-IPSS	Change in Q_{max}, mL/s	Change in Nocturia, Voids/Night
Carraro *et al.* [157]	1996				180			
		S. repens	320	467		-5.39	2.68	-0.74
		Finasteride	5	484		-5.92	3.26	-0.69
Grasso *et al.* [162]	1995				21			
		S. repens	320	31		NR	2.8	-1.0
		Alfuzosin	7.5	32		NR	4.7	-1.0
Debruyne *et al.* [163]	2002				360			
		S. repens	320	349		-5.73	1.52	-1.07
		Tamsulosin	0.4	354		-5.12	1.56	-0.96

▶ **FIGURE 3-42.** Comparison of the effects of *Serenoa repens* with those of other medical therapies for symptomatic benign prostatic hyperplasia. A few clinical studies have attempted to compare the effects of saw palmetto with the 5α-reductase inhibitor finasteride as well as with the α-adrenergic receptor antagonists alfuzosin and tamsulosin. Results from these studies have suggested that saw palmetto may have some efficacy in increasing the maximum urine flow rate (Q_{max}). Compared with finas-teride, saw palmetto appears to provide a similar response in urologic symptom scores and flow measures. However, the reader is advised to remember that the response to finasteride has been followed over months and not weeks. Thus, the validity of this comparison is not without concern. AUA-IPSS—American Urological Association–International Prostate Symptom Score; NR—not recorded

Adverse Effects of Phytotherapy: Comparison Between Saw Palmetto and Tamsulosin

Adverse Effect	Saw Palmetto, %	Tamsulosin, %
Rhinitis	8.6	12.1
Headache	8	10.5
Dizziness	2.9	1.7
Fatigue	1.7	1.4
Asthenia	1.1	1.4
Hypotension (postural)	1.1	<1
Dry mouth	<1	<1
Ejaculation disorders	<1	4.2
Decrease in libido	<1	1.1

▶ **FIGURE 3-43.** Adverse effects of phytotherapy: a comparison between saw palmetto and tamsulosin. Clinical studies have demonstrated a low frequency of side effects attributed to the use of saw palmetto for the treatment of benign prostatic hyperplasia. Adverse effects due to saw palmetto (*Serenoa repens*) were generally mild and comparable with placebo. *S. repens* has a decreased rate of side effects compared with tamsulosin and other more traditional therapies, such as finasteride [161] (*see* Fig. 3-24). The rate of erectile dysfunction caused by *S. repens* is significantly reduced when compared with tamsulosin or finasteride. Serious complications did not occur more frequently in the saw palmetto group. Acute urinary retention occurred at the same rate in both the saw palmetto and tamsulosin groups.

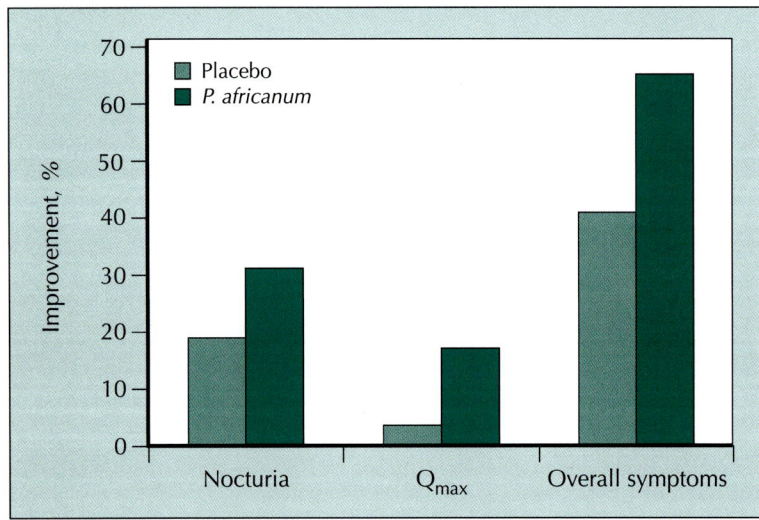

▶ **FIGURE 3-44.** African prune tree extract (*Pygeum africanum*) for the treatment of patients with benign prostatic hyperplasia (BPH). *P. africanum* is derived from the African plum tree [147]. It has been used in Europe since the middle of the 20th century for the treatment of genitourinary symptoms. The mechanism of action of *P. africanum* is not known. However, it has been postulated that the active components contained within the extract include phytosterols, especially β-sitosterols, as well as long-chain fatty alcohols. In animal studies, these compounds are believed to modulate bladder contractility, decrease inflammation, and decrease the production of leukotrienes [164].

The graph represents the data obtained from one randomized control trial of 263 patients that compared the effects of African plum tree extract to placebo. The data demonstrate that *P. africanum* has significant improvement in urinary symptoms when treated with plum tree extract compared with placebo [165]. Results from a meta-analysis of clinical studies of *P. africanum* indicate that it modestly but significantly improves urologic symptoms and urinary flow rates [166]. Further research involving multicenter, randomized-controlled, placebo-controlled studies will be required to determine its long-term effectiveness and treatment for urinary complaints related to BPH. Q_{max}—maximum urine flow rate.

Clinical Trials of Cernilton

Study	Year	Daily Doses, n	Patients, n	Study Duration, wks	Change in Flow Rate, mL/s Cernilton	Placebo/Drug†	Improvement in Nocturia Frequency, % Cernilton	Placebo/Drug†
Maekawa et al.	1981	4	192	12	1.65	1.23†	24	20†
Becker and Ebeling	1988	6	103	12	0.12	0.10	69*	37
Buck et al.	1990	4	60	24	0.20	0.30	50	30
Dutkiewicz	1996	3–6	89	16	3.02	1.64†	NR	NR†*

†These studies are controlled with other active substances. Maekawa et al. compared Cernilton with African prune tree extract and Dutkiewicz compared Cernilton with Paraprost. NR—not recorded.

▶ **FIGURE 3-45.** Randomized or controlled clinical trials of Cernilton (Graminex, Saginaw, MI), a derivative of the rye grass pollen (*Secale cereale*), for the treatment of benign prostatic hyperplasia (BPH). Cernilton, prepared from the rye grass pollen, is another phytotherapy used for the treatment of BPH. In the United States, Cernilton is used by approximately 5000 men daily [167]. One dose of Cernilton contains 60 mg of water-soluble compounds and approximately 3 mg of acetone-soluble compounds. The acetone-soluble fraction contains the β-sterols, which are believed to be the active components of the extract responsible for the antiandrogen and muscle-relaxing properties.

A systematic review of the literature demonstrated that Cernilton has the ability to decrease the frequency of nocturia and significantly reduce the postvoid residual volume in patients with BPH. Cernilton had no more effect than placebo or active controls on urinary flow measures [168]. Overall, it remains to be determined whether Cernilton has efficacy in the treatment of BPH. Future randomized-controlled, placebo-controlled multicenter studies are required to determine this effectiveness.

CONCLUSION: MEDICAL THERAPY FOR THE TREATMENT OF BENIGN PROSTATIC HYPERPLASIA

Benign prostatic hyperplasia (BPH) is a common complaint that increases with aging. As the prostate enlarges, it may cause clinical symptoms because it obstructs the urinary outlet by its larger physical size (static component) and increased smooth muscle tone (dynamic component). Treatment intervention for clinical BPH has mostly been directed toward the alleviation of bothersome lower urinary tract symptoms (LUTS). However, more recent attention has been focused on the prevention of BPH related to disease progression.

The decision to institute medical therapy as a treatment for BPH begins with an appropriate assessment and examination of the patient. In the United States, the finding of a small, smooth prostate in an individual with bothersome LUTS invokes the use of an α-adrenergic receptor antagonist. As the cost of selective α-adrenergic receptor antagonists decreases, their use as primary therapies for BPH will increase. Combination therapy with an α-adrenergic receptor antagonist and a 5α-reductase inhibitor should be used for patients who present with bothersome LUTS and a large prostate. This combined therapy will be directed at relieving the acute LUTS as well as preventing BPH progression. In addition, it is now suggested that patients with few bothersome LUTS but large prostates should be started on monotherapy with a 5α-reductase inhibitor to prevent BPH progression. Official recommendations on the use of phytotherapy have not been instituted because of numerous problems with study design and the lack of control groups, a mechanism of action, overall quality control, and regulation of production.

Taken together, medical therapy for bothersome LUTS has evolved along with our comprehension of the underlying pathophysiology of BPH. Current therapies are relatively effective in treating both the symptomatology and the progression of BPH. Future medical therapeutic agents will be directed toward alleviating both the irritative and the obstructive voiding symptoms of BPH, halting the disease progression, and minimizing adverse effects of the pharmaceutical agents themselves.

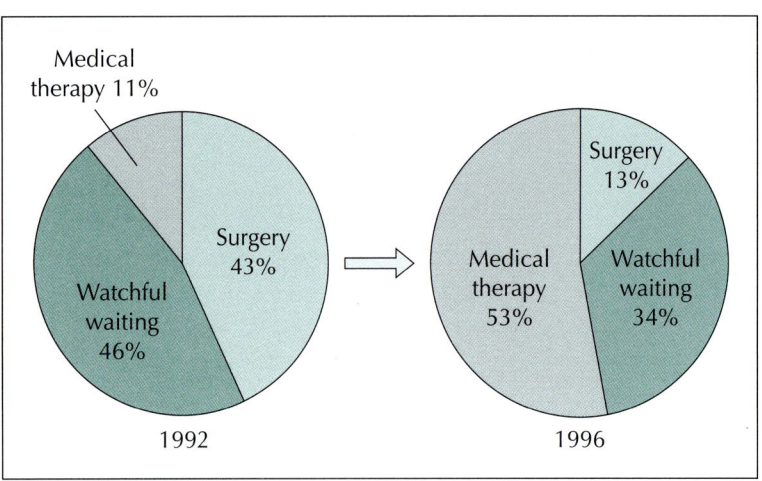

▶ **FIGURE 3-46.** Treatment trends for benign prostatic hyperplasia (BPH): impact of medical therapy during the past decade. Despite the overall aging of the population and the progressively increasing number of men enrolled in the Medicare program, a recent review of the US Medicare database revealed a continual decline in the annual number of prostatectomies and surgical therapies performed for BPH [16]. In 1994, 147,300 prostatectomies were performed; but in 2000, only 88,132 were performed. This decline coincides with a progressive annual increase in the number of men choosing medical therapy for BPH [169]. By 2000, there were 4.5 million visits to urologists for symptoms related to BPH, and more than 2.1 million prescriptions were written for α-blockers [170].

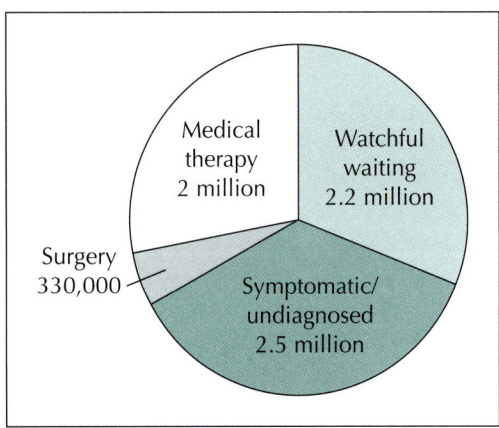

▶ **FIGURE 3-47.** Prevalence of medical therapy and treatment trends for benign prostatic hyperplasia (BPH). BPH will remain the predominant disease that urologists treat. As the average life span continues to increase, the number of potential patients with symptomatic BPH will continue to rise. The statistics show that approximately 6 million men suffer from clinical BPH. Because of its noninvasiveness, medical therapy will continue to be the most commonly used initial intervention for the treatment of BPH.

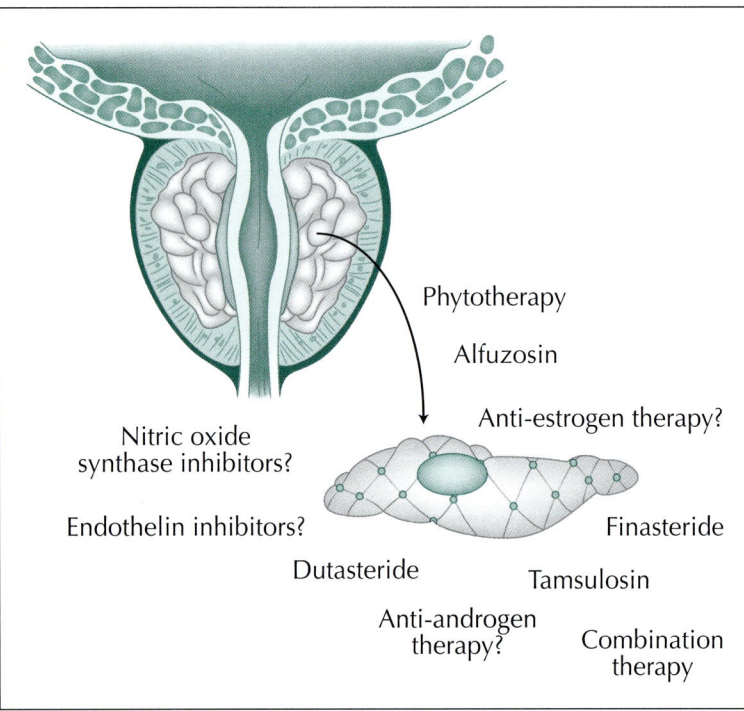

▶ **FIGURE 3-48.** Future drug targets for the treatment of benign prostatic hyperplasia (BPH). The current therapies described in this chapter are effective therapies for the treatment of BPH. However, many of the drugs used today are associated with adverse effects, are not selective for prostate adrenoreceptors, have multiple-times-a-day dosing, and are a financial burden. The ideal agents would provide relief for bothersome lower urinary tract symptoms, prevent the progression of BPH, allow for once-daily dosing to increase compliance, have a rapid onset of action, be selective, have minimal side effects, and be affordable. In addition, new pharmaceuticals will be developed as our understanding of the molecular mechanisms that govern BPH increases. One potential drug target includes nitric oxide synthetase inhibitors. Studies have demonstrated a reduction in the nitrergic innervation in BPH [171]. Nitric oxide is involved in smooth muscle relaxation, and replacement of nitric oxide may help alleviate some of the symptoms of BPH. In addition, endothelin receptors may be a future target as they have been shown to regulate tension in prostatic smooth muscle [172–174]. However, no matter which types of drugs are used, medical therapy will continue to play an increasing role in the treatment and prevention of benign prostatic hyperplasia.

1. Lee C, Kozlowski JM, Grayhack JT: Etiology of benign prostatic hyperplasia. *Urol Clin North Am* 1995, 22:237–246.

2. Lee C, Kozlowski JM, Grayhack JT: Intrinsic and extrinsic factors controlling benign prostatic growth. *Prostate* 1997, 31:131–138.

3. Partin AW, Oesterling JE, Epstein JI, *et al.*: Influence of age and endocrine factors on the volume of benign prostatic hyperplasia. *J Urol* 1991, 145:405–409.

4. McVary KT, McKenna KE, Lee C: Prostate innervation. *Prostate Suppl* 1998, 8:2–13.

5. Garraway WM, Collins GN, Lee RJ: High prevalence of benign prostatic hypertrophy in the community. *Lancet* 1991, 338:469–471.

6. Bosch JL, Hop WC, Kirkels WJ, Schroder FH: The International Prostate Symptom Score in a community-based sample of men between 55 and 74 years of age: prevalence and correlation of symptoms with age, prostate volume, flow rate and residual urine volume. *Br J Urol* 1995, 75:622–630.

7. Bosch JL, Hop WC, Kirkels WJ, Schroder FH: Natural history of benign prostatic hyperplasia: appropriate case definition and estimation of its prevalence in the community. *Urology* 1995, 46(3 Suppl A):34–40.

8. Oesterling JE: Benign prostatic hyperplasia. Medical and minimally invasive treatment options. *N Engl J Med* 1995, 332:99–109.

9. Bruskewitz R: Management of symptomatic BPH in the US: who is treated and how? *Eur Urol* 1999, 36(Suppl 3):7–13.

10. Gosling JA, Dixon JS: Structure of trabeculated detrusor smooth muscle in cases of prostatic hypertrophy. *Urol Int* 1980, 35:351–355.

11. Di Silverio F, Gentile V, Pastore AL, *et al.*: Benign prostatic hyperplasia: what about a campaign for prevention? *Urol Int* 2004, 72:179–188.

12. O'Leary MP: Lower urinary tract symptoms/benign prostatic hyperplasia: maintaining symptom control and reducing complications. *Urology* 2003, 62(3 Suppl 1):15–23.

13. McConnell JD, Barry MJ, Bruskewitz RC: Benign prostatic hyperplasia: diagnosis and treatment. Agency for Health Care Policy and Research. *Clin Pract Guidel Quick Ref Guide Clin* 1994, Feb.:1–17.

14. Baine WB, Yu W, Summe JP, Weis KA: Epidemiologic trends in the evaluation and treatment of lower urinary tract symptoms in elderly male Medicare patients from 1991 to 1995. *J Urol* 1998, 160(3 Pt 1):816–820.

15. Gushchin GL, Jones CA, Nyberg LM: Decline in the surgical treatment of benign prostatic hyperplasia among black and white men in the United States: 1980 to 1994 [abstract]. *J Urol* 1997, 157:311.

16. Wasson JH, Bubolz TA, Lu-Yao GL, *et al.*: Transurethral resection of the prostate among medicare beneficiaries: 1984 to 1997. For the Patient Outcomes Research Team for Prostatic Diseases. *J Urol* 2000, 164:1212–1215.

17. McNeal JE, Redwine EA, Freiha FS, Stamey TA: Zonal distribution of prostatic adenocarcinoma. Correlation with histologic pattern and direction of spread. *Am J Surg Pathol* 1988, 12:897–906.

18. Berry SJ, Coffey DS, Walsh PC, Ewing LL: The development of human benign prostatic hyperplasia with age. *J Urol* 1984, 132:474–479.

19. Malloy BJ, Price DT, Price RR, *et al.*: Alpha1-adrenergic receptor subtypes in human detrusor. *J Urol* 1998, 160(3 Pt 1):937–943.

20. Eri LM, Svindland A: Can prostate epithelial content predict response to hormonal treatment of patients with benign prostatic hyperplasia? *Urology* 2000, 56:261–265.

21. Girman CJ, Jacobsen SJ, Tsukamoto T, *et al.*: Health-related quality of life associated with lower urinary tract symptoms in four countries. *Urology* 1998, 51:428–436.

22. Roberts RO, Rhodes T, Panser LA, *et al.*: Natural history of prostatism: worry and embarrassment from urinary symptoms and health care-seeking behavior. *Urology* 1994, 43:621–628.

23. Stoevelaar HJ, van de Beek C, Nijs HG, *et al.*: The symptom questionnaire for benign prostatic hyperplasia: an ambiguous indicator for an ambiguous disease. *Br J Urol* 1996, 77:181–185.

24. Guess HA: Benign prostatic hyperplasia: antecedents and natural history. *Epidemiol Rev* 1992, 14:131–153.

25. Wennberg JE, Mulley AG Jr, Hanley D, *et al.*: An assessment of prostatectomy for benign urinary tract obstruction. Geographic variations and the evaluation of medical care outcomes. *JAMA* 1988, 259:3027–3030.

26. McPherson K, Wennberg JE, Hovind OB, Clifford P: Small-area variations in the use of common surgical procedures: an international comparison of New England, England, and Norway. *N Engl J Med* 1982, 307:1310–1314.

27. Guess HA, Jacobsen SJ, Girman CJ, *et al.*: The role of community-based longitudinal studies in evaluating treatment effects. Example: benign prostatic hyperplasia. *Med Care* 1995, 33(4 Suppl):AS26–AS35.

28. Jacobsen SJ, Girman CJ, Guess HA, *et al.*: Natural history of prostatism: longitudinal changes in voiding symptoms in community dwelling men. *J Urol* 1996, 155:595–600.

29. Barry MJ, Fowler FJ Jr, Bin L, *et al.*: The natural history of patients with benign prostatic hyperplasia as diagnosed by North American urologists. *J Urol* 1997, 157:10–14; discussion 14–15.

30. Anderson JB, Roehrborn CG, Schalken JA, Emberton M: The progression of benign prostatic hyperplasia: examining the evidence and determining the risk. *Eur Urol* 2001, 39:390–399.

31. Partin AW: Etiology of benign prostatic hyperplasia. In *Prostatic Diseases*. Edited by Lepor H. Philadelphia: WB Saunders Co; 2000: 95–105.

32. Isaacs JT, Coffey DS: Changes in dihydrotestosterone metabolism associated with the development of canine benign prostatic hyperplasia. *Endocrinology* 1981, 108:445–453.

33. McConnell JD, Akakura K, Bartsch G, *et al.*: Hormonal treatment of benign prostatic hyperplasia. In *The 2nd International Consultation on Benign Prostatic Hyperplasia (BPH), Proceedings 2*. Edited by Cockett ATK, Khoury S, Aso Y, *et al.* Paris: Scientific Communication International; 1993:417.

34. Brooks JR, Berman D, Glitzer MS, *et al.*: Effect of a new 5 alpha-reductase inhibitor on size, histologic characteristics, and androgen concentrations of the canine prostate. *Prostate* 1982, 3:35–44.

35. Geller J: Effect of finasteride, a 5 alpha-reductase inhibitor on prostate tissue androgens and prostate-specific antigen. *J Clin Endocrinol Metab* 1990, 71:1552–1555.

36. McConnell JD, Wilson JD, George FW, *et al.*: Finasteride, an inhibitor of 5 alpha-reductase, suppresses prostatic dihydrotestosterone in men with benign prostatic hyperplasia. *J Clin Endocrinol Metab* 1992, 74:505–508.

37. Vermeulen A, Giagulli VA, De Schepper P, Buntinx A: Hormonal effects of a 5 alpha-reductase inhibitor (finasteride) on hormonal levels in normal men and in patients with benign prostatic hyperplasia. *Eur Urol* 1991, 20(Suppl 1):82–86.

38. Coffey DS: The molecular biology, endocrinology and physiology of the prostate and seminal vesicles. In *Campbell's Urology*. Edited by Walsh PC, Gittes RF, Perlmutter AD, *et al.* Philadelphia: WB Saunders Co; 1992:221–266.

39. Schroeder FH, Westerhof M, Bosch RJ, Kurth KH: Benign prostatic hyperplasia treated by castration or the LH-RH analogue buserelin: a report on 6 cases. *Eur Urol* 1986, 12:318–321.

40. Cabot AT: The question of castration for enlarged prostate. *Ann Surg* 1896, 24:265–309.

41. White JW: The results of double castration in hypertrophy of the prostate. *Ann Surg* 1895, 22:1–80.

42. Walsh PC, Madden JD, Harrod MJ, *et al.*: Familial incomplete male pseudohermaphroditism, type 2. Decreased dihydrotestosterone formation in pseudovaginal perineoscrotal hypospadias. *N Engl J Med* 1974, 291:944–949.

43. Imperato-McGinley J, Guevro L, Gauteri T, Petersen RE: Steroid 5a-reductase deficiency in a man: an inherited form of pseudohermaphroditism. *Science.* 1974, 186:1213–1215.

44. Imperato-McGinley J, Gauteri T, Zirinsky K, *et al.*: Prostate visualization studies in males, homozygous and heterozygous with 5a-reductase deficiency. *J Clin Endocrinol Metab.* 1992, 75:1022–1026.

45. Coffey DS: The endocrine control of normal and abnormal growth of the prostate. In *Urologic Endocrinology*. Edited by Rajfer J. Philadelphia: WB Saunders Co; 1986:170–193.

46. Gormley GJ, Stoner E, Bruskewitz RC, *et al.*: The effect of finasteride in men with benign prostatic hyperplasia. The Finasteride Study Group. *N Engl J Med* 1992, 327:1185–1191.

47. McConnell JD, Bruskewitz R, Walsh P, *et al.*: The effect of finasteride on the risk of acute urinary retention and the need for surgical treatment among men with benign prostatic hyperplasia. Finasteride Long-Term Efficacy and Safety Study Group. *N Engl J Med* 1998, 338:557–563.

48. Boyle P, Gould AL, Roehrborn CG: Prostate volume predicts outcome of treatment of benign prostatic hyperplasia with finasteride: meta-analysis of randomized clinical trials. *Urology* 1996, 48:398–405.

49. Arrighi HM, Metter EJ, Guess HA, Fozzard JL: Natural history of benign prostatic hyperplasia and risk of prostatectomy. The Baltimore Longitudinal Study of Aging. *Urology* 1991, 38(1 Suppl):4–8.

50. Boyle P, Severi G, Giles GG: The epidemiology of prostate cancer. *Urol Clin North Am* 2003, 30:209–217.

51. Oesterling JE, Jacobsen SJ, Chute CG, *et al.*: Serum prostate-specific antigen in a community-based population of healthy men. Establishment of age-specific reference ranges. *JAMA* 1993, 270:860–864.

52. Lieber MM, Jacobsen SJ, Roberts RO, *et al.*: Prostate volume and prostate-specific antigen in the absence of prostate cancer: a review of the relationship and prediction of long-term outcomes. *Prostate* 2001, 49:208–212.

53. Guess HA, Heyse JF, Gormley GJ, *et al.*: Effect of finasteride on serum PSA concentration in men with benign prostatic hyperplasia. Results from the North American phase III clinical trial. *Urol Clin North Am* 1993, 20:627–636.

54. Guess HA, Heyse JF, Gormley GJ: The effect of finasteride on prostate-specific antigen in men with benign prostatic hyperplasia. *Prostate* 1993, 22:31–37.

55. Lange PH: Is the prostate pill finally here? *N Engl J Med* 1992, 327:1234–1236.

56. Stoner E: Three-year safety and efficacy data on the use of finasteride in the treatment of benign prostatic hyperplasia. *Urology* 1994, 43:284–292; discussion 292–294.

57. Oesterling JE, Roy J, Agha A, *et al.*: Biologic variability of prostate-specific antigen and its usefulness as a marker for prostate cancer: effects of finasteride. The Finasteride PSA Study Group. *Urology* 1997, 50:13–18.

58. Thompson IM, Goodman PJ, Tangen CM, *et al.*: The influence of finasteride on the development of prostate cancer. *N Engl J Med* 2003, 349:215–224.

59. Shirakawa T, Okada H, Acharya B, *et al.*: Messenger RNA levels and enzyme activities of 5 alpha-reductase types 1 and 2 in human benign prostatic hyperplasia (BPH) tissue. *Prostate* 2004, 58:33–40.

60. Gisleskog PO, Hermann D, Hammarlund-Udenaes M, Karlsson MO: A model for the turnover of dihydrotestosterone in the presence of the irreversible 5 alpha-reductase inhibitors GI198745 and finasteride. *Clin Pharmacol Ther* 1998, 64:636–647.

61. Thigpen AE, Davis DL, Milatovich A, *et al.*: Molecular genetics of steroid 5 alpha-reductase 2 deficiency. *J Clin Invest* 1992, 90:799–809.

62. Evans HC, Goa KL. Dutasteride. *Drugs Aging* 2003, 20:905–916; discussion 917–918.

63. Roehrborn CG, Boyle P, Nickel JC, *et al.*: Efficacy and safety of a dual inhibitor of 5-alpha-reductase types 1 and 2 (dutasteride) in men with benign prostatic hyperplasia. *Urology* 2002, 60:434–441.

64. Roehrborn CG, Marks LS, Fenter T, *et al.*: Efficacy and safety of dutasteride in the four-year treatment of men with benign prostatic hyperplasia. *Urology* 2004, 63:709–715.

65. Boyle PP, Siami P, Wachs BH, *et al.*: Effect of dutasteride on the risk of acute urinary retention and the need for surgical treatment. *J Urol* 2002, 167:373.

66. Gabrilove JL, Levine AC, Kirschenbaum A, Droller M: Effect of long-acting gonadotropin-releasing hormone analog (leuprolide) therapy on prostatic size and symptoms in 15 men with benign prostatic hypertrophy. *J Clin Endocrinol Metab* 1989, 69:629–632.

67. Eri LM, Tveter KJ: A prospective, placebo-controlled study of the luteinizing hormone-releasing hormone agonist leuprolide as treatment for patients with benign prostatic hyperplasia. *J Urol* 1993, 150(2 Pt 1):359–364.

68. Stone NN, Ray PS, Smith JA, *et al.*: A double-blind randomized controlled study of the effect of flutamide on benign prostatic hypertropy: clinical efficacy [abstract]. *J Urol* 1989, 141:240A.

69. Eri LM, Tveter KJ: A prospective, placebo-controlled study of the antiandrogen Casodex as treatment for patients with benign prostatic hyperplasia. *J Urol* 1993, 150:90–94.

70. Coffey DS, Walsh PC: Clinical and experimental studies of benign prostatic hyperplasia. *Urol Clin North Am* 1990, 17:461–475.

71. Moore RJ, Gazak JM, Wilson JD: Regulation of cytoplasmic dihydrotestosterone binding in dog prostate by 17 beta-estradiol. *J Clin Invest* 1979, 63:351–357.

72. Berry SJ, Strandberg JD, Saunders WJ, Coffey DS: Development of canine benign prostatic hyperplasia with age. *Prostate* 1986, 9:363–373.

73. Barrack ER, Berry SJ: DNA synthesis in the canine prostate: effects of androgen and estrogen treatment. *Prostate* 1987, 10:45–56.

74. Tunn UW, Goldschmidt AJ: Aromatase inhibitors in the medical treatment of benign prostatic hypertrophy [in French]. *J Urol (Paris)* 1993, 99:307.

75. Habenicht UF, Tunn UW, Senge T, *et al.*: Management of benign prostatic hyperplasia with particular emphasis on aromatase inhibitors. *J Steroid Biochem Mol Biol* 1993, 44:557–563.

76. Gingell JC, Knonagel H, Kurth KH, Tunn UW: Placebo controlled double-blind study to test the efficacy of the aromatase inhibitor atamestane in patients with benign prostatic hyperplasia not requiring operation. The Schering 90.062 Study Group. *J Urol* 1995,154(2 Pt 1):399–401.

77. el Etreby MF: Atamestane: an aromatase inhibitor for the treatment of benign prostatic hyperplasia. A short review. *J Steroid Biochem Mol Biol* 1993, 44:565–572.

78. *1998 Physician's Desk Reference,* edn 52. Montvale, NJ: Medical Economics Company; 1998.

79. Roehrborn CG, Schwinn DA: Alpha1-adrenergic receptors and their inhibitors in lower urinary tract symptoms and benign prostatic hyperplasia. *J Urol* 2004, 171:1029–1035.

80. Lepor H, Laddu A: Terazosin in the treatment of benign prostatic hyperplasia: the United States experience. *Br J Urol* 1992, 70(Suppl 1):2–9.

81. Furuya S, Kumamoto Y, Yokoyama E, *et al.*: Alpha-adrenergic activity and urethral pressure in prostatic zone in benign prostatic hypertrophy. *J Urol* 1982, 128:836–839.

82. Yokoyama E, Furuya S, Kumamoto Y: Quantitation of alpha-1 and beta adrenergic receptor densities in the human normal and hypertrophied prostate [in Japanese]. *Nippon Hinyokika Gakkai Zasshi* 1985, 76:325–337.

83. Kobayashi S, Tang R, Shapiro E, Lepor H: Characterization and localization of prostatic alpha 1 adrenoceptors using radioligand receptor binding on slide-mounted tissue section. *J Urol* 1993, 150:2002–2006.

84. Caine M, Perlberg S, Shapiro A: Phenoxybenzamine for benign prostatic obstruction. Review of 200 cases. *Urology* 1981, 17:542–546.

85. Caine M, Perlberg S, Meretyk S: The use of alpha-adrenergic blockers in benign prostatic obstruction. *Br J Urol* 1978, 48:551–554.

86. Abrams P, Hollister P, Lawrence J, *et al.*: Bladder outflow obstruction treated with phenoxybenzamine. Preliminary note. *Br J Urol* 1982, 54:530.

87. Abrams PH, Shah PJ, Stone R, Choa RG: Bladder outflow obstruction treated with phenoxybenzamine. *Prog Clin Biol Res* 1981, 78:269–275.

88. Piascik MT, Perez DM: Alpha1-adrenergic receptors: new insights and directions. *J Pharmacol Exp Ther* 2001, 298:403–410.

89. Tseng-Crank J, Kost T, Goetz A, *et al.*: The alpha 1C-adrenoceptor in human prostate: cloning, functional expression, and localization to specific prostatic cell types. *Br J Pharmacol* 1995, 115:1475–1485.

90. DiSanto ME, Wein AJ, Chacko S: Lower urinary tract physiology and pharmacology. *Curr Urol Rep* 2000, 1:227–234.

91. Lepor H: Alpha 1-adrenoceptor selectivity: clinical or theoretical benefit? *Br J Urol* 1995, 76(Suppl 1):57–61.

92. Price DT, Schwinn DA, Lomasney JW, *et al.*: Identification, quantification, and localization of mRNA for three distinct alpha 1 adrenergic receptor subtypes in human prostate. *J Urol* 1993, 150(2 Pt 1):546–551.

93. Beduschi MC, Beduschi R, Oesterling JE: Alpha-blockade therapy for benign prostatic hyperplasia: from a nonselective to a more selective alpha1A-adrenergic antagonist. *Urology* 1998, 51:861–872.

94. Broten T, Scott A, Siegl PKS, *et al.*: Alpha-1 adrenoreceptor blockade inhibits detrusor instability in rats with bladder outlet obstruction [abstract]. *FASEB J* 1998, 12:445A.

95. Smith MS, Schambra UB, Wilson KH, *et al.*: Alpha1-adrenergic receptors in human spinal cord: specific localized expression of mRNA encoding alpha1-adrenergic receptor subtypes at four distinct levels. *Brain Res Mol Brain Res* 1999, 63:254–261.

96. Schwinn DA: The role of alpha1-adrenergic receptor subtypes in lower urinary tract symptoms. *BJU Int* 2001, 88(Suppl 2):27–34; discussion 49–50.

97. Lyseng-Williamson KA, Jarvis B, Wagstaff AJ: Tamsulosin: an update of its role in the management of lower urinary tract symptoms. *Drugs* 2002, 62:135–167.

98. Michel MC, Flannery MT, Narayan P: Worldwide experience with alfuzosin and tamsulosin. *Urology* 2001, 58:508–516.

99. Chapple CR: Alpha-adrenergic blocking drugs in bladder outflow obstruction: what potential has alpha 1-adrenoceptor selectivity? *Br J Urol* 1995, 76(Suppl 1):47–55.

100. Lee M: Alfuzosin hydrochloride for the treatment of benign prostatic hyperplasia. *Am J Health Syst Pharm* 2003, 60:1426–1439.

101. Fabricius PG, Weizert P, Dunzendorfer U, *et al.*: Efficacy of once-a-day terazosin in benign prostatic hyperplasia: a randomized, double-blind placebo-controlled clinical trial. *Prostate Suppl* 1990, 3:85–93.

102. Lepor H, Auerbach S, Puras-Baez A, *et al.*: A randomized, placebo-controlled multicenter study of the efficacy and safety of terazosin in the treatment of benign prostatic hyperplasia. *J Urol* 1992, 148:1467–1474.

103. Lepor H, Meretyk S, Knapp-Maloney G: The safety, efficacy and compliance of terazosin therapy for benign prostatic hyperplasia. *J Urol* 1992, 147:1554–1557.

104. Di Silverio F: Use of terazosin in the medical treatment of benign prostatic hyperplasia: experience in Italy. *Br J Urol* 1992, 70(Suppl 1):22–26.

105. Brawer MK, Adams G, Epstein H: Terazosin in the treatment of benign prostatic hyperplasia. Terazosin Benign Prostatic Hyperplasia Study Group. *Arch Fam Med* 1993, 2:929–935.

106. Debruyne FM, Witjes WP, Fitzpatrick J, *et al.*: The international terazosin trial: a multicentre study of the long-term efficacy and safety of terazosin in the treatment of benign prostatic hyperplasia. The ITT Group. *Eur Urol* 1996, 30:369–376.

107. Elhilali MM, Ramsey EW, Barkin J, *et al.*: A multicenter, randomized, double-blind, placebo-controlled study to evaluate the safety and efficacy of terazosin in the treatment of benign prostatic hyperplasia. *Urology* 1996, 47:335–342.

108. Lepor H, Williford WO, Barry MJ, *et al.*: The efficacy of terazosin, finasteride, or both in benign prostatic hyperplasia. Veterans Affairs Cooperative Studies Benign Prostatic Hyperplasia Study Group. *N Engl J Med* 1996, 335:533–539.

109. Roehrborn CG, Oesterling JE, Auerbach S, *et al.*: The Hytrin Community Assessment Trial study: a one-year study of terazosin versus placebo in the treatment of men with symptomatic benign prostatic hyperplasia. HYCAT Investigator Group. *Urology* 1996, 47:159–168.

110. Holme I, Fauchald P, Rugstad HE, Stokke HP: Preliminary results of the Norwegian doxazosin postmarketing surveillance study: a twelve-week experience. *Am Heart J* 1991, 121(1 Pt 2):260–267.

111. Gillenwater JY, Mobley DL: A sixteen week, double-blind, placebo-controlled, dose-titration study using doxazosin tablets for the treatment of benign prostatic hyperplasia (BPH) in normotensive males: a multicenter study group [abstract]. *J Urol* 1993, 153(suppl):273A.

112. Janknegt RA, Chapple CR: Efficacy and safety of the alpha-1 blocker doxazosin in the treatment of benign prostatic hyperplasia. Analysis of 5 studies. Doxazosin Study Groups. *Eur Urol* 1993, 24:319–326.

113. Chapple CR, Carter P, Christmas TJ, *et al.*: A three month double-blind study of doxazosin as treatment for benign prostatic bladder outlet obstruction. *Br J Urol* 1994, 74:50–56.

114. Fawzy A, Braun K, Lewis GP, *et al.*: Doxazosin in the treatment of benign prostatic hyperplasia in normotensive patients: a multicenter study. *J Urol* 1995, 154:105–109.

115. Gillenwater JY, Conn RL, Chrysant SG, *et al.*: Doxazosin for the treatment of benign prostatic hyperplasia in patients with mild to moderate essential hypertension: a double-blind, placebo-controlled, dose-response multicenter study. *J Urol* 1995, 154:110–115.

116. Kirby RS: Doxazosin in benign prostatic hyperplasia: effects on blood pressure and urinary flow in normotensive and hypertensive men. *Urology* 1995, 46:182–186.

117. Roehrborn CG, Siegel RL: Safety and efficacy of doxazosin in benign prostatic hyperplasia: a pooled analysis of three double-blind, placebo-controlled studies. *Urology* 1996, 48:406–415.

118. Abrams P, Schulman CC, Vaage S: Tamsulosin, a selective alpha 1c-adrenoceptor antagonist: a randomized, controlled trial in patients with benign prostatic 'obstruction' (symptomatic BPH). The European Tamsulosin Study Group. *Br J Urol* 1995, 76:325–336.

119. Schulman CC, Cortvriend J, Jonas U, *et al.*: Tamsulosin, the first prostate-selective alpha 1A-adrenoceptor antagonist. Analysis of a multinational, multicentre, open-label study assessing the long-term efficacy and safety in patients with benign prostatic obstruction (symptomatic BPH). European Tamsulosin Study Group. *Eur Urol* 1996, 29:145–154.

120. Chapple CR, Wyndaele JJ, Nordling J, *et al.*: Tamsulosin, the first prostate-selective alpha 1A-adrenoceptor antagonist. A meta-analysis of two randomized, placebo-controlled, multicentre studies in patients with benign prostatic obstruction (symptomatic BPH). European Tamsulosin Study Group. *Eur Urol* 1996, 29:155–167.

121. Lepor H: Phase III multicenter placebo-controlled study of tamsulosin in benign prostatic hyperplasia. Tamsulosin Investigator Group. *Urology* 1998, 51:892–900.

122. Lepor H: Long-term evaluation of tamsulosin in benign prostatic hyperplasia: placebo-controlled, double-blind extension of phase III trial. Tamsulosin Investigator Group. *Urology* 1998, 51:901–906.

123. Narayan P, Tewari A: A second phase III multicenter placebo controlled study of 2 dosages of modified release tamsulosin in patients with symptoms of benign prostatic hyperplasia. United States 93-01 Study Group. *J Urol* 1998, 160:1701–1706.

124. Narayan P, Bruskewitz R: A comparison of two phase III multicenter, placebo-controlled studies of tamsulosin in BPH. *Adv Ther* 2000, 17:287–300.

125. Michel MC, Bressel HU, Mehlburger L, Goepel M: Tamsulosin: real life clinical experience in 19,365 patients. *Eur Urol* 1998, 34(Suppl 2):37–45.

126. Jardin A, Bensadoun H, Delauche-Cavallier MC, Attali P: Alfuzosin for treatment of benign prostatic hypertrophy. The BPH-ALF Group. *Lancet* 1991, 337:1457–1461.

127. Buzelin JM, Hebert M, Blondin P: Alpha-blocking treatment with alfuzosin in symptomatic benign prostatic hyperplasia: comparative study with prazosin. The PRAZALF Group. *Br J Urol* 1993, 72:922–927.

128. Hansen BJ, Nordling J, Mensink HJ, *et al.*: Alfuzosin in the treatment of benign prostatic hyperplasia: effects on symptom scores, urinary flow rates and residual volume. A multicentre, double-blind, placebo-controlled trial. ALFECH Study Group. *Scand J Urol Nephrol Suppl* 1994, 157:169–176.

129. Schulman CC, De Sy W, Vandendris M, *et al.*: Belgian multicenter clinical study of alfuzosin, a selective alpha 1-blocker, in the treatment of benign prostatic hyperplasia. The Alfuzosin Belgian Group. *Acta Urol Belg* 1994, 62:15–21.

130. Buzelin JM, Delauche-Cavallier MC, Roth S, *et al.*: Clinical uroselectivity: evidence from patients treated with slow-release alfuzosin for symptomatic benign prostatic obstruction. *Br J Urol* 1997, 79:898–904; discussion 904–906.

131. Buzelin JM, Roth S, Geffriaud-Ricouard C, Delauche-Cavallier MC: Efficacy and safety of sustained-release alfuzosin 5 mg in patients with benign prostatic hyperplasia. ALGEBI Study Group. *Eur Urol* 1997, 31:190–198.

132. van Kerrebroeck P, Jardin A, Laval KU, van Cangh P: Efficacy and safety of a new prolonged release formulation of alfuzosin 10 mg once daily versus alfuzosin 2.5 mg thrice daily and placebo in patients with symptomatic benign prostatic hyperplasia. ALFORTI Study Group. *Eur Urol* 2000, 37:306–313.

133. Roehrborn CG: Efficacy and safety of once-daily alfuzosin in the treatment of lower urinary tract symptoms and clinical benign prostatic hyperplasia: a randomized, placebo-controlled trial. *Urology* 2001, 58:953–959.

134. Roehrborn CG, Van Kerrebroeck P, Nordling J: Safety and efficacy of alfuzosin 10 mg once-daily in the treatment of lower urinary tract symptoms and clinical benign prostatic hyperplasia: a pooled analysis of three double-blind, placebo-controlled studies. *BJU Int* 2003, 92:257–261.

135. Wilt TJ, Howe W, MacDonald R: Terazosin for treating symptomatic benign prostatic obstruction: a systematic review of efficacy and adverse effects. *BJU Int* 2002, 89:214–225.

136. Dunn CJ, Matheson A, Faulds DM: Tamsulosin: a review of its pharmacology and therapeutic efficacy in the management of lower urinary tract symptoms. *Drugs Aging* 2002, 19:135–161.

137. McConnell JD, Roehrborn CG, Bautista OM, *et al.*: The long-term effect of doxazosin, finasteride, and combination therapy on the clinical progression of benign prostatic hyperplasia. *N Engl J Med* 2003, 349:2387–2398.

138. Bautista OM, Kusek JW, Nyberg LM, *et al.*: Study design of the Medical Therapy of Prostatic Symptoms (MTOPS) trial. *Control Clin Trials* 2003, 24:224–243.

139. Kirby RS, Roehrborn C, Boyle P, *et al.*: Efficacy and tolerability of doxazosin and finasteride, alone or in combination, in treatment of symptomatic benign prostatic hyperplasia: the Prospective European Doxazosin and Combination Therapy (PREDICT) trial. *Urology* 2003, 61:119–126.

140. Denis L, McConnell JD, Khoury S, *et al.*: Recommendation of the International Scientific Committee: The evaluation and treatment of lower urinary tract symptoms (LUTS) suggestive of benign prostatic obstruction. In *Proceedings of the Fourth International Consultation on Benign Prostatic Hyperplasia*. Edited by Denis L, Griffiths K, Deans KG, Khoury S, *et al.* Plymouth, UK: Health Publications, Ltd; 1998: 158–183.

141. Fukatsu A, Ono Y, Ito M, *et al.*: Relationship between serum prostate-specific antigen and calculated epithelial volume. *Urology* 2003, 61:370–374.

142. Roehrborn CG, Oesterling JE, Olson PJ, Padley RJ: Serial prostate-specific antigen measurements in men with clinically benign prostatic hyperplasia during a 12-month placebo-controlled study with terazosin. HYCAT Investigator Group. Hytrin Community Assessment Trial. *Urology* 1997, 50:556–561.

143. Girman CJ, Panser LA, Chute CG, *et al.*: Natural history of prostatism: urinary flow rates in a community-based study. *J Urol* 1993, 150:887–892.

144. Roberts RO, Jacobsen SJ, Jacobson DJ, *et al.*: Longitudinal changes in peak urinary flow rates in a community based cohort. *J Urol* 2000, 163:107–113.

145. Jacobsen SJ, Jacobson DJ, Girman CJ, *et al.*: Treatment for benign prostatic hyperplasia among community dwelling men: the Olmsted County study of urinary symptoms and health status. *J Urol* 1999, 162:1301–1306.

146. Krzeski T, Kazon M, Borkowski A, *et al.*: Combined extracts of *Urtica dioica* and *Pygeum africanum* in the treatment of benign prostatic hyperplasia: double-blind comparison of two doses. *Clin Ther* 1993, 15:1011–1020.

147. Lowe FC, Fagelman E: Phytotherapy in the treatment of benign prostatic hyperplasia. *Curr Opin Urol* 2002, 12:15–18.

148. Lowe FC: Phytotherapy in the management of benign prostatic hyperplasia. *Urology* 2001, 58(6 Suppl 1):71–76; discussion 76–77.

149. Boccafoschi C, Annoscia S: Confronto fra estratto di *Serenoa repens* e placebo mediate prova clinica controllata in pazienti con adenomatosi prostatica. *Urologia* 1983, 50:1257–1268.

150. Emili E, Lo Cigno M, Petrone U: Risultati clinici su un nuovo farmaco nella terapia dell'ipertofia della prostata (Permixon). *Urologia* 1983, 50:1042–1048.

151. Champault G, Patel JC, Bonnard AM: A double-blind trial of an extract of the plant *Serenoa repens* in benign prostatic hyperplasia. *Br J Clin Pharmacol* 1984, 18:461–462.

152. Cukier J, Ducassou J, Le Guillou M, *et al.*: Permixon versus placebo: resultats d'une etude multicentrique. *Ther Pharmacol Clin* 1985, 4:15–21.

153. Tasca A, Barulli M, Cavazzana A, *et al.*: Trattamento della sintomatologia ostruttiva da adenoma prostatico con estratto di *Serenoa repens*. *Minerva Urol Nefrol* 1985, 37:87–91.

154. Reece-Smith H, Memon A, Smart CJ, Dewbury K: The value of permixon in benign prostatic hypertrophy. *Br J Urol* 1986, 58:36–40.

155. Carbin BE, Larsson B, Lindahl O: Treatment of benign prostatic hyperplasia with phytosterols. *Br J Urol* 1990, 66:639–641.

156. Descotes JL, Rambeaud JJ, Deschaseaux P, Faure G: Placebo-controlled evaluation of the efficacy and tolerability of Permixon in benign prostatic hyperplasia after the exclusion of placebo responders. *Clin Drug Invest* 1995, 5:291–297.

157. Carraro JC, Raynaud JP, Koch G, *et al*.: Comparison of phytotherapy (Permixon) with finasteride in the treatment of benign prostate hyperplasia: a randomized international study of 1098 patients. *Prostate* 1996, 29:231–240; discussion 241–242.

158. Braeckman J, Denis L, de Lavel J, *et al*.: A double-blind, placebo-controlled study of the plant extract *Serenoa repens* in the treatment of benign hyperplasia of the prostate. *Eur J Clin Res* 1997, 9:247–259.

159. Willetts KE, Clements MS, Champion S, *et al*.: *Serenoa repens* extract for benign prostate hyperplasia: a randomized controlled trial. *BJU Int* 2003, 92:267–270.

160. Lowe FC, Ku JC: Phytotherapy in treatment of benign prostatic hyperplasia: a critical review. *Urology* 1996, 48:12–20.

161. Boyle P, Robertson C, Lowe F, Roehrborn C: Updated meta-analysis of clinical trials of *Serenoa repens* extract in the treatment of symptomatic benign prostatic hyperplasia. *BJU Int* 2004, 93:751–756.

162. Grasso M, Montesano A, Buonaguidi A, *et al*.: Comparative effects of alfuzosin versus *Serenoa repens* in the treatment of symptomatic benign prostatic hyperplasia. *Arch Esp Urol* 1995, 48:97–103.

163. Debruyne F, Koch G, Boyle P, *et al*.: Comparison of a phytotherapeutic agent (Permixon) with an alpha-blocker (tamsulosin) in the treatment of benign prostatic hyperplasia: a 1-year randomized international study. *Eur Urol* 2002, 41:497–506; discussion 506–507.

164. Wilt T, Ishani A, Mac Donald R, *et al*.: *Pygeum africanum* for benign prostatic hyperplasia. *Cochrane Database Syst Rev.* 2002:CD001044.

165. Barlet A, Albrecht J, Aubert A, *et al*.: Efficacy of *Pygeum africanum* extract in the medical therapy of urination disorders due to benign prostatic hyperplasia: evaluation of objective and subjective parameters. A placebo-controlled double-blind multicenter study [in German]. *Wien Klin Wochenschr* 1990, 102:667–673.

166. Ishani A, MacDonald R, Nelson D, *et al*.: *Pygeum africanum* for the treatment of patients with benign prostatic hyperplasia: a systematic review and quantitative meta-analysis. *Am J Med* 2000, 109:654–664.

167. Wilt TJ, Ishani A, Rutks I, MacDonald R: Phytotherapy for benign prostatic hyperplasia. *Public Health Nutr* 2000, 3(4A):459–472.

168. MacDonald R, Ishani A, Rutks I, Wilt TJ: A systematic review of Cernilton for the treatment of benign prostatic hyperplasia. *BJU Int* 2000, 85:836–841.

169. Borth CS, Beiko DT, Nickel JC: Impact of medical therapy on transurethral resection of the prostate: a decade of change. *Urology* 2001, 57:1082–1085.

170. Pharmaceutical pricing update: prescription audit. *Med Ad News* 2000, 19:40.

171. Takeda M, Tang R, Shapiro E, *et al*.: Effects of nitric oxide on human and canine prostates. *Urology* 1995, 45:440–446.

172. Kobayashi S, Tang R, Wang B, *et al*.: Localization of endothelin receptors in the human prostate. *J Urol* 1994, 151:763–766.

173. Kobayashi S, Tang R, Wang B, *et al*.: Binding and functional properties of endothelin receptor subtypes in the human prostate. *Mol Pharmacol* 1994, 45:306–311.

174. Langenstroer P, Tang R, Shapiro E, *et al*.: Endothelin-1 in the human prostate: tissue levels, source of production and isometric tension studies. *J Urol* 1993, 150:495–499.

175. Jacobsen SJ, Girman CJ, Lieber MM: Natural history of benign prostatic hyperplasia. *Urology* 2001, 58:5–16.

Minimally Invasive Therapies for Benign Prostatic Hyperplasia: Transurethral Microwave Thermotherapy and Needle Ablation

4

Bob Djavan,
Matthias Waldert,
Michael Marberger,
& Reginald C. Bruskewitz

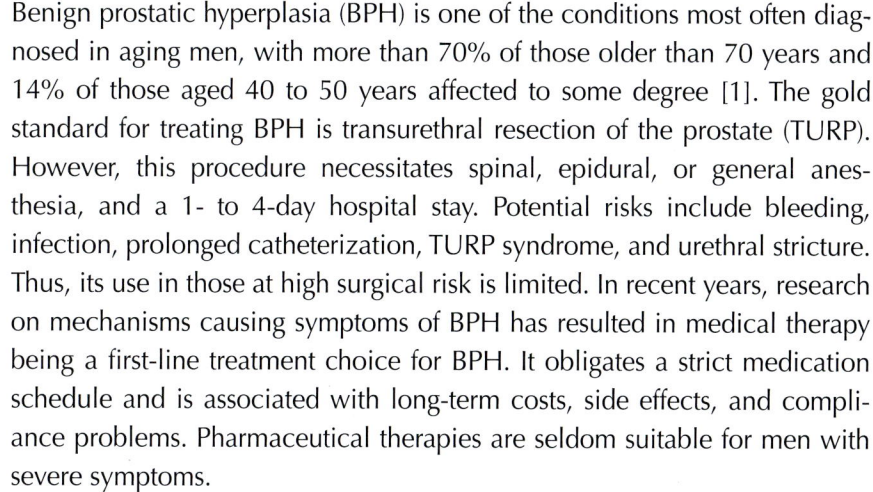

Benign prostatic hyperplasia (BPH) is one of the conditions most often diagnosed in aging men, with more than 70% of those older than 70 years and 14% of those aged 40 to 50 years affected to some degree [1]. The gold standard for treating BPH is transurethral resection of the prostate (TURP). However, this procedure necessitates spinal, epidural, or general anesthesia, and a 1- to 4-day hospital stay. Potential risks include bleeding, infection, prolonged catheterization, TURP syndrome, and urethral stricture. Thus, its use in those at high surgical risk is limited. In recent years, research on mechanisms causing symptoms of BPH has resulted in medical therapy being a first-line treatment choice for BPH. It obligates a strict medication schedule and is associated with long-term costs, side effects, and compliance problems. Pharmaceutical therapies are seldom suitable for men with severe symptoms.

The aim of minimally invasive therapies is to provide alternatives to pharmacotherapy and TURP. To date, thermoablation has been the underlying principle of all the minimally invasive devices that have been introduced. Heat can be applied in different ways. In the presurgical era, recommendations included hot sitz baths and rectal as well as urethral rinses with warm or even hot water. Microwaves and radio waves applied rectally or transurethrally were not used to deliver heat to the prostate until the late 1980s. Transurethral delivery later evolved into thermotherapy, *ie*, transurethral microwave thermotherapy (TUMT), by which microwaves are applied by the transurethral route.

Currently, minimally invasive therapies for BPH that can rival surgical resection and medical therapy include TUMT and transurethral needle ablation. Unlike surgical debulking procedures, the minimally invasive therapies require a postoperative period for resolution of effects before alleviation of symptoms. The ability to provide therapy without general or regional anesthesia, and even ambulatory procedures performed in the office, are realistic expectations for these two therapies. High-energy targeted microwave thermotherapy is now the most valuable minimally invasive device that meets subjective and objective outcome goals as well as minimal invasiveness in terms of anesthesia requirements. These treatment options are not necessarily alternatives to TURP, but they offer adequate alternatives to medical therapy and drugs.

Effect of Heat on Normal Prostate Tissue

Temperature	Tissue Effect	Therapy
37°	None	Fever
42° to 44°	No histologic changes	Hyperthermia
45° to 50°	Minimal changes	Thermotherapy
60°	Protein denaturization	Thermocoagulation
100° +	Coagulation and vaporization	Thermoablation

▶ **FIGURE 4-1.** Effects of heat on normal prostate tissue. Any treatment aiming at tissue ablation in the prostate should strive to achieve temperatures higher than 45°C. Treatments that achieve temperatures lower than 45°C have proven ineffective and incapable of creating permanent tissue change [2].

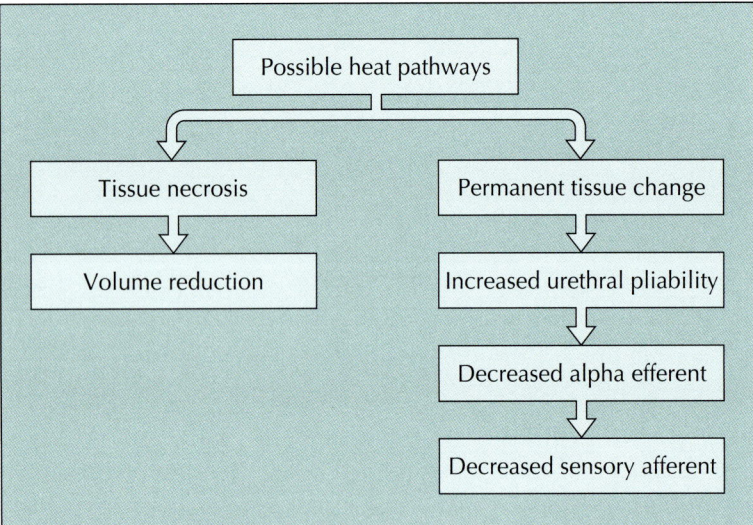

▶ **FIGURE 4-2.** The possible effects and pathways of prostate tissue heating. Coagulation necrosis is believed to act by permanent tissue volume reduction and permanent changes in tissue composition and function, resulting in increased urethral pliability, a reduction in efferent neuromuscular elements, and a reduction in sensory neural elements in the affected and then regenerated areas [3].

TRANSURETHRAL MICROWAVE THERMOTHERAPY

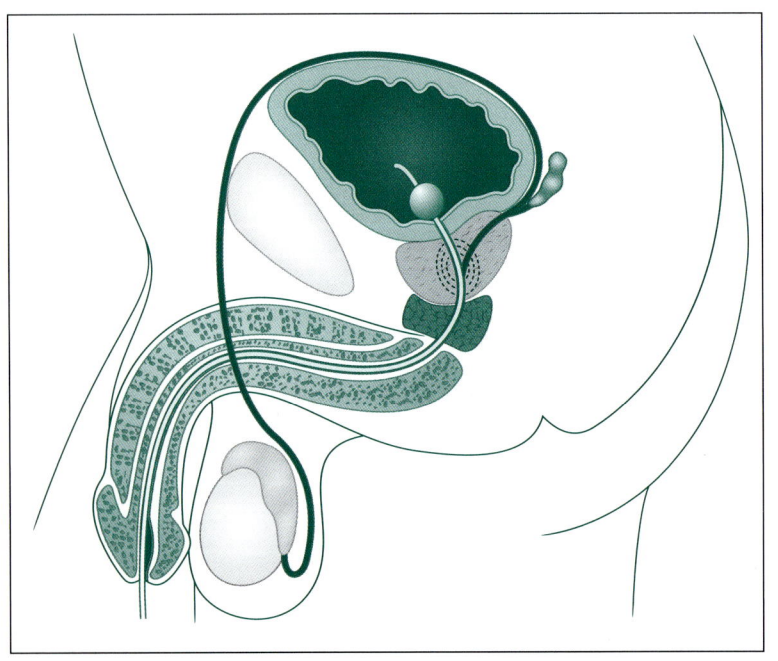

▶ **FIGURE 4-3.** Devices used for transurethral microwave thermotherapy (TUMT). The devices used for TUMT have a microwave heat applicator embedded in a transurethral catheter. Microwave energy transmitted through an intraurethral antenna results in heat-induced coagulative necrosis of prostate tissue (*ie*, heating the prostate in excess of 45°C), sparing the urethra and anatomic structures outside the target. TUMT is a combination of radiative heating through the microwave antenna and conductive cooling through channels in the catheter. The conductive cooling of the immediate urethral lining and the first few millimeters of periurethral tissue prevents both necrosis and pain sensation in the patient. Today, TUMT results in intraprostatic temperatures ranging from 45° to 80°C with no statistically significant heating of the surrounding tissues of the urethra, rectum, and external sphincter.

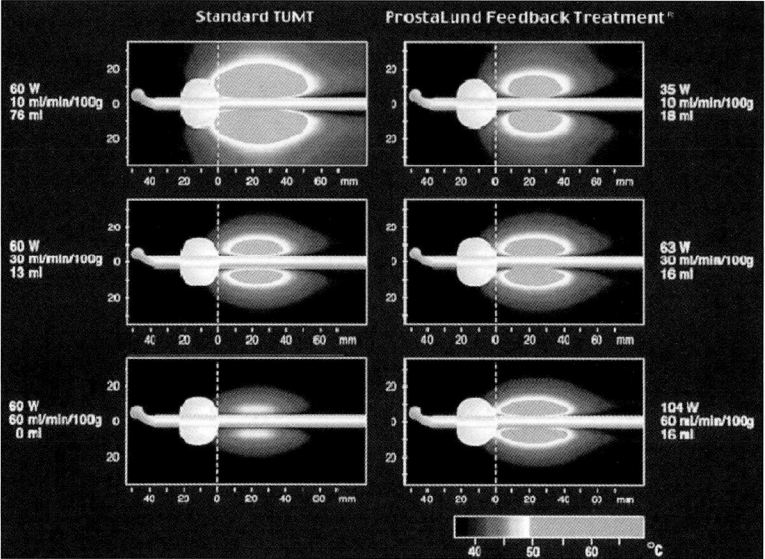

▶ **FIGURE 4-4.** (*See Color Plate*) Distribution of temperatures in transurethral microwave thermotherapy (TUMT). Using different frequencies ranging from 95 to 1296 MHz, temperatures in excess of 45°C can be achieved. The actual distribution of temperatures inside the prostatic gland depending on its size and the TUMT system used is shown. The distribution of temperatures differs considerably depending on anatomy and histologic composition.

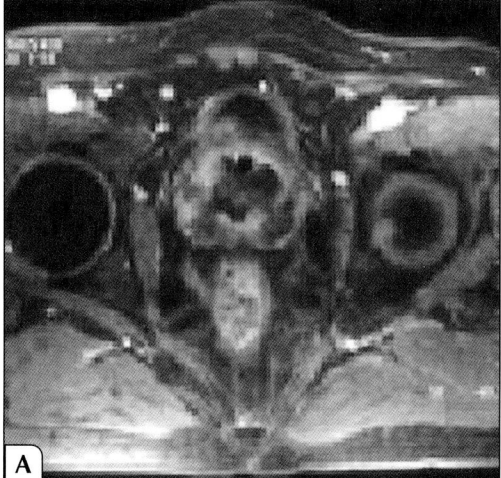

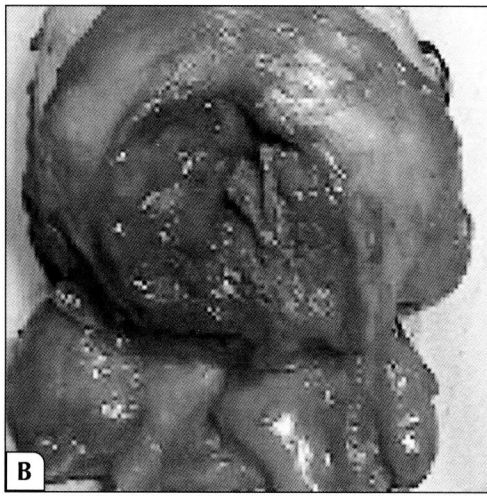

▶ **FIGURE 4-5.** Prostatic shrinkage at the prostate base after transurethral microwave thermotherapy (ProstaLund, Culver City, CA). The magnetic resonance image (**A**) and pathologic specimen (**B**) indicate a necrotic area in the prostate circumferentially surrounding the urethra.

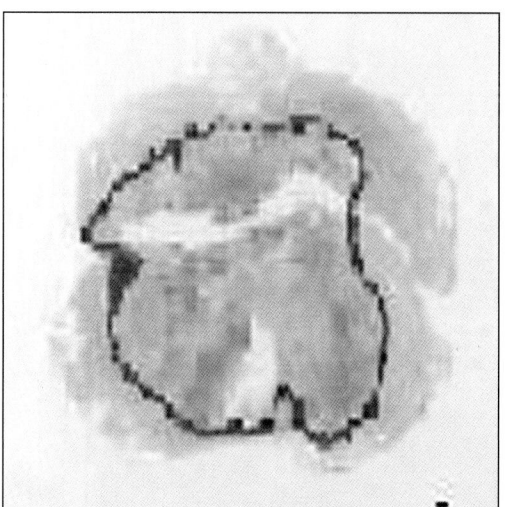

▶ **FIGURE 4-6.** (*See Color Plate*) Whole-mount histologic section taken from the prostate base after transurethral microwave thermotherapy (TUMT). The red *dotted line* indicates the area of heat-induced necrosis.

Minimally Invasive Therapies for Benign Prostatic Hyperplasia: Transurethral Microwave Thermotherapy and Needle Ablation

55

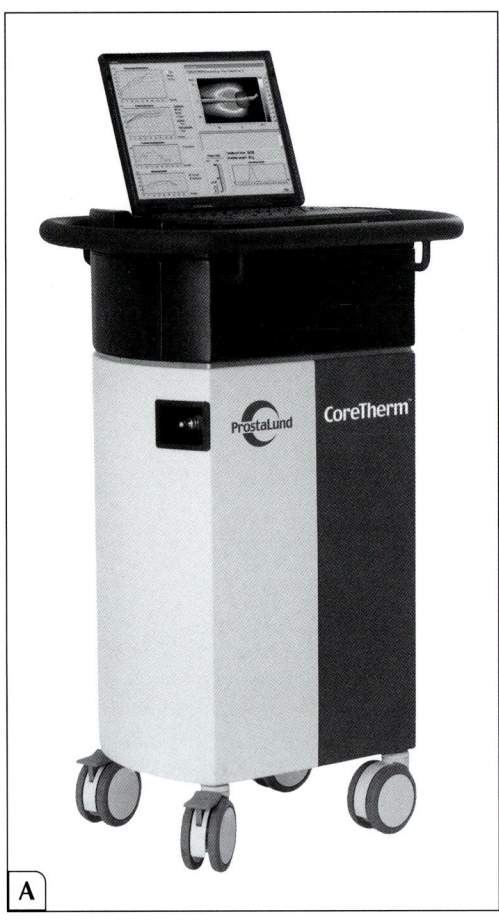

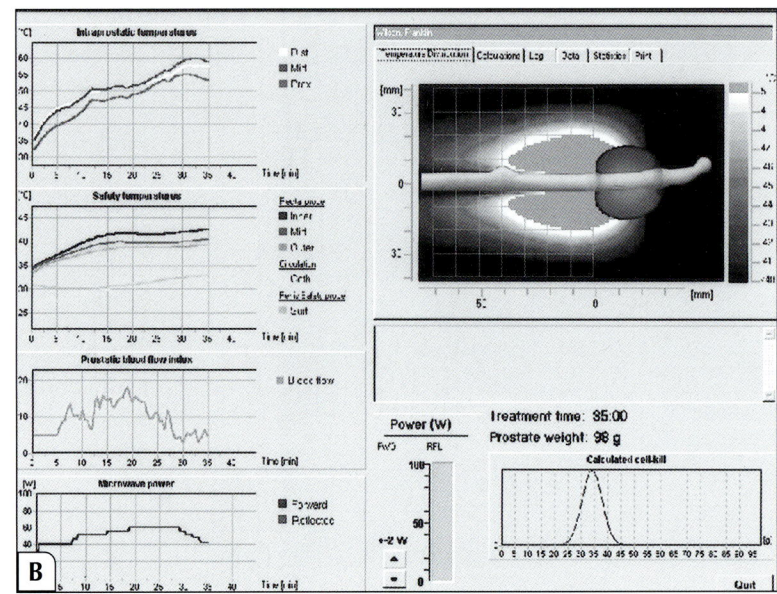

▶ **FIGURE 4-7.** Transurethral microwave thermotherapy (TUMT) device. All TUMT devices have a microwave power generator, a keyboard for data entry, and a computer screen to display treatment parameters in real time and to provide the means to adjust temperatures, energies, and coolant flow. **A,** The CoreTherm (ProstaLund, Culver City, CA). **B,** The CoreTherm's screen picture and displayed treatment parameters.

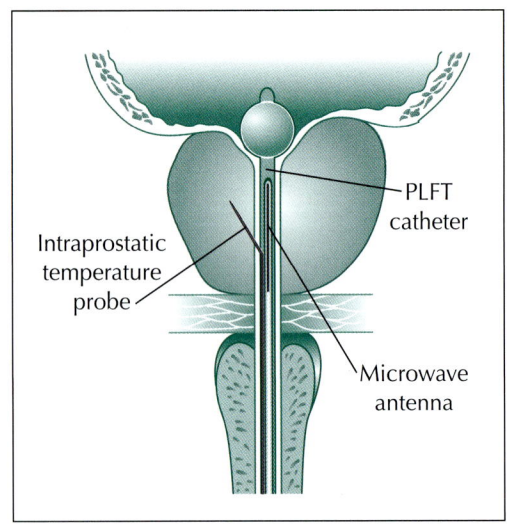

▶ **FIGURE 4-8.** A typical treatment catheter. All devices use an anchoring balloon to secure the catheter at the bladder neck. The microwave antenna is surrounded by a chamber, allowing perfusion with chilled water for urethral cooling. Cooling parameters vary from device to device. Some catheters (not the one shown in the figure) feature a channel to drain the urine during treatment time. The CoreTherm catheter (ProstaLund, Culver City, CA) shown here also features an intraprostatic temperature probe for measuring intraprostatic treatment temperature. PLFT—ProstaLund feedback treatment.

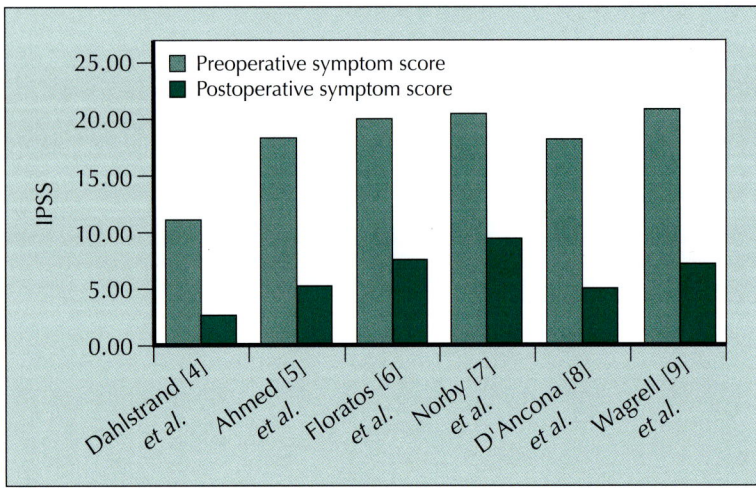

▶ **FIGURE 4-9.** Pre- and posttreatment symptom scores of patients treated with either the Prostatron (Urologix, Minneapolis, MN) or ProstaLund (Culver City, CA) transurethral microwave thermotherapy (TUMT) device. All these studies were randomized, controlled trials comparing TUMT with transurethral resection of the prostate. The results of the TUMT groups are shown in the graph. These results are based on data from 322 patients who underwent TUMT as an outpatient procedure [4–9].

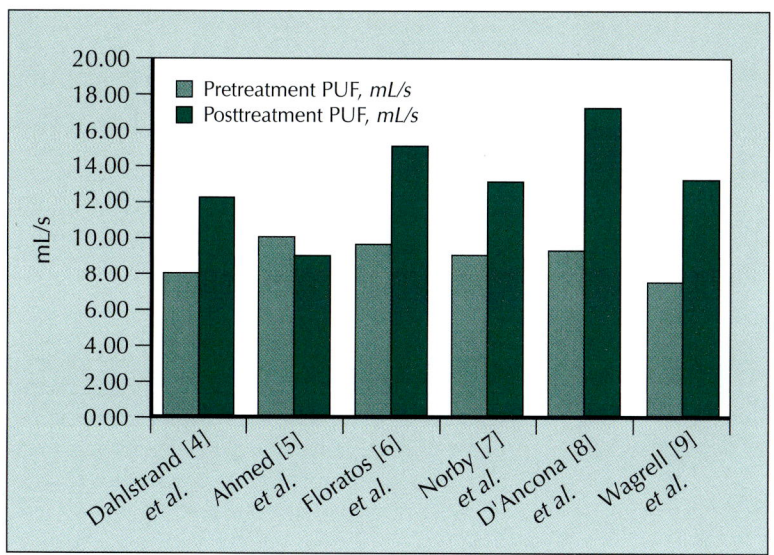

▶ **FIGURE 4-10.** Pre- and posttreatment peak urinary flow (PUF) rates in milliliters per second for the six studies mentioned in Figure 4-9. Only two of these studies reported a mean PUF that was greater than 15 mL/s. Ahmed *et al.* [5] found that transurethral microwave thermotherapy did not improve PUF [4–9].

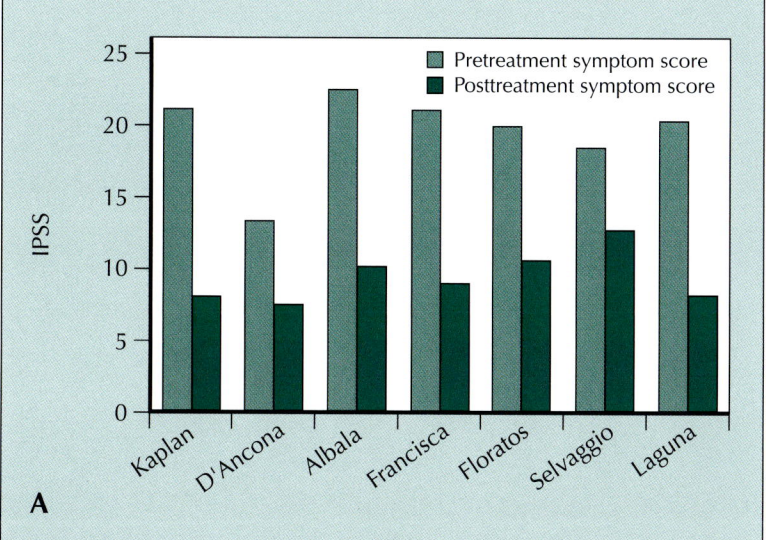

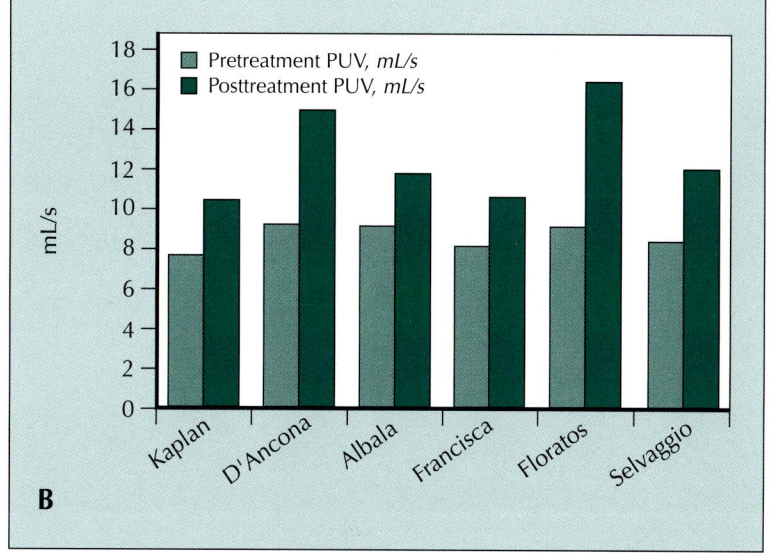

▶ **FIGURE 4-11.** Long-term efficacy and durability of microwave treatment. Published long-term improvement in symptom score (**A**) and peak urinary volume (**B**; PUV) is outlined. Patient follow-up was up to 60 months. However, durability may be a bit of a misnomer in this and other studies analyzing long-term efficacy. These analyses were done in patients who remained in the study. It stands to reason that these represent the best data. In most studies, less than half the initial group of men treated is analyzed at 5 year [6,8,10–14].

Morbidity After TUMT	
Hospitalization time	0 days
Acute urinary retention	15%
Transfusion	1.5%
Urinary tract infections	9%
Posttreatment irritative voiding symptoms	51%
Significant hematuria	2%
Incontinence	2%
Intraoperative morbidity	3%
Secondary procedure	12%
Retrograde ejaculation	2%
Erectile dysfunction	8.7%
Treatment failure	18%
Strictures	2%
Secondary procedure	12%
Invasive treatment at 5 years	13.6%

▶ **FIGURE 4-12.** Morbidity of transurethral microwave thermotherapy (TUMT). Values for each variable are expressed as estimated mean value of pooled analysis where applicable. Morbidities of TUMT are consistent with other minimally invasive, heat-delivering therapies of the prostate. Postoperative catheterization times varied widely, not only because of the different indications for treatment, but also because of the different aims of the individual trials. Most of the trials that treated patients who were not in urinary retention involved mean catheterization times of 3 to 7 days [15,16].

Minimally Invasive Therapies for Benign Prostatic Hyperplasia: Transurethral Microwave Thermotherapy and Needle Ablation

57

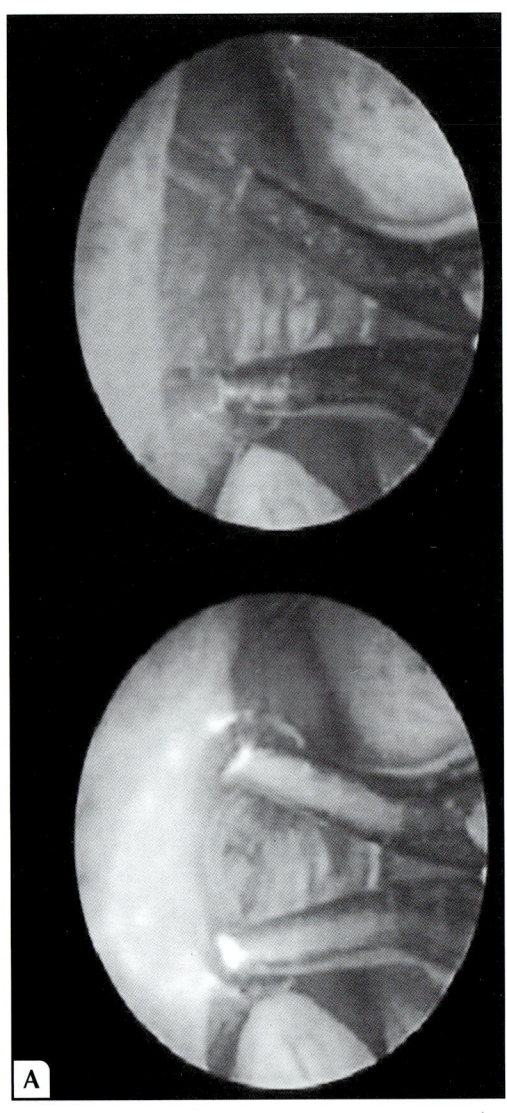

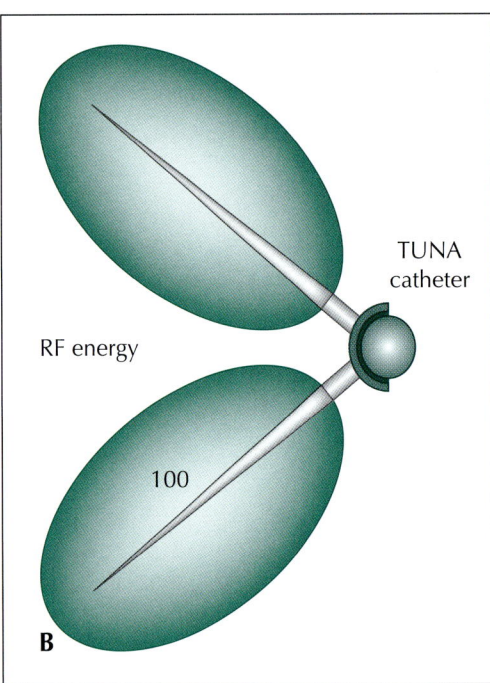

▶ **FIGURE 4-13.** Transurethral needle ablation (TUNA) of the prostate. **A and B,** TUNA uses a low-level radiofrequency (RF) generator operator frequency of 415 KHz. The energy is delivered under visual control in selected areas of the prostate by means of endoscopic needle placement. This procedure achieves well-demarcated RF heating (90° to 110°C) through two needles inserted into the prostate. Preservation of the urethral mucosa is the major advantage of TUNA. Outlet obstruction improves because of the retraction of necrotic tissue and scar. Frequency of the RF waves causes agitation of tissue particles and ions, creating heating of the tissue. The resulting lesion is elliptic and centered around the exposed needle electrode.

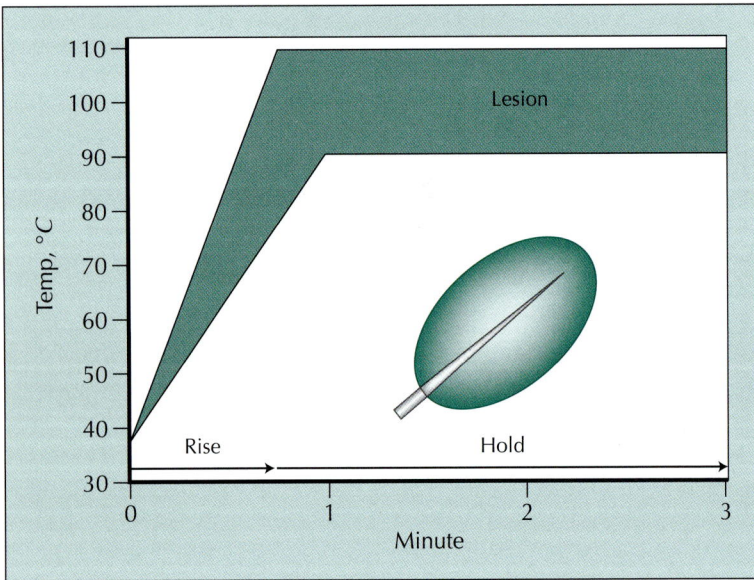

▶ **FIGURE 4-14.** Temperature buildup and maintenance over treatment time. The automated radiofrequency generator is programmed to achieve the best possible result.

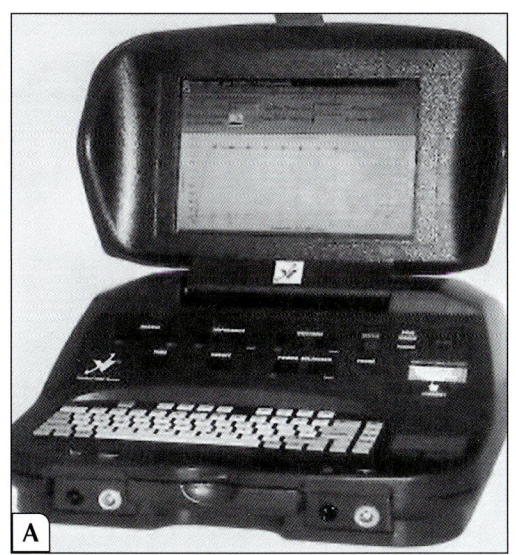

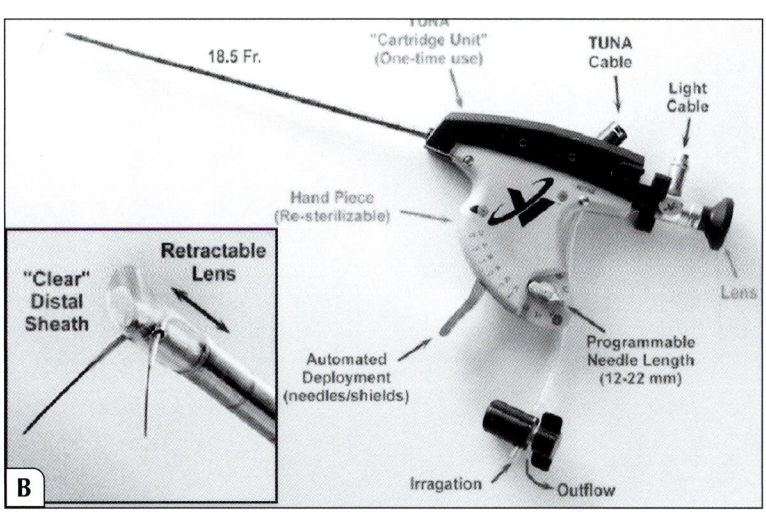

▶ **FIGURE 4-15.** The transurethral needle ablation (TUNA) system. The TUNA system consists of a radiofrequency generator (**A**) with an adjacent keyboard for data entry. The monitor allows monitoring of urethral, prostatic, and rectal temperatures in real time. The TUNA catheter (**B**) is fitted with two extending needles 40° from each other. The operator avoids destruction of the prostatic capsule by placement of needles under visual control, controlling needle length with extendible Teflon shields and varying generator wattage. Integrated thermocouples monitor urethral temperature to prevent urethral damage.

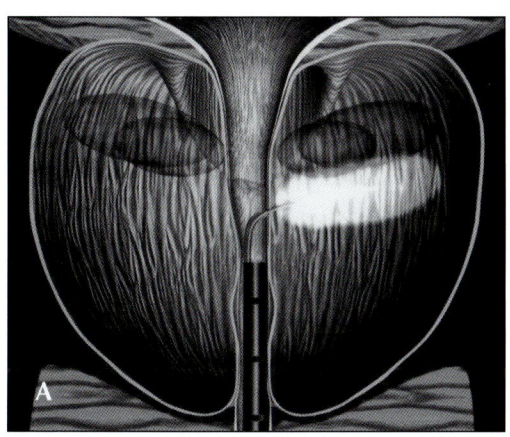

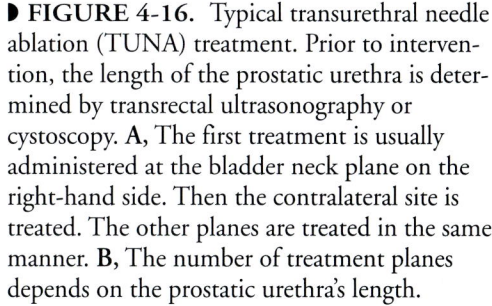

B. Treatment Planes in TUNA

Prostatic Urethra Length, cm	Treatment Planes
< 4	2
4–5	3
> 5	4

▶ **FIGURE 4-16.** Typical transurethral needle ablation (TUNA) treatment. Prior to intervention, the length of the prostatic urethra is determined by transrectal ultrasonography or cystoscopy. **A,** The first treatment is usually administered at the bladder neck plane on the right-hand side. Then the contralateral site is treated. The other planes are treated in the same manner. **B,** The number of treatment planes depends on the prostatic urethra's length.

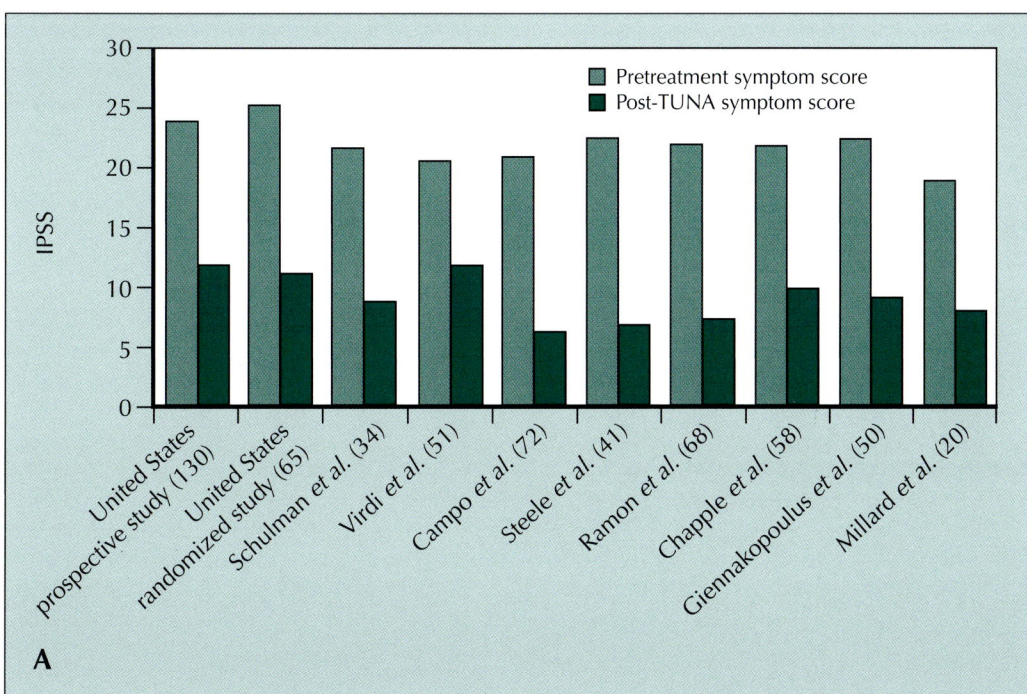

▶ **FIGURE 4-17.** Worldwide clinical experience with transurethral needle ablation (TUNA) of the prostate; summary of the changes in (**A**) International Prostate Symptom Score (IPSS) and (**B**) peak urinary flow rate after 12 months of follow-up.

(*Continued on next page*)

Minimally Invasive Therapies for Benign Prostatic Hyperplasia: Transurethral Microwave Thermotherapy and Needle Ablation

59

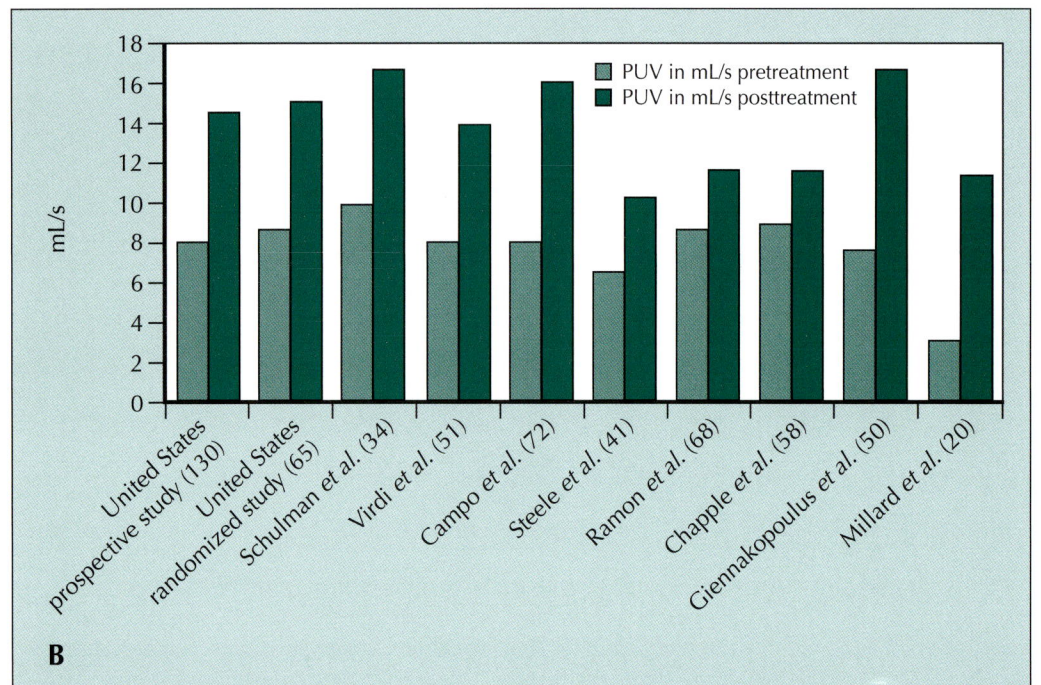

B

▶ **FIGURE 4-17.** (*Continued*) Patient numbers are indicated within the parentheses after each author's name. All these studies showed a statistically significant decrease in IPSS and peak urinary volume (PUV) 12 months after treatment. (*Adapted from* Tunuguntla and Evans [17].)

A. Comparison of Pretreatment and Long-Term Follow-up of Patients Treated With TUNA

Parameter	Baseline	Long-Term Follow-up	P Value
Number of patients	188	131	
Q_{max}, mean, mL/s	8.6	12.1	< 0.001
Residual volume, mean, mL	179	121	< 0.001
IPSS, mean	20.9	8.7	< 0.001
Quality-of-life score, mean	4.9	2.2	< 0.001

B. Percentage of Patients Who Improved by 50% After TUNA

Parameter	Patients Who Improved by 50%
Q_{max}	24%
Mean residual volume	72%
IPSS	78%
Quality of life score	77%

▶ **FIGURE 4-18.** Summary of the results in clinical outcome up to 5 years after treatment with transurethral needle ablation (TUNA) from three European centers. **A,** Comparison between pretreatment and long-term follow-up data of treated patients in whom follow-up was available (131). These 131 available patients had not been treated either surgically or with drugs after the TUNA treatment. One hundred twenty-one patients had a 5-year follow-up, 10 patients had a 4-year follow-up. **B,** Percentage of patients who improved by 50% after TUNA at long-term follow-up compared with baseline values (n = 131) [18]. IPSS—International Prostate Symptom Score; Q_{max}—maximal flow rate

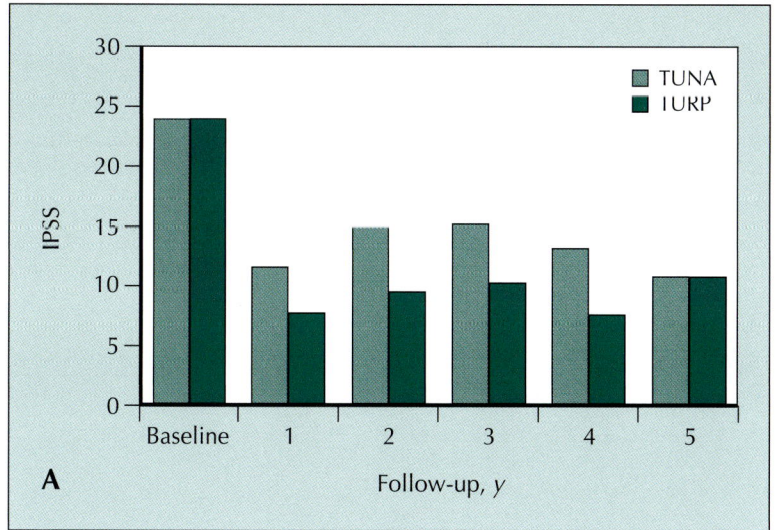

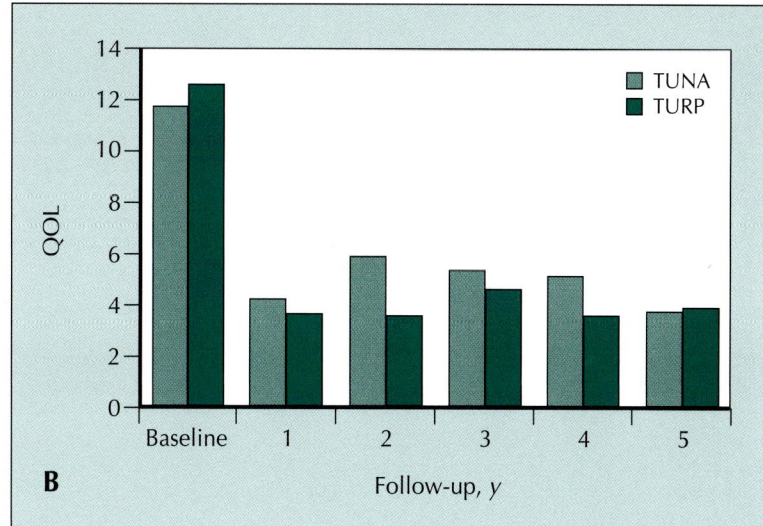

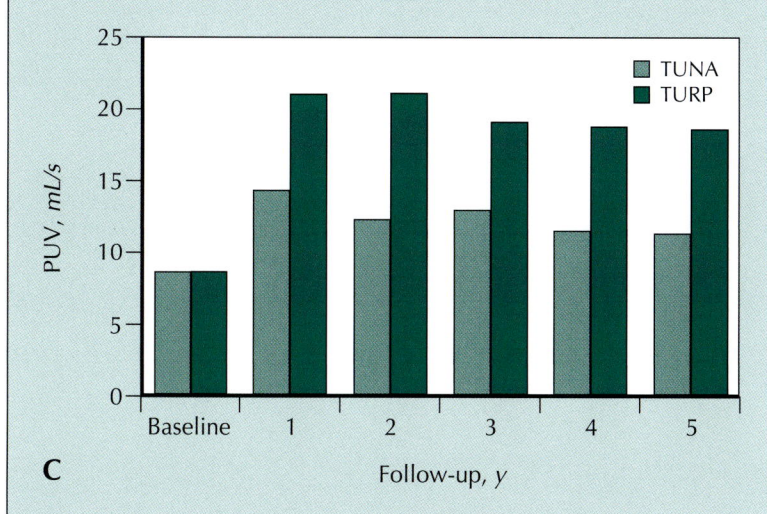

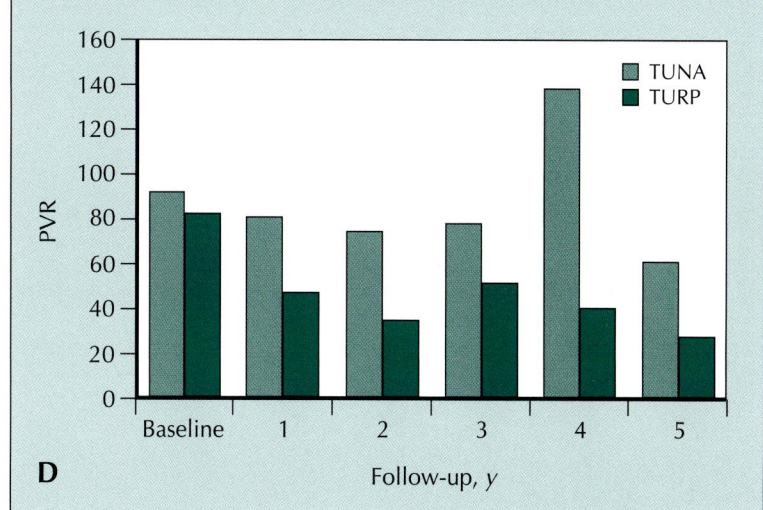

▶ **FIGURE 4-19.** Transurethral needle ablation (TUNA) versus transurethral resection of the prostate (TURP) . A total of 121 patients were enrolled in a prospective study; 65 were treated with TUNA and 56 were treated with TURP. The figures show the baseline characteristics and the 1-, 2-, 3-, 4-, and 5-year results. International Prostate Symptom Score (IPSS; **A**) and quality of life (QoL; **B**) measured the subjective response, whereas peak urinary volume (PUV; **C**) and postvoid residual (PVR; **D**) measured the objective response to treatment. Mean patient age was 66.1 years, and mean American Urological Association symptom score was 24 and 24.1. Five-year data show a significant improvement from baseline in the two cohorts. The improvement was greater for TURP than for TUNA. The improvement in QoL for TUNA and TURP remained durable throughout the study course. When comparing TUNA with TURP, there was a statistically significant difference in QoL only at year 2. Both TUNA and TURP demonstrated a significant improvement in PUV at each interval compared with baseline, the patients treated with TURP showing a greater improvement than those treated with TUNA; the difference was statistically significant at each interval. PVR did not statistically significantly decrease in the TUNA cohort. The change in PVR for TURP was greater at each time point [19].

Minimally Invasive Therapies for Benign Prostatic Hyperplasia: Transurethral Microwave Thermotherapy and Needle Ablation

61

REFERENCES

1. Walsh PC: Benign prostatic hyperplasia. In *Campbell's Urology*, edn 6. Edited by Walsh PC, Retik AB, Stamey TA, Vaughan ED. Philadelphia: WB Saunders, 1992;1007–1027.

2. Larson BT, Bostwick DG, Corica AG: Histological changes of minimally invasive procedures for the treatment of benign prostatic hyperplasia and prostate cancer: clinical implications. *J Urol* 2003, 170:12–19.

3. Perlmutter AP, Perachino M: Mechanism of microwave thermotherapy. *World J Urol* 1998, 16:82–88.

4. Dahlstrand C, Walden M, Geirsson G, Pettersson S: Transurethral microwave thermotherapy versus transurethral resection for symptomatic benign prostatic obstruction: a prospective randomized study with a 2-year followup. *Br J Urol* 1995, 76:614–618.

5. Ahmed M, Bell T, Lawrence WT, *et al.*: Transurethral microwave thermotherapy (Prostatron version 2.5) compared with transurethral resection of the prostate for the treatment of benign prostatic hyperplasia: a randomized, controlled, parallel study. *Br J Urol* 1997, 79:181–185.

6. Floratos DL, Kiemeney LA, Rossi C, *et al.*: Long-term followup of randomized transurethral microwave thermotherapy versus transurethral prostatic resection study. *J Urol* 2001, 165:1533–1538.

7. Norby B, Nielsen HV, Frimodt-Moller PC: Transurethral interstitial laser coagulation of the prostate and transurethral microwave thermotherapy vs transurethral resection or incision of the prostate: results of a randomized, controlled study in patients with symptomatic benign prostatic hyperplasia. *BJU Int* 2002, 90:853–862.

8. D'Ancona FC, Francisca EA, Witjes WP, *et al.*: Transurethral resection of the prostate vs high-energy thermotherapy of the prostate in patients with benign prostatic hyperplasia: long-term results. *Br J Urol* 1998, 81:259–264.

9. Wagrell L, Schelin S, Nordling J, *et al.*: Feedback microwave thermotherapy versus TURP for clinical BPH—a randomized controlled multicenter study. *Urology* 2002, 60:292–299.

10. Kaplan S, Blute M, Bruskewitz RC, *et al.*: Long term efficacy and durability in 345 patients treated with transurethral microwave thermotherapy for benign prostatic hyperplasia: five year results [abstract]. *J Urol* 2002, 167:297.

11. Albala D, Andriole G, Davis BE, *et al.*: Transurethral microwave thermotherapy (TUMT) using the Thermatrx TMx-2000; durability exhibited in a study comparing TUMT with a sham procedure in patients with benign prostatic hyperplasia (BPH) [abstract]. *J Urol* 2003, 169:465.

12. Francisca EA, d'Ancona FC, Meuleman EJ, *et al.*: Sexual function following high energy microwave thermotherapy: results of a randomized controlled study comparing transurethral microwave thermotherapy to transurethral prostatic resection. *J Urol* 1999, 161:486–492.

13. Selvaggio O, Ditonno P, Battaglia M, *et al.*: Long term results (4 years) of high-energy transurethral microwave. *Eur Urol* 2003, 2:102-106.

14. Laguna P, van Hest P, Smelov V, *et al.*: Efficacy and durability of the 30 minutes high energy TUMT protocol in 213 patients [abstract]. *J Endourol* 2002, 15:38.

15. AUA Practice Guidelines Committee: AUA guideline on management of benign prostatic hyperplasia (2003). Chapter 1: diagnosis and treatment recommendations. *J Urol* 2003, 170:530–547.

16. Gonzalez RR, Te AE: How do transurethral needle ablation of the prostate and transurethral microwave thermotherapy compare with transurethral prostatectomy? *Curr Urol Rep.* 2003; 4:297–306.

17. Tunuguntla HS, Evans CP: Minimally invasive therapies for benign prostatic hyperplasia. *World J Urol* 2002, 20: 197-206.

18. Zlotta AR, Giannakopoulos X, Maehlum O *et al*: Long- term evaluation of transurethral needle ablation of the prostate (TUNA) for treatment of symptomatic benign prostatic hyperplasia: Clinical outcome up to five years from three centers. *Eur Urol* 2003, 44: 89-93.

19. Hill B, Belville W, Bruskewitz R, *et al.*: Transurethral needle ablation versus transurethral resection of the prostate for treatment of symptomatic benign prostatic hyperplasia. *J Urol* 2004, 6:2336–2341.

Laser Prostatectomy

5

*Ricardo R. Gonzalez,
Jaspreet S. Sandhu,
Richard K. Lee,
& Alexis E. Te*

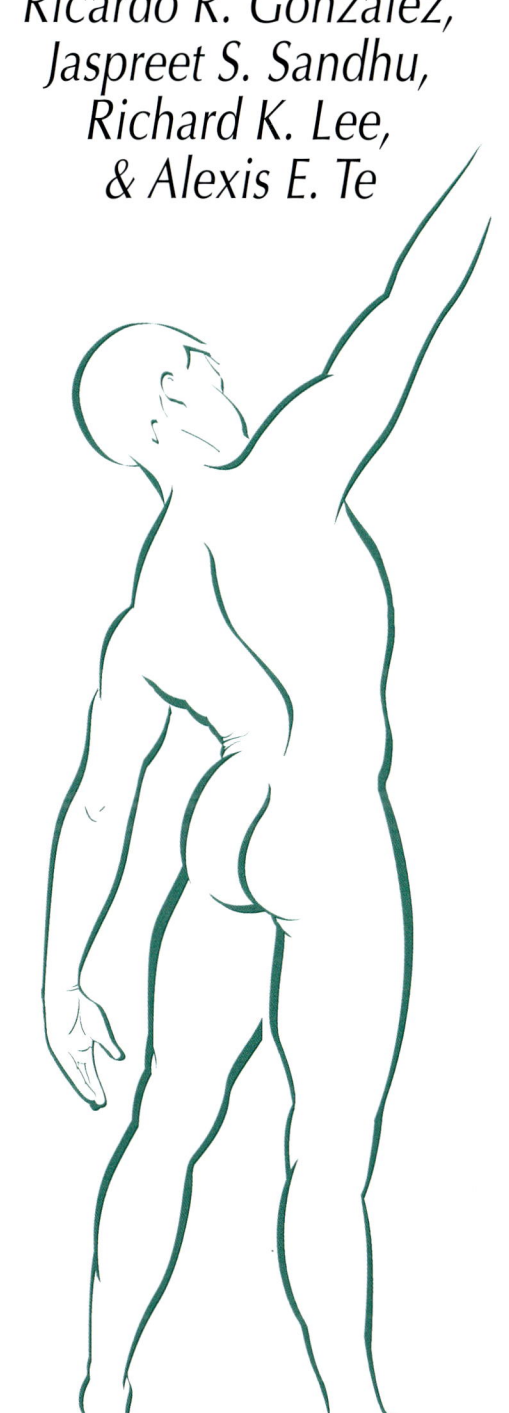

Since their introduction into the field of urology approximately two decades ago, lasers have undergone an evolution from theory to practical application. One of the more recent applications lies in the treatment of benign prostatic hyperplasia, or BPH, via laser prostatectomy.

The gold standard for treatment of BPH used to lie with electrocautery-based transurethral resection of the prostate (TURP). TURP, however, is fraught with complications and side effects, including fluid absorption, electrolyte imbalance, perioperative bleeding, and inadequate resection. These problems have led to the search for safer, more effective alternatives for treatment. Laser therapy has several advantages over standard TURP, including technical simplicity and the minimization of complications such as intraoperative fluid absorption, bleeding, retrograde ejaculation, and impotence. Patients also require a shorter hospital stay and recover more quickly. The lack of bleeding and irrigant absorption also theoretically allows laser prostatectomy to treat larger glands with less physiologic stress, suggesting a role for laser therapy in patients with a high burden of coexisting medical disease. Recent estimates suggest that up to 40% of practicing urologists are in fact already performing laser prostatectomies on patients with symptomatic BPH, and this number is certain to keep increasing.

Laser energy can be delivered through small semiflexible fibers that pass through standard endoscopes. Depending on the laser's physical characteristics, lasers can achieve coagulation (at temperatures around 60ºC) or vaporization (at temperatures above 100ºC). Although easy to perform, laser techniques that depend on coagulative necrosis to produce a delayed clinical improvement are falling out of favor because of prolonged irritative voiding symptoms and the need for prolonged urine drainage. In contrast, standard TURP is directly being challenged for its title of gold standard by vaporization techniques—including holmium laser enucleation of the prostate and photoselective vaporization prostatectomy—which remove obstructing prostate tissue immediately with minimal side effects and maximum clinical improvement.

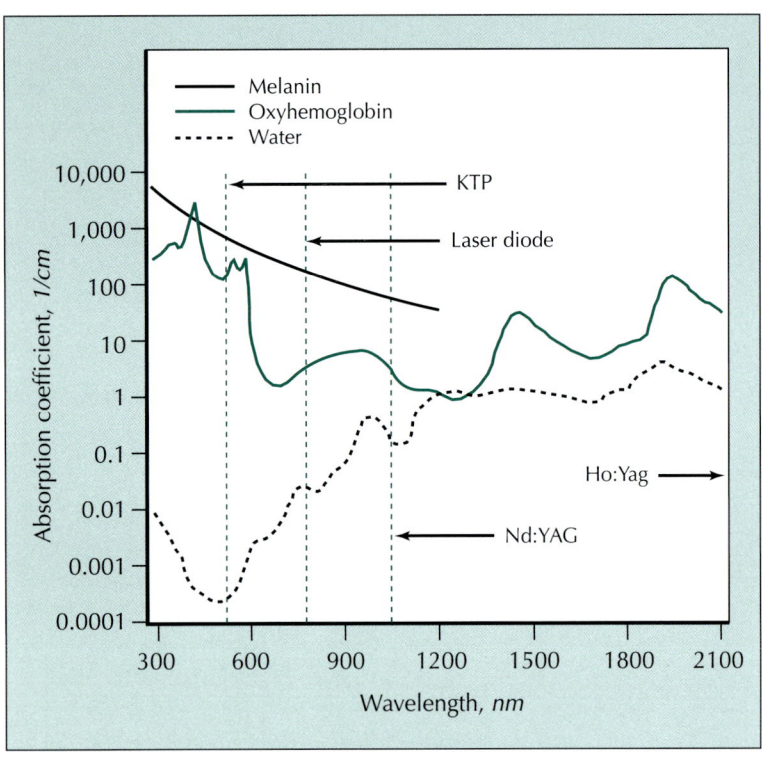

▶ FIGURE 5-1. Laser physics. Different laser wavelengths are absorbed by water, oxyhemoglobin, and melanin. The figure demonstrates the absorption characteristic for each wavelength in a given medium of absorption. The absorption coefficient is plotted as a function of the wavelength, and the absorption coefficient for a given material is plotted on the graph. A high absorption coefficient means the given laser wavelength is well absorbed in the selected medium. A low absorption corresponds with a greater degree of transparency, allowing the light to go through the medium without absorption.

The potassium-titanyl-phosphate (KTP) laser beam at a wavelength of 532 nm is fully transmitted through the aqueous irrigant but highly absorbed by oxyhemoglobin in the tissue. This allows KTP laser energy to get selectively absorbed by tissue with high oxyhemoglobin content, such as prostatic tissue. This results in vaporization that is focused and efficient in prostate tissue; for this reason, the KTP laser procedure is referred to as photoselective vaporization of the prostate.

In contrast, the holmium:yttrium aluminum garnet (Ho:YAG) laser energy is absorbed more by water, in the endoscopic irrigant, than by the tissue. Energy absorption by the irrigant forms a vapor bubble around the laser fiber tip. Tissue disruption depends on the photomechanical interaction of this vapor bubble with the tissue. This interaction results in a microexplosion, causing a "jackhammer" effect that can tear tissue apart or break a stone. The Ho:YAG laser requires close contact with the target tissue and is an efficient laser scalpel. Because neodymium:yttrium aluminum garnet (Nd:YAG) and diode lie have similarly high absorption coefficients for water, oxyhemoglobin, and melanin, this translates into excellent and deeper absorption into tissue.

Note: The vertical scale is logarithmic, *ie*, each grid line is equivalent to a change in the absorption coefficient by one order of magnitude (factor 10).

LASER-TISSUE INTERACTIONS

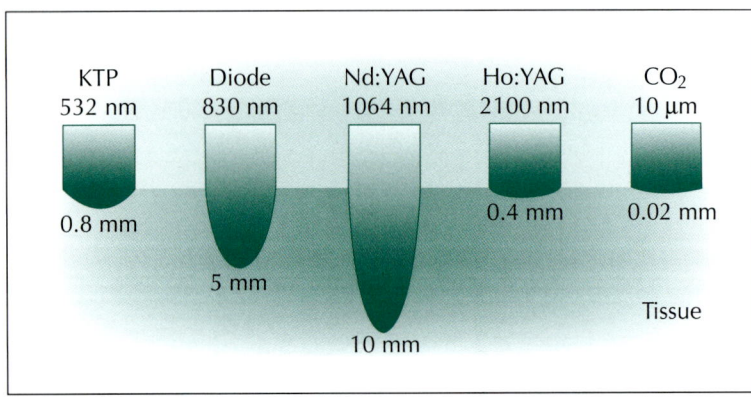

▶ FIGURE 5-2. Laser tissue penetration. Laser energies penetrate tissues differently. Laser energy that is not reflected or scattered off the surface of the tissue subsequently penetrates the tissue. The depth of penetration by laser energy depends on the wavelength, absorption coefficient, and composition of the receiving tissue. The figure depicts different penetration depths of various laser wavelengths into prostatic tissue. Penetration is often described by "extinction length," the depth of penetration of an incident beam beyond which only 10% of the initial beam energy is left, *ie*, 90% absorption. Therefore, after one extinction length, 10% of the beam will penetrate further, whereas after two extinction lengths, 1% of the beam will penetrate further, and so on. In this figure, because of a longer extinction length, neodymium:yttrium aluminum garnet (Nd:YAG) energy penetrates the tissue twice as deep as the diode laser, 10 times more than the potassium-titanyl-phosphate (KTP) laser, and so forth. Ho:YAG—holmium:yttrium aluminum garnet

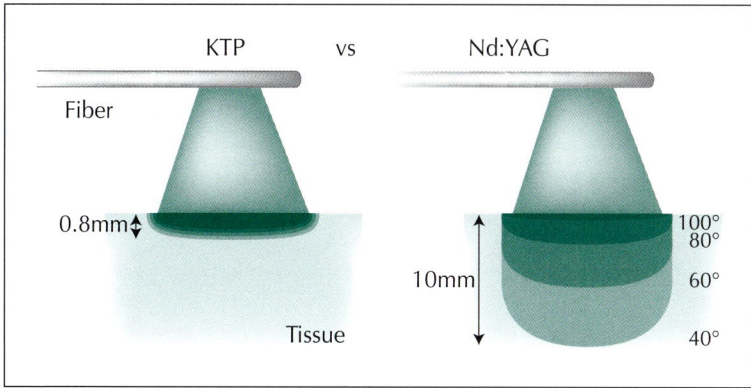

FIGURE 5-3. Laser tissue absorption. Laser energy is absorbed by tissue and thermally converted to produce tissue effects. Absorption of laser energy is often described by "absorption length," the depth of tissue through which 63% of the incident beam energy is absorbed. It is important to note that the different components of living tissue absorb different types of laser energy wavelengths in variable fashions. Water, constituting 75% to 85% of soft tissue, absorbs potassium-titanyl-phosphate (KTP) laser energy very poorly and transmits deeper into tissue, resulting in deep penetration of laser beam into tissue. In contrast, holmium:yttrium aluminum garnet energy is very well absorbed by water, resulting in less penetration and increased surface vaporization. Pigments such as hemoglobin, bilirubin, and melanin absorb neodymium:yttrium aluminum garnet (Nd:YAG) energy moderately well, and as a result, tissue proteins absorb Nd:YAG energy moderately well. Finally, carbon, an abundant constituent of all living tissue, is a strong absorber of all wavelengths of laser energy because of its black color characteristic. The figure represents prostatic tissue absorption and subsequent penetration by KTP and Nd:YAG laser energy. The selective absorption of KTP energy by hemoglobin in the prostate allows limited penetration that results in thermal conversion that is more superficial than that of Nd:YAG.

Photothermal Conversion

Temperature Threshold, °C	Biologic Effect
37	Body temperature
45	Hyperthermia
60	Coagulation
100	Vaporization
150	Carbonization
300	Melting

FIGURE 5-4. Photothermal conversion. The predominant mechanism of laser-induced tissue effect is the thermal conversion of laser energy, or photothermolysis, which results in the elevation of target tissue temperature. Laser tissue effects may be subsequently categorized as either coagulation (*ie*, photopyrolysis) followed by delayed tissue sloughing, or vaporization (*ie*, photovaporolysis), resulting in immediate tissue ablation.

The overall rate of tissue ablation is determined by the rate of laser energy deposition into tissue, which in turn is driven by the laser light wavelength (λ). In laser prostatectomy, one attempts to quickly deliver a sufficient amount of energy per unit volume of tissue to bring cells to vaporization temperature. If the cells are brought only to coagulation temperature, they then become half as penetrable to laser energy, thus increasing backscatter and surrounding coagulation and thereby halting the forward progress of ablation. This directly implies that applying laser light energy at lower power densities for increasing periods of time will result only in a greater depth of coagulation and possible periprostatic injury rather than creation of a channel defect.

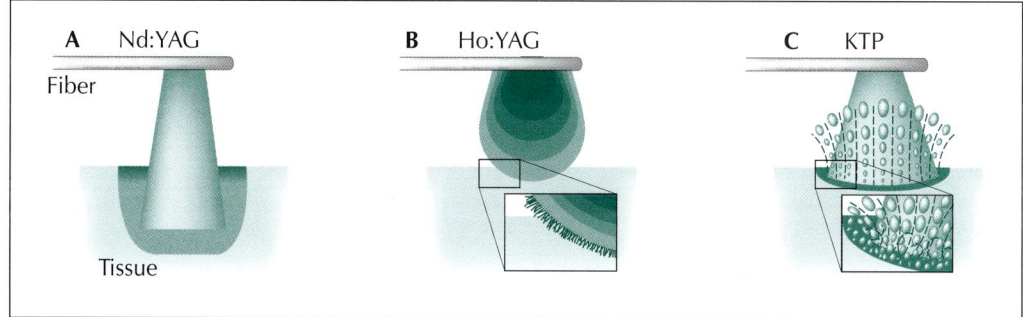

FIGURE 5-5. Laser-induced tissue effects. **A,** Coagulation, as is achieved with the neodymium:yttrium aluminum garnet (Nd:YAG) laser, represents the process of raising the temperatures of organic compounds to the point of molecular breakdown, usually greater than 50°C. Once tissue has been coagulated and further laser energy is applied, absorption does not appear to be affected but scattering may be doubled. The backscatter and reflection cause greater diversion of energy and therefore a wider and longer zone of coagulation. This may be useful if a limited depth of penetration with a wider width of laser effect is desired. For therapy of benign prostatic hyperplasia, however, the use of coagulation alone makes the procedure imprecise and it can be especially hazardous when working close to the external urethral sphincter.

B, Compared with the Nd:YAG laser's coagulative effect, the holmium:yttrium aluminum garnet (Ho:YAG) laser wavelength penetrates less than 500 μm into tissue, is highly absorbed in water, and can be used for tissue cutting and vaporization. Because of the high absorption in water, a vapor bubble is formed in front of the optical fiber during each laser pulse, consuming part of the laser energy. The bubble produces an initial photomechanical effect tearing the tissue apart, followed by a tissue vaporization effect occurring in the vapor environment of the bubble that is associated with superficial coagulation of the target tissue. The high absorption of the Ho:YAG laser beam in the aqueous irrigant implies that close contact between the optical fiber and the tissue must be constantly maintained for efficient tissue vaporization effect.

C, Vaporization refers to the change from solid to gaseous state of a material. Human tissue requires approximately 2500 J/g to change its temperature from 37°C to 100°C. Unlike the Nd:YAG wavelength, the potassium-titanyl-phosphate (KTP) wavelength is selectively absorbed by hemoglobin, which acts as an intracellular chromophore. KTP laser energy is transparently delivered through a fluid medium such as water into the cell, where it is absorbed by hemoglobin, then rapidly heated, leading to rapid vaporization of tissue. With KTP photoselective vaporization of the prostate, gaseous vapors and tissue proteins that are converted to smoke are washed away with irrigation. The kinetic energy of escaping vapor causes miniexplosions within tissue, further adding to the mechanical rupture of membranes.

Commonly Used Laser Techniques

Technique	Abbreviation	Energy Source	Power, W	Effect
Visual/endoscopic laser ablation of the prostate	VLAP, ELAP, LAP	Nd:YAG 1064 nm, low-power density, wide-beam, noncontact, side-firing fiber	40–60	Deep coagulation and some immediate tissue disruption
Holmium laser enucleation of the prostate	HoLEP	Ho:YAG 2100 nm via end- or side-firing fiber with contact or near-contact	100	Incision used to excise prostate lobes, subsequently requiring morcellation in the bladder for removal
Holmium laser ablation of the prostate	HoLAP	Ho:YAG 2100 nm via bare end- or side-firing fiber with near-contact	100	Vaporization used for immediate tissue disruption with minimal coagulation effect
Photoselective vaporization of the prostate	PVP	KTP 532 nm via side-firing fiber with near-contact	80	Vaporization used for immediate tissue disruption with minimal coagulation effect
Interstitial laser coagulation	ILC	Diode 830 nm or Nd:YAG 1064 nm via bare or modified fiber	2–20	Deep localized coagulation with minimal immediate tissue disruption

▶ **FIGURE 5-6.** The laser prostatectomy techniques in common practice today. Ho:YAG—holmium:yttrium aluminum garnet; KTP—potassium-titanyl-phosphate; Nd:YAG—neodymium:yttrium aluminum garnet.

NEODYMIUM:YTTRIUM ALUMINUM GARNET LASER

•• VISUAL LASER ABLATION OF THE PROSTATE ••

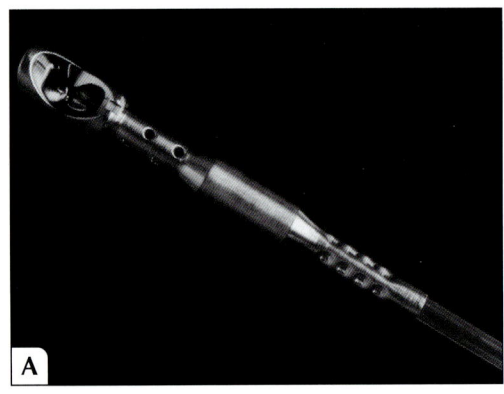
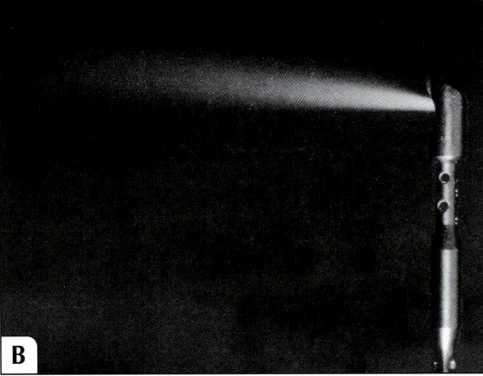
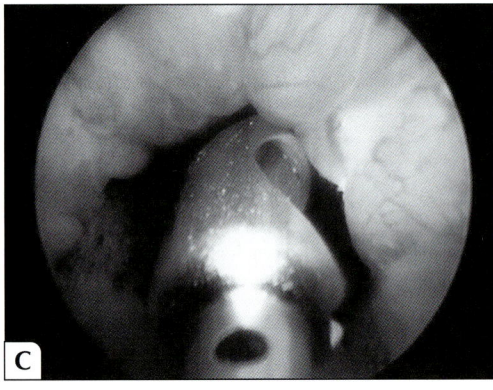

▶ **FIGURE 5-7.** Neodymium:yttrium aluminum garnet (Nd:YAG) for visual laser ablation of the prostate. The Nd:YAG 1064-nm wavelength is well suited for transmission through flexible fibers, which are easily manipulated through standard urologic endoscopes and applied under direct vision [1]. This allows for visually guided prostatic irradiation. **A,** Distal reflecting mirror of the side-firing Nd:YAG laser delivery fiber for prostatic irradiation (Urolase; CR Bard and Trimedyne, Covington, GA). **B,** This fiber allows the laser beam to be aimed directly at the lateral or median lobe of the prostate under direct vision. **C,** Visual cystoscopic appearance of the laser fiber in use. The fiber is directed at obstructing tissue and held in place during the irradiation. (*Images courtesy of* John N. Kabalin, MD)

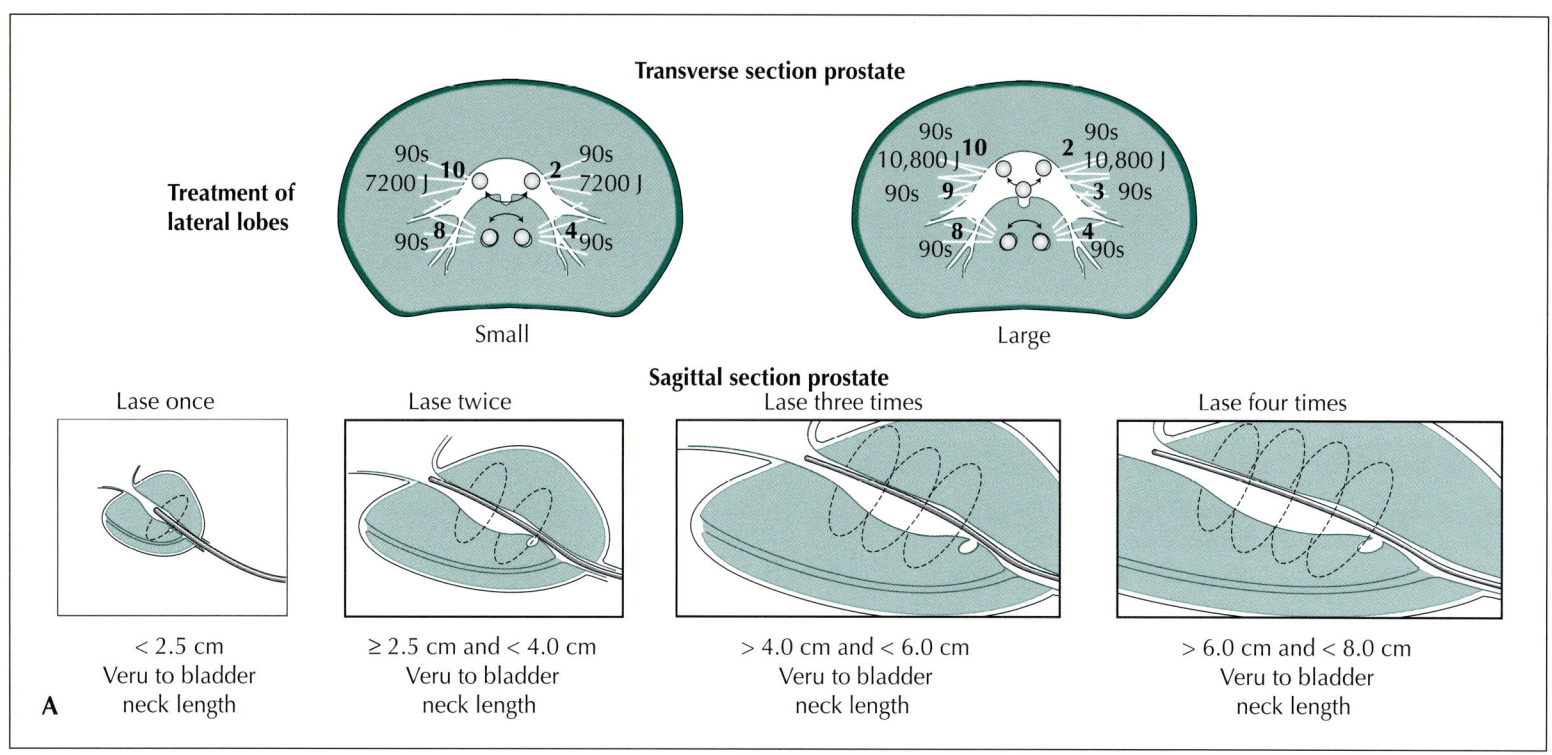

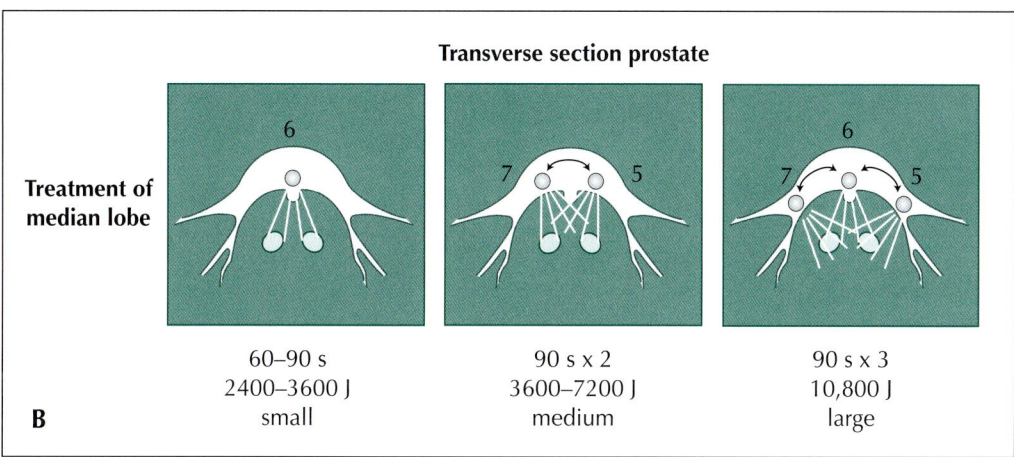

FIGURE 5-8. Technique for performing visual laser ablation of the prostate. Prostatectomy using neodymium:yttrium aluminum garnet (Nd:YAG) laser typically is performed under regional or general anesthesia. A cystoscope of relatively small caliber (≤ 22 French) accommodates almost all side-firing laser fibers used for Nd:YAG laser prostatectomy. Because Nd:YAG laser coagulation seals blood vessels, preventing both bleeding and intraoperative fluid absorption (and thus, transurethral resection syndrome), sterile water or saline irrigation commonly is used. Room temperature irrigation dissipates the heat more effectively, and thus is preferred over warm irrigation. In the spot-coagulation technique described by Kabalin [2], the Nd:YAG laser fiber is held in close approximation, without touching the obstructing benign prostatic hyperplasia (BPH) tissue. Laser energy is applied for a minimum of 60 to 90 seconds, and power settings between 40 and 60 W are used, depending on the degree of divergence of the emitting laser fiber. If the laser is applied without causing tissue char, the depth of coagulation necrosis is approximately 1.5 cm. Areas of coagulation necrosis eventually undergo dissolution and pass in the urinary stream over several weeks.

A, All obstructing lateral lobe BPH tissue is sequentially irradiated with multiple spot laser energy applications. A typical treatment consists of spot laser energy application at 2- and 4-o'clock positions (left lateral lobe) and 8- and 10-o'clock positions (right lateral lobe) in the transverse plane. For larger prostates with greater anteroposterior dimensions, further spot laser applications may be needed no more than 1.5 cm apart to ensure treatment of all tissue. For larger, longer prostates, spot laser energy applications are repeated in sequential transverse planes every 1.5 cm along the length of the gland from bladder neck to the veru montanum, until all obstructing lateral lobe BPH is irradiated.

B, The median lobe is similarly treated with spot laser energy applications. For larger median lobes, multiple spot laser treatments across the breadth of the median lobe (no more than 1.5 cm apart) are performed until all obstructing median lobe BPH is irradiated. (*Images courtesy of John N. Kabalin, MD*)

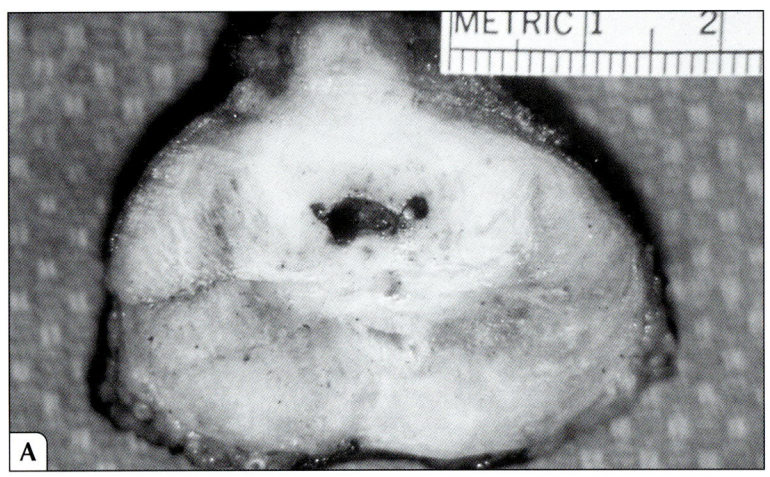 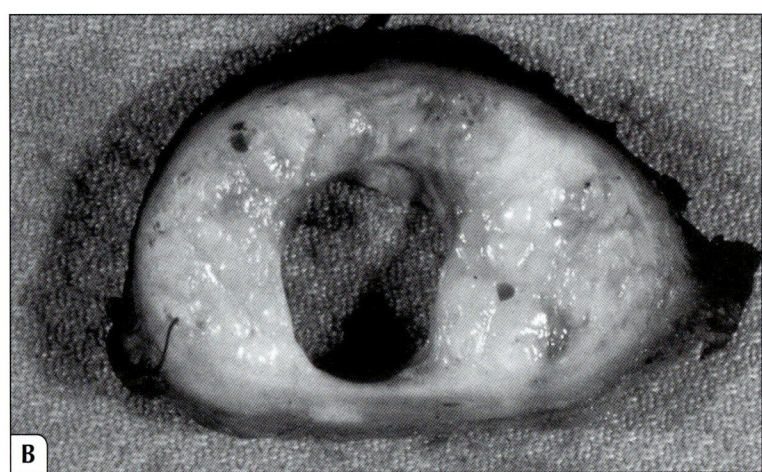

▶ **FIGURE 5-9.** Acute and chronic neodymium:yttrium aluminum garnet (Nd:YAG) tissue effects. The acute and chronic tissue effects of Nd:YAG laser spot applications have been demonstrated in vivo by Kabalin *et al.* [3]. **A,** A transverse section through a human prostate removed immediately after Nd:YAG laser spot applications. The transition zone shows extensive coagulation necrosis. **B,** A transverse section through a human prostate removed 1 year after Nd:YAG laser spot applications. The transition zone slough is complete, leaving a large laser defect.(*Images courtesy of* John N. Kabalin, MD)

VLAP Outcomes						
Parameter	**Preoperative (n)**	**1 y**	**2 y**	**3 y**	**4 y**	**≥ 5 y**
Peak flow rate, *mL/s*	6.7 (220)	17.8 (196)	18.7 (180)	18 (167)	16 (127)	16.6 (98)
Postvoid residual, *mL*	159	52	53	51	54	50
International Prostate Symptom Score	22	7.0	7.3	7.2	7.4	7.5

▶ **FIGURE 5-10.** Visual laser ablation of the prostate (VLAP): outcomes. Long-term outcomes reported by a single institution in 230 consecutive men who underwent VLAP with a median follow-up of 36 months [4]. Several studies have supported VLAP as an effective treatment for benign prostatic hyperplasia (BPH) with minimal morbidity [4–6]. However, despite low morbidities reported by investigators, the VLAP procedure developed a reputation for long-term dysuria and urinary retention requiring extended postoperative catheterization or drainage with a suprapubic tube [7]. VLAP was limited in its ability to effectively treat BPH with effective durability; although the neodymium:yttrium aluminum garnet laser was capable of reaching power outputs as high as 120 W in continuous-wave mode, its predominant coagulative effect on tissue led to sloughing and slow resorption, resulting in prolonged postoperative catheterization and dysuria. (*Adapted from* Carter *et al.* [7].)

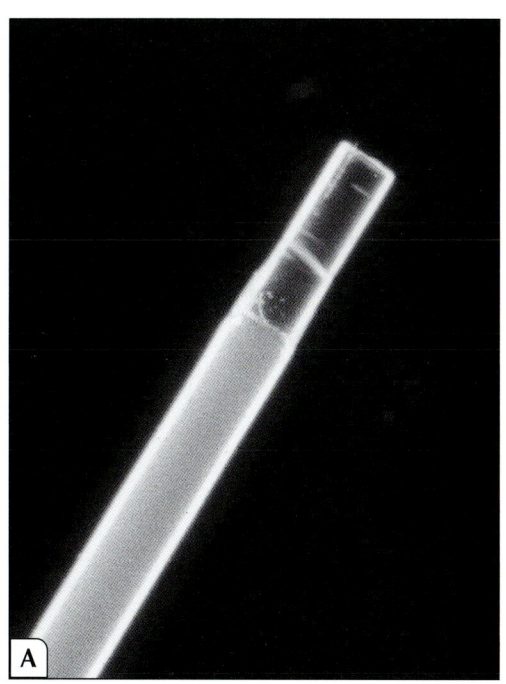

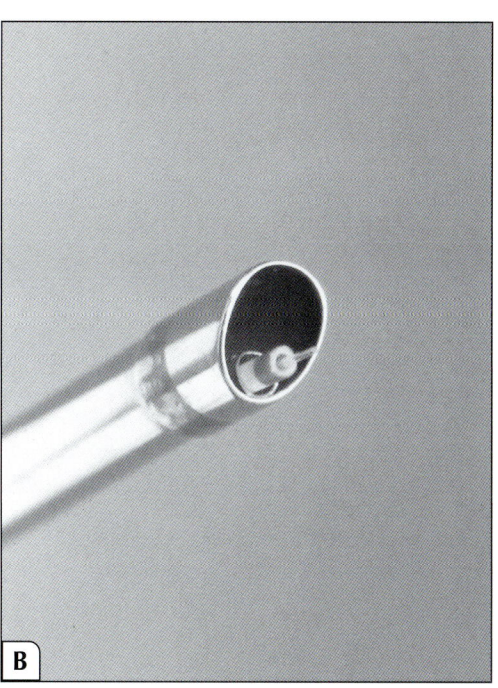

▶ **FIGURE 5-11.** Tools used with the holmium:yttrium aluminum garnet (Ho:YAG) laser. Shown are the tools used for Ho:YAG laser prostatectomy. The Ho:YAG 2100-nm wavelength penetrates less than 500 μm into tissue, is highly absorbed in water, and can be used for tissue cutting and vaporization. Because of the high absorption in water, a vapor bubble is formed in front of the optical fiber during each laser pulse, consuming part of the laser energy. The bubble explosion produces an initial photomechanical effect tearing the tissue apart, followed by a tissue coagulation effect occurring within the vapor environment of the bubble that is associated with superficial coagulation of the target tissue. The high absorption of the Ho:YAG laser beam in the aqueous irrigant implies that close contact between the optical fiber and the tissue must be constantly maintained for efficient tissue vaporization effect.

A, Holmium laser resection and enucleation of the prostate is most commonly performed with a 550-μm bare end-firing flexible laser fiber, although side-firing fibers are also available for this wavelength. The pulsed Ho:YAG laser is typically set at 80 to 100 W to maximize efficiency in incision.

B, A 26-French continuous-flow resectoscope that incorporates a fixed channel to minimize movement and vibration distally is used. Normal saline is used for irrigation.(*Images courtesy of* John N. Kabalin, MD)

•• HOLMIUM LASER ENUCLEATION OF THE PROSTATE ••

A. Enucleation of Middle Lobe

Step	Description
1	Incise posterior bladder neck deeply at 5- and 7-o'clock positions, extending them along the prostatic urethra to the veru montanum
2	Connect these incisions in front of the veru montanum
3	Work retrograde, back toward the bladder neck, with a combination of laser incision and blunt dissection with tip of resectoscope, undermining and excising the median lobe

▶ **FIGURE 5-12.** Steps in holmium laser enucleation of the prostate (HoLEP) [8]. **A** and **B,** Enucleation of the middle lobe (steps 1 through 3). Prior to complete lobe enucleation, which requires subsequent tissue morcellation, the surgeon may consider dividing the lobe into smaller pieces using the same holmium:yttrium aluminum garnet laser. This technique is known as holmium laser resection of the prostate (HoLRP) [9,10]. Despite not requiring an additional transurethral tissue morcellator, HoLRP is far less efficient and not practical for large glands.

(*Continued on next page*)

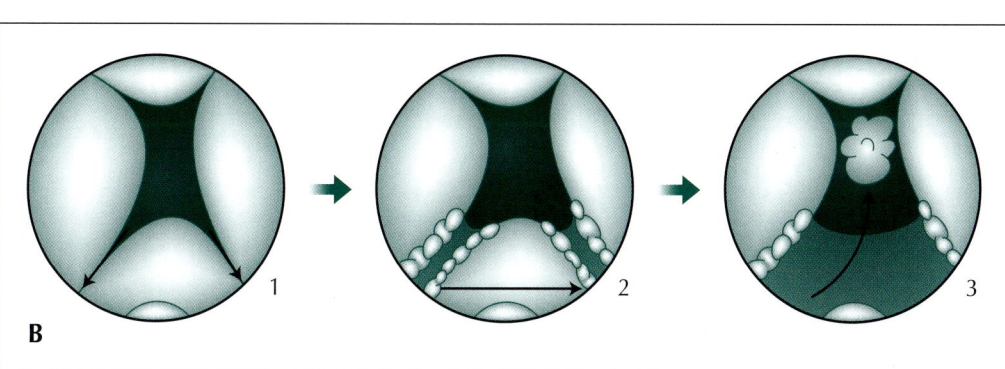

C. Enucleation of Lateral Lobes

Step	Description
4	Make a lateral apical incision on the right, extending from the 7-o'clock position circumferentially toward the 9-o'clock position, detaching the distal apex from the inner surface of the sphincter.
5	Lateral lobe, inferior separation: Undermine the right lateral lobe, always pointing the fiber in the direction of the capsule, working toward the bladder neck. It is important to work along broad planes and not in a deep, narrow "hole."
6	Make a 12-o'clock incision by rotating the scope 180° and cutting to the capsule from the bladder neck to the level of the veru montanum.
7	Lateral lobe, superior separation: Undermine the superior aspect of the lobe, working mainly from the bladder neck distally.
8	Superior apical attachment incision: Withdrawing the resectoscope to the level of the sphincter allows visualization of the remaining bridge of tissue attaching the lateral lobe on its apical end. Judiciously incise the mucosa at this point, cutting from the apex toward the bladder neck until the lateral lobe is enucleated and pushed into the bladder.
9	Repeat steps 4–8 (omitting step 6) in a mirror-image fashion on the left side until the left lobe is enucleated and pushed into the bladder.
10	A standard tissue morcellator with reciprocating blades can be introduced transurethrally through a 27-French nephroscope for removal of the enucleated prostatic lobes. To reduce the risk of bladder injury, tissue morcellation can be done within the prostatic fossa.

▶ **FIGURE 5-12.** (*Continued*) **C** and **D**, Enucleation of the lateral lobes (steps 4 through 10). HoLEP is a technically challenging procedure with a steep learning curve, requiring an estimated 20 cases to learn in the hands of an experienced resectionist [8]. (*Adapted from* Gilling *et al.* [9].)

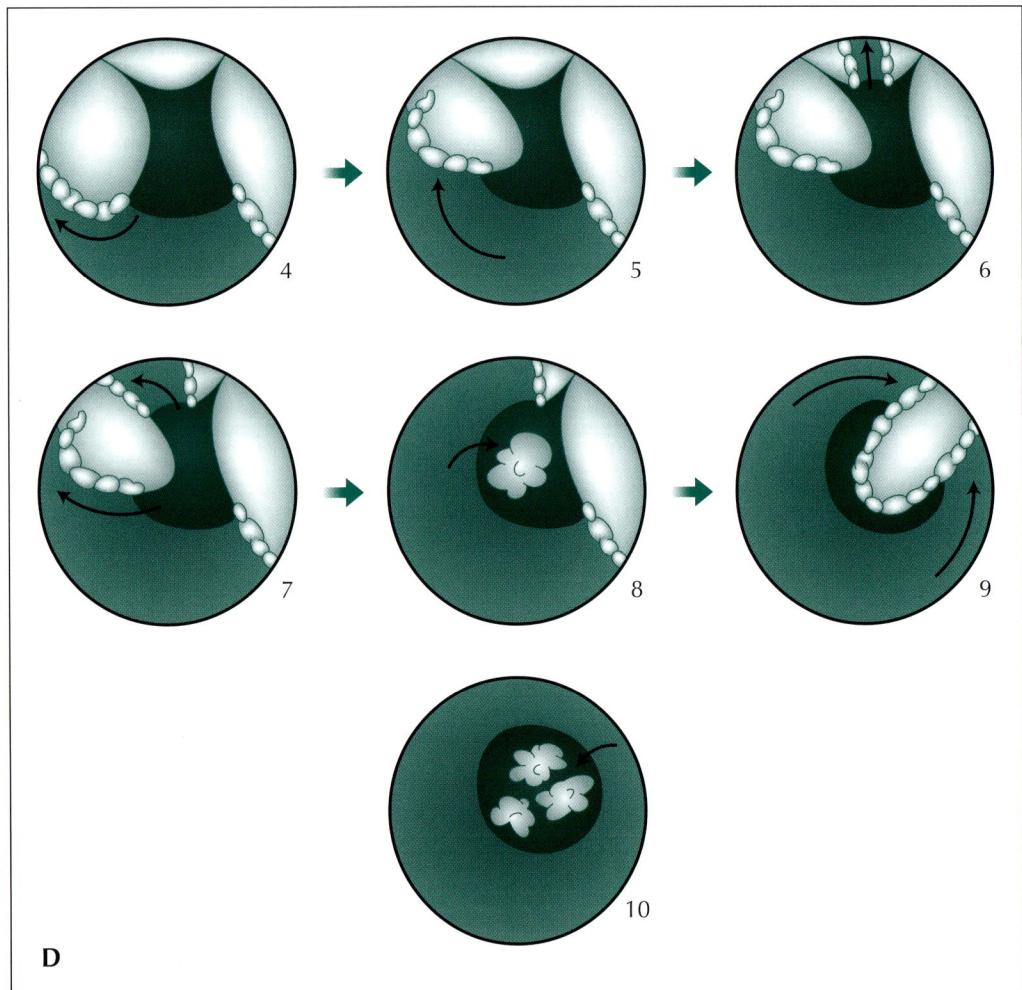

D

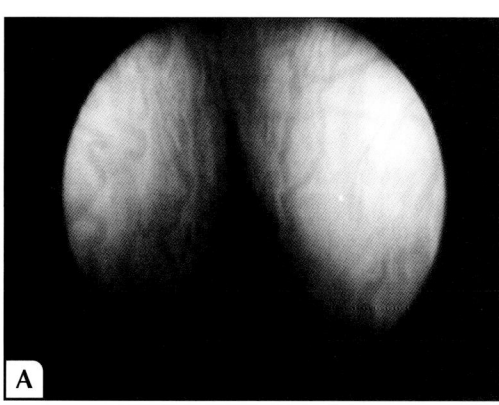

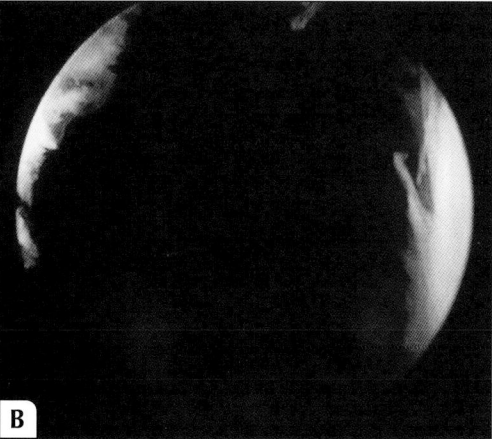

▶ **FIGURE 5-13.** Complete hemostatic holmium:yttrium aluminum garnet laser removal of all obstructing prostatic tissue. **A,** Preoperative view of obstructing prostatic tissue. **B,** Immediate hemostatic postoperative view of unobstructed prostatic fossa after holmium enucleation. (*Images courtesy of* John N. Kabalin, MD)

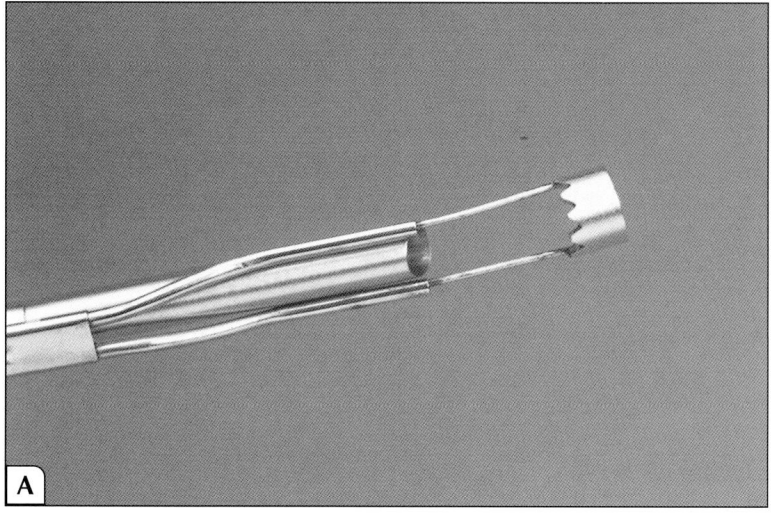

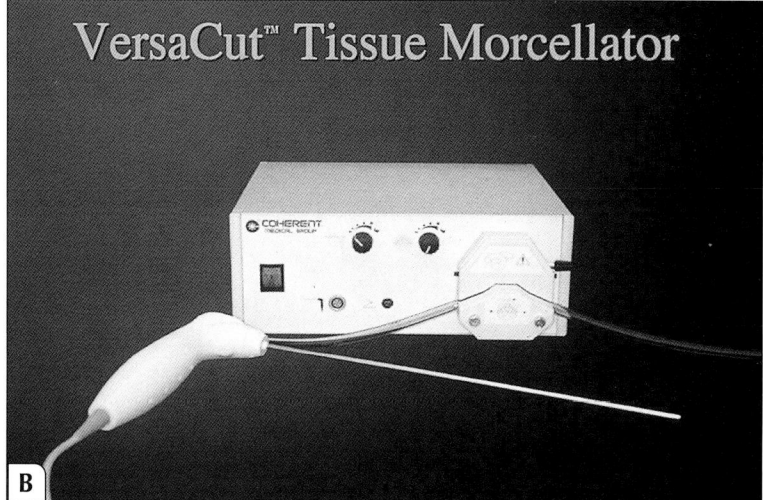

▶ **FIGURE 5-14.** Tools for excising prostate tissue segments. **A,** During holmium laser resection of the prostate, larger pieces of tissue can be grasped with a special loop designed to fit a standard resectoscope working element and can be used to grab and extract tissue from the bladder. **B,** During holmium laser enucleation of the prostate, enucleated prostate tissue is drawn into the reciprocating blades of a specially designed morcellator (Coherent Versacut Morcellator; Luminis, Palo Alto, CA) that uses concurrent high-powered suction. This allows simultaneous aspiration through the hollow lumen of the inner blade and collection in a sieve. Care must be taken not to insert the tip of the morcellator more than 1 to 2 cm beyond the tip of the nephroscope, and the tip must be visible at all times. A distended bladder is needed to keep the bladder mucosa from being drawn into the blades, causing serious bladder injuries by quickly stripping mucosa off the detrusor. A morcellator efficiency of up to 5 to 10 g/minute is routine [11]. (*Images courtesy of* John N. Kabalin, MD)

A. HoLEP Versus TURP: Adverse Events

Event	HoLEP, n (%)	TURP, n (%)
Initial follow-up		
Bladder mucosal injury*	10 (18.2)	0
Reintervention for bleeding	1 (1.7)	1 (2.2)
Transurethral resection syndrome	0	1 (2.2)
Early acute urinary retention	3 (5.3)	1 (2.2)
Dysuria (burning)†	33 (58.9)	13 (29.5)
Transient urge incontinence	25 (44)	17 (38.6)
6–12-month follow-up		
Urethral stricture	1 (1.7)	4 (7.4
Stress incontinence	1 (1.7)	1 (2.2)

*P = 0.0012
†P = 0.0002

B. HoLEP Versus TURP: Perioperative Data

Parameter	HoLEP, mean	TURP, mean	P Value
Operative time, *min*	74	57	< 0.05
Resected weight, *g*	36.08	25.4	< 0.05
Catheterization time, *h*	31	57.8	< 0.001
Hospital stay, *h*	59	85.8	< 0.001

Data from Montorsi et al. [12]

C. HoLEP Versus TURP: 1-Year Follow-up Data

Parameter	HoLEP, mean	TURP, mean	P Value
Peak flow rate, *mL/s*			
Preoperative	8.2	7.8	0.61
12-month postoperative	25.1	24.7	0.25
International Prostate Symptom Score			
Preoperative	21.6	21.9	0.83
12-month postoperative	4.1	3.9	0.58

Data from Montorsi et al. [12]

> **FIGURE 5-15.** Holmium laser enucleation of the prostate (HoLEP): outcomes. **A,** HoLEP versus transurethral resection of the prostate (TURP): adverse events in a prospective, randomized trial in 100 consecutive men with obstructive benign prostatic hyperplasia [12]. Because normal saline is used for irrigation, transurethral resection syndrome is not a complication of HoLEP. In contrast, bladder mucosal injury is more likely with HoLEP secondary to the need for tissue morcellation for removal of the enucleated prostate. Additionally, initial dysuria is more common in HoLEP patients, although there is no difference in voiding symptoms between TURP and HoLEP by 1 month post surgery [12]. A separate review of complications of 206 HoLEP procedures by Kuo *et al.* [13] reported similar findings. Specifically, they reported five clot retention episodes (2.4%), five urethral strictures (2.4%), eight bladder neck contractures (3.9%), and 16 patients requiring recatheterization (7.8%). Of interest, 20 of the 206 patients (9.7%) were found to have incidental adenocarcinoma of the prostate [13]. **B,** Perioperative data. **C,** One-year follow-up data. (*Adapted from* Montsori *et al.* [12].)

•• HOLMIUM LASER ABLATION OF THE PROSTATE ••

HoLAP Outcomes

Parameter	Preoperative	3 mo	7 y
Patients, *n*	79	79	34
Peak flow rate, *mL/s*	9.2	14.5	16.8
International Prostate Symptom Score	18.8	8.3	10

> **FIGURE 5-16.** Holmium laser ablation of the prostate (HoLAP): outcomes. Gilling *et al.* [14] first described the use of the holmium:yttrium aluminum garnet laser in a side-firing mode, described as holmium laser ablation of the prostate. The first studies of HoLAP described successful early removal of catheters and good clinical outcomes with this "vaporizing" wavelength, either alone or combined with the neodymium:yttrium aluminum garnet laser. Long-term outcomes from the initial series of 79 consecutive men who underwent HoLAP are summarized in the table [15].

Although the laser was able to achieve vaporization, removal of large tissue volumes was tedious and long given that true vaporization occurred in thin layers with a relatively thin underlying coagulation zone. Because of this, HoLAP has been relegated to a procedure suited only for smaller glands [16].

More recently, a 100-W side-firing holmium laser system has been released and is being promoted as an ablative treatment for small glands. However, it is a new technology that will still require scrutiny and long-term assessment. (*Adapted from* Gilling *et al.* [14].)

•• POTASSIUM-TITANYL-PHOSPHATE PHOTOSELECTIVE •• VAPORIZATION PROSTATECTOMY

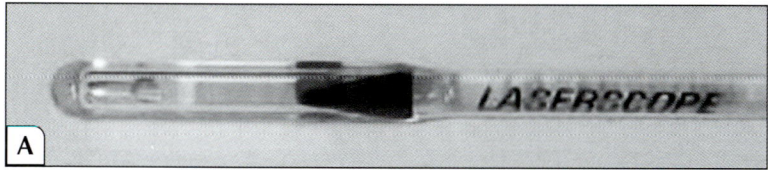

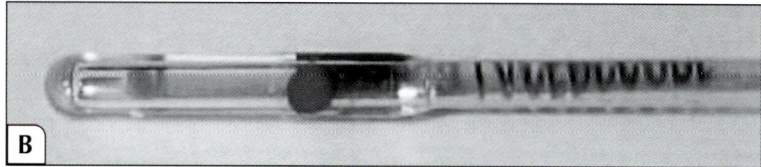

▶ **FIGURE 5-17.** Tools used with the potassium-titanyl-phosphate (KTP) laser. Doubling the frequency of pulsed neodymium:yttrium aluminum garnet (Nd:YAG) laser energy with a KTP crystal led to the creation of a 532-nm wavelength laser with substantially different tissue interaction properties compared with its parent [17]. Unlike the Nd:YAG wavelength, the KTP wavelength is selectively absorbed by hemoglobin, which acts as an intracellular chromophore. KTP laser energy is transparently delivered through a fluid medium such as water into the cell, where it is absorbed by hemoglobin, then rapidly heated, leading to rapid vaporization of tissue. This, in addition to the wavelength's short optical penetration into tissue, confines high-power laser energy to a superficial layer of prostatic tissue that is vaporized rapidly and hemostatically with only a 1- to 2-mm rim of coagulation. These selective characteristics led to the use of the KTP laser in prostatectomy being coined as "photoselective vaporization of the prostate".

Photoselective vaporization of the prostate is currently performed with an 80-W KTP side-firing laser (Laserscope; Greenlight PV, San Jose, CA) system through a 23-French continuous-flow cystoscope with normal saline as the irrigant. The Laserscope side-firing laser fiber has special markings on the tip to facilitate its safe use. When the blue arrow (**A**) is visualized, it indicates that the KTP laser beam fires from the opposite side of the telescope. The red octagonal "stop sign" (**B**) prompts the user to rotate the fiber to the proper lasing position.

Steps in Photoselective Vaporization Prostatectomy

Step	Description
1	Starting at the median lobe, vaporize using a sweeping "painting" motion to the level of the transverse fibers of the prostatic capsule.
2	Remove tissue from the bladder neck to the veru montanum.
3	Continue with the same technique while rotating to each lateral lobe.
4	Remove tissue from the bladder neck to the veru montanum bilaterally.
5	Continue with technique, rotating 180° for the anterior lobe.
6	At the end of the procedure, inspect the bladder and prostate for effective hemostasis.

Note: The laser fiber should be maintained at a near-contact position for the most effective vaporization. Bubbling is the result of the vaporization, and its visualization is an important sign of effective vaporization. Increasing the laser spot size (decreasing power density) by increasing the distance between the fiber and the tissue may result in more coagulation when appropriate.

▶ **FIGURE 5-18.** Photoselective vaporization of the prostate (PVP): technique. PVP is technically easy to perform, especially compared with holmium laser enucleation of the prostate, as described in Figure 5-12. The procedure may be performed with a range of anesthetics, from a local prostate block with intravenous sedation, to a regional anesthetic, to general anesthesia. PVP may be performed in high-risk patients, such as those anticoagulated with heparin, warfarin, nonsteroidal anti-inflammatory drugs, or aspirin. Often, no postoperative irrigation is required, and catheter time is relatively short. Many patients do not even require postoperative catheters. The table summarizes the steps involved in PVP [18].

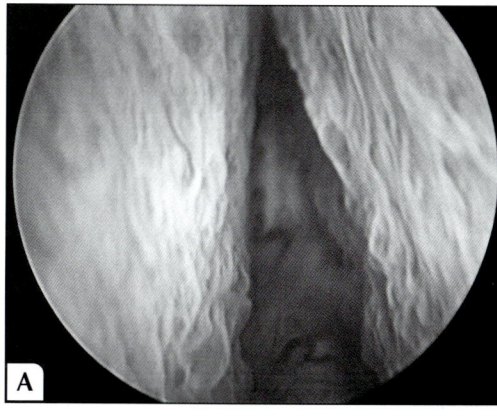

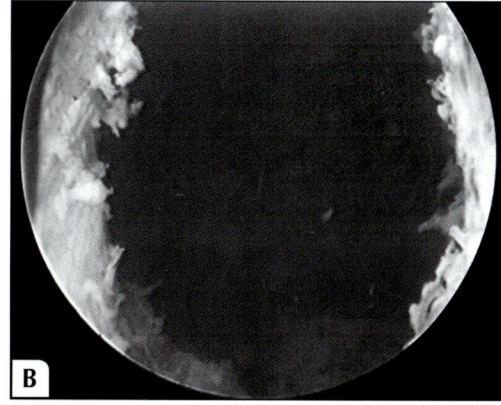

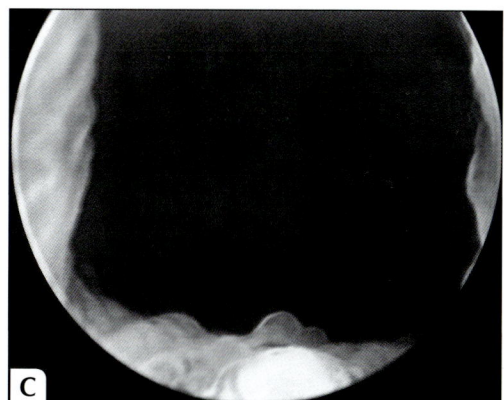

▶ **FIGURE 5-19.** Endoscopic views of the prostate before and after photoselective vaporization of the prostate (PVP). **A,** Preoperative view of trilobar prostatic obstruction. **B,** Immediate postoperative view after PVP. Note the hemostasis achieved with the potassium-titanyl-phosphate laser. **C,** Three-month postoperative view showing no obstructing prostatic tissue and reepithelialized prostatic urethra.

PVP Outcomes

Parameter	Preoperative	1 mo	3 mo	6 mo	1 y
Patients, n	200	156	104	87	42
Peak flow rate, mL/s	8.5	19.4	19.3	20.9	16.6
International Prostate Symptom Score	18.4	10.7	8.9	7.4	7.9
Postvoid residual, mL	178	77	69	75	91

▶ **FIGURE 5-20.** Photoselective vaporization of the prostate (PVP): outcomes. The largest series reported to date was presented by Te *et al.* [19], who studied the first 200 consecutive men treated with PVP between 2002 and 2004. Results from that trial are summarized in the table. Mean preoperative prostate volume by ultrasound was 89.6 ± 48 mL (range 22 to 274 mL) and mean age was 69 ± 10.1 years (range 44 to 103 mL). Forty-five patients were in retention. Mean operative time per procedure was 96 ± 65 minutes. Anesthesia included intravenous sedation with perineal prostate block (*n* = 76), spinal anesthesia (*n* = 62), and general anesthesia (*n* = 62). All patients except five were discharged within 23 hours without significant complications. Serum sodium did not change significantly. Similar results confirming PVP as a safe, effective treatment for benign prostatic hyperplasia were published in a US multicenter prospective trial [20]. (*Adapted from* Te *et al.* [20].)

Complications of PVP

Complication	First Year Incidence, n (%)
Prolonged dysuria	13 (9.4)
Transient hematuria	12 (8.6)
Transient urge incontinence	9 (6.5)
Urinary tract infection (culture confirmed)	3 (2.2)
Urinary retention (requiring short-term recatheterization)	7 (5)
Bladder neck contracture	2 (1.4)
Urethral stricture	1 (0.7)
Epididymitis	1 (0.7)
Impotence	0
Reoperation for symptoms[+]	0

▶ **FIGURE 5-21.** Complications of photoselective vaporization of the prostate (PVP) in the first US multicenter prospective trial. In 139 men treated at six major US medical centers with 1-year follow-up, reported morbidities were generally minor and are summarized in the table [20]. The two bladder neck contractures (1.4%) occurred in patients with urodynamically proven bladder dysfunction. No postoperative erectile dysfunction was reported from patients who were potent preoperatively. At 1 year, no reoperation for persistent or recurring symptoms following treatment was observed.

In this series of 139 men, 75 reported being sexually active preoperatively. No adverse impact of PVP was evident on sexual activity or function. However, retrograde ejaculation was reported in 27 of 75 sexually active men (36%) at 1 year.

PVP in Anticoagulated Men

Anticoagulant	Patients, n
Warfarin	8
Aspirin	14
Clopidogrel	2

▶ **FIGURE 5-22.** Photoselective vaporization of the prostate (PVP) in anticoagulated men. Of the series described in Figure 5-20, 58 patients were on anticoagulants. A recent report detailed the use of PVP in the first 24 of these men [21]. Men on warfarin discontinued the drug 2 days prior to surgery and restarted it the day after the procedure. Clopidogrel and aspirin were not discontinued.

Mean preoperative prostate volume was 78 mL (range 34 to 164 mL). Mean age was 75 years. Nine men (38%) were in urinary retention. Eight patients (33%) had a previous myocardial infarction. Seven men (29%) had cerebrovascular disease, and seven (29%) had peripheral vascular disease. Mean operative time was 101 minutes. No perioperative transfusions were required. All men were discharged within 23 hours without significant complications. Twenty-two men (92%) were discharged without a catheter. Serum sodium and hematocrit did not change significantly (140.5 mmol/L and 39.0% to 139.5 mmol/L and 38.3%). Similar to results from PVP series of patients not on anticoagulants, International Prostate Symptom Score decreased to 13.2, 10.9, 9.7, and 11.1 at 1, 3, 6, and 12 months, respectively, from 18.7 preoperatively. Peak flow rate increased from 9.0 mL/s preoperatively to 15.7, 16.3, 21.7, and 22.4 mL/s at 1, 3, 6, and 12 months, respectively [21]. No patients had clinically significant hematuria postoperatively and none developed clot retention.

PVP for Men With Large Prostates

Parameter	Preoperative	1 mo	3 mo	6 mo	1 y
Patients, n	64	57	42	42	25
Peak flow rate, mL/s	7.9	16.4	16.2	20.6	18.9
International Prostate Symptom Score	18.4	9.9	8.6	7.2	6.7
Postvoid residual, mL	152	78	78	67	109

▶ **FIGURE 5-23.** Photoselective vaporization of the prostate (PVP) for men with large prostates. PVP has been shown to be safe and effective in the treatment of men with large prostates (> 60 mL) [22]. A total of 64 men with symptomatic benign prostatic hyperplasia and large-volume prostates underwent photoselective laser vaporization of the prostate between May 2002 and September 2003. Medical therapy had failed in all men, and 18 presented with urinary retention. PVP was performed with an 80-W potassium-titanyl-phosphate side-firing laser system through a 23-French continuous-flow cystoscope with normal saline as the irrigant.

Mean preoperative prostate volume was 101 mL (range 60 to 247 mL). The average age and American Society of Anesthesiology (ASA) class were 70.1 years and 2.2. Mean operative time per procedure was 121 minutes. Anesthesia included intravenous sedation and prostate block (n = 28), spinal anesthesia (n = 28), and general anesthesia (n = 8). No transfusions were required. Average length of stay was 0.9 days. Twelve patients (19%) were discharged the same day, and 62 (97%) by postoperative day 1. The serum sodium level did not change significantly. Two patients needed staged procedures, two had self-limited postoperative urinary retention, four developed retrograde ejaculation, and one developed clot retention postoperatively that resolved after irrigation. Three patients (5%) needed reoperation for return of symptoms within 1 year [21].

A. Steps in PVP-VIT for Large Prostates

Step	
1	Starting at the median lobe, create a midline "incision" from the trigone to the veru montanum.
Note:	*The vaporization is not done as traditionally defined, with large slow, sweeping motions. Instead use quick sweeping motions and proximal-distal movement of the fiber to create the grooves. The fact that bubbles are still being created confirms that efficient vaporization is occurring.*
2	Create a lateral groove on one side of the median lobe, aiming just lateral to the ipsilateral ureteral orifice. Deepen this groove until it is level from the veru montanum to the trigone.
3	Vaporize the tissue between these two grooves with larger, sweeping motions. Small fragments of tissue can be "excised" between these two grooves and swept by irrigation into the bladder. These can be removed later with an Ellick evacuator.
4	Repeat this procedure on the contralateral side until the median lobe is completely removed.
	Lateral Lobes
5	Use the same technique to create incisions at 11 o'clock and 1 o'clock from the bladder neck to the level of the veru montanum.
6	Vaporize the tissue between the upper incision and the inferior prostatic fossa with larger, sweeping motions. Small fragments of tissue can be "excised" between these two grooves and swept by irrigation into the bladder. These can be removed later with an Ellick evacuator.
7	Once both lateral lobes have been vaporized, the anterior prostate should be vaporized between the 11-o'clock and 1-o'clock incisions from the level of the bladder neck to the veru montanum.
8	Finally, right and left apical tissue should be carefully vaporized with the cystoscope positioned at—but looking away from—the veru montanum. Care should be taken to avoid backscatter that may injure the ejaculatory ducts if they are in close proximity.
9	At the end of the procedure, inspect the bladder and prostate for effective hemostasis.

▶ **FIGURE 5-24.** Photoselective vaporization of the prostate vaporization-incision technique (PVP-VIT) for large prostates. PVP is effective but time consuming for the treatment of men with large (> 60 mL), obstructing prostates. **A** and **B**, Steps in the PVP-VIT—a novel method for vaporizing larger prostates in a more time-effective manner. This technique also ensures adequate removal of tissue through the use of anatomic landmarks. The same potassium-titanyl-phosphate laser equipment and setting at 80 W are used, and postoperative care is identical.

(*Continued on next page*)

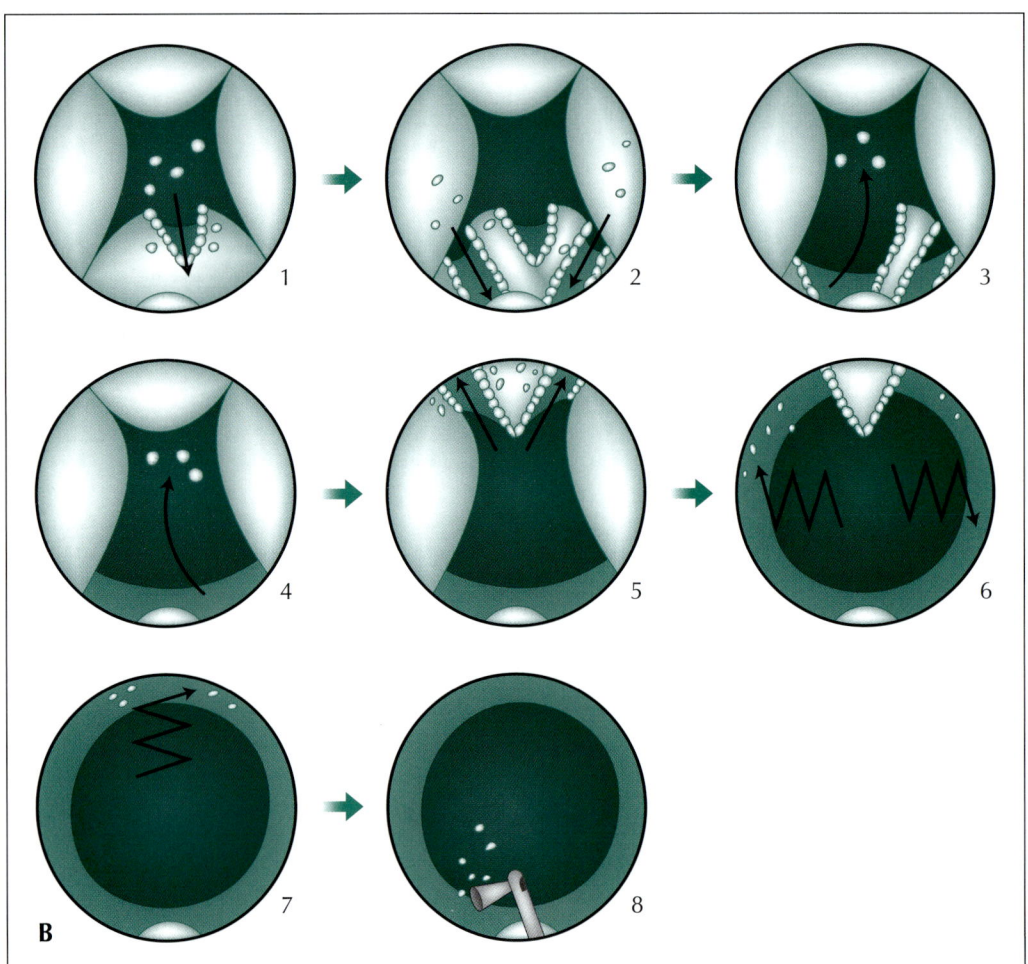

FIGURE 5-24. (*Continued*) The first 20 patients who underwent PVP-VIT had an average prostate volume of 123 mL. The procedure took an average time of 135 minutes, equating to roughly 1.10 min/mL. This compares to an average volume of 101 mL and a time of 1.24 min/mL during our previous large-gland series [21,22]. Early results indicate that the International Prostate Symptom Score decreased by 9.7 points and maximum flow rates increased by 6.1 mL/s at 1 month and 10.3 points and 11.7 mL/s at 3 months. There continues to be no development of dilutional hyponatremia, and no blood transfusions have been needed to date [23].

INTERSTITIAL LASER COAGULATION OF THE PROSTATE

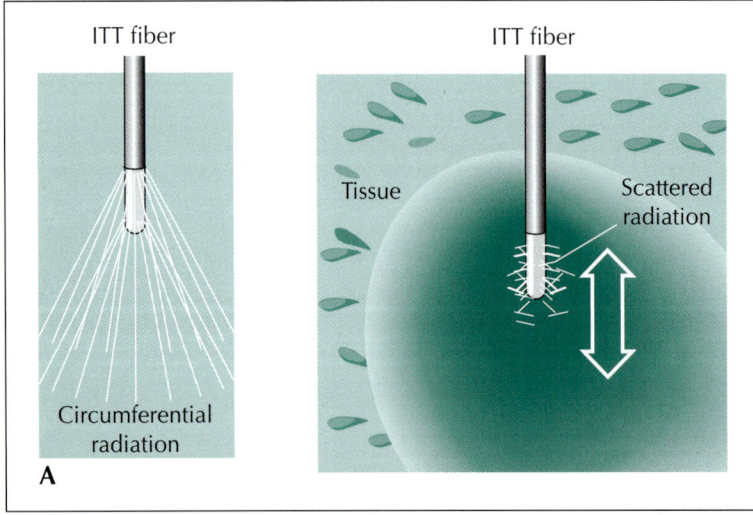

FIGURE 5-25. Interstitial laser coagulation (ILC) of the prostate. ILC is performed using specialized laser delivery fibers that are inserted transurethrally directly into the obstructing benign prostatic hyperplasia (BPH) tissue. These interstitial thermal therapy (ITT) fibers are designed to emit diffuse laser radiation circumferentially along the distal segment of the fiber. A neodymium:yttrium aluminum garnet or semiconductor diode laser is typically used to perform ILC. In contrast to the free-beam laser prostatectomy approaches described previously, ILC selectively targets BPH tissue deep to the prostatic urethral surface, attempting to spare the urethral mucosa. **A,** Using a diffusing ITT laser fiber buried within the BPH adenoma, a timed laser application is performed with radiation of laser energy and resulting thermal effects, creating a zone of coagulation necrosis within the prostate.

(*Continued on next page*)

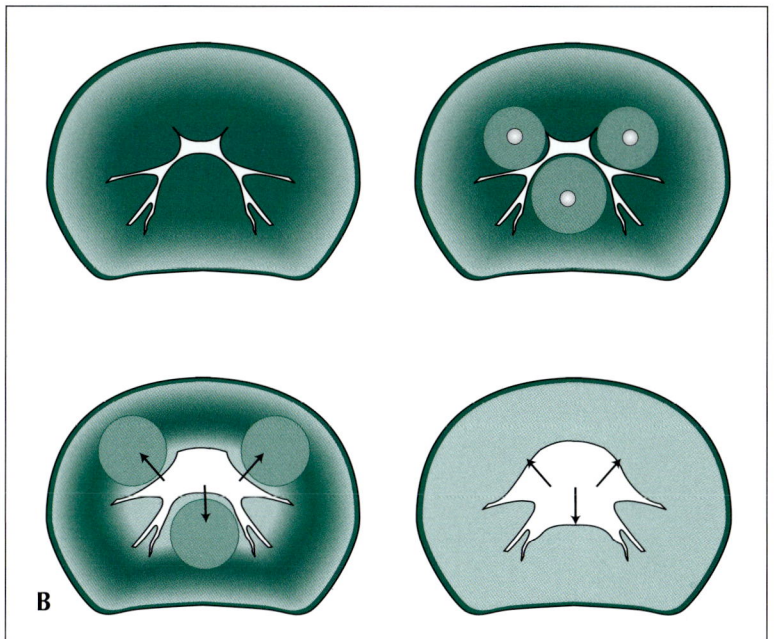

▶ **FIGURE 5-25.** (*Continued*) **B,** Multiple interstitial laser applications
are repeated, depending on the size of the prostate, encompassing obstructive medial lobe and lateral lobe tissue. During the next several weeks, the
resulting zones of coagulation necrosis undergo involution with gradual
reduction in prostate volume to relieve bladder outlet obstruction. (*Images
courtesy of* John N. Kabalin, MD)

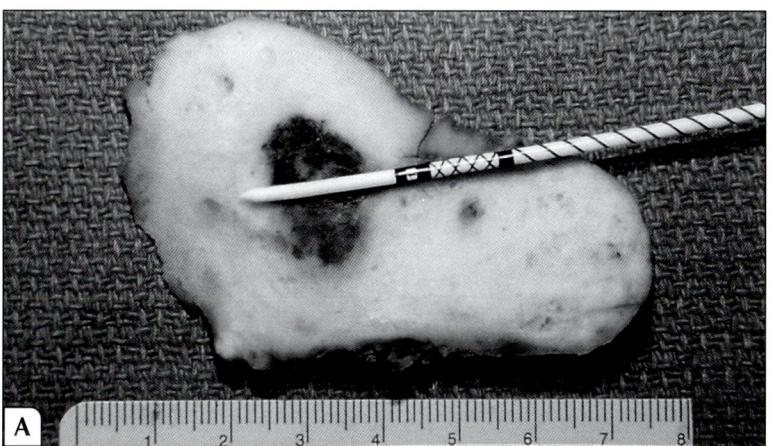

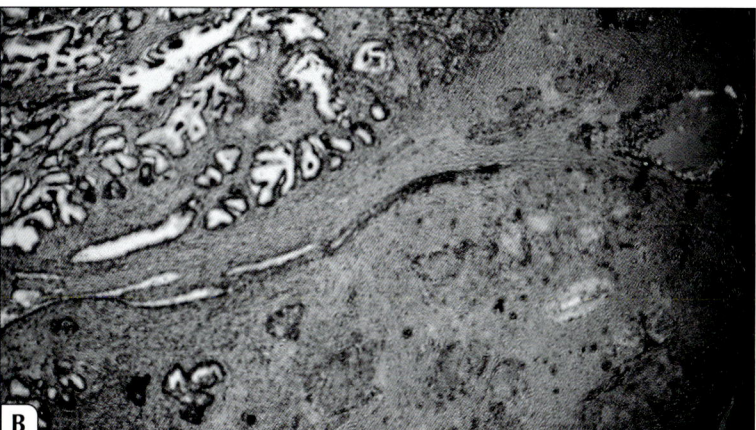

▶ **FIGURE 5-26.** Interstitial laser coagulation (ILC)-induced coagulation
necrosis; regions of coagulation necrosis in a prostatectomy specimen. **A,** An
open prostatectomy specimen removed 5 days after ILC with the laser fiber
positioned to recreate treatment conditions. The *dark area* represents coagulation and hemorrhagic necrosis. The coagulation zone correlates with the
predicted region of treatment based on the diffusing delivery fiber. **B,** A

photomicrograph demonstrating the necrosis grossly identified in *panel A.*
The lower half demonstrates necrosis. Note the sharp demarcation between
the treated zone and the untreated benign prostatic hyperplasia tissue.
Indigo interstitial fiber (Indigo Medical, Cincinnati, OH) shown in *panel A.*
(*Images courtesy of* John N. Kabalin, MD)

Complications of Interstitial Laser Coagulation of the Prostate in 239 Men With 1-Year Postoperative Follow-up

	Incidence, n(%)
Acute complications	
Significant hemorrhage/transfusion	1 (0.4)
Transurethral resection syndrome	0 (0)
Prostatic perforation/extravasation	0 (0)
Urinary tract infection/epididymitis	6 (2.5)
Long-term complications	
Stress urinary incontinence	1 (0.4)
Urethral stricture	9 (3.8)
Bladder neck contracture	4 (1.7)
Reoperation for residual tissue	23 (9.6)

▶ **FIGURE 5-27.** Complications of interstitial laser coagulation (ILC) of the
prostate in 239 men with 1-year postoperative follow-up. ILC of the prostate is
typically performed as an outpatient procedure. Postoperatively, patients experience significant prostatic edema and require catheter drainage of the bladder
for at least several days after treatment. Although acute complications associated with ILC therapy are uncommon, the long-term reoperation rate for
residual benign prostatic hyperplasia tissue is relatively high compared with
other operative techniques. (*Data from* Muschter and Hofstetter [24].)

Voiding Outcomes of ILC of the Prostate

Parameter	Preoperative (n = 239)	Postoperative		
		3 mo (n = 239)	6 mo (n = 216)	12 mo (n = 198)
Peak flow rate, mL/s	7.7	16.3	17.9	17.8
Postvoid residual, mL	151	32	18	19
International Prostate Symptom Score	25.4	8.1	6.1	6.1

▶ **FIGURE 5-28.** Interstitial laser coagulation (ILC): outcomes. ILC is capable of producing good voiding outcomes with a minimally invasive approach. However, there is great variability in published results, possibly because of different technical approaches to ILC [25]. Persistent postoperative irritative symptoms, as well as the need for prolonged catheterization, have made methods that employ coagulative necrosis (*ie*, ILC and visual laser ablation of the prostate) less favorable options when compared with ablative procedures such as holmium laser enucleation of the prostate and photoselective vaporization of the prostate. (*Data from* Muschter and Hofstetter [24].)

REFERENCES

1. Johnson DE, Levinson AK, Greskovitch FJ, *et al.*: Transurethral laser prostatectomy using a right angle delivery system. *SPIE Proceedings* 1991, 1421:36–41.

2. Kabalin JN: Laser prostatectomy performed with a right angle firing Nd:YAG laser fiber at 40 watts power setting. *J Urol* 1993, 150:95–99.

3. Kabalin JN, Terris MK, Mancianti ML, *et al.*: Dosimetry studies utilizing the Urolase right angle firing Nd:YAG laser fiber in the human prostate. *Lasers Surg Med* 1996, 18:72–80.

4. Sengor F, Gurdal M, Tekin A, *et al.*: Neodymium:YAG visual laser ablation of the prostate: 7 years of experience with 230 patients. *J Urol* 2002, 167:184–187.

5. Kabalin JN, Gill HS, Bite G, Wolfe V: Comparative study of laser versus electrocautery prostatic resection: 18-month followup with complex urodynamic assessment. *J Urol* 1995, 153:94–97.

6. Kabalin JN, Bite J, Doll S: Neodymium: YAG laser coagulation prostatectomy: 3 years of experience with 227 patients. *J Urol* 1996, 155:181–185.

7. Carter A, Sells H, Speakman M, *et al.*: Quality of life changes following KTP/Nd:YAG laser treatment of the prostate and TURP. *Eur Urol* 1999, 36:92–98.

8. El-Hakim A, Elhilali MM: Holmium laser enucleation of the prostate can be taught: the first learning experience. *BJU Int* 2002, 90:863–869.

9. Gilling PJ, Cass CB, Creswell MD, Fraundorfer MR: Holmium laser resection of the prostate: preliminary results of a new method for the treatment of benign prostatic hyperplasia. *Urology* 1996, 47:48–51.

10. Kabalin JN: Holmium:YAG laser prostatectomy: results of US pilot study. *J Endourol* 1996, 10:453–457.

11. Gilling PJ: Holmium laser enucleation of the prostate for glands larger than 100 g: an endourologic alternative to open prostatectomy. *J Endourol* 2000, 14:529–531.

12. Montorsi F, Naspro R, Salonia A, *et al.*: Holmium laser enucleation versus transurethral resection of the prostate: results from a 2-center, prospective, randomized trial in patients with obstructive benign prostatic hyperplasia. *J Urol* 2004, 172(5 Pt 1):1926–1929.

13. Kuo RL, Paterson RF, Siqueira TM Jr, *et al.*: Holmium laser enucleation of the prostate: morbidity in a series of 206 patients. *Urology* 2003, 62:59–63.

14. Gilling P, Cass C, Malcolm A, Fraundorfer M: Combination holmium and Nd:YAG laser ablation of the prostate: initial clinical experience. *J Endourol* 1995, 9:151–153.

15. Tan AH, Gilling PJ, Kennett KM, *et al.*: Long-term results of high-power holmium laser vaporization (ablation) of the prostate. *BJU Int.* 2003, 92:707–709.

16. Patterson RF, Lingeman JE: Holmium laser prostatectomy. *Curr Urol Rep* 2001, 2:269–276.

17. Kuntzman RS, Malek R, Barrett DM, Bostwick DG: Potassium-titanyl-phosphate laser vaporization of the prostate: a comparative functional and pathologic study in canines. *Urology* 1996, 48:575–583.

18. Gonzalez RR, Te AE: Photoselective vaporization of the prostate with the 80 watt quasicontinuous KTP laser for the treatment of benign prostatic hyperplasia. Video presented at American College of Surgeons, Cine Clinics, Clinical Congress. New Orleans, LA; October 12, 2004.

19. Te AE, Sandhu JS, Reddy B, *et al.*: The first 200 patients treated with high-power KTP photoselective laser vaporization prostatectomy: the New York Presbyterian experience. To be presented at the American Urological Association Annual Meeting. San Antonio, TX; May 21–26, 2005.

20. Te AE, Malloy TR, Stein BS, *et al.*: Photoselective vaporization of the prostate for the treatment of benign prostatic hyperplasia: 12-month results from the first United States multicenter prospective trial. *J Urol* 2004, 172(4 Pt 1):1404–1408.

21. Sandhu JS, Ng CK, Gonzalez RR, *et al.*: Photoselective vaporization prostatectomy in anticoagulated men. *J Endourol* 2004, 18(suppl 1):A3–A246.

22. Sandhu JS, Ng C, Vanderbrink BA, *et al.*: High-power potassium-titanyl-phosphate photoselective laser vaporization of prostate for treatment of benign prostatic hyperplasia in men with large prostates. *Urology* 2004, 64:1155–1159.

23. Sandhu JS, Te AE: Photoselective vaporization of the prostate—the vaporization incision technique (VIT) for large volume prostates. Video to be presented at the American Urological Association Annual Meeting. San Antonio, TX; May 21–26, 2005.

24. Muschter R, Hofstetter A: Technique and results of interstitial laser coagulation. *World J Urol* 1995, 13:109–114.

25. Muschter R, Gilling AP: Lasers for median lobe hyperplasia. *Curr Urol Rep* 2001, 2:306–310.

Transurethral Resection and Incision of the Prostate, and Open Prostatectomy for Benign Prostatic Hyperplasia

6

Jeetesh Bhardwa,
Roger S. Kirby,
& Rolf P. Muschter

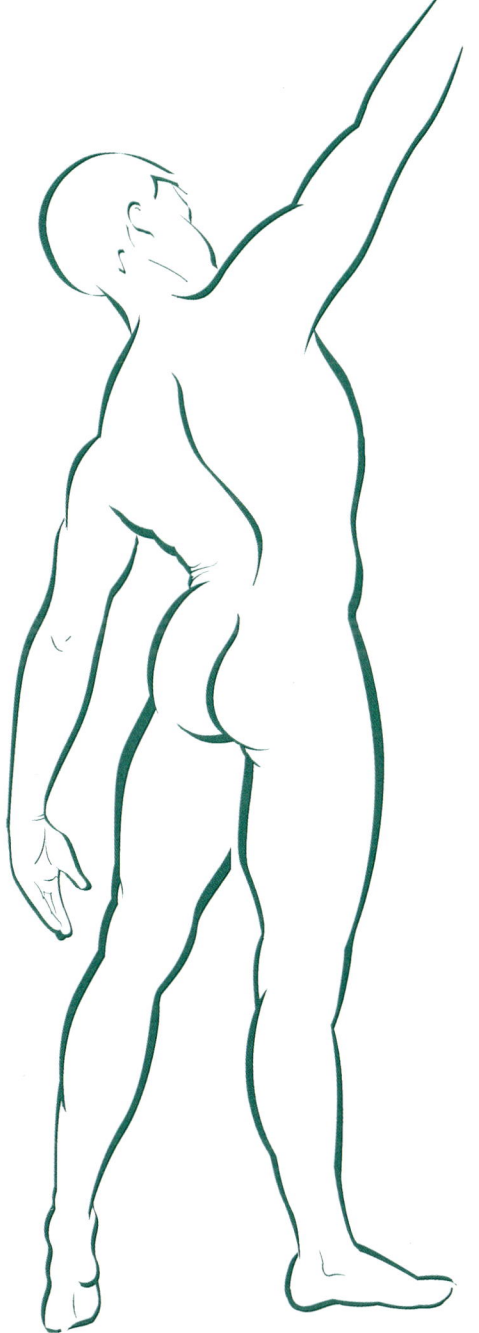

The most common surgical procedures for benign prostatic hyperplasia (BPH) are still transurethral (electro-) resection of the prostate (TURP) and transurethral incision of the prostate (TUIP). Newer technologies, however, increasingly challenge their position as the gold standard therapy for BPH. Development of the early resectoscope depended on many scientific advances, such as the cystoscope, the incandescent lamp, and the vacuum tube, which made possible the development of an electrosurgical unit for coagulation and cutting of tissue. Modern transurethral resection and incision are based on improved materials and engineering, fiberoptic light sources, rod lens systems, video cameras, and high-tech electrosurgery generators. Open prostatectomy also improved with the developments of modern surgery, such as anesthesia, blood transfusion, and antibiotics. Common techniques employ the perineal, retropubic, and suprapubic transvesical approachs.

Certain complications of BPH are considered a definite requirement for surgical intervention. These complications are acute refractory urinary retention, recurrent urinary tract infection, recurrent hematuria, bladder stones, and renal insufficiency secondary to obstructing BPH.

TURP and TUIP remain the gold standard operations for treating bladder outflow obstruction due to BPH. However, the number of TURPs performed has declined significantly. This is partly the result of the emergence of new technologies, such as lasers, and the refinement in procedures such as microwave therapy and ultrasound needle ablation, which has led these procedures to gain ground on the more traditional operations as well inroads made by pharmacotherapy in the treatment of lower urinary tract symptoms (LUTS).

Many urologists have accepted these newer approaches as they solve some of the problems posed by TURP and TUIP. The newer procedures have a shorter length of inpatient stay associated with them; they also require a shorter duration of anesthesia and can often be done under local or regional anesthesia or sedation. These factors therefore make procedures such as laser prostatectomy, microwave therapy, and needle ablation more appealing.

The morbidity and mortality of TURP are quite low but still exist, as described below. Figures in parentheses denote complication rates according to the National Prostatectomy Audit carried out in the United Kingdom [1]. Perioperative complications included:

- Bleeding leading to the operation being halted (0.7%)
- Cardiorespiratory problems (1.4%)
- Rectal perforation and extravasation (0.5%)
- Conversion to open prostatectomy (0.2%)

Early postoperative complications included:

- Urinary tract infection (2.7%)
- Return to theater due to bleeding (0.6%)
- Chest infection, septicemia (2.2%)
- Cardiorespiratory problems (1.9%)
- TURP syndrome (0.5%)
- Failure of a trial without a catheter, necessitating sending the patient home with a catheter (9.2%)

Late postoperative complications included:

- Difficulty in micturition due to clots (10%)
- Epididymitis (5%)
- Intervention by general practitioner, including prescription for antibiotics (32%)
- Retrograde ejaculation (68%)
- Erectile dysfunction (31%)
- Urinary incontinence (6%)
- Urethral strictures (3.1%)

The overall mortality rate for TURP was 1% at 30 days and 3.4% at 90 days.

Following TURP, about 64% of patients report an improvement in symptoms; however, up to a quarter of all men who undergo TURP fail to report any significant change in their symptomatology as measured by American Urological Association symptom scores or quality-of-life/bother scores.

The question that is now being put to urologists is, Given that the rate of major inpatient complications following TURP is 10% and more than 35% of patients develop some complications after discharge, should TURP be reserved for men with retention, bladder stones, and recurrent urinary stones and should symptomatic patients with LUTS be offered treatment only with less-invasive therapies, such as those mentioned above?

The TUIP procedure is best performed in smaller glands with a minimal amount of lateral lobe tissue and a high posterior lip of the bladder. In such cases, it is a safe and effective method, with its main advantages being reductions in operative time, bleeding, and incidence of retrograde ejaculation.

Open prostatectomy certainly removes more completely all adenomatous tissue and achieves the best clinical results with the lowest retreatment rate; however, it has a considerable morbidity rate and a small mortality rate. Conversely, TURP in patients with very large glands (ie, > 100 g) may be associated with significant fluid absorption, intraoperative bleeding, and intraoperative and immediate postoperative complications. Therefore, the open procedure usually is reserved for patients with larger glands (ie, > 100 g). The decision whether to do a TURP or open prostatectomy depends on the urologist's surgical skills in resecting larger glands.

POSITIONING FOR SURGERY

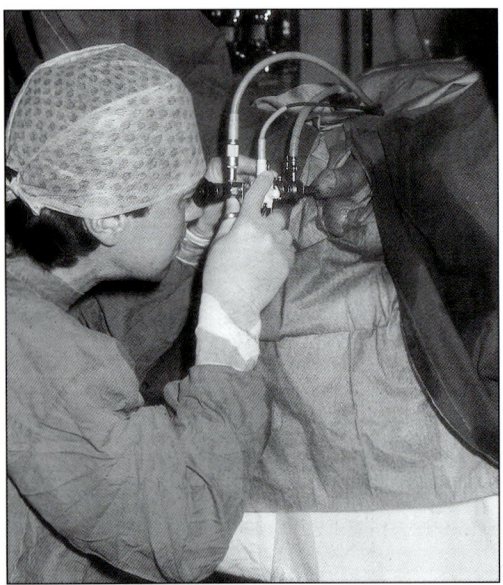

▶ **FIGURE 6-1.** Patient positioning and operating room equipment for performing transurethral resection and incision of the prostate. The patient is on the operating table in a lithotomy position.

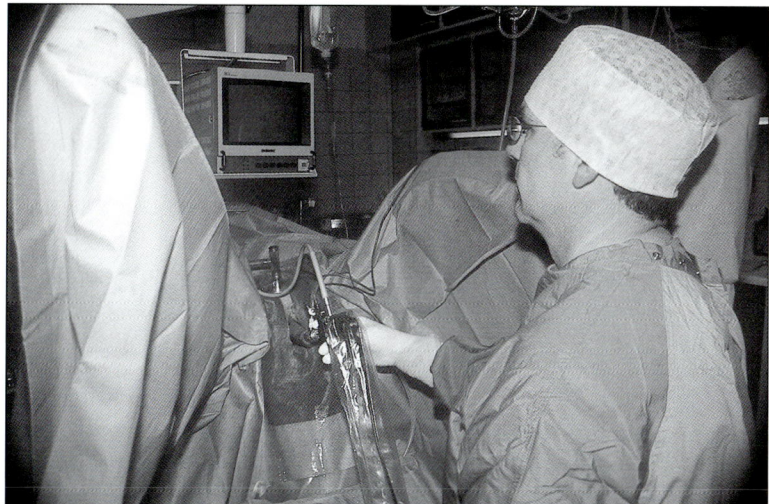

▶ **FIGURE 6-2.** Position of the surgeon performing a video-assisted transurethral resection of the prostate.

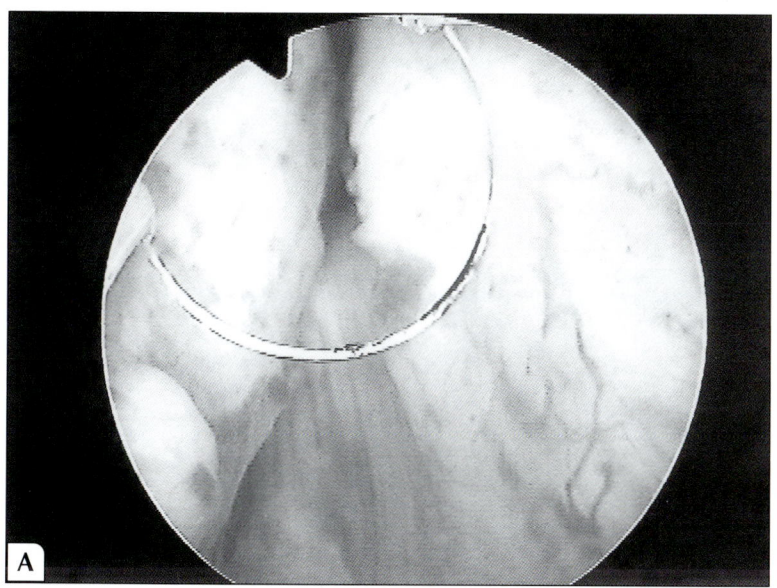

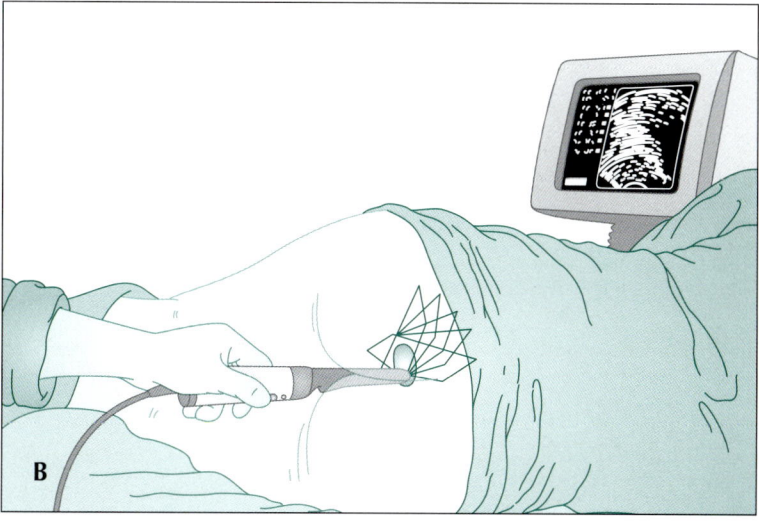

▶ **FIGURE 6-3. A,** Endoscopic view of benign prostatic hyperplasia (BPH). This view before resection shows the relationship of the prostate lobes to the bladder and verumontanum and the size of the loop.

B, Patient positioning in transrectal ultrasound scan of the prostate. Although transrectal ultrasound is not routinely used in the management of BPH, it is more accurate than digital rectal examination in determining prostate size.

C, A large intravesical component of the prostate. The size of such a prostate would be underestimated by digital rectal examination. It is the median lobe of the prostate that causes the most severe symptoms, and it may lead to urinary retention by acting as a flap valve over the bladder neck.

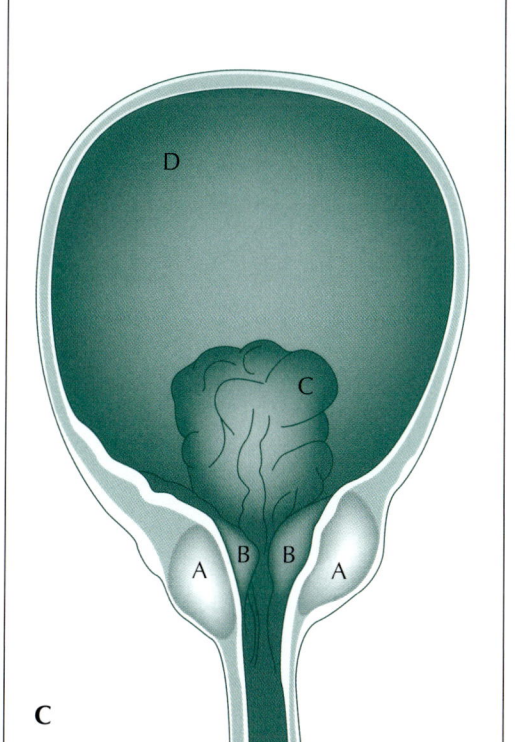

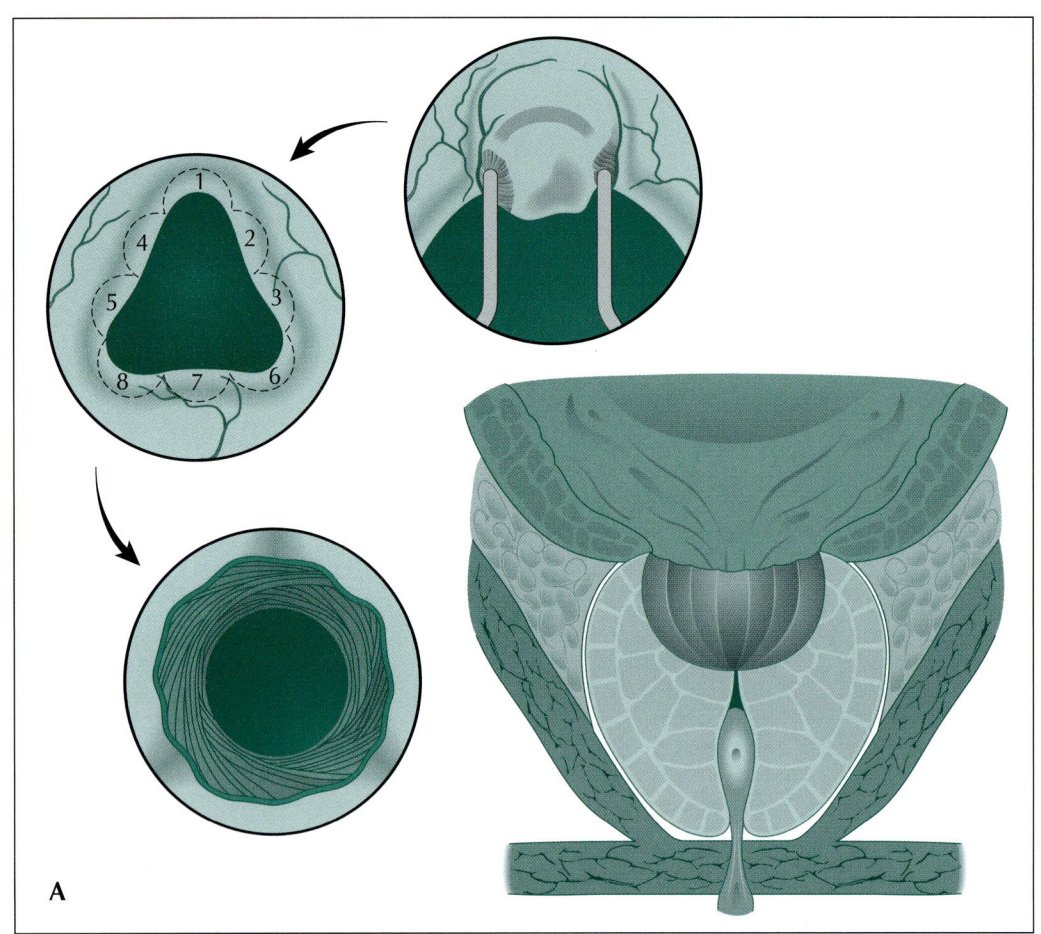

▶ **FIGURE 6-4.** Transurethral resection of the prostate (TURP): stage 1. **A,** Schematic representation of stage 1. There are a number of ways of resecting the prostate, but all should be done in a step-by-step, orderly fashion to control the bleeding so that a precise anatomic dissection of the adenoma can be done. The Nesbit three-staged technique is illustrated here. The bladder is distended with approximately 100 mL of fluid to demarcate more clearly the prostate, the bladder neck, and the bladder wall. An initial cut is made anteriorly at 12 o'clock with the resectoscope loop. The incision is carried deeply until the seemingly circular fibers of the bladder neck are exposed. The resection is carried to approximately the 3 o'clock position, and bleeding points are carefully controlled. The resection is then continued counterclockwise from 12 to 9 o'clock, in a similar fashion. The resection is completed from the 3 to 9 o'clock position. **B,** Deep anterior cut at 12 o'clock. **C,** First incision of the anterior part of the right side lobe. **D,** Incompletely resected prostatic fossa at the end of stage 1 of TURP.

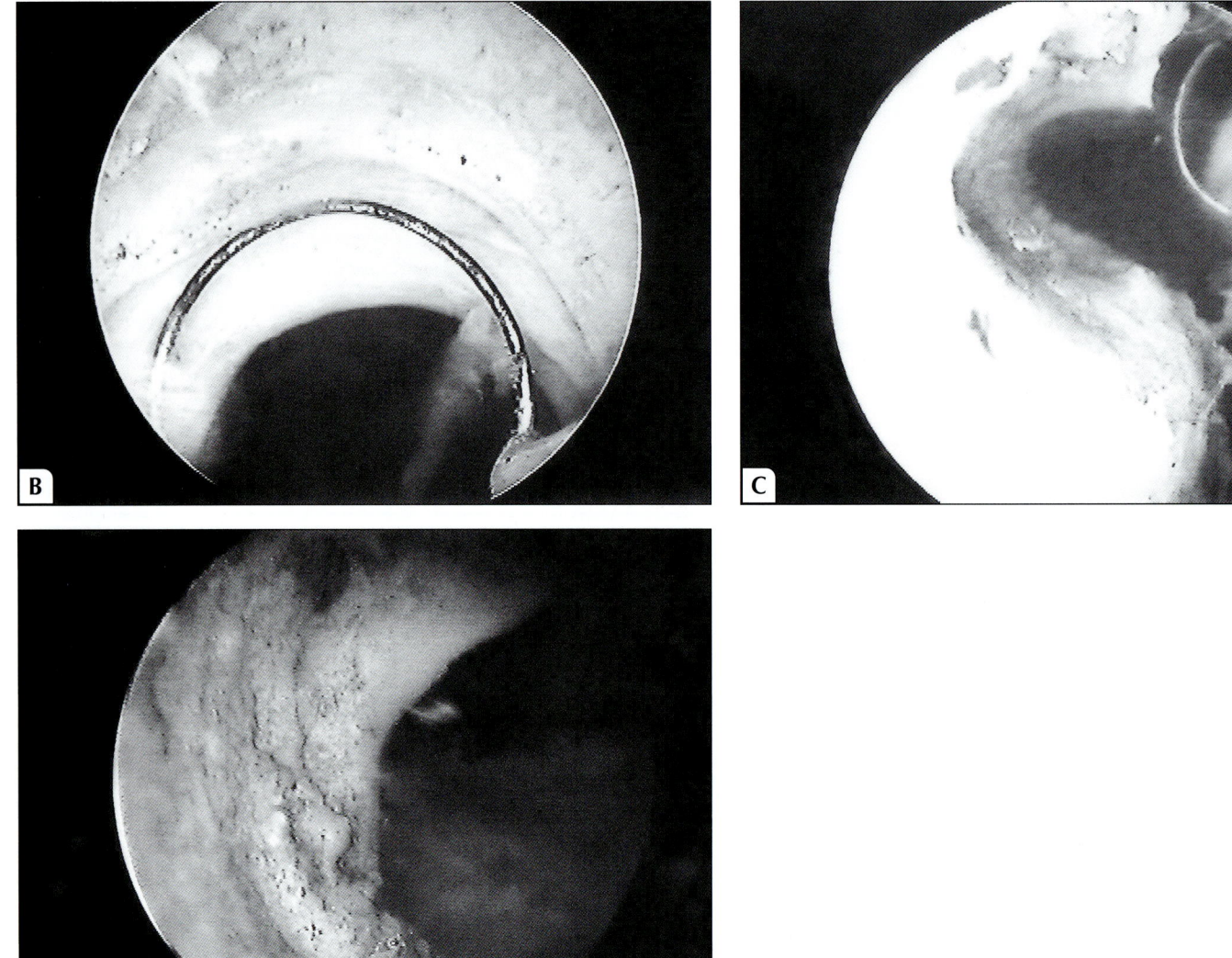

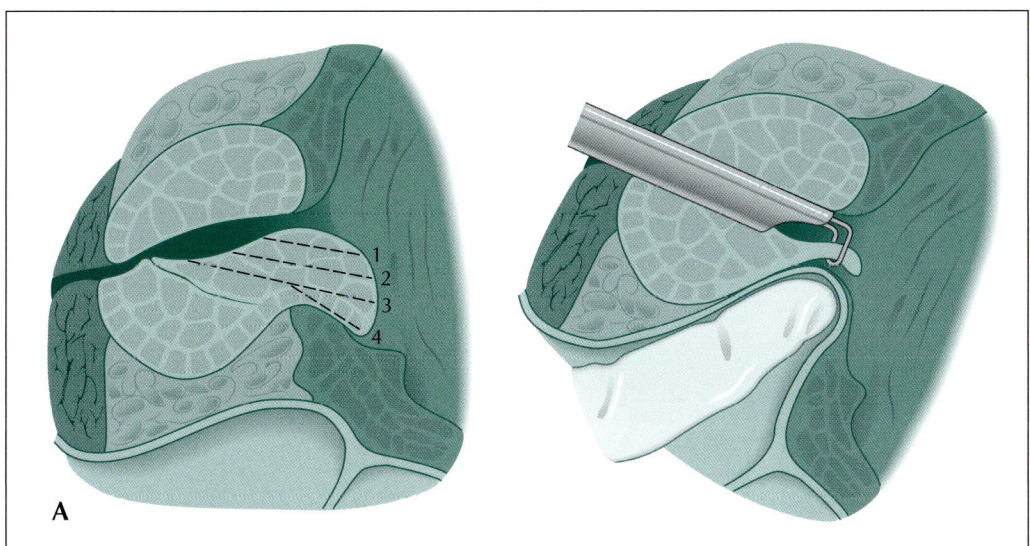

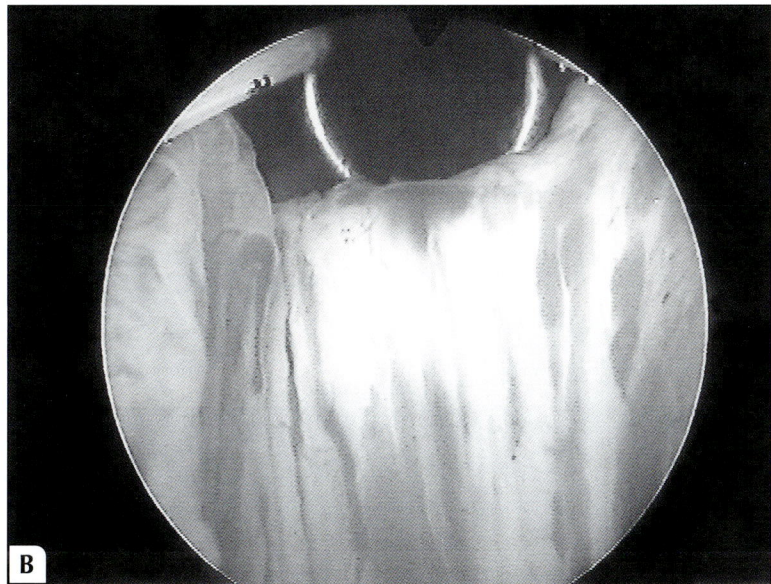
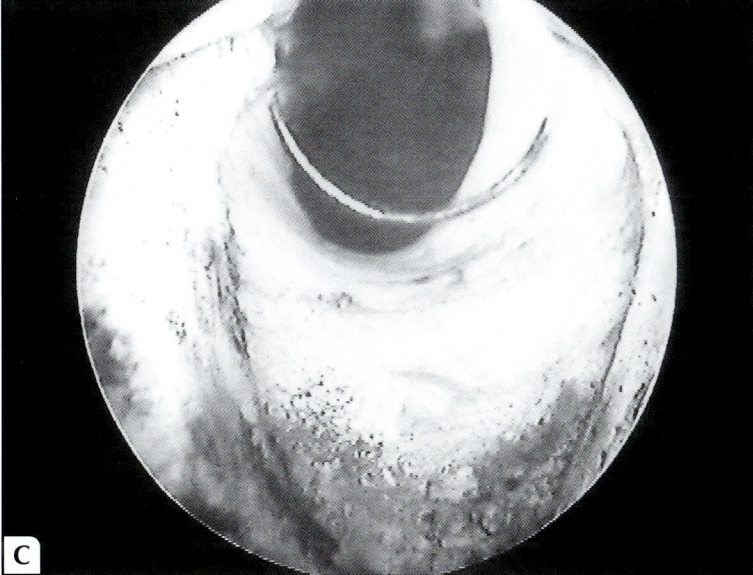

▶ **FIGURE 6-5.** Resecting the median lobe. **A,** Schematic representation. The median lobe is resected by going back and forth from left to right then right to left and resecting it level by level (1 to 4, *left*). At this point, manipulation of the prostate floor and median lobe with the finger in an O'Connor rectal sheath (*right*) facilitates the resection. If the anatomy of the gland is that of a primary vesical neck contracture, or what has been called a "median bar," one or two incisions at 6 o'clock or at 5 and 7 o'clock are made through the bladder neck at the end of the procedure if the neck is very prominent. **B,** Endoscopic view of the median bar before transurethral resection. **C,** Resection of the median lobe in the 6 o'clock position down to the capsule.

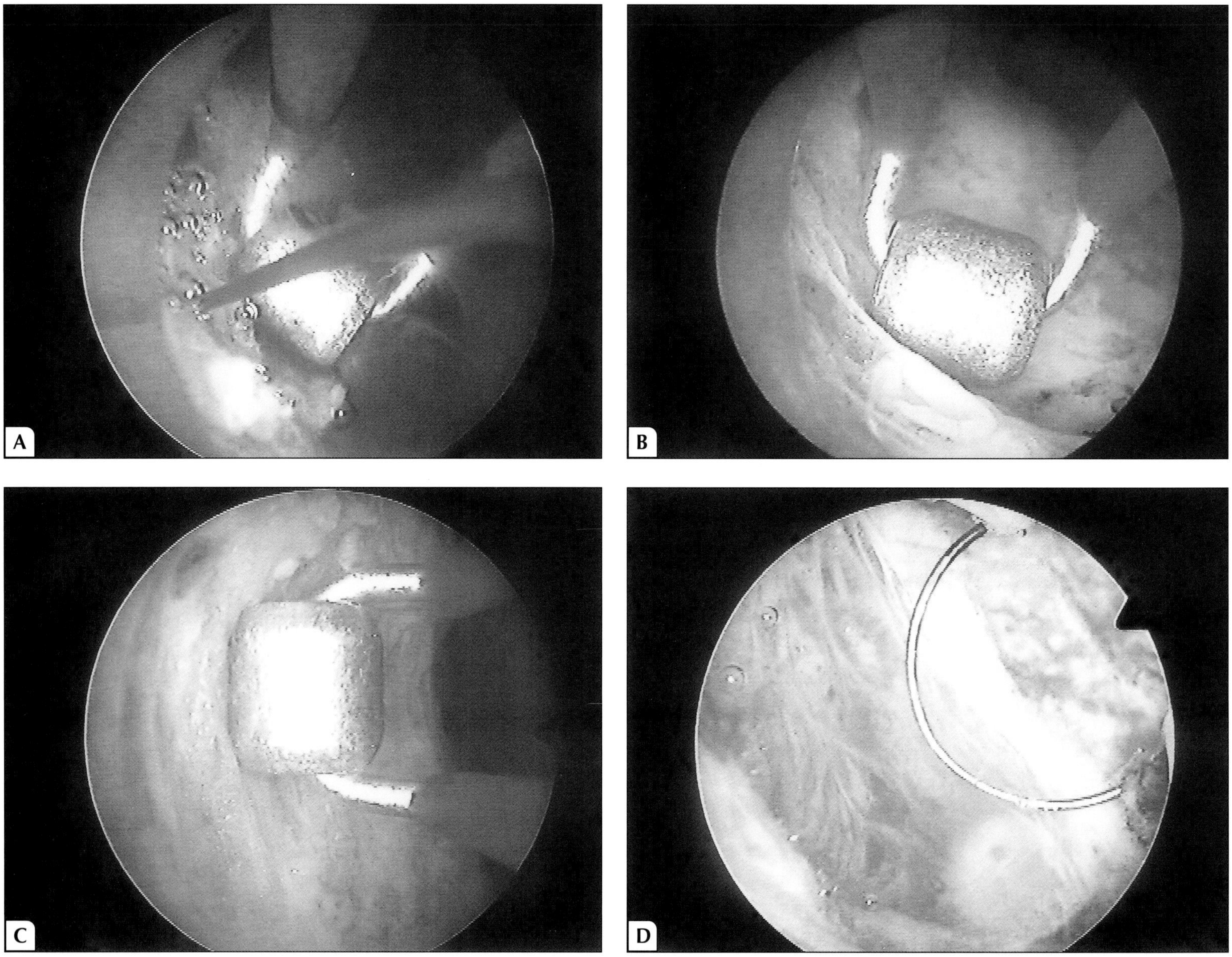

▶ **FIGURE 6-8.** Transurethral prostatectomy continued. **A,** Surgical land-marks for transurethral prostatectomy. Note the arterial bleeding point. Control of bleeding is done by coagulation, *eg,* using a ball-shaped electrode. **B,** Venous sinus exposed. Venous bleeding appears cloudlike when the water flow is reduced. **C,** Globules of fat protruding. **D,** Perforation of the surgical capsule. If there has been extensive resection of the prostatic capsule, it will be necessary to terminate the operation because of excessive absorption of fluid into the periprostatic tissue and venous complexes.

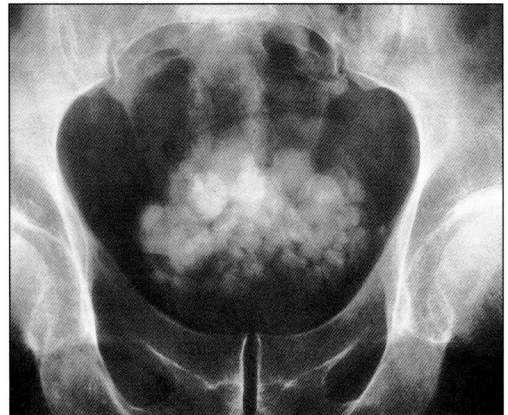

▶ **FIGURE 6-9.**
Bladder stones. Bladder stones in the male are usually caused by outflow obstruction and are an indication of the need for surgery in the form of either endoscopic or open prostatectomy. Bladder stones themselves can be dealt with either endoscopically or by open means.

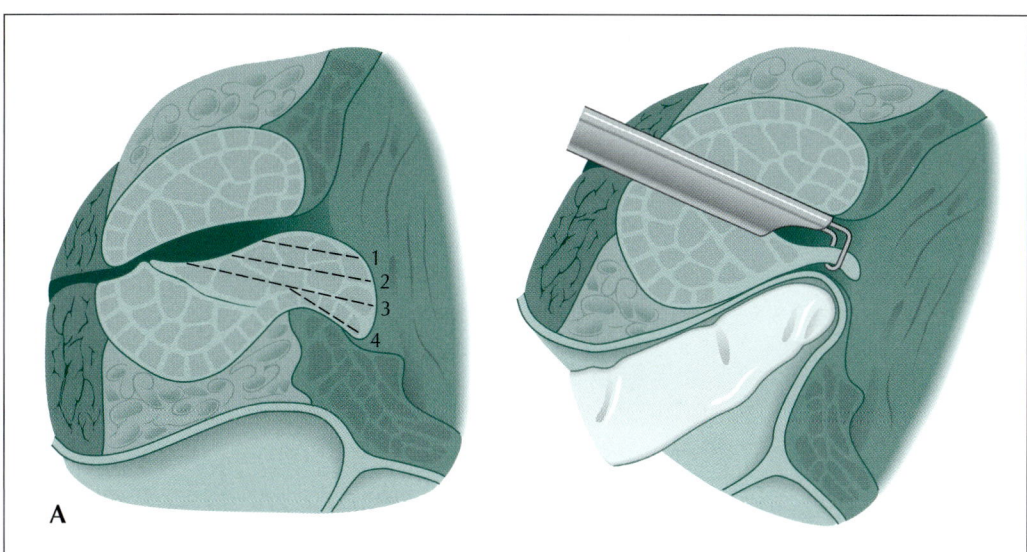

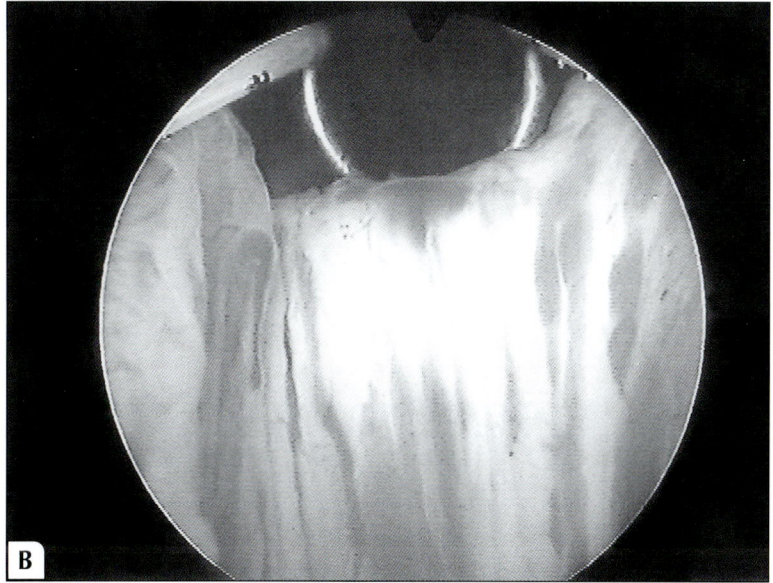

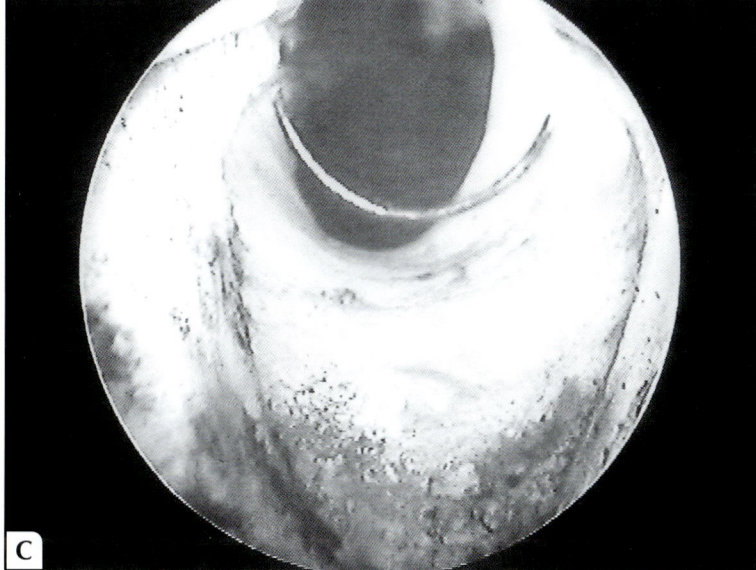

▶ **FIGURE 6-5.** Resecting the median lobe. **A,** Schematic representation. The median lobe is resected by going back and forth from left to right then right to left and resecting it level by level (1 to 4, *left*). At this point, manipulation of the prostate floor and median lobe with the finger in an O'Connor rectal sheath (*right*) facilitates the resection. If the anatomy of the gland is that of a primary vesical neck contracture, or what has been called a "median bar," one or two incisions at 6 o'clock or at 5 and 7 o'clock are made through the bladder neck at the end of the procedure if the neck is very prominent. **B,** Endoscopic view of the median bar before transurethral resection. **C,** Resection of the median lobe in the 6 o'clock position down to the capsule.

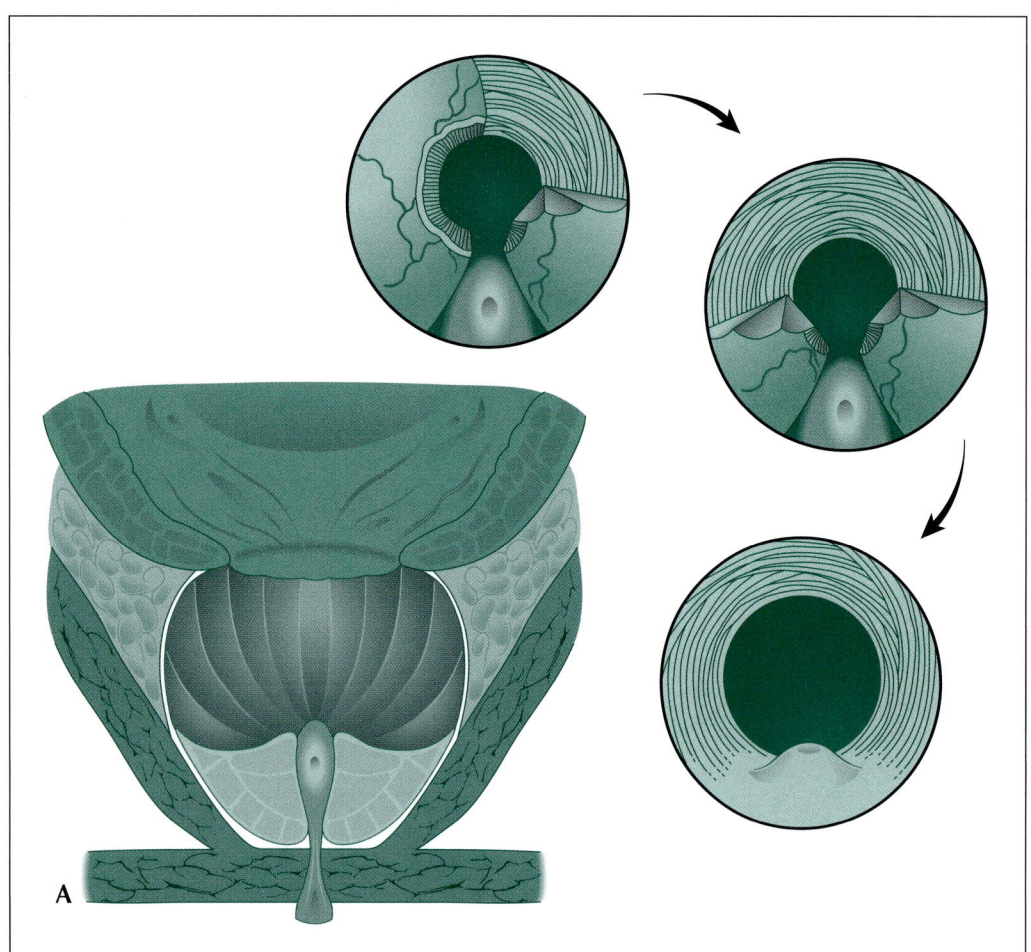

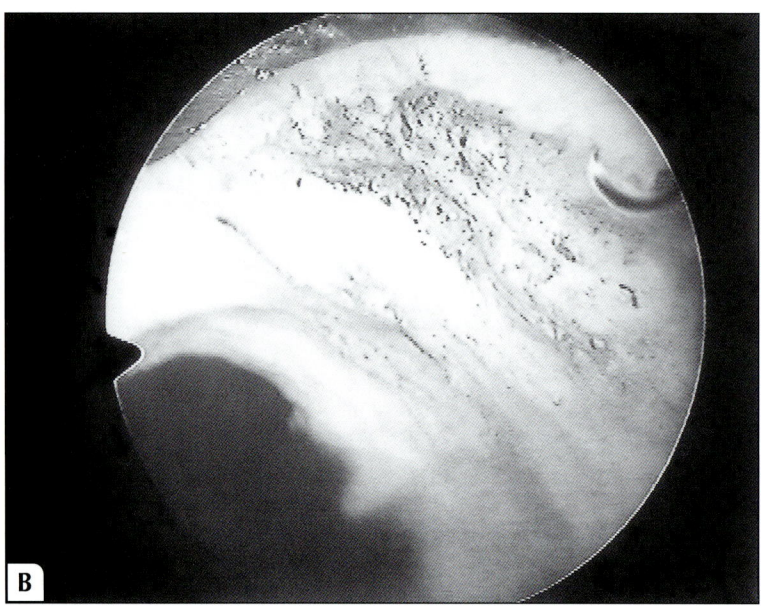

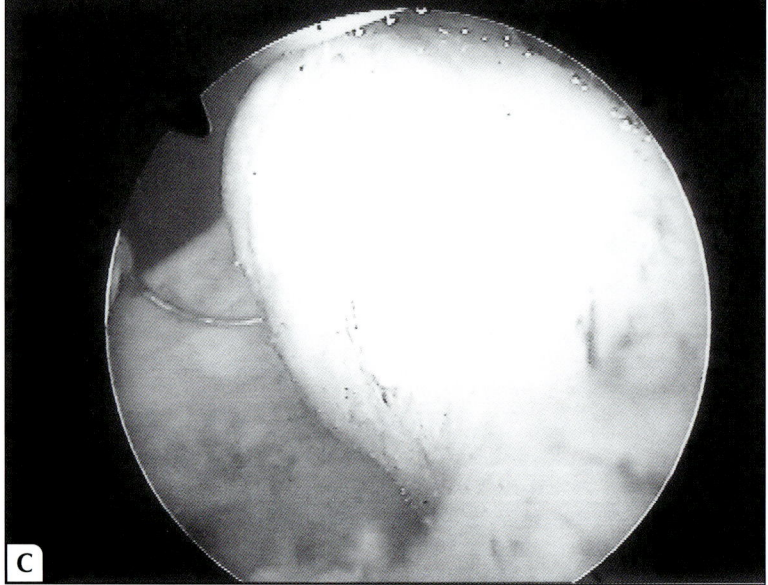

▶ **FIGURE 6-6.** Transurethral resection of the prostate: stage 2.
A, Schematic representation. Depending on the length of the prostatic fossa, the resectoscope is placed in front of the verumontanum and the resection is begun at the 12 o'clock position. Resection is done again by quadrants, first from 12 to 3 o'clock, with bleeding points controlled as necessary. Resection is carried down until the surgical capsule of the prostate is identified. The quadrant from 12 to 9 o'clock is resected. When resecting the two posterior quadrants, the resection is usually taken down

from the 9 o'clock to the 7 o'clock position, resecting most of the bulk of the lateral lobe. It is moved to the other posterior quadrant, which is resected similarly from 3 to 5 o'clock. The floor is resected last, if required, manipulating the tissue with the finger in the O'Connor sheath. Fibers readily identified on the roof and sides of the prostate usually are not as apparent on the floor. **B,** Resection at the 12 o'clock position. **C,** Beginning of the resection of the posterior quadrant of the left lobe.

(*Continued on next page*)

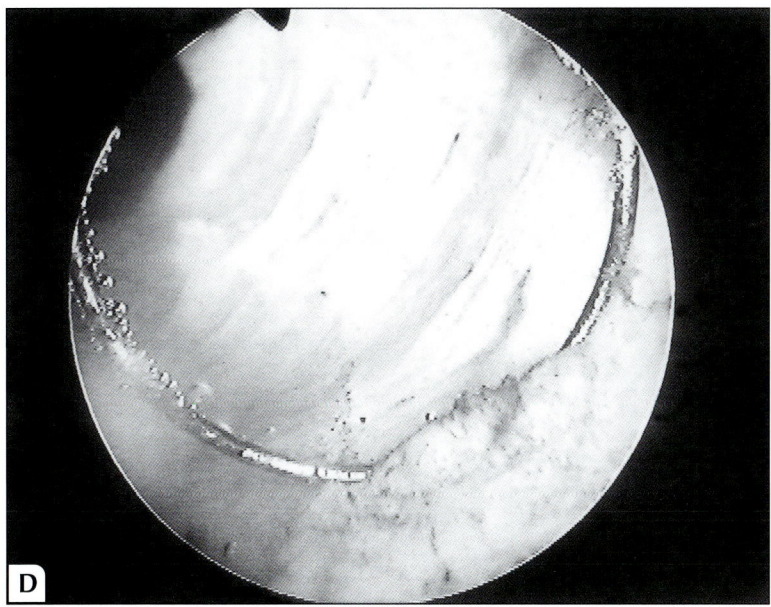

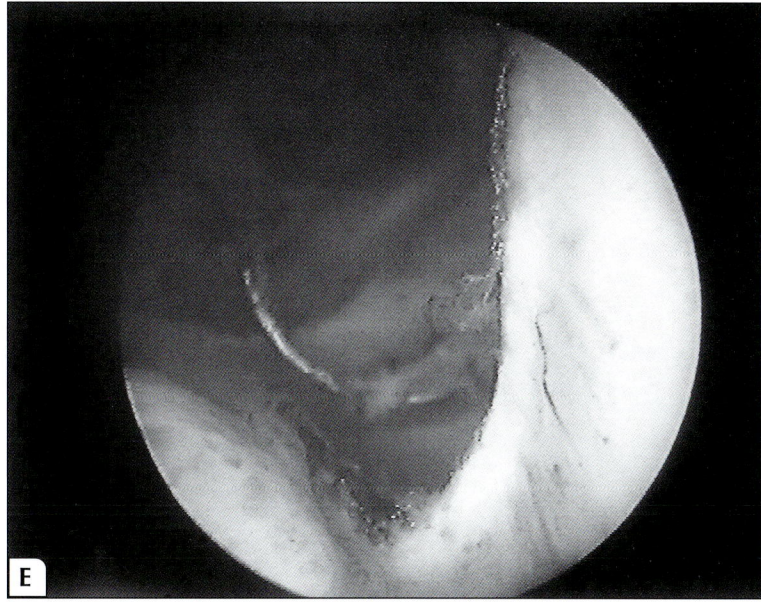

▶ **FIGURE 6-6.** (*Continued*) **D,** Resection of the posterior quadrant of the left lobe until the surgical capsule is identified. **E,** View of the prostatic fossa at the end of stage 2. Apical tissue is not completely resected.

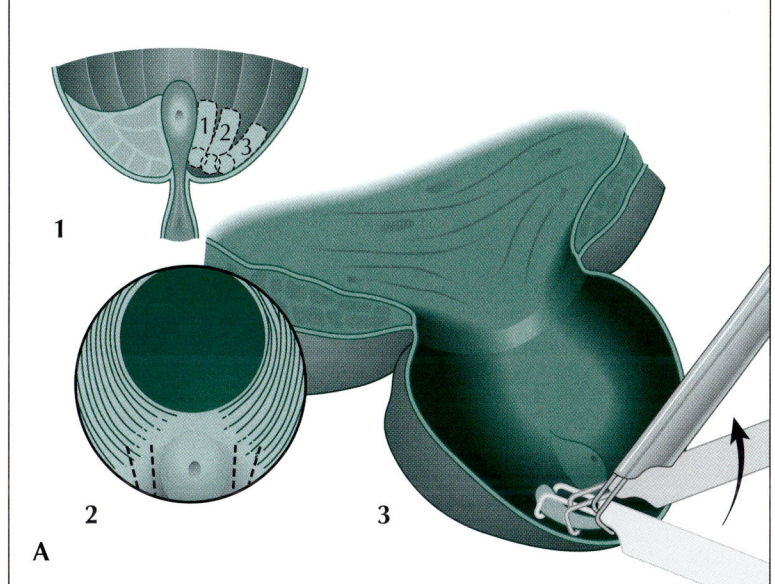

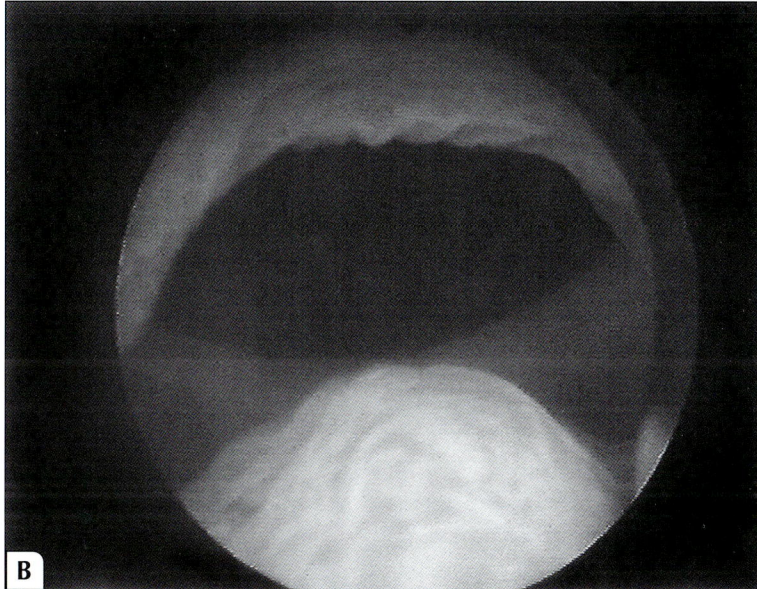

▶ **FIGURE 6-7.** Transurethral resection of the prostate: stage 3. **A,** Schematic representation. The external sphincter and the verumontanum are identified. The tissue lying next to the verumontanum at the 5 and 7 o'clock positions is removed carefully with the resectoscope. The resection now is begun at the apex, proceeding from 7 to 12 o'clock. Use of a lateral-to-medial sweep of the resectoscope loop in response to the concavity of the gland can be helpful as adenomatous tissue is removed. Care must be taken not to advance the scope inward or, more significantly,

not to retract the scope out during the resection, thereby inadvertently injuring the external sphincter. The resection is then carried out similarly from 5 to 12 o'clock. Bleeding is carefully controlled. In a larger gland, the lateral lobe tissue of the apex may project beyond the verumontanum into the sphincter area. In such cases, it is advisable to leave a thin rim of apical prostatic tissue rather than risk inadvertently resecting the sphincter.

B, Endoscopic view of the verumontanum, the sphincter, and the empty prostatic fossa at the end of stage 3 of the transurethral resection.

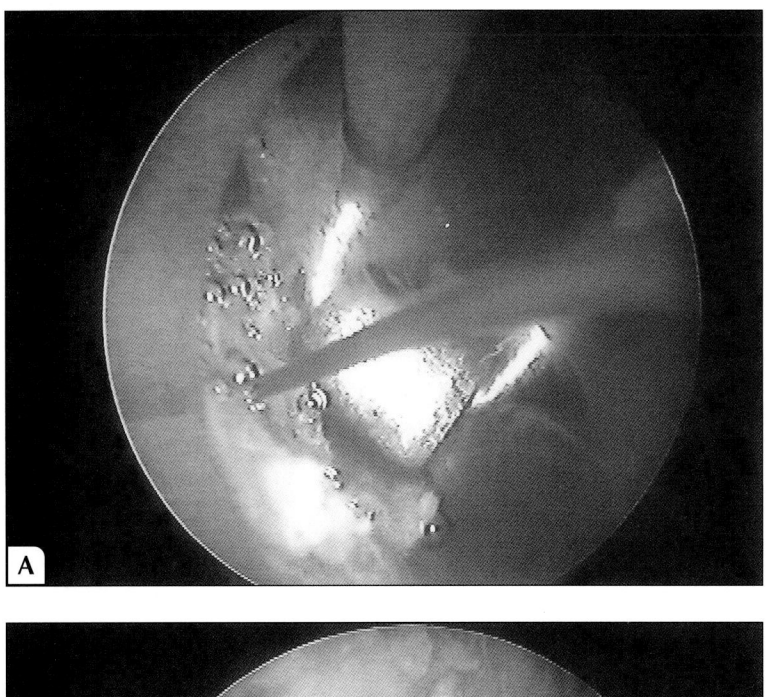

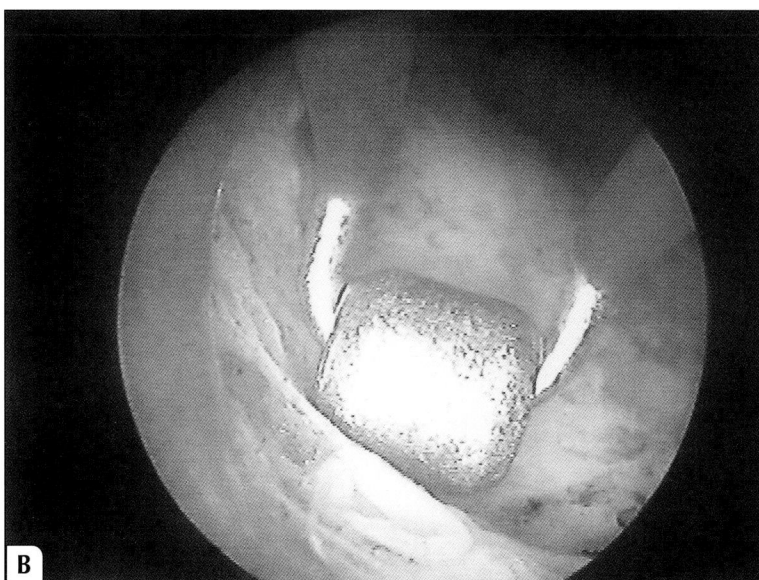

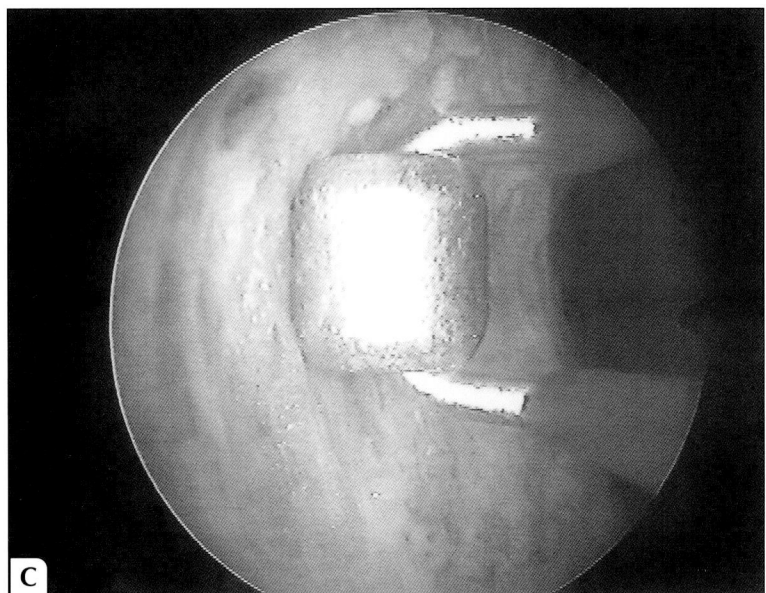

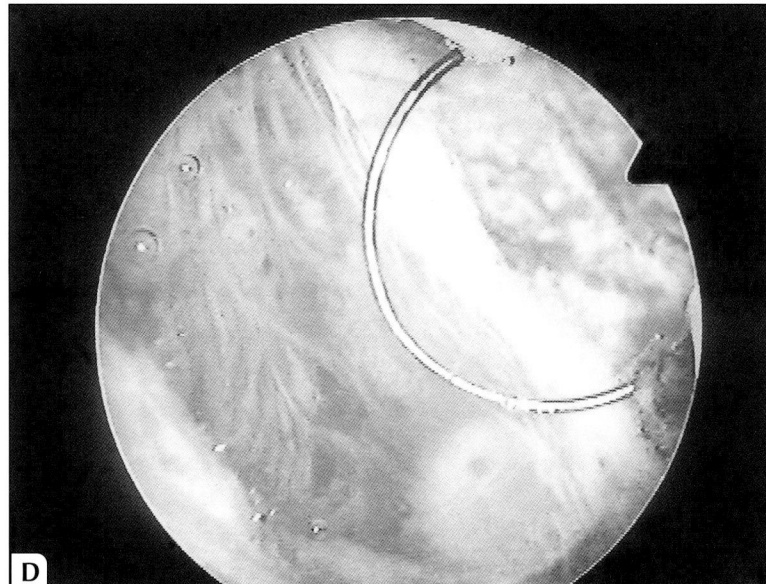

▶ **FIGURE 6-8.** Transurethral prostatectomy continued. **A,** Surgical landmarks for transurethral prostatectomy. Note the arterial bleeding point. Control of bleeding is done by coagulation, *eg,* using a ball-shaped electrode. **B,** Venous sinus exposed. Venous bleeding appears cloudlike when the water flow is reduced. **C,** Globules of fat protruding. **D,** Perforation of the surgical capsule. If there has been extensive resection of the prostatic capsule, it will be necessary to terminate the operation because of excessive absorption of fluid into the periprostatic tissue and venous complexes.

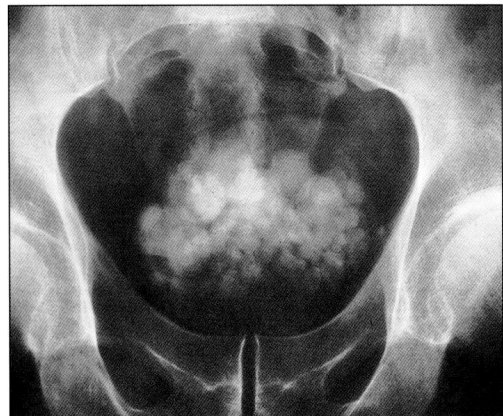

▶ **FIGURE 6-9.**
Bladder stones. Bladder stones in the male are usually caused by outflow obstruction and are an indication of the need for surgery in the form of either endoscopic or open prostatectomy. Bladder stones themselves can be dealt with either endoscopically or by open means.

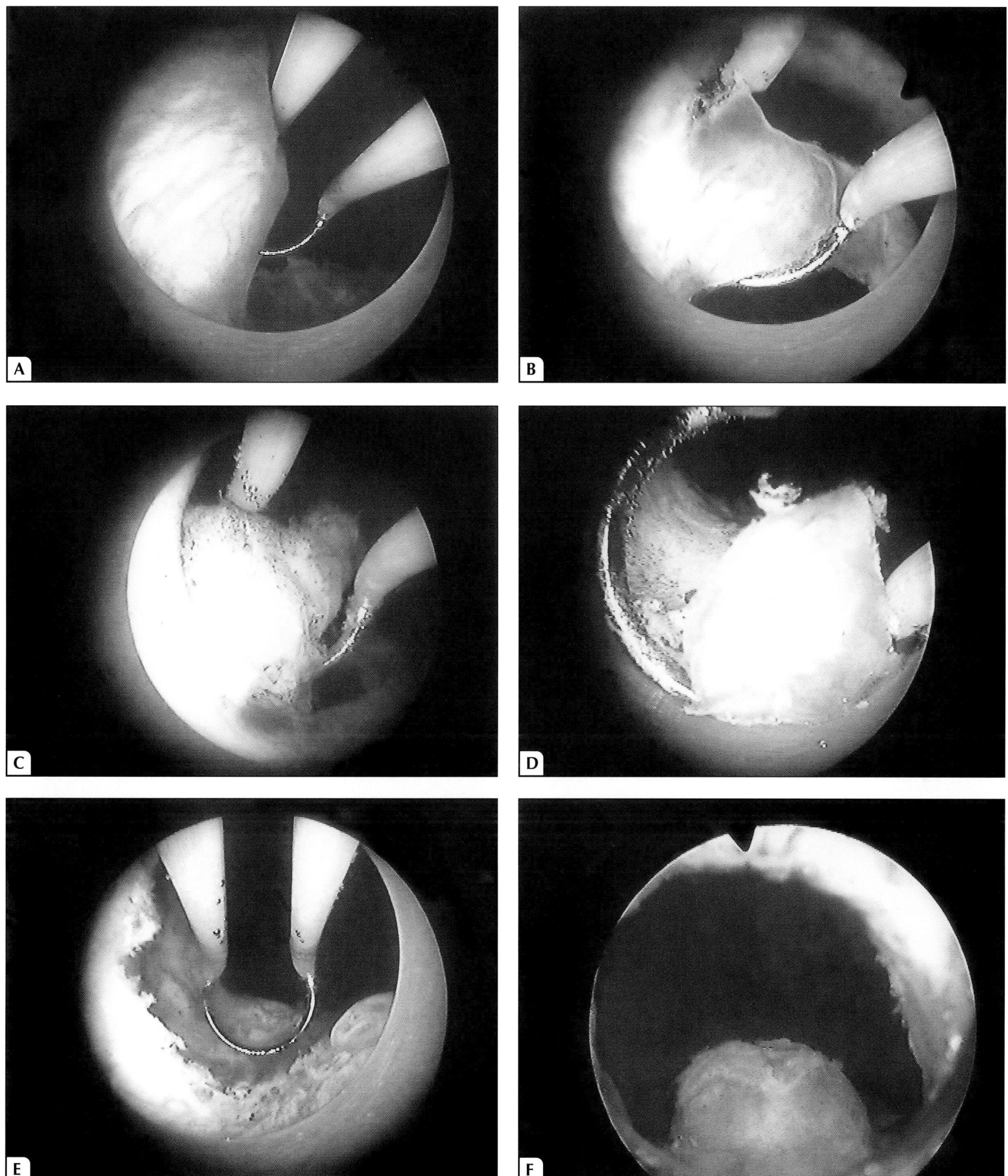

▶ **FIGURE 6-10.** Modified transurethral resection of the prostate using a "thick loop" for better hemostasis. The increased mass of the loop slows down cutting speed but improves coagulation. During resection, some of the tissue water is vaporized. **A** to **D,** Resection of the apex right side lobe. **E,** Resection of prostate almost completed. **F,** This endoscopic view shows the verumontanum, the sphincter, and the empty prostatic fossa at the end of resection.

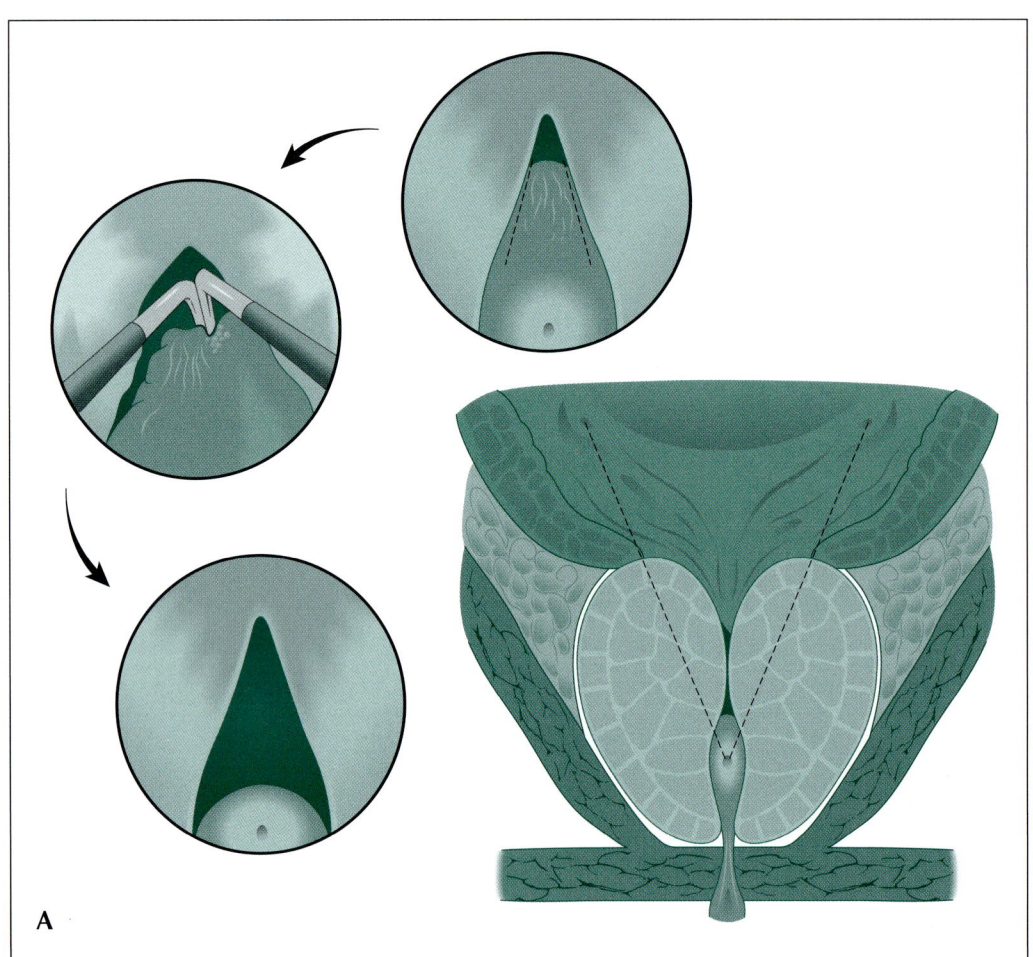

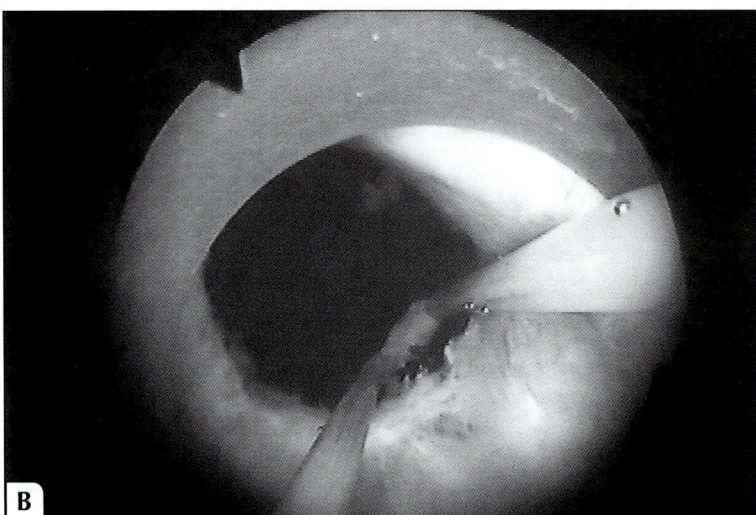

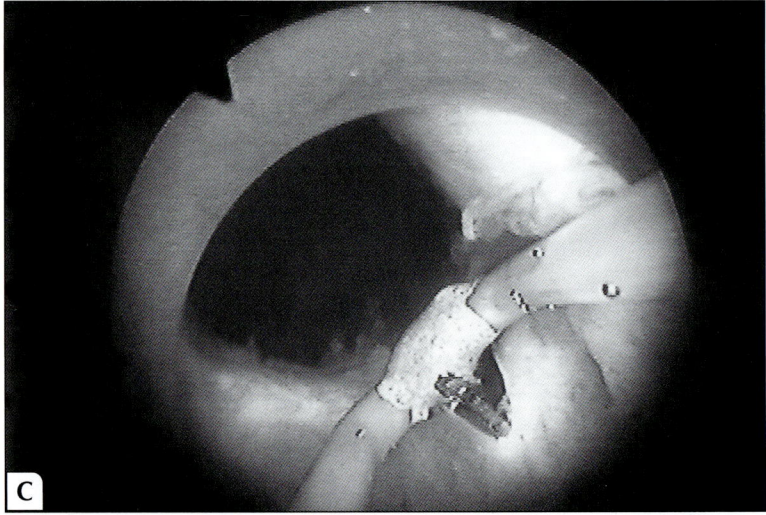

▶ **FIGURE 6-11.** Transurethral incision of the prostate (TUIP): schematic representation. **A,** TUIP is started at the right ureteral orifice and continued through the bladder neck. The depth through the bladder neck should expose the shiny, filmy fibers at the vesical-prostate junction. The incision is then carried through the floor of the prostate down to the capsule. A corresponding incision is carried out similarly from the left ureteral orifice to the verumontanum. Bleeding is carefully controlled. **B** to **D,** Endoscopic view of transurethral incision of the prostate in the 5 o'clock position.

(*Continued on next page*)

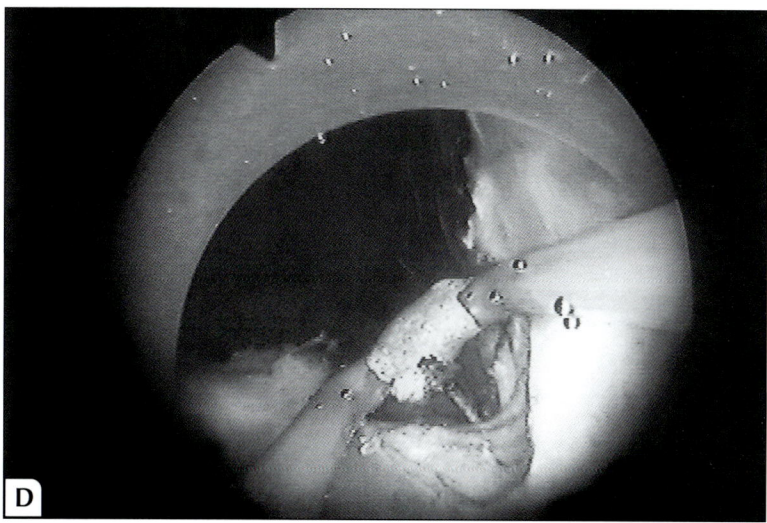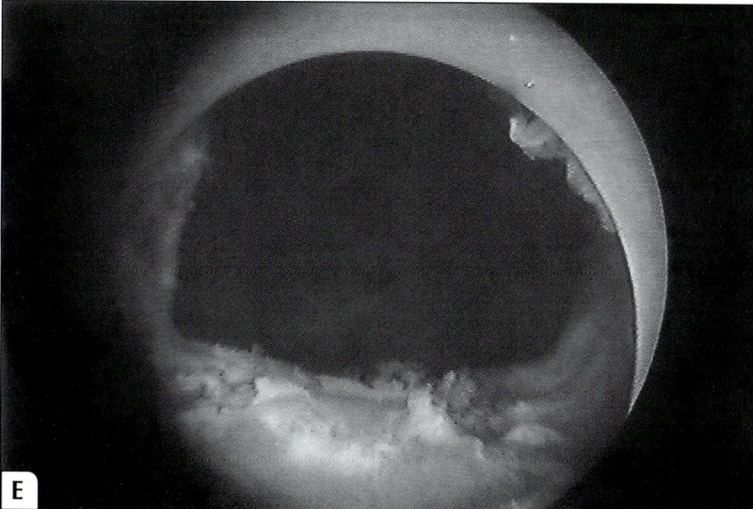

▶ **FIGURE 6-11.** (*Continued*) Cuts are consecutive. E, Endoscopic view of the open bladder outlet at the end of transurethral incision of the prostate.

CLINICAL OUTCOMES OF TRANSURETHRAL RESECTION OF THE PROSTATE

Treatment Outcomes From Recent Studies on Transurethral Resection of the Prostate

Study	IPSS		Q_{max}	
	Baseline	**Postoperative**	**Baseline**	**Postoperative**
Anson *et al.* [2]	18.2	5.1	10.0	21.8
Borboroglu *et al.* [3]	23.8	6.4	ND	ND
Carter *et al.* [4]	19.8	5.9	ND	ND
Cowles *et al.* [5]	20.8	7.5	9.5	16.5
Dixon *et al.* [6]	20.5	7.7	8.8	14.7
Fay *et al.* [7]	22.5	8.6	8.8	18.9
Francisca *et al.* [8]	20.8	3.2	7.9	23.5
Gilling *et al.* [9]	23.0	4.3	9.1	20.4
Kabalin *et al.* [10]	18.8	6.4	9.0	21.2
Kaplan *et al.* [11]	18.3	6.1	8.3	19.6
Karanjavala *et al.* [12]	19.0	4.5	9.5	19.7
Keoghane *et al.* [13]	19.4	6.5	11.4	12.7
Keoghane *et al.* [14]	20.2	7.0	9.0	14.0
Küpeli *et al.* [15]	21.6	5.2	9.2	19.7
Mottet *et al.* [16]	23.7	4.7	7.7	17.6
Muschter *et al.* [17]	21.1	3.5	8.9	25.6
Oesterling *et al.* [18]	24.0	8.6	8.8	20.8
Patel *et al.* [19]	23.3	3.2	7.5	22.6
Uchida *et al.* [20]	21.3	3.3	8.0	21.1

▶ **FIGURE 6-12.** Treatment outcomes of the transurethral resection of the prostate (TURP) arms of recent studies comparing TURP with minimally invasive treatment modalities demonstrating overall excellent improvements of symptoms and urinary flow rates. IPSS—International Prostate Symptom Score.

A. Complications of Transurethral Resection of the Prostate

Study	Mortality, %	Morbidity, %	Blood Transfusion, %	Hospital Stay, d
Borboroglu et al. [3] (n = 520, 1991–1998, 42-mo follow-up, resected weight 18.8 g)	0	2.5 (intraoperative) 10.8 (early postoperative) 8.5 (late) 2.5 (repeat TURP)	0.4	2.4
Uchida et al. [21] (n = 1941, 1985–1996, resected weight 23 g)	0.05	9.5 (overall)	6.1	
Uchida et al. [21] (n = 1930, 1971–1985, resected weight 26 g)	0.2	17 (overall)	20	
Fourcade et al. [22] (n = 410, 1996, resected weight 25.3 g)		8.5 (UTI) 6.5 (urethral stenosis)	2.4	
Mebust et al. [23] (n = 3885, 1989, resected weight 22 g)	0.1	24.9	6.4	5 (in 78% of patients)
Barba et al. [24] (n = 1000, 1990–1994, resected weight 37 g)		7.9 (sodium substitution) 8.5 (postoperative revision)	16.5	7.7

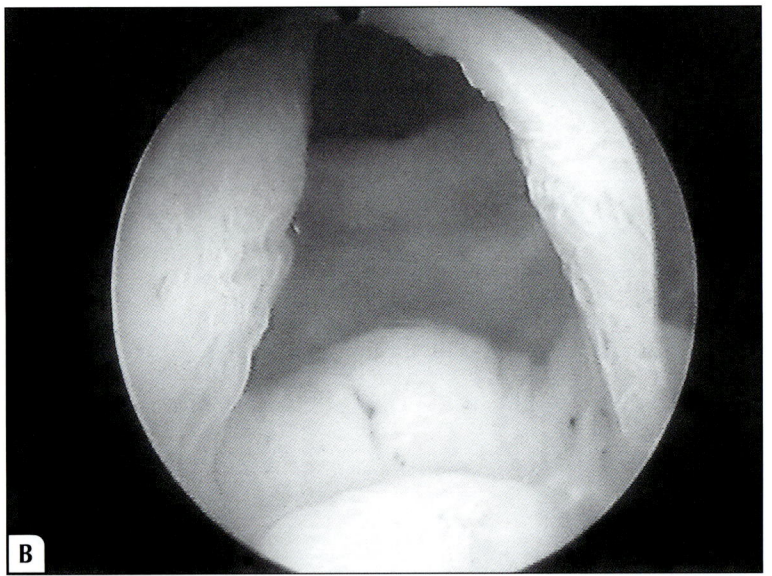

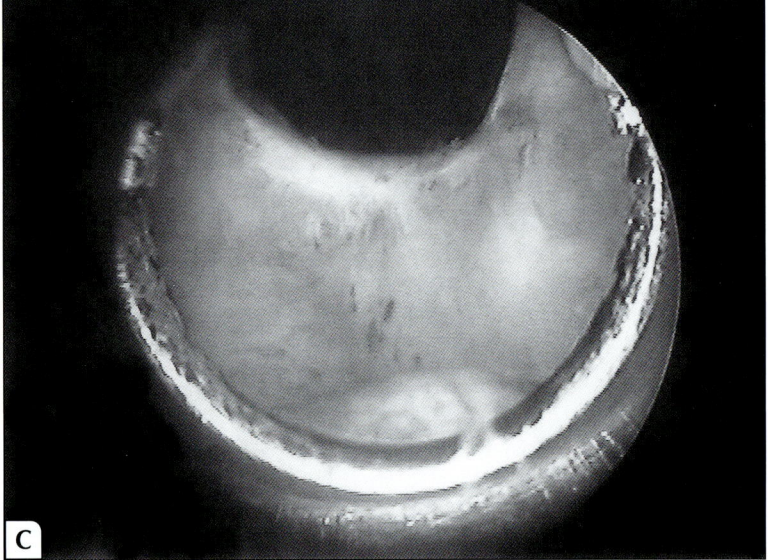

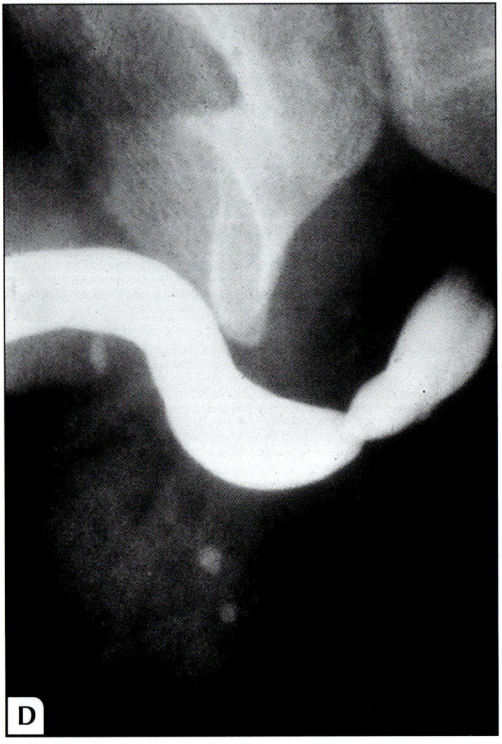

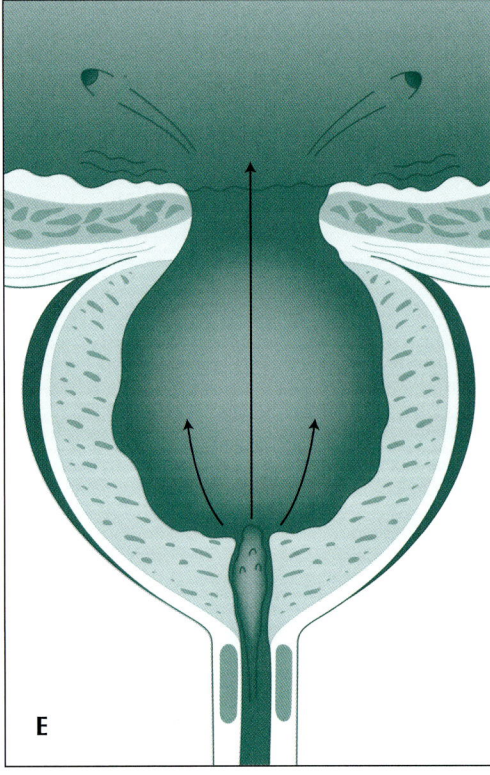

▶ **FIGURE 6-13.** Various complications of transurethral resection of the prostate (TURP) are shown here. **A,** Complications of transurethral resection of the prostate. **B,** Insufficient clinical outcome. **C,** Bladder neck stricture. **D,** Urethral stricture. **E,** Retrograde ejaculation.

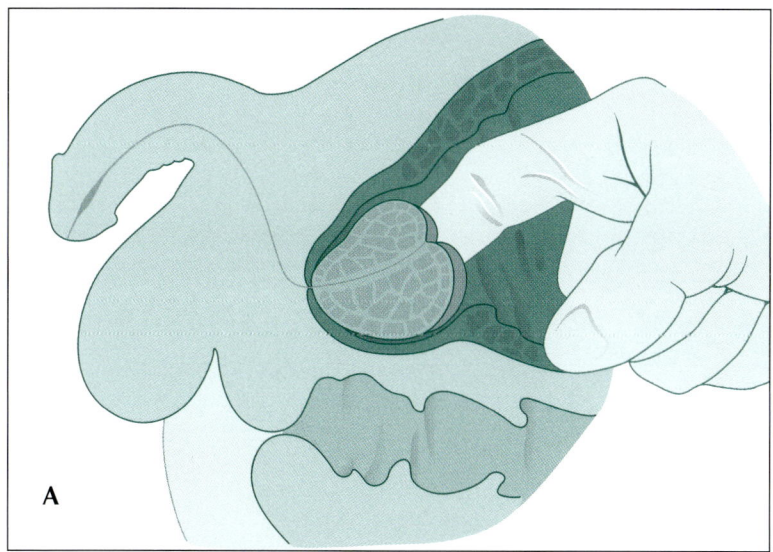

A

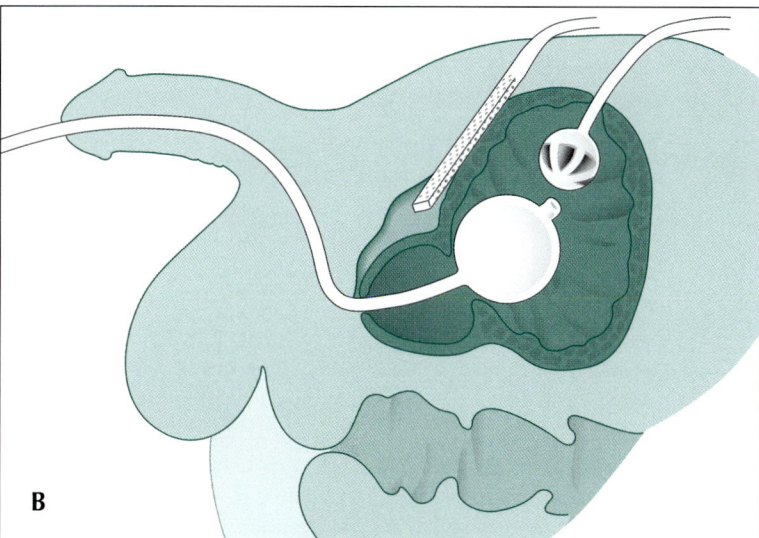

B

▶ **FIGURE 6-14.** Blunt enucleation of the prostate. **A,** After skin incision and separation of the muscles in the midline, the retropubic space is exposed. If a wider exposure is needed, the tendinous insertion of the rectus on the pubis can be partially incised and reapproximated at the end of the procedure. Classically, a suprapubic or transvesical prostatectomy is performed through a midline bladder incision. The incision starts just cephalad to the bladder neck. Alternatively, a transverse incision approximately 1 cm above the bladder neck may be used. The combined incision is in the midline of the bladder and extends into the capsule of the prostate. With extension into the muscle of the prostate, it may be necessary to place a deep stitch into the capsule of the prostate to control bleeding from the dorsal vein complex. Blunt enucleation of the prostate is begun by cutting through the anterior commissure of the prostate. The surgeon then finds the plane between the compressed prostatic capsule and the adenoma. Alternatively, the surgeon may incise the mucosa overlying the prostate at the vesical junction and bluntly or sharply find the plane between the adenoma and surgical capsule. The adenoma is then enucleated. The apex can then be pinched off as it meets the prostatic urethra. Care must be taken not to distract the apex cephalad and inadvertently damage the more distal portion of the external sphincter mechanism. If the vertical incision has been extended into the prostatic capsule, the urethra can be divided from the prostate more precisely with better exposure of the area. A warm, moist gauze pack is placed firmly in the prostatic fossa to tamponade venous bleeding after a transvesical prostatectomy. Figures-of-Eight absorbable sutures are placed at 5 and 7 o'clock to control bleeding from major arterial branches to the prostate. Bleeding within the fossa is controlled via individual suture ligatures of 3-0 chromic, or, alternatively, bleeding points can be cauterized using the ball electrode. Bleeding from the prostatic fossa may also be controlled by using a pull-out suture of heavy nonabsorbable suture to pursestring the bladder neck. With a pursestring pulled tight to approximate the bladder neck, a Foley catheter is snugged up to the bladder neck.

B, A suprapubic tube (*eg,* 26-F Malecot) is placed through the dome of the bladder after the bleeding is controlled. An indwelling urethral catheter is left to permit through-and-through irrigation to wash out clots. A suction drain is left in the space of Retzius. The bladder is closed in two layers using 2-0 absorbable running suture on the mucosa and interrupted 0 absorbable suture on the serosa and muscular area.

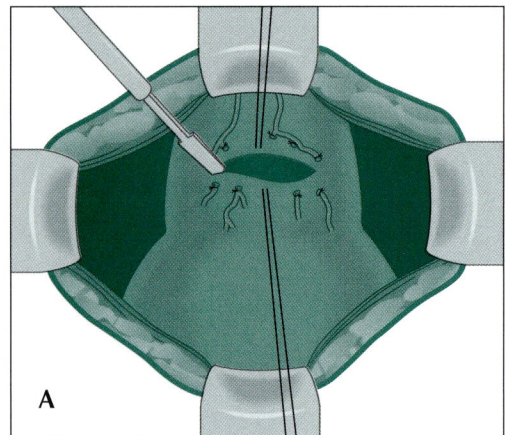

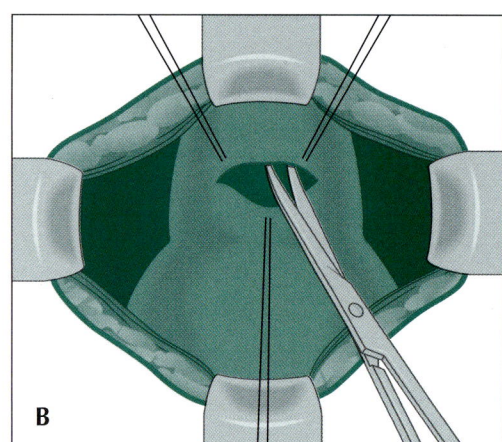

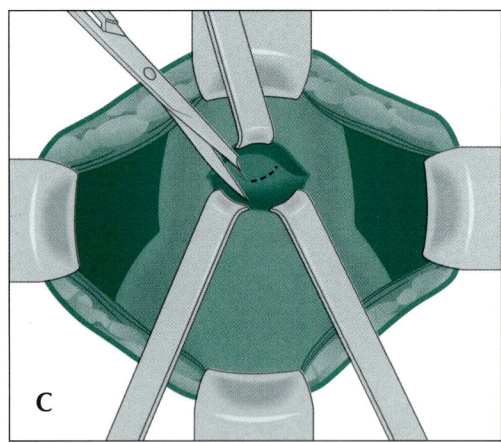

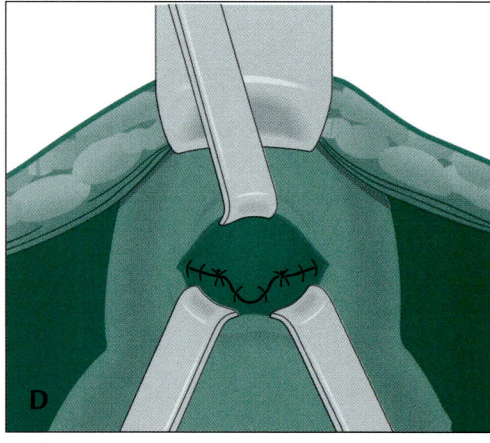

▶ **FIGURE 6-15.** Schematic representation. **A,** Incision of the prostate capsule. A transverse capsular incision is made through the prostate midway between the apex of the prostate and bladder neck. Stay sutures are used to elevate the surgical capsule, exposing the adenoma. Venous capsular bleeders are suture ligated or cauterized as necessary.

B, Sharp dissection of the adenoma. A plane between the capsule and the adenoma is identified and, using curved scissors, the adenoma is sharply dissected away from the surgical capsule of the prostate. The urethral mucosa attachment can be transected with scissors and careful dissection of the lateral lobes of the prostate accomplished. The adenoma is then grasped with a tenaculum and dissection carried out sharply, removing the adenoma up to the bladder neck. At this point, the mucosa at the bladder neck is sharply incised and the adenoma removed. Figure-eight 0 chromic sutures are placed at 5 and 7 o'clock in the bladder neck to control arterial bleeding.

C, Wedge resection of bladder neck. After retropubic prostatectomy, a V-shaped wedge of bladder neck may be removed if the bladder neck appears to be partially obstructed. **D,** Closure of wedge resection of the bladder neck. After a wedge of bladder neck is removed, the bladder mucosa is advanced over the cut edge and secured to the prostatic fossa. This may prevent a secondary vesical neck contracture. Bleeding within the prostatic capsule is controlled with suture ligatures and cautery as needed. If bleeding is insignificant at this point, a suprapubic tube may be unnecessary. A three-way catheter is inserted into the bladder for continuous irrigation with normal saline in the postoperative period. The capsule of the prostate is closed with interrupted 0 absorbable sutures. A suction drain is placed into the retropubic space and brought out through a separate stab wound in the anterior abdominal wall. The abdominal fascia and skin are closed in the usual manner.

REFERENCES

1. Neal DE: The National Prostatectomy Audit. *Br J Urol* 1997, 79:69–75.

2. Anson KM, Nawrocki J, Buckley J, *et al.*: A multicenter, randomized, prospective study of endoscopic laser ablation versus transurethral resection of the prostate. *Urology* 1995, 46:305–310.

3. Borboroglu PG, Kane CJ, Ward JF, *et al.*: Immediate and postoperative complications of transurethral prostatectomy in the 1990s. *J Urol* 1999, 162:1307–1310.

4. Carter A, Sells H, Speakman M, *et al.*: Quality of life changes following KTP/Nd:YAG laser treatment of the prostate and TURP. *Eur Urol* 1999, 36:92–98.

5. Cowles RS, Kabalin JN, Childs S, *et al.*: A prospective randomized comparison of transurethral resection to visual laser ablation of the prostate for the treatment of benign prostatic hyperplasia. *Urology* 1995, 46:155–160.

6. Dixon CM: A comparison of transurethral prostatectomy with visual laser ablation of the prostate using the Urolase right-angle fiber for the treatment of BPH. *World J Urol* 1995, 13:126–129.

7. Fay R, Chan SL, Kahn R, *et al.*: Initial results of a randomized trial comparing interstitial laser coagulation therapy to transurethral resection of the prostate. *J Urol* 1997, 157:41.

8. Francisca EAE, d'Ancona FCH, Hendriks JCM, *et al.*: A randomized study comparing high-energy TUMT to TURP: quality-of-life-results. *Eur Urol* 2000, 38:569–575.

9. Gilling PJ, Mackey M, Cresswell M, *et al.*: Holmium laser versus transurethral resection of the prostate: a randomized prospective trial with 1-year follow-up. *J Urol* 1999, 162:1640–1644.

10. Kabalin JN, Gill HS, Bite G, Wolfe V: Comparative study of laser versus electrocautery prostatic resection: 18-month followup with complex urodynamic assessment. *J Urol* 1995, 153:94–97.

11. Kaplan SA, Laor E, Fatal M, Te AE: Transurethral resection of the prostate versus transurethral electrovaporization of the prostate: a blinded, prospective comparative study with 1-year followup. *J Urol* 1998, 159:454–458.

12. Karanjavala JD, Buckley JF: Prostatic laser ablation versus transurethral resection of the prostate. *Br J Urol* 1997, 79:818–819.

13. Keoghane SR, Lawrence KC, Gray AM, *et al.*: A double-blind randomized controlled trial and economic evaluation of transurethral resection vs contact laser vaporization for benign prostatic enlargement: a 3-year follow-up. *BJU Int* 2000, 85:74–78.

14. Keoghane SR, Sullivan ME, Doll HA, *et al.*: Five-year data from the Oxford laser prostatectomy trial. *BJU Int* 2000, 86:227–228.

15. Küpeli S, Baltaci S, Soygur T, *et al.*: A prospective randomized study of transurethral resection of the prostate and transurethral vaporization of the prostate as a therapeutic alternative in the management of men with BPH. *Eur Urol* 1998, 34:15–18.

16. Mottet N, Anidjar M, Bourdon O, *et al.*: Randomized comparison of transurethral electroresection and holmium:YAG laser vaporization for symptomatic benign prostatic hyperplasia. *J Endourol* 1999, 13:127–130.

17. Muschter R, Whitfield H: Interstitial laser therapy of benign prostatic hyperplasia. *Eur Urol* 1999, 35:147–154.

18. Oesterling JE, Issa MM, Roehrborn CG, *et al.*: Long-term results of a prospective, randomised clinical trial comparing TUNA to TURP for the treatment of symptomatic BPH. *J Urol* 1997, 157:328.

19. Patel A, Fuchs GJ, Gutierrez-Aceves J, *et al.*: Prostate heating patterns comparing electrosurgical transurethral resection and vaporization: a prospective randomized study. *J Urol* 1997, 157:169–172.

20. Uchida T, Egawa S, Iwamura M, *et al.*: A non-randomized comparative study of visual laser ablation and transurethral resection of the prostate in benign prostatic hyperplasia. *Int J Urol* 1996, 3:108–111.

21. Uchida T, Ohori M, Soh S, *et al.*: Factors influencing morbidity in patients undergoing transurethral resection of the prostate. *Urology* 1999, 53:98–105.

22. Fourcade RO, Vallancien G: Morbidity of endoscopic resection of the prostate: a prospective study with 3-months follow-up. *Progr Urol* 2000, 10:48–52.

23. Mebust WK, Holtgrewe HL, Cockett ATK, *et al.*, and the Writing Committee: Transurethral prostatectomy: immediate and postoperative complications: a cooperative study of 13 participating institutions evaluating 3,885 patients. *J Urol* 1989, 141:243–247.

24. Barbra M, Leyh H, Fischer H, Hartung R: Perioperative morbidity of transurethral resection of the prostate (TURP). *Urology* 1998, 37:S20.

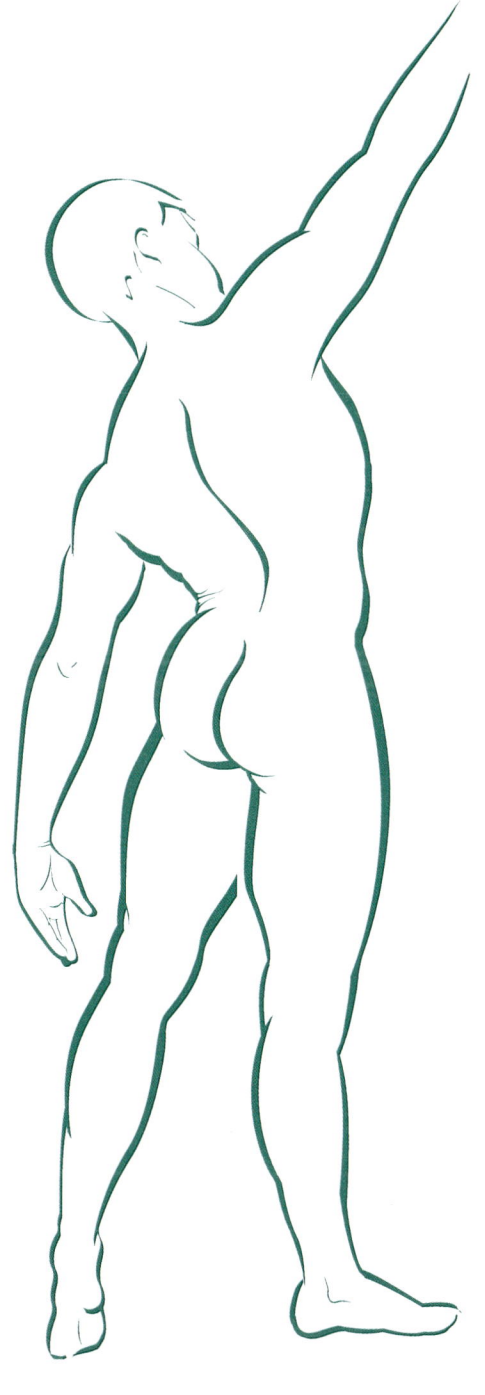

Prostatitis: Definition and Clinical Approaches

7

John N. Krieger

We tell our medical students that the prostate is easy. There are only three problems: 1) prostate cancer (CaP), which is a common cause of death among adult men; 2) benign prostatic hyperplasia (BPH), which is also a common cause of morbidity among adult men and represents an indication for considerable medical and surgical therapy; and 3) prostatitis. Prostatitis also causes considerable morbidity and loss of productivity, and is a frequent cause of visits to physicians in the United States [1–4]. Of the three conditions, prostatitis is by far the least well understood. Perhaps the problem with prostatitis is that we do not have a good abbreviation!

There are several definitions of prostatitis. One of the real problems is that it matters very much which literature one is reviewing. The definition is remarkably different depending on how one approaches this problem. There are different definitions in the pathology literature, in the urology literature, in the infertility literature, and in clinical practice. These definitions include histologic and traditional urologic, based on presence or absence of infection, and the standard clinical definition. The aims of this chapter are to 1) examine many of these definitions, 2) to explain the new consensus classification of prostatitis, and 3) to outline current approaches to diagnosis and treatment.

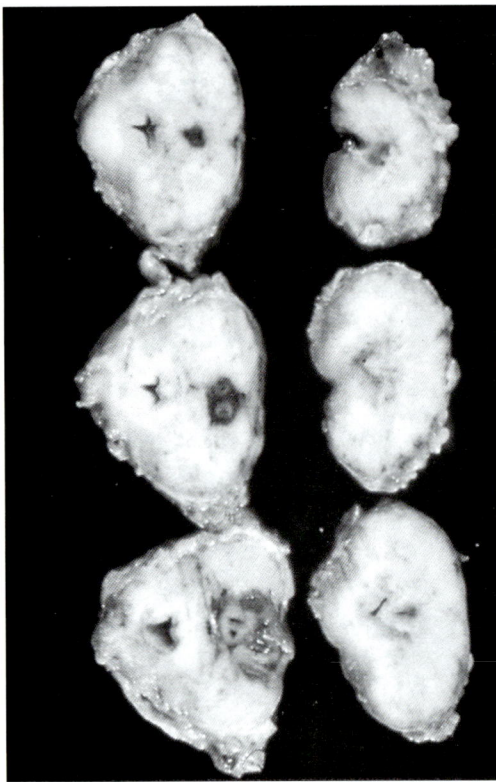

▶ **FIGURE 7-1.** Step-sections of a "normal prostate" from the bladder base through the urethra. Note that there is a focus of gross inflammation apparent in this specimen, illustrating that areas of pathologic prostatitis are commonly seen in autopsy material.

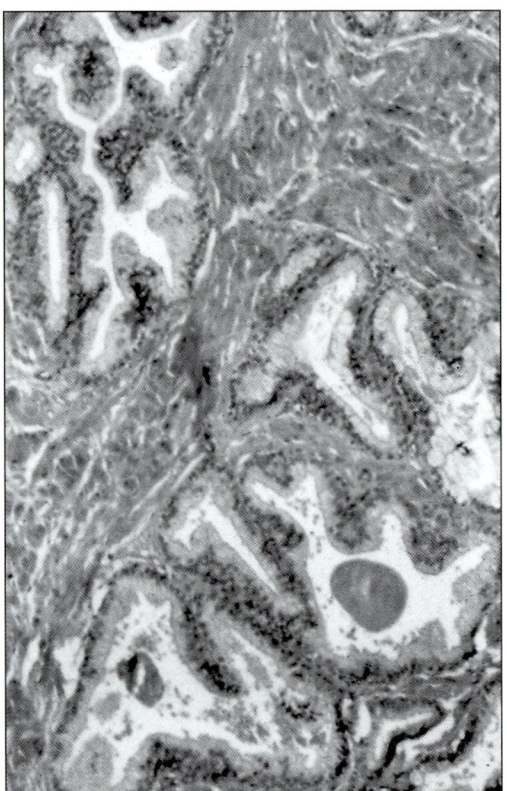

▶ **FIGURE 7-2.** Normal prostate showing the typical histologic appearance of benign-appearing glands and stroma. Note the corpora amylacea.

Histopathologic Criteria for Prostatitis Diagnosis

Examination of tissue
    Prostate cancer
    Benign prostatic hypertrophy
    Definition and categorization of prostatitis
    Inflammatory infiltrates
        Presence
        Characteristics

▶ **FIGURE 7-3.** Criteria for prostatitis diagnosis. In pathology, diagnosis of prostatitis is based on the histologic picture. Pathologists seldom have access to clinical history, physical examination, or microbiologic findings. Thus, diagnosis of prostatitis by pathologists is based entirely on histopathologic criteria.

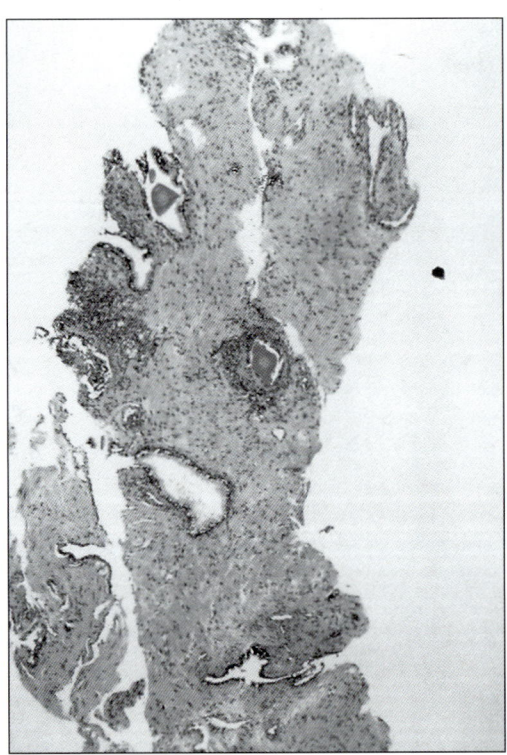

▶ **FIGURE 7-4.** Typical low-power view of a prostate chip from a transurethral resection specimen showing areas of obvious inflammation. This image represents a very unusual patient from the pathologic perspective—because of the documented clinical history and microbiologic data. The patient is a 67-year-old man with acute urinary tract obstruction due to acute bacterial infection with *Escherichia coli* (>10^6 cfu/mL). Bladder drainage and antimicrobial agents resolved his infection. Unfortunately, he was unable to resume normal voiding. Several weeks later we performed a transurethral resection of the prostate, which resolved his bladder outflow obstruction.

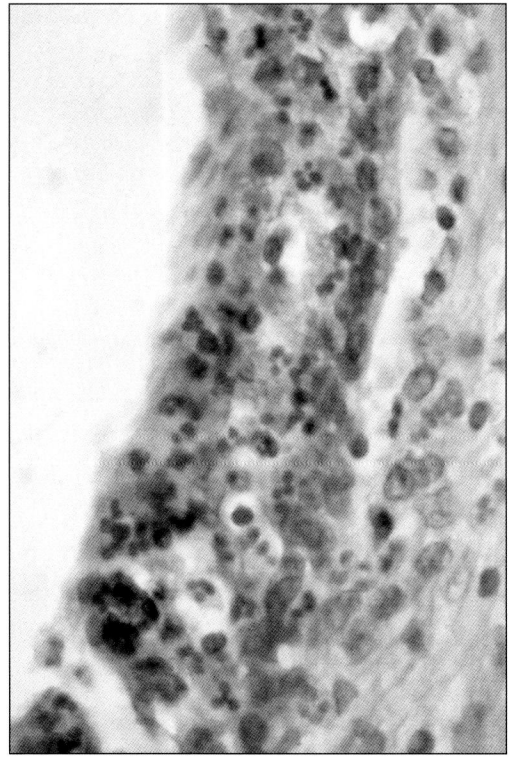

◗ **FIGURE 7-5.** High-power view showing an acute inflammatory infiltrate. The pathologic diagnosis was acute prostatitis.

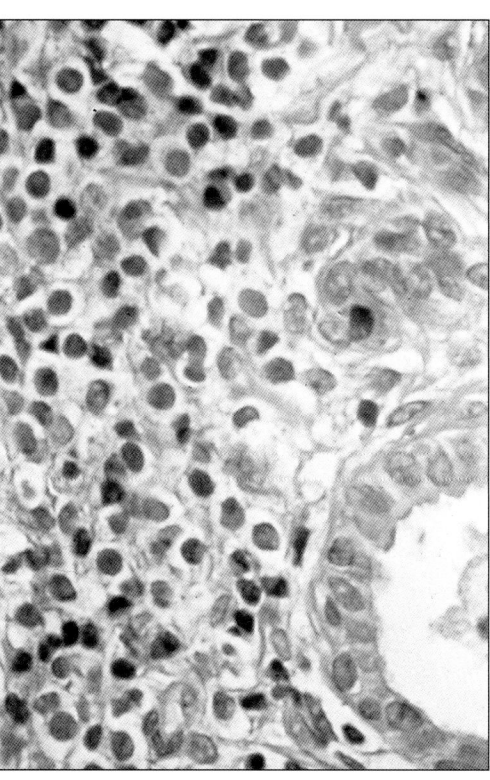

◗ **FIGURE 7-6.** Another case with a chronic inflammatory infiltrate. The pathologic diagnosis was chronic prostatitis.

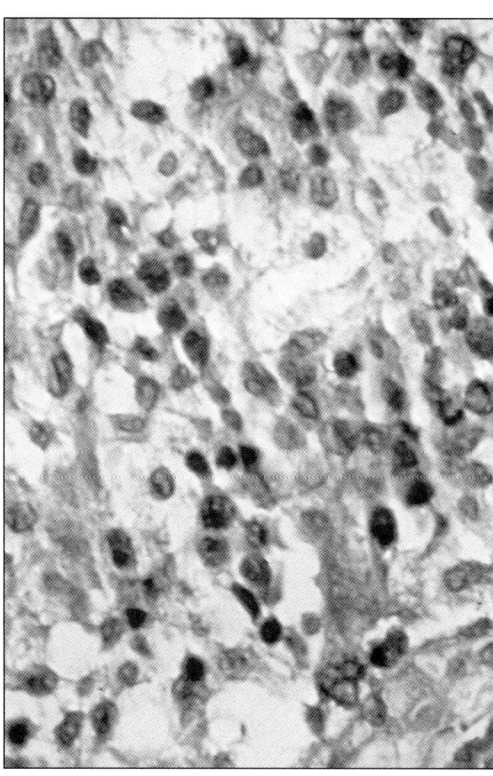

◗ **FIGURE 7-7.** A case of eosinophilic prostatitis with characteristic red-staining eosinophils predominating in the inflammatory infiltrate. These cases are often associated with allergic reactions.

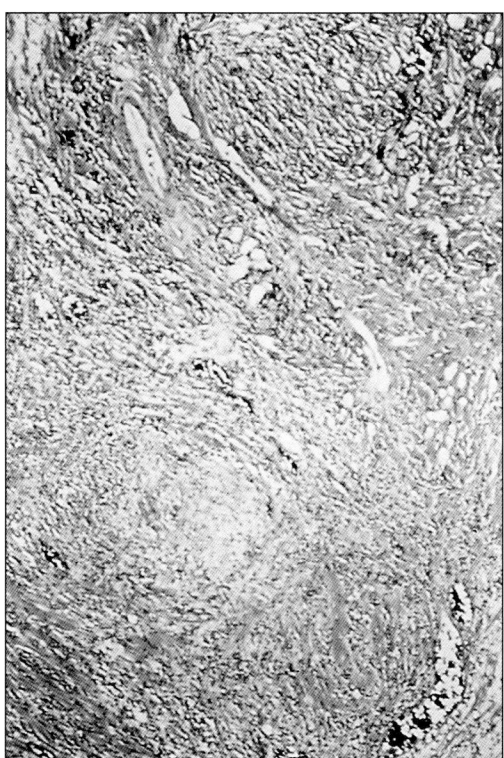

◗ **FIGURE 7-8.** Pathologic diagnosis of granulomatous prostatitis. Granulomatous prostatitis is the characteristic histologic reaction of the prostate to a variety of different causes. Many cases are idiopathic, including this one.

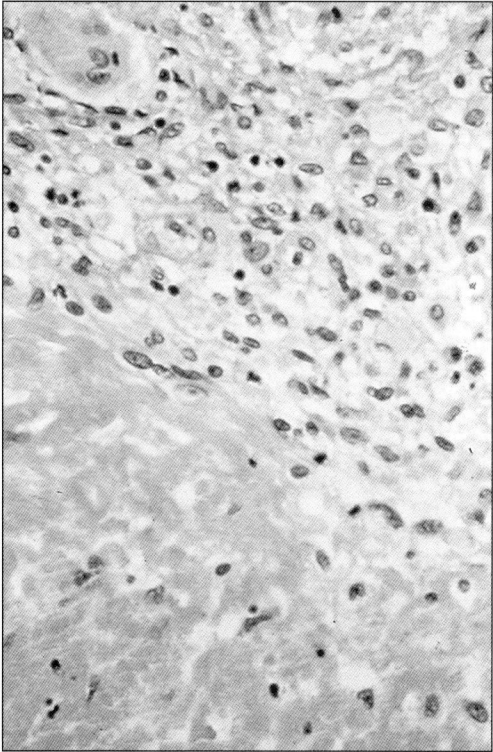

◗ **FIGURE 7-9.** Granulomatous prostatitis due to tuberculosis. Other cases of granulomatous prostatitis are related to urologic surgery or to specific infections, such as tuberculosis, bacille Calmette-Guérin therapy, or fungal infections. Note the caseous necrosis and Langerhan's giant cells.

Problems with the Pathologic Definition and Classification of Prostatitis

Population
Inflammation or infection may be focal
Not well correlated with clinical findings
Many men with no history of prostatitis have histologic findings
 of prostatitis

FIGURE 7-10. Problems with the pathologic definition and classification of prostatitis. First, the population studied is approximately 20 years older than the typical population of patients with symptoms of chronic prostatitis. Second, step-sections of prostates removed at autopsy show that inflammation and infection may be focal, affecting some areas of the prostate but not other areas. Third, the pathologic diagnoses and findings have not been well correlated with clinical findings. In the older literature, pathology has rarely been found to be helpful in the clinical management of patients with prostatitis symptoms. Fourth, in our practice many men with no history of prostatitis who undergo prostatectomy for benign or malignant disease have histologic findings of prostatitis.

Prostate Histopathology in Chronic Prostatitis

Study	Patients, n	Prostate Biopsies, n	Patient Characteristics
True *et al.* [5]	97	368	All had symptoms of chronic prostatitis Negative evaluation for infection Negative clinical evaluation

FIGURE 7-11. Results of a recent study on prostate histopathology in chronic prostatitis [5]. Recent studies demonstrate another fundamental problem with the pathological definition of prostatitis [5]. This study evaluated more than 368 transperineal prostate biopsy specimens from 97 patients with symptoms of chronic prostatitis. None of these patients had evidence of infection following an extensive microbiologic evaluation. None had evidence of structural or functional abnormalities of the lower genitourinary tract. The surprising finding was that only 38% of these patients had inflammation in their prostate biopsies. Further, of the patients with histologic evidence of inflammation, most had only modest inflammatory infiltrates.

The Traditional Definition of Prostatitis

Meares-Stamey (research definition)
 Lower urinary tract localization
 VB1, VB2, EPS, VB3 (cultures or microscopy)
Four clinical syndromes
 Acute bacterial prostatitis
 Chronic bacterial prostatitis
 Nonbacterial prostatitis
 Prostatodynia

FIGURE 7-12. The traditional definition of prostatitis. The traditional definition used in the urology literature has been based on the Meares-Stamey definition and classification [6–8]. This research definition is based on careful lower urinary tract localization studies, which include examination of the following: VB1 (voided bladder 1 or first-void urine), VB2 (voided bladder 2, or midstream urine), expressed prostatic secretions (EPS), and VB3 (voided bladder 3, or postmassage urine), using quantitative cultures and microscopy. The four clinical syndromes that have classically been described are listed in this figure.

Distinctions Among the Four Clinical Syndromes of Prostatitis

Syndrome	Symptoms	EPS Leukocytes	Bacteriuria	Physical Examination
Acute bacterial	+	+	+	+
Chronic bacterial	+	+	+	
Nonbacterial	+	+		
Prostatodynia	+			

FIGURE 7-13. Distinctions among the four clinical syndromes of prostatitis. Acute bacterial prostatitis is associated with characteristic symptoms of acute urinary tract infection. On occasion, the patient may be septic and present with a systemic illness. The physical examination is frequently impressive with local bladder tenderness, an exquisitely tender and tense prostate on rectal examination, and occasionally signs of systemic infection. The patient has bacteriuria defined as presence of uropathogens in the midstream urine. The expressed prostatic secretions (EPS) have leukocytes and pathogenic bacteria.

Chronic bacterial prostatitis is characterized by recurrent symptoms of acute urinary tract infection. There are increased numbers of leukocytes in the prostatic secretions, and uropathogens are present episodically in the midstream urine. The physical examination may or may not be impressive. The characteristic clinical feature of chronic bacterial prostatitis is recurrent urinary tract infections caused by the same bacterial species.

In contrast, nonbacterial prostatitis and prostatodynia are not associated with bacteriuria. These patients are symptomatic. The distinction between nonbacterial prostatitis and prostatodynia is based on the presence of increased numbers of EPS leukocytes in patients with nonbacterial prostatitis, but not in patients with prostatodynia.

Characteristics of Acute Bacterial Prostatitis

Systemic symptoms of tissue-invasive infection ("flu")
  Malaise, myalgias, fever
Urinary tract symptoms of bacteriuria
  Frequency, dysuria, and obstructive voiding
  Physical examination finds "tense," exquisitely tender prostate
Responds dramatically to antimicrobial therapy

▶ **FIGURE 7-14.** Characteristics of acute bacterial prostatitis. Acute bacterial prostatitis is associated with systemic symptoms of a tissue-invasive infection. The patient may present with a flu-like syndrome characterized by malaise, myalgias, and fever. The patient will have urinary tract symptoms of bacteriuria characterized by increased urinary frequency, dysuria, and often obstructed voiding. On physical examination the prostate may be "tense" and exquisitely tender. Fortunately, these patients respond dramatically to appropriate antimicrobial therapy for recognized uropathogens. Many agents that do not get into the prostate under noninflamed conditions work very well in this syndrome. This is usually not a difficult or subtle diagnosis.

Characteristics and Treatment of Chronic Bacterial Prostatitis

Recurrent bacteriuria in adult men
Often asymptomatic between episodes of bacteriuria
Treatment strategies
  Antimicrobials that penetrate prostate
  Curative: long course, full dose
  Suppressive: continuous, low dose

▶ **FIGURE 7-15.** Characteristics of chronic bacterial prostatitis. Chronic bacterial prostatitis is the most common cause of recurrent bacteriuria in adult men. It is noteworthy that these patients may be totally asymptomatic between acute episodes of bacteriuria.

There are a number of treatment strategies using antimicrobial agents that penetrate the prostatic parenchyma. One can use curative treatment strategies, meaning a long course (in my practice, 6 weeks to 3 months) of full-dose antimicrobial therapy, usually using a drug such as fluoroquinolone or trimethoprim-sulfamethoxazole. This regimen will cure 30% to 50% of patients. For patients who cannot be cured, one can use a strategy of suppression with continuous low-dose therapy using nightly or every-other-night dosing of a low-dose agent to suppress bladder bacteriuria. This is the US Food and Drug Administration's definition of prostatitis, but it represents very few patients seen in clinical practice.

Diagnosis Localization Cultures in Some Cases of Chronic Bacterial Prostatitis

Organism	VB1	VB2	EPS	VB3
Escherichia coli	1200	1200	15,000	4400
E. coli	0	0	4000	110
E. coli	100	200	2700	110
E. coli	240	140	2700	270
E. coli	0	0	100	0
Pseudomonas aeruginosa	0	0	50,000	300
Enterobacter cloacae	0	0	1500	10

▶ **FIGURE 7-16.** Diagnostic localization cultures in some cases of chronic bacterial prostatitis [9]. In each case the patient had recurrent episodes of bacteriuria caused by the same organism that we localized to the prostate using the four-glass test. Many of these patients required more than one study for definitive localization. Note that these organisms are all recognized uropathogens. These seven patients all had gram-negative rod infections. It is possible to have a gram-positive result, but it is important to document recurrent episodes of bacteriuria caused by that organism. The characteristic localization pattern is a 10-fold increase when the VB3 sample is compared with the VB1 sample. If that criterion fails, one can compare the expressed prostatic secretion (EPS) sample with the VB1. VB1—voided bladder 1; VB2—voided bladder 2; VB3—voided bladder 3.

Problems with the Urologic Definition of Prostatitis

Represents < 10% of all bacterial prostatitis cases (acute or chronic)
  Studies concern a small subset of patients
  Only group of interest to US FDA for drug development
Localization seldom done in clinical practice
  Laboratory problems
  Subtleties in technique
  Usually negative or not helpful

▶ **FIGURE 7-17.** Problems with the urologic definition of prostatitis. First and foremost, this definition represents less than 10% of bacterial prostatitis seen in clinical practice. Much of the literature concerns a very small subset of highly selected patients. Localization studies, although described very carefully and thoroughly in research settings, are seldom done in clinical practice. This is for a number of reasons, such as problems setting up the laboratory studies and subtleties in technique. However, most clinicians believe that these studies are usually negative and thus are not particularly helpful or cost-effective for most patients. In contrast, the US FDA uses bacterial localization as the criterion for treatment studies for prostatitis. US FDA—US Food and Drug Administration.

Assumptions Made by the Traditional Definition

Nonbacterial prostatitis indicates a physical problem
  Fastidious microorganisms
    (many classified as bacteria, *eg, Chlamydia trachomatis*)
Inflammatory disorder (noninfectious)
Allergy
Stones
Other organic pathology

> **FIGURE 7-18.** Assumptions implicit in the traditional urologic definition of prostatitis. The first is that patients with nonbacterial prostatitis have a physical problem, such as the presence of fastidious microorganisms. Many of these potential organisms are classified as bacteria, such as *Chlamydia trachomatis* [9]. Thus, nonbacterial prostatitis is in fact a misnomer. Others have suggested that nonbacterial prostatitis is an inflammatory disorder that may be noninfectious [10]. Other theories in the literature are that nonbacterial prostatitis is related to allergy, prostate stones, a variant of interstitial cystitis, or other organic pathology, such as voiding dysfunction or reflux of sterile urine into the prostatic ducts [10–17].

Causes of Prostatodynia

Neuromuscular: genitourinary diaphragm
  "Pelvic floor tension myalgia"
Primary voiding disturbance
  Bladder neck obstruction
  External sphincter spasm
  Treatment includes TURP, TUIP, cystoprostatectomy, hyperthermia, diazepam, α-blockers
Primary psychologic disturbances

> **FIGURE 7-19.** Prostatodynia. The syndrome of prostatodynia has been ascribed to a variety of causes, such as neuromuscular dysfunction of the genitourinary diaphragm. Some suggest that this is "pelvic floor tension myalgia" [10]. Others suggest that this is a primary voiding disturbance with abnormalities at the bladder neck or external sphincter spasm. Treatment recommendations include transurethral resection or incision of the prostate. Other procedures described in the recent literature include cystoprostatectomy, hyperthermia, and use of α-blockers. Such treatments may help some patients, although our clinic is full of patients in whom such therapies failed. Still other authors suggest that there is a primary psychologic disturbance in these patients, and that "psychiatric counseling should be seriously pursued, because these patients have serious personality disturbances and defects in sexual identification" [7]. TUIP—transurethral incision of the prostate; TURP—transurethral resection of the prostate.

Experiential Findings Regarding Prostatitis and Prostatodynia

Symptoms similar in nonbacterial prostatitis and prostatodynia
EPS findings variable
Fastidious organisms isolated from both populations
Both groups are often frustrated, depressed
  Psychologic abnormalities common among patients with chronic diseases associated with pain
  Gastric ulcer and *Helicobacter pylori*

> **FIGURE 7-20.** Experiential findings regarding prostatitis and prostatodynia. In our experience, symptoms are often similar in patients with nonbacterial prostatitis and prostatodynia. Further, findings in the prostatic fluid of individual men may be variable [13]. We have isolated fastidious organisms from both populations. Both groups of men are often frustrated and depressed [14,15]. Their quality of life is impaired substantially [16]. However, psychologic abnormalities are very common among patients with chronic diseases associated with pain, and one must not forget that gastric ulcer, once ascribed to personality disorders, now is recognized as an infectious disease. EPS—expressed prostatic secretion.

Another Definition of Prostatitis Based on the Fertility Literature

Seminal fluid analysis
Various terms in addition to prostatitis
  Leukocytospermia
  Pyosemia
  Prostatoseminal vesiculitis
  Epididymo-prostato-vesiculitis
  Male accessory gland infection
  Seminal inflammation (preferred)

> **FIGURE 7-21.** Still another definition of prostatitis is used in the fertility literature. This definition is based on identification of inflammation in the seminal fluid. Various terms are used in this literature in addition to prostatitis [17].

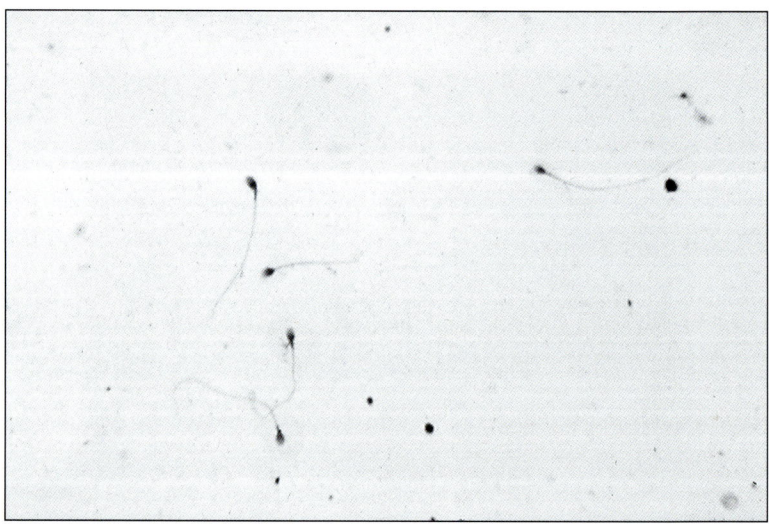

> **FIGURE 7-22.** A normal seminal fluid specimen that has been stained with Papanicolaou stain. Sperm and a few leukocytes are shown.

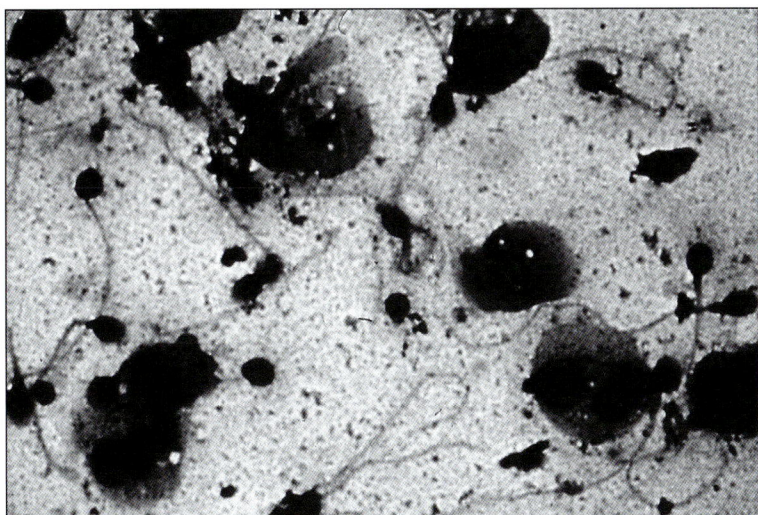

▶ **FIGURE 7-23.** A seminal fluid sample with increased numbers of polymorphonuclear leukocytes. Note that the slide is stained with Bryan-Leishman's stain to facilitate differentiation of leukocytes from sperm forms. Cells with pink cytoplasm are leukocytes, whereas cells with gray cytoplasm are germ cells.

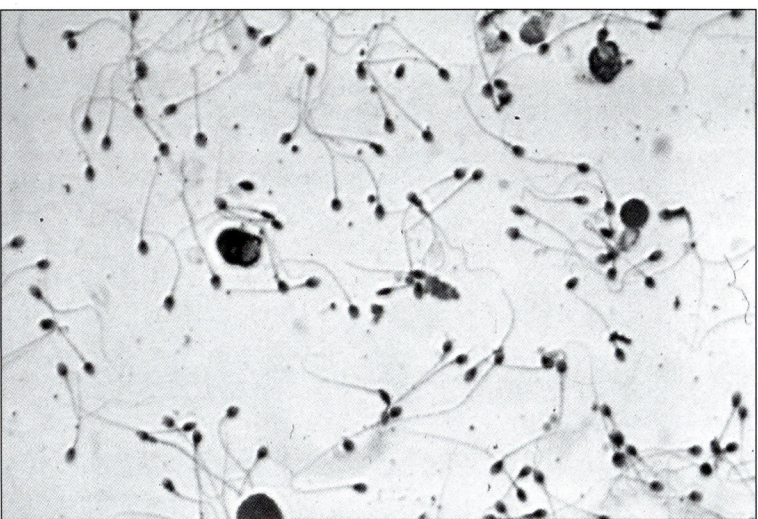

▶ **FIGURE 7-24.** A monoclonal antibody-stained preparation (HLe1), illustrating that the inflammatory cells are indeed leukocytes.

Problems with the Andrology Definition of Prostatitis

Populations studied
Methods
   Staining: distinguish leukocytes from sperm
   Definition of inflammation
      > 10^6 leukocytes per milliliter of semen
      > 6 leukocytes per 100 sperm
Possible relationship of leukocytospermia to:
   Infection
   Infertility

▶ **FIGURE 7-25.** Problems with the andrology definition of prostatitis. The first problem is the populations studied, which are predominantly patients with infertility as their chief complaint, not prostatitis. A second problem concerns the methods. Many studies used "round cell" counts in unstained specimens. Staining is necessary to distinguish leukocytes from sperm. Third, there have been varying definitions of inflammation (numbers or concentrations of leukocytes) used in this literature. Fourth, the question of the relationship between leukocytospermia and either infection or infertility is incompletely defined.

Other problems include the fact that leukocytes in semen can come from multiple sites besides the prostate. Most studies in this literature, however, seldom evaluate other sites, such as the urethra or expressed prostatic secretions, for presence of inflammation. Many studies lack data on patients' symptoms or physical findings. Finally, limited data correlate seminal fluid analysis findings with either findings in the prostatic secretions or with histology of the prostate.

Standard Clinical Definition of Prostatitis

Based on symptoms
Limited laboratory evaluation
Repeated courses of empirical therapy

▶ **FIGURE 7-26.** The clinical definition of prostatitis. Stamey [7] describes this definition as "a wastebasket of clinical ignorance used to describe any condition associated with prostatic inflammation or prostatic symptoms . . . most commonly diagnosed in patients who have no history of bladder infection despite the presence of perineal aching, low back pain, or urinary discomfort."

The standard clinical definition of prostatitis is based entirely on symptoms. Most patients undergo limited laboratory evaluation. In contrast, they have repeated courses of empirical therapy using a variety of agents. This does have one overriding advantage: the clinical definition does address what patients actually suffer from.

Genitourinary Symptoms of Chronic Prostatitis

General agreement in literature
   Certain pain symptoms common, *ie*, perineal, back, and genital
Marked disagreement regarding:
   Voiding complaints
   Sexual dysfunction

▶ **FIGURE 7-27.** The genitourinary symptoms of chronic prostatitis. Careful review of the literature found general agreement on the presence of certain pain symptoms, such as perineal, back, and genital pain [18]. However, there was marked disagreement on the prevalence of voiding complaints and sexual dysfunction.

Problems With the Clinical Definition of Prostatitis

Characteristic symptoms poorly defined
No diagnostic physical finding or laboratory test
Therapy is entirely empirical and often unsatisfactory

▶ **FIGURE 7-28.** Problems with the clinical definition of prostatitis. The model used for benign prostatic hyperplasia (BPH) may prove valuable. In the new BPH model, the American Urological Association symptom score proved critical for developing new therapies, although we still do not completely understand the cause of BPH.

Genitourinary Symptoms of Prostatitis

Stress and psychologic abnormalities common
Patients present to urologists with somatic symptoms
Concentrated on the urogenital complaints
  Pain complaints
  Voiding complaints
  Sexual dysfunction

▶ **FIGURE 7-29.** Genitourinary symptoms of prostatitis. What we do know about the genitourinary symptoms of prostatitis is that stress and psychologic abnormalities are very common. Many of these patients present to urologists with somatic symptoms; therefore, we and others have concentrated on developing instruments that evaluate the genitourinary complaints of these patients. We found that most complaints can be classified as either pain complaints, voiding complaints, or sexual dysfunction complaints [18]. To summarize, prostatitis causes considerable morbidity. It is neglected in terms of research and new clinical initiatives compared with the other prostate diseases. Although there are at least four definitions, none of them works well for the great majority of patients.

A. Aspects of the Working Definition of "Chronic Prostatitis"

Symptoms: pain complaints are primary component
Closer to patient presentation and clinical practice
New synonym for chronic prostatitis: CPPS

▶ **FIGURE 7-30.** Consensus working definition of "chronic prostatitis." As a first step in addressing these problems, a new working definition for chronic prostatitis was developed by an expert panel convened by the National Institute of Diabetes and Digestive and Kidney Diseases (NIDDK) [19]. **A,** This new definition, which has yet to be validated, concentrated on patients' symptoms using pain complaints as a primary component. In this respect it is much closer to patient presentation and clinical practice. In addition there is a new synonym for chronic prostatitis: chronic pelvic pain syndrome (CPPS).

B, Exclusion criteria. These criteria include duration less than 3 months, presence of genitourinary cancers such as transitional cell carcinoma (TCC), carcinoma in situ (CIS), or carcinoma of the prostate. Other exclusions include presence of active stone disease, because a distal ureteral stone or crystaluria can cause lower tract symptoms. Presence of active infection,

B. Automatic Exclusion Criteria for Chronic Prostatitis

Duration < 3 mo
Genitourinary cancer (*eg*, TCC, CIS, prostate cancer)
Active stone disease
Active infection
  Bacteriuria, herpes, genitourinary tuberculosis
Gastrointestinal disorders
  Inflammatory bowel disease
  Perirectal disease (*eg*, fissure, fistula)
Radiation/chemical cystitis
Acute urethritis
Acute epididymitis
Acute orchitis
Urethral stricture
Neurologic disease affecting bladder

such as bacteriuria, herpes, or genitourinary tuberculosis, presence of genitourinary disease, such as inflammatory bowel disease or perirectal disease such as fissure or fistula, also exclude patients from the NIDDK definition. Other automatic exclusions are also listed in this figure.

A. Symptomatic Prostatitis Syndromes

Bacterial prostatitis
   Acute and chronic
Chronic prostatitis
   CPPS or "abacterial" prostatitis

B. Aspects of Acute and Chronic Bacterial Prostatitis

Acute
   Bacteriuria
      Uropathogens
   Possible systemic illness
Chronic
   Recurrent episodes of bacteriuria
   Organism "localizes" to prostate

C. Chronic Prostatitis or Chronic Pelvic Pain Syndrome

Inflammatory
   Leukocytes in EPS, semen, VB3
Noninflammatory
   No leukocytes

▶ **FIGURE 7-31.** Prostatitis syndromes. The National Institute of Diabetes and Digestive and Kidney Diseases consensus classification of prostatitis considers prostatitis syndromes as either symptomatic or asymptomatic. **A,** The symptomatic prostatitis syndromes include bacterial prostatitis, either acute or chronic, and chronic prostatitis or chronic pelvic pain syndrome (CPPS), also known as "abacterial" prostatitis. **B,** Aspects of acute and chronic bacterial prostatitis. Acute bacterial prostatitis is characterized by presence of bacteriuria caused by recognized uropathogens. Some patients may have a systemic illness. The hallmark of chronic bacterial prostatitis is recurrent episodes of bacteriuria caused by the same organism that localizes to the prostate on segmented cultures. **C,** The third syndrome is chronic prostatitis or chronic pelvic pain syndrome, which has an inflammatory subtype, characterized by presence of leukocytes in prostatic secretions, semen, or postmassage urine, and a noninflammatory subtype, characterized by absence of leukocytes. EPS—expressed prostatic secretions; VB3—voided bladder 3.

Characteristics of Asymptomatic Inflammatory Prostatitis

Increased PSA level
Histology indicates prostatitis
Infertility is only symptom

▶ **FIGURE 7-32.** Asymptomatic inflammatory prostatitis. Finally, there is a category termed "asymptomatic inflammatory prostatitis." For example, an asymptomatic patient presents with an increased prostate-specific antigen (PSA) and this leads to a biopsy. The most common noncancer diagnosis is prostatitis. There are also patients with infertility, who have no symptoms other than their infertility, and have prostatitis based on seminal fluid findings. Such patients are characterized as having asymptomatic inflammatory prostatitis.

The New Consensus Classification of Prostatitis Syndromes

Acute bacterial prostatitis
Chronic bacterial prostatitis
Chronic prostatitis or CPPS
   Inflammatory
   Noninflammatory
Asymptomatic inflammatory prostatitis

▶ **FIGURE 7-33.** Summary of the new classification of prostatitis syndromes. CPPS—chronic pelvic pain syndromes.

A. Outline of the National Institutes of Health–Chronic Prostatitis Symptom Index (NIH-CPSI)

Nine questions
Four domains
   Pain or discomfort: four items
   Urination: two items
   Impact of symptoms: two items
   Quality of life: one item
Total score

B. NIH-CPSI Pain and Discomfort Scale

In the last week, have you experienced any pain or discomfort in the following areas:
   Perineum
   Testicles
   Tip of penis
   Below the waist, in your pubic or bladder area
In the last week, have you experienced:
   Pain or burning with urination
   Pain or discomfort during or after sexual climax

C. NIH-CPSI Frequency of Pain and Discomfort Scale

How often have you had pain or discomfort in any of these areas over the past week? (0–5 scale)
Which number best describes your *average* pain or discomfort on the days that you have had it, over the last week? (0–10 scale)

▶ **FIGURE 7-34.** The National Institutes of Health–Chronic Prostatitis Symptom Index (NIH-CPSI). To help provide a tool for patient evaluation and development of clinical protocols, a symptom index was developed and validated [20]. **A,** Outline of the NIH-CPSI. The symptom index consists of nine questions (items) covering four domains. Thus, it is possible to calculate a total score and scores for each domain. **B,** The pain or discomfort domain evaluates presence of pain in several locations and during urination and during or after ejaculation. **C,** The frequency that patients experience pain or discomfort and the average pain or discomfort level.

(Continued on next page)

D. NIH-CPSI Urination Scale

How often have you had a sensation of not emptying your bladder completely after you finished urinating, over the last week? (0–5 scale)

How often have you had to urinate again < 2 h after you finished urinating, over the last week? (0–5 scale)

E. NIH-CPSI Impact of Symptoms Scale

How much have your symptoms kept you from doing the kinds of things you would usually do, over the last week? (0–3 scale)

How much did you think about your symptoms, over the last week? (0–3 scale)

F. NIH-CPSI Quality of Life Scale

If you were to spend the rest of your life with your symptoms just the way they have been during the last week, how would you feel about that? (0–6 scale)

▶ **FIGURE 7-34.** (*Continued*) D, Urination scale. The urination scale contains two items that evaluate the sensation of bladder emptying and the need to urinate again within 2 hours of the previous micturition. **E,** Impact of symptoms scale. This scale contains two items that evaluate how much the patient's symptoms kept him from doing his usual activities and how much he thinks about his symptoms. **F,** The quality of life scale consists of one item. The combination of the consensus classification for prostatitis syndromes with the NIH-CPSI instrument has provided a new framework for patient evaluation and assessment of symptoms.

Epidemiology of Prostatitis: Ideal Study Characteristics

Population based
Clear case definition
Standard survey strategy
Sufficient size

▶ **FIGURE 7-35.** Epidemiology of prostatitis. The ideal study should have four characteristics. First, it should be population based, not a "cherry-picked" series of highly selected cases. Second, there should be a clear case definition that bears some relationship to clinical practice. The usual practice is to employ a more restrictive case definition than the one usually employed in practice. This allows most clinicians to agree that "the cases in the series are truly cases," recognizing that some patients in practice would be excluded from the study. Third, there should be a standard population survey strategy. Finally, the ideal series should include sufficient numbers of cases to provide statistical power for the primary outcome and for important secondary analyses. Fortunately, a number of recent studies have many of these characteristics [21].

Prevalence Studies: United States

Study	Population	Number	Age, y	Prevalence, %
Moon, 1997 [22]	Wisconsin National Guard	184 men	20–49	5
Roberts, 1998 [23]	Olmsted County, MN	2115 men	40–79	9
Collins, 1998 [3]	U.S. National Ambulatory Care Survey	58,955 visits	>18	Urology: 8 Primary care: 1
Roberts, 2002 [24]	Olmsted County, MN	1.541	40–79	2.2

▶ **FIGURE 7-36.** Prevalence studies from the United States. The table summarizes recent population-based epidemiologic studies from the United States [4, 22–24]. These studies evaluated from 184 to almost 59,000 participants. The prevalence of prostatitis-like symptoms ranged from 2.2% to 9% among community-dwelling men.

Prevalence Studies: Asia

Study	Country	Subjects, n	Age, y	Prevalence, %
Tan, 2002 [25]	Singapore	1087	21–70	2.7
Kunishima, 2002	Japan	502	20–79	5
Cheah, 2003 [26]	Malaysia	3147	20–50	8.7

▶ **FIGURE 7-37.** Prevalence studies from Asia. The table summarizes population-based survey studies from various Asian countries [21,25,26]. These studies evaluated from 500 to more than 3000 participants. The prevalence of prostatitis-like symptoms ranged from 2.7% to 8.7%, reflecting different populations, case definitions, and survey methods.

Prevalence: Europe and Canada

Study	Country	Subjects, n	Age, y	Prevalence, %
Mehik, 2000 [27]	Finland (Oulu and Lapland provinces)	1832	20–59	"Lifetime prevalence" (incidence), 14.2
Nickel, 2001 [2]	Canada (Lennox and Addington counties)	868	20–74	9.7

▶ **FIGURE 7-38.** Prevalence studies from Europe and Canada. The table summarizes two population-based survey studies from northern Europe [27] and Canada [2]. The Finnish study of 1832 men reported a "lifetime prevalence" of prostatitis-like symptoms of 14.2%. The Canadian study of 868 patients of family practitioners in eastern Canada reported a 9.7% prevalence of prostatitis-like symptoms.

Prostatitis May Increase BPH Risk

Collins, 2002 [28]: U.S. health care
    professionals
31,681 men without CaP
16% with prostatitis history
OR for BPH: 7.7 for men with prostatitis
    history

▶ **FIGURE 7-39.** Prostatitis may increase benign prostatic hypertrophy (BPH) risk. New data suggest that prostatitis may be a risk factor for development of other prostate disorders. For example, in the U.S. health care professionals follow-up cohort study of 31,681 men without prostate cancer (CaP), the prevalence of a self-reported history of prostatitis was 16% [28]. Men reporting a history BPH had 7.7-fold greater odds of a history of prostatitis.

Prostatitis May Increase CaP Risk

Dennis, 2002 [29]: meta-analysis
    Increased CaP risk with a prostatitis history
    OR, 1.6 overall
    OR, 1.8 in population-based case-control studies
Roberts, 2004 [30]: medical records review
    409 CaP cases, 803 age-matched controls
    Any type of prostatitis: OR, 1.7 for CaP
    Acute prostatitis: OR, 2.5
    Chronic bacterial prostatitis: OR, 1.6
    Chronic pelvic pain syndrome: OR, 0.9

▶ **FIGURE 7-40.** Prostatitis may increase prostate cancer (CaP) risk. Other studies suggest that a history of prostatitis may be associated with an increased risk of CaP. Meta-analysis of pooled epidemiologic data suggests that there is an increased risk among men with a history of prostatitis (OR, 1.6), particularly with population-based case-control studies (OR, 1.8) [29]. These data are consistent with recent medical records of histologically proven CaP cases that were each age matched to two control subjects [30]. There was an increased risk of CaP among men with history of any type of prostatitis (OR, 1.7; 95% CI, 1.1–2.6) or acute prostatitis (OR, 2.5; 95% CI, 1.3–4.7). The mean time from the most recent episode of acute prostatitis to the diagnosis of CaP was 12.2 years.

Possible Links

Chronic inflammation
    Frequent in biopsy, radical prostatectomy,
        and BPH specimens
    Proliferative inflammatory atrophy
    Proinflammatory and anti-inflammatory
        factors
    Germline variants of genes associated with
        inflammation may modulate CaP risk

▶ **FIGURE 7-41.** Possible links. Numerous potential mechanisms have been proposed to explain how prostatitis may increase the risk for subsequent development of other prostate disorders [31,32]. Chronic inflammation is a leading candidate as a mechanism linking prostatitis with prostate cancer (CaP). Inflammation has long been linked to cancers with an infectious etiology, such as stomach, liver, and colon cancers, in patients with inflammatory bowel disease. Inflammation is frequently identified in prostate biopsies, prostatectomy specimens, and tissue resected for treatment of benign prostatic hyperplasia. Genetic data have implicated variants of several genes associated with the immunologic aspects of inflammation in modulating prostate cancer risk. BPH–benign prostatic hyperplasia.

Prostatitis Epidemiology

Important cause of morbidity worldwide
    Prevalence: 2%–10% in adult men
    Lifetime incidence: 15% (1 study)
    Patient visits (1 study)
        8% to urologists
        1% to primary care practitioners
    Preliminary data suggest prostatitis increases:
        BPH risk
        CaP risk

▶ **FIGURE 7-42.** Prostatitis epidemiology. In summary, prostatitis represents an important cause of morbidity worldwide. The prevalence of symptoms appears to be in the 2% to 10% range in varied populations. Symptoms of prostatitis are responsible for a substantial proportion of patient visits to both urologists and primary care practitioners. Finally, epidemiologic data suggest potential links between prostatitis and both prostate cancer (CaP) and benign prostatic hyperplasia (BPH).

Treatment of Prostatitis

Clear
  Acute bacterial
  Chronic bacterial
Fuzzy
  Chronic prostatitis/chronic pelvic pain
  syndrome
  Asymptomatic inflammatory

▶ **FIGURE 7-43.** Treatment of prostatitis. Treatment strategies are clear for acute bacterial prostatitis and for chronic bacterial prostatitis. In contrast, there is considerable controversy and confusion about the optimal approaches for managing patients with chronic prostatitis/chronic pelvic pain syndrome and for asymptomatic inflammatory prostatitis.

Acute/Chronic Bacterial Prostatitis

Antibiotics
Depending on culture and sensitivity testing
First choice: fluoroquinolone
Second choice:
  trimethoprim-sulfamethoxazole

▶ **FIGURE 7-44.** Treatment of acute and chronic bacterial prostatitis. Antimicrobial therapy is clearly indicated for patients with documented bacterial infections of the prostate [33,34]. Therapy should be directed based on culture and sensitivity testing. In general, the first choice is a fluoroquinolone and the second choice is trimethoprim-sulfamethoxazole.

CP/CPPS Treatment

No proven therapy
Quality of treatment trials improving
  dramatically
Likely important to distinguish populations
  Amount and types of previous therapy
  Duration of clinical symptoms
  Other prognostic factors?

▶ **FIGURE 7-45.** Treatment of chronic prostatitis/chronic pelvic pain syndrome (CP/CPPS). Unfortunately, there is no proven therapy for these patients. Several references are provided to suggest the scope of theories and agents that have been investigated [35–43]. The most important aspect is that the quality of prostatitis treatment studies has improved dramatically in the past decade. It is also clear that it will likely prove critical to distinguish different populations for therapy. Factors that appear likely to be important in distinguishing populations for different therapies include the amount and types of previous therapy, duration and characteristics of symptoms, and other undefined factors.

CP/CPPS: Promising Approaches

Antibiotics
α-Blockers
Pain therapies
Anti-inflammatory therapies
Phytotherapy
Combination therapy

▶ **FIGURE 7-46.** Chronic prostatitis/chronic pelvic pain syndrome (CP/CPPS) promising treatment approaches. In our opinion, the literature currently supports a number of promising approaches for patients with CP/CPPS. These approaches include antibiotics [35], α-blockers [35,36,40], pain therapies [37,43], anti-inflammatory therapy [43], phytotherapy [44], and combinations of these approaches [41]. Currently, none of these approaches has been proven definitively [38].

Asymptomatic Inflammatory Prostatitis

Do we need to treat?
Potential benefits:
  Decreased need for prostate biopsies to evaluate increased PSA
  Potential to decrease BPH or CaP risk
  Potential to increase fertility
Potential disadvantages:
  No proven therapy
  Potential toxicity of therapy for asymptomatic patients

▶ **FIGURE 7-47.** Treatment of asymptomatic inflammatory prostatitis. The first question is, Do we really need to treat these patients? Potential benefits of treatment include the possibility of decreasing the rate of unnecessary prostate biopsies for evaluation of elevated prostate-specific antigen (PSA) values, the theoretic possibility of decreasing subsequent development of benign prostatic hyperplasia (BPH) or prostate cancer (CaP), and the potential to increase fertility for patients presenting with infertility. There are very real concerns about treating these asymptomatic patients. These concerns include the facts that there are no proven therapies and that all treatments recommended to date have adverse effects that are of concern to patients who have no symptoms.

REFERENCES

1. Alexander RB, Trissel D: Chronic prostatitis: results of an Internet survey. *Urology* 1996, 48:568–574.

2. Nickel JC, Downey J, Hunter D, *et al.*: Prevalence of prostatitis-like symptoms in a population based study using the National Institutes of Health chronic prostatitis symptom index. *J Urol* 2001, 165:842–845.

3. Collins MM, Stafford RS, O'Leary MP, *et al.*: How common is prostatitis? A national survey of physician visits. *J Urol* 1998, 159:1224–1228.

4. Krieger JN: How common is prostatitis? [editorial]. *J Urol* 1998, 159:1228.

5. True LD, Berger RE, Rothman I, *et al.*: Prostate histopathology and the chronic prostatitis/chronic pelvic pain syndrome: a prospective biopsy study. *J Urol* 1999, 162: 2014–2018.

6. Meares E Jr, Stamey TA: Bacteriologic localization patterns in bacterial prostatitis and urethritis. *Invest Urol* 1968, 5:492–518.

7. Stamey T: *Urinary Infections in Males: Pathogenesis and Treatment of Urinary Tract Infections.* Baltimore: Williams & Wilkins; 1980:342.

8. Krieger JN, McGonagle LA: Diagnostic considerations and interpretation of microbiological findings for evaluation of chronic prostatitis. *J Clin Microbiol* 1989, 27:2240–2244.

9. Krieger JN, Egan KJ: Comprehensive evaluation and treatment of 75 men referred to chronic prostatitis clinic. *Urology* 1991, 38:11–19.

10. Krieger J: Prostatitis syndromes. In *Sexually Transmitted Diseases*, edn 2. Edited by Holmes K, Sparling P, Mardh P-A. New York: McGraw-Hill; 1998.

11. Nickel JC, Johnston B, Downey J, *et al.*: Pentosan polysulfate therapy for chronic nonbacterial prostatitis (chronic pelvic pain syndrome category IIIA): a prospective multicenter clinical trial. *Urology* 2000, 56:413–417.

12. Alexander RB, Brady F, Ponniah S: Autoimmune prostatitis: evidence of T cell reactivity with normal prostatic proteins. *Urology* 1997, 50:893–899.

13. Wright ET, Chmiel JS, Grayhack JT, *et al.*: Prostatic fluid inflammation in prostatitis. *J Urol* 1994, 152:2300–2303.

14. Egan KJ, Krieger JL: Chronic abacterial prostatitis: a urological chronic pain syndrome? *Pain* 1997, 69:213–218.

15. Egan KJ, Krieger JN: Psychological problems in chronic prostatitis patients with pain. *Clin J Pain* 1994, 10:218–226.

16. McNaughton-Collins M, Pontari MA, O'Leary MP, *et al.*: Quality of life is impaired in men with chronic prostatitis: the Chronic Prostatitis Collaborative Research Network. *J Gen Intern Med* 2001, 16:656–662.

17. Krieger JN, Berger RE, Ross SO, *et al.*: Seminal fluid findings in men with nonbacterial prostatitis and prostatodynia. *J Androl* 1996, 17:310–318.

18. Krieger JN, Egan KJ, Ross SO, *et al.*: Chronic pelvic pains represent the most prominent urogenital symptoms of "chronic prostatitis." *Urology* 1996, 48:715–722.

19. Krieger JN, Nyberg L Jr, Nickel JC: NIH consensus definition and classification of prostatitis. *JAMA* 1999, 282:236–237.

20. Litwin MS, McNaughton-Collins M, Fowler FJ Jr, *et al.*: The National Institutes of Health chronic prostatitis symptom index: development and validation of a new outcome measure. Chronic Prostatitis Collaborative Research Network. *J Urol* 1999, 162:369–375.

21. Krieger JN, Riley DE, Cheah PY, *et al.*: Epidemiology of prostatitis: new evidence for a world-wide problem. *World J Urol* 2003, 21:70–74.

22. Moon TD: Questionnaire survey of urologists and primary care physicians' diagnostic and treatment practices for prostatitis. *Urology* 1997, 50:543–547.

23. Roberts RO, Lieber MM, Rhodes T, *et al.*: Prevalence of a physician-assigned diagnosis of prostatitis: the Olmsted County Study of Urinary Symptoms and Health Status Among Men. *Urology* 1998, 51:578–584.

24. Roberts RO, Jacobson DJ, Girman CJ, *et al.*: Prevalence of prostatitis-like symptoms in a community based cohort of older men. *J Urol* 2002, 168:2467–2471.

25. Tan JK, Png DJ, Liew LC, *et al.*: Prevalence of prostatitis-like symptoms in Singapore: a population-based study. *Singapore Med J* 2002, 43:189–193.

26. Cheah PY, Liong ML, Yuen KH, *et al.*: Chronic prostatitis: symptom survey with follow-up clinical evaluation. *Urology* 2003, 61:60–64.

27. Mehik A, Hellstrom P, Lukkarinen O, *et al.*: Epidemiology of prostatitis in Finnish men: a population-based cross-sectional study. *BJU Int* 2000, 86:443–448.

28. Collins MM, Meigs JB, Barry MJ, *et al.*: Prevalence and correlates of prostatitis in the health professionals follow-up study cohort. *J Urol* 2002, 167:1363–1366.

29. Dennis LK, Lynch CF, Torner JC: Epidemiologic association between prostatitis and prostate cancer. *Urology* 2002, 60:78–83.

30. Roberts RO, Bergstralh EJ, Bass SE, *et al.*: Prostatitis as a risk factor for prostate cancer. *Epidemiology* 2004, 15:93–99.

31. Platz EA, De Marzo AM: Epidemiology of inflammation and prostate cancer. *J Urol* 2004, 171(2 Pt 2):S36–S40.

32. Palapattu GS, Sutcliffe S, Bastian PJ, *et al.*: Prostate carcinogenesis and inflammation: emerging insights. *Carcinogenesis* 2004 [Epub ahead of print].

33. Naber KG, Bergman B, Bishop MC, *et al.*: EAU guidelines for the management of urinary and male genital tract infections. Urinary Tract Infection (UTI) Working Group of the Health Care Office (HCO) of the European Association of Urology (EAU). *Eur Urol* 2001, 40:576–588.

34. Wagenlehner FM, Naber KG: Fluoroquinolone antimicrobial agents in the treatment of prostatitis and recurrent urinary tract infections in men. *Curr Urol Rep* 2004, 5:309–316.

35. Alexander RB, Propert KJ, Schaeffer AJ, *et al.*: Ciprofloxacin or tamsulosin in men with chronic prostatitis/chronic pelvic pain syndrome: a randomized, double-blind trial. *Ann Intern Med* 2004, 141:581–589.

36. Cheah PY, Liong ML, Yuen KH, *et al.*: Initial, long-term, and durable responses to terazosin, placebo, or other therapies for chronic prostatitis/chronic pelvic pain syndrome. *Urology* 2004, 64:881–886.

37. Chen R, Nickel JC: Acupuncture ameliorates symptoms in men with chronic prostatitis/chronic pelvic pain syndrome. *Urology* 2003, 61:1156–1159; discussion 1159.

38. McNaughton-Collins M, Mac Donald R, Wilt T: Interventions for chronic abacterial prostatitis. *Cochrane Database Syst Rev* 2001, CD002080.

39. McNaughton-Collins M, Wilt T: Allopurinol for chronic prostatitis. *Cochrane Database Syst Rev* 2000, CD001041.

40. Mehik A, Alas P, Nickel JC, *et al.*: Alfuzosin treatment for chronic prostatitis/chronic pelvic pain syndrome: a prospective, randomized, double-blind, placebo-controlled, pilot study. *Urology* 2003, 62:425–429.

41. Nickel JC, Downey J, Ardern D, *et al.*: Failure of a monotherapy strategy for difficult chronic prostatitis/chronic pelvic pain syndrome. *J Urol* 2004, 172:551–554.

42. Nickel JC, Downey J, Clark J, *et al.*: Levofloxacin for chronic prostatitis/chronic pelvic pain syndrome in men: a randomized placebo-controlled multicenter trial. *Urology* 2003, 62:614–617.

43. Nickel JC, Pontari M, Moon T, *et al.*: A randomized, placebo controlled, multicenter study to evaluate the safety and efficacy of rofecoxib in the treatment of chronic nonbacterial prostatitis. *J Urol* 2003, 169:1401–1405.

44. Shoskes DA: Phytotherapy in chronic prostatitis. *Urology* 2002, 60(6 Suppl):35–37; discussion 37.

Prostate-specific Antigen and Related Markers of Prostatic Disease

8

Brett S. Carver,
Thomas Steuber,
& Hans Lilja

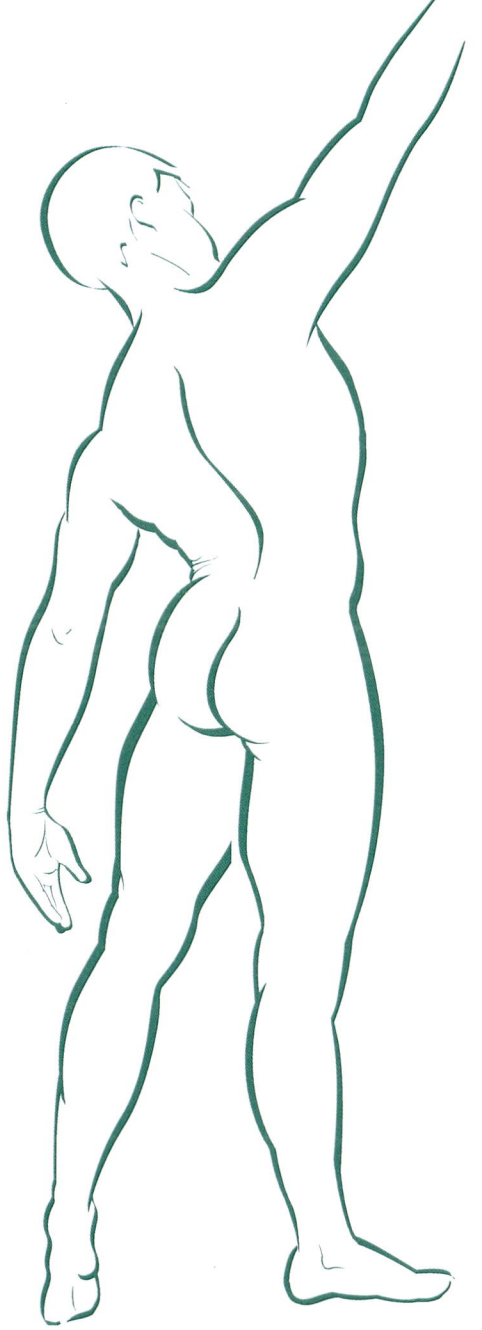

The human kallikrein (hK) family, located on chromosome 19, encodes prostate-specific antigen (PSA [or hK3]), hK2, hK4, and hK15 (prostin), as well as other serine proteases. Human glandular kallikrein 3 (hK3), commonly known as PSA, and human glandular kallikrein 2 (hK2) represent the most widely studied and clinically important members of the human glandular kallikrein family. Because of their restricted tissue expression patterns with high abundance in human prostate glands, PSA and hK2 have been thoroughly evaluated as candidate biomarkers for benign and malignant prostatic disease. Since its clinical introduction as a serum marker for the detection and staging of prostate cancer, PSA has had a profound and dramatic impact on the diagnosis and management of prostate cancer, and more recently, of benign prostatic hyperplasia. Through the intensive study of PSA, and the related kallikrein molecular markers (hK2), researchers have continued to improve and refine the usefulness of these markers.

Several isoforms of PSA have recently been introduced into clinical practice to help refine the specificity of serum PSA testing. These include free PSA, complexed PSA, and nicked PSA, each demonstrating improved ability to discriminate benign from cancerous disease over serum PSA level alone. In addition, investigators have demonstrated the utility of PSA density and PSA velocity in prostate cancer diagnosis.

Numerous models have been developed that predict for prostate cancer diagnosis, pathologic stage, and disease recurrence following treatment for prostate cancer. In all these models, serum PSA level plays a central role, demonstrating its dramatic utility as a marker for prostate cancer. Recent investigators have reported an increasing role of hK2 as a marker for prostatic disease. Several studies have demonstrated that hK2 is an independent predictor for prostate cancer detection and disease recurrence following radical prostatectomy.

In this chapter, we review the kallikrein gene family; the biology of PSA, the most well-characterized protein in this family; and the role of PSA and hK2 in prostate cancer diagnosis and staging.

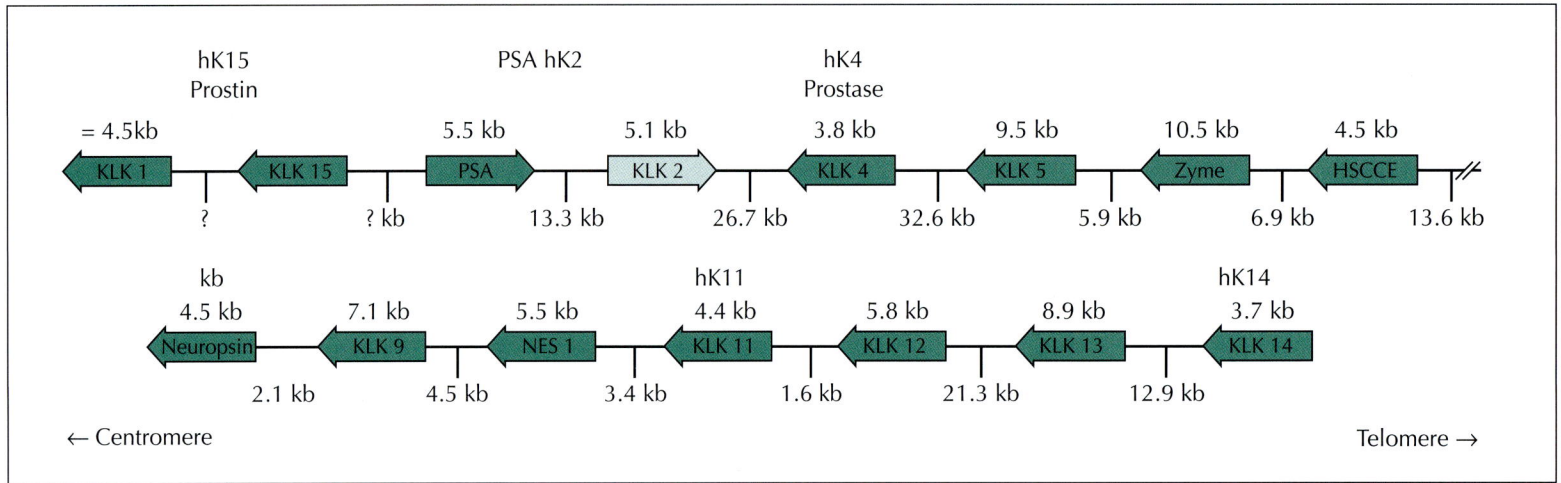

FIGURE 8-1. The human kallikrein (hK) gene locus. The hK gene locus is located on chromosome 19q13.3 to 13.4, spanning a region of 300 kb. The kallikrein family, located on chromosome 19, includes 15 characterized genes. Of these, prostate-specific antigen (PSA), hK2, hK4 (prostase), and hK15 (prostin) are expressed with abundance in prostatic tissue. Although their precise roles in the detection and progression of prostate cancer remain incompletely defined, they have enhanced diagnostic effects and may well provide information leading to more-effective therapies [1,2]. (*Adapted from* Lilja [1].)

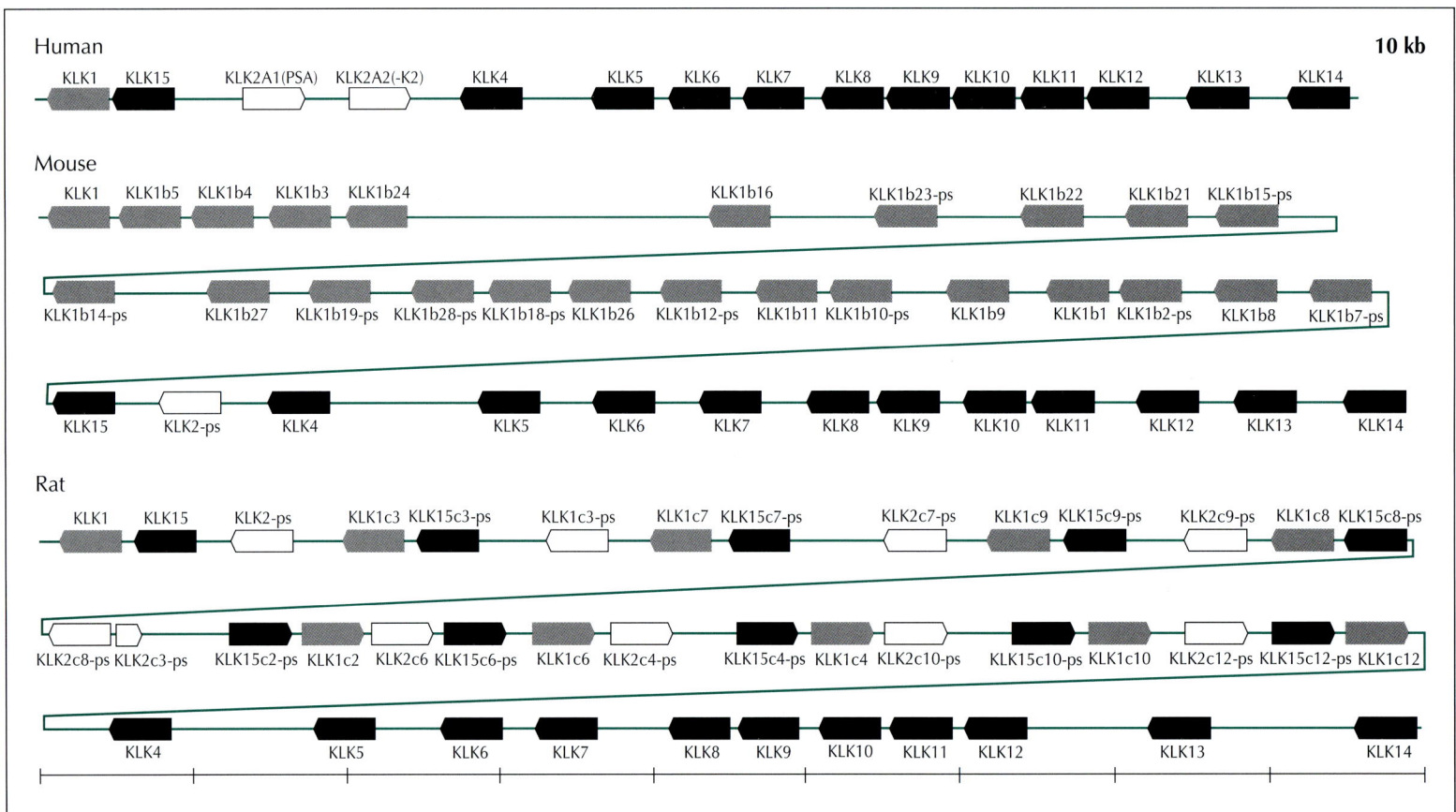

FIGURE 8-2. Evolutionarily conserved regions of the kallikrein gene locus; the glandular kallikrein loci of the human, the mouse, and the rat. The *arrows* indicate the location of the individual genes and the direction of transcription. The relative distances between the genes are drawn to scale, but the sizes of the genes are not. The *arrows* represent KLK1 paralogs (gray), KLK2 paralogs (white), and KLK4 to 15 (black). The boundaries of the duplicated regions of the rat are depicted at the *bottom*, and a *scale bar* (in kilobases) is shown at the *top right*. Although the vast majority of the kallikrein gene locus appears to be evolutionarily conserved across species, it has been noted that in the region of the prostate-specific antigen (PSA) and hK2 genes, a group of pseudogenes occupies these loci. Thus far, with the exception of old-world primates and the dog, no functional PSA or hK2 gene has been identified in other species. In the dog, the gene encoding the prostatic arginine esterase was identified as an ortholog to the progenitor of the PSA and hK2 genes, and it carries the same conserved androgen-responsive elements directing prostate transcription as these genes. This is highly interesting with respect to animal models of benign prostatic hyperplasia and prostate adenocarcinoma, diseases that have been described only in humans and dogs [3,4]. (*Adapted from* Olsson *et al.* [3,4].)

Common Structural Features of the Human Kallikrein Genes and Proteins

All genes are formed of five coding exons, and most of them have one or more extra 5′ untranslated exons. The first coding exon always contains a 5′ untranslated region, followed by the methionine start codon, located ~50 bp away from the end of the exon. The stop codon is always located ~156 bp from the beginning of the last coding exon.

Exon sizes are very similar or identical.

The intron phases of the coding exons (ie, the position where the intron starts in relation to the last codon of the previous exon) are conserved in all genes. The pattern of the intron phase is always I–II–I–O.

The positions of the residues of the catalytic triad of serine proteases are conserved, with the histidine always occurring near the end of the second coding exon, the aspartate in the middle of the third coding exon, and the serine residue at the beginning of the fifth coding exon.

All kallikrein proteins are synthesized as pre/propeptides with a signal peptide of ~17–20 amino acids at the amino terminus, followed by an activation peptide of ~4–9 amino acids (with the exception of hK5), followed by the mature (enzymatically active) protein.

The amino acid of the substrate-binding pocket is either aspartate, indicating trypsinlike specificity (11 enzymes), or another amino acid (probably conferring chymotryptic [PSA] or other activity).

Most, if not all, genes are under steroid hormone regulation.

All proteins contain 10–12 cysteine residues that will form 5–6 disulfide bonds. The positions of the cysteine residues are also fully conserved.

▶ **FIGURE 8-3.** Common structural features of the kallikrein genes and proteins. Similarities exist with regard to gene structure and function across the members of the kallikrein gene family. The protein products of these genes also share a high degree of homology with regard to protein structure, processing, and function [5]. PSA—prostate-specific antigen. (*Adapted from* Diamandis *et al.* [5].)

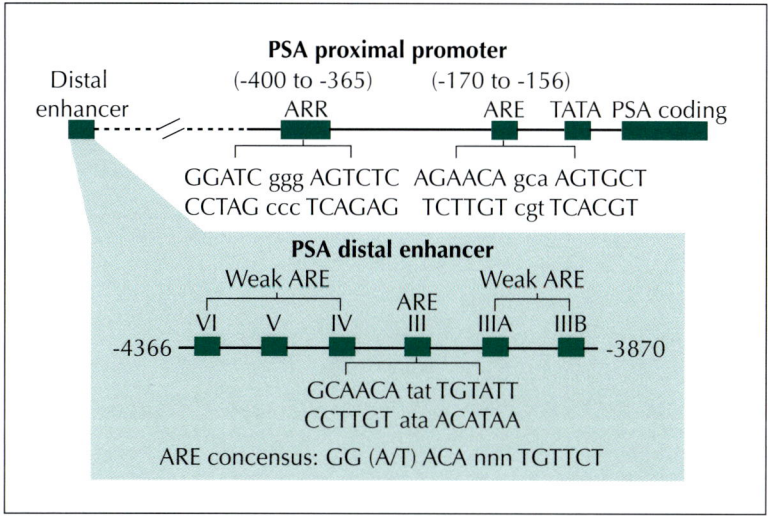

▶ **FIGURE 8-4.** Transcriptional regulation of the prostate-specific antigen (PSA) gene. Transcription of the PSA gene is positively regulated by the androgen receptor (AR), and PSA has been extensively studied as a model androgen-regulated gene. The AR is a steroid hormone receptor that binds as a homodimer to specific DNA sequences termed androgen-responsive elements (AREs), and a consensus ARE is located upstream from the transcriptional start site of the PSA gene. The AR can also bind weakly to sites that differ from the strong consensus ARE, and such a weak nonconsensus ARE (termed ARR) has been identified. Further studies have mapped the region responsible for high-level androgen-stimulated PSA expression to a fragment of about 450 bp, located approximately 4.2 kb upstream of the transcriptional start site, termed the PSA distal enhancer. This region contains a single strong consensus ARE (ARE III), but binding studies have demonstrated the presence of multiple additional weak nonconsensus AREs. The cooperative binding of multiple ARs to this region likely accounts for its strong androgen-dependent activity [2,6–8].

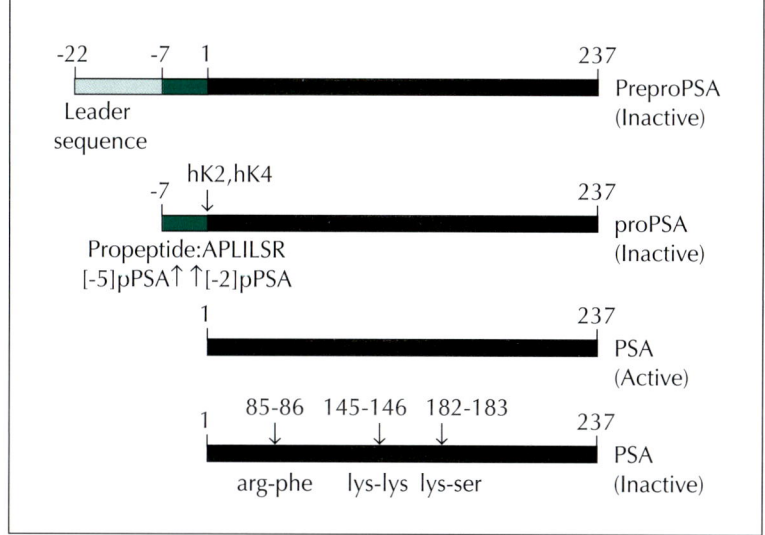

▶ **FIGURE 8-5.** Posttranscriptional processing of prostate-specific antigen (PSA). PSA is synthesized with a 17–amino acid leader sequence (preproPSA) that is cleaved cotranslationally to generate an inactive 244–amino acid precursor protein (proPSA). Cleavage of the N-terminal seven amino acids from proPSA generates the active enzyme, which has five intrachain disulfide bonds, a single asparagine-linked oligosaccharide, and a mass of 33 kD. This proPSA cleavage normally occurs between the arginine at position 7 and isoleucine at position 8, with the isoleucine becoming the N-terminus of the mature active protein. This site can be readily digested by trypsin, but the major activating enzyme in vivo is hK2, which has a trypsin-like activity and is expressed predominantly by prostate secretory epithelium. PSA may also be activated by other prostate kallikreins, including prostase (hK4) [2,9,10].

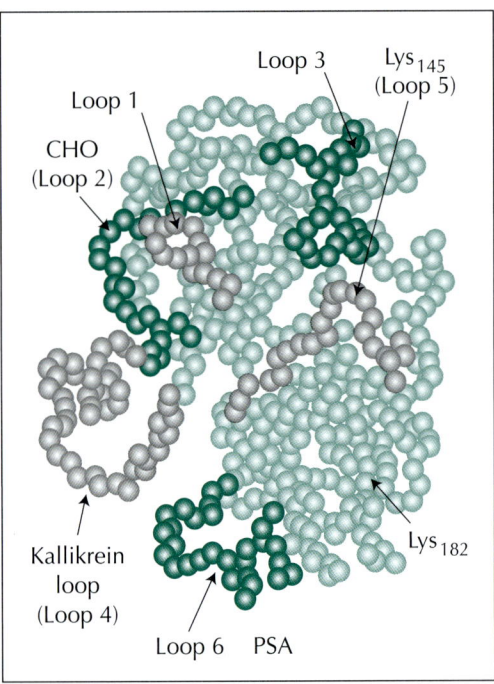

Loop 1
Loop 3
Lys₁₄₅ (Loop 5)
CHO (Loop 2)
Kallikrein loop (Loop 4)
Loop 6   PSA
Lys₁₈₂

▶ **FIGURE 8-6.** Molecular model of prostate-specific antigen (PSA; backbone structure only) demonstrating the six loops as described by Bridon and Dowell [11]. The major form of PSA in the seminal fluid is a single-chain glycoprotein with a polypeptide backbone of approximately 26 kd consisting of 237 amino acid residues. PSA manifests chymotrypsin-like proteolytic enzyme activity, hydrolyzing the peptide bonds of the carboxy-terminal at certain tyrosine and leucine residues. PSA activity is unique, however, in that it is ineffective at hydrolysis of peptide bonds that are most sensitive to the action of chymotrypsin. The enzyme activity of PSA is believed to be mainly directed against the major gel-forming proteins—semenogelin I and II—and fibronectin in freshly ejaculated semen. Proteolysis of these proteins induces liquefaction of semen, which results in the subsequent release of progressively motile spermatozoa. The catalytic triad (H41, D96, S189) is located in the center of the protein near loop 1 [11,12]. (*Adapted from* Bridon *et al.* [12].)

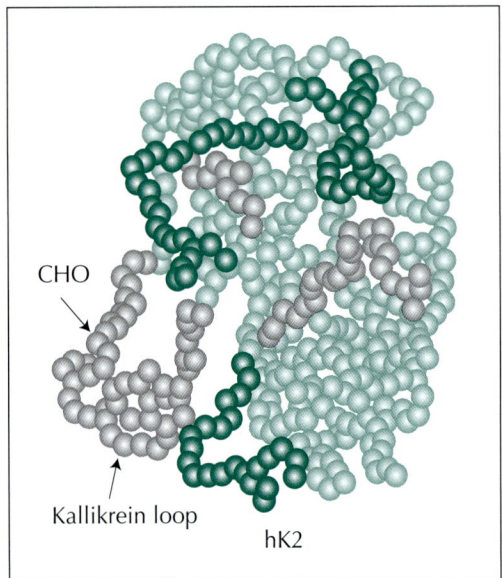

CHO
Kallikrein loop
hK2

▶ **FIGURE 8-7.** Molecular model of hK2. Molecular model of hK2 (backbone structure only) demonstrating the six loops as described by Bridon and Dowell [11]. Prostate-specific antigen (PSA) and hK2 share approximately 80% identity in primary protein structure. Like PSA, hK2 is a glycoprotein containing 237 amino acids, with a calculated mass of 26.2 kD based on amino acid sequence, but with an actual mass of 28.5 kD as determined by mass spectroscopy. Unlike PSA, hK2 displays the trypsinlike specificity common to most members of the kallikrein family of proteases. hK2 is highly selective for cleavage at arginine residues. Although hK2 can cleave semenogelin proteins with an activity that is comparable to PSA's, because the level of hK2 in the seminal fluid is only approximately 1% that of PSA, its physiologic role remains unclear. The catalytic triad (H41, D96, S189) is located in the center of the protein near loop 1 [11,13]. (*Adapted from* Bridon *et al.* [12].)

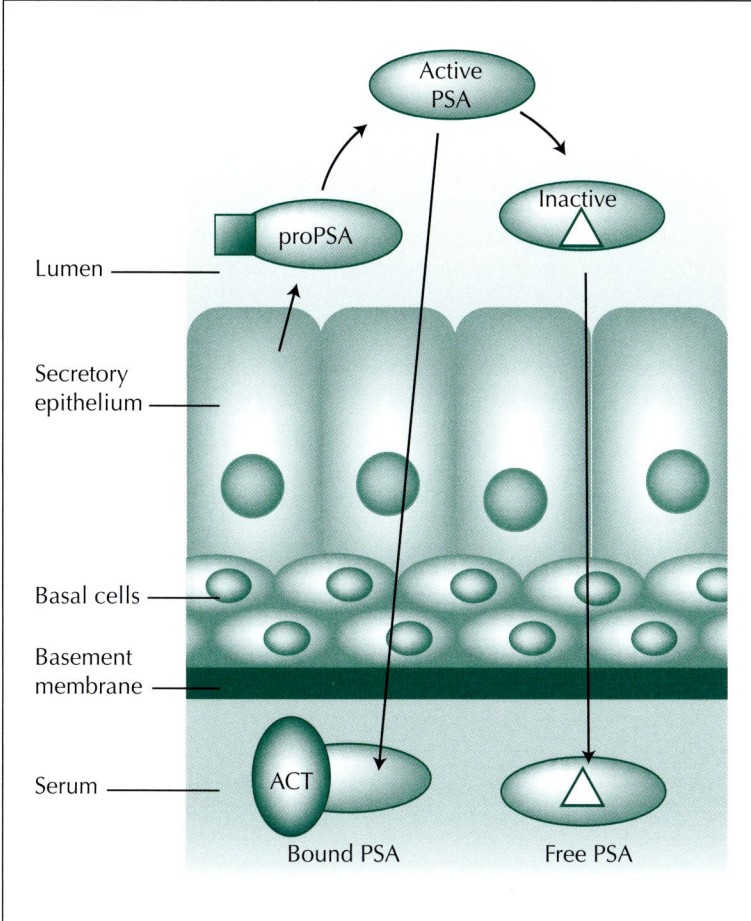

FIGURE 8-8. Prostate-specific antigen (PSA) synthesis and secretion in a normal prostatic epithelium. Model of PSA biosynthesis in normal prostate epithelium. Normal secretory epithelium, surrounded by basal cells and a basement membrane, secretes proPSA into the lumen, where the propeptide is removed by hK2 to generate active PSA. A fraction of this active PSA may diffuse into the circulation, where it is rapidly bound by protease inhibitors (primarily α_1-antichymotrypsin [ACT]). The active PSA also undergoes proteolysis in the lumen to generate inactive PSA, which may enter the bloodstream and circulate in an unbound state (free PSA) [2].

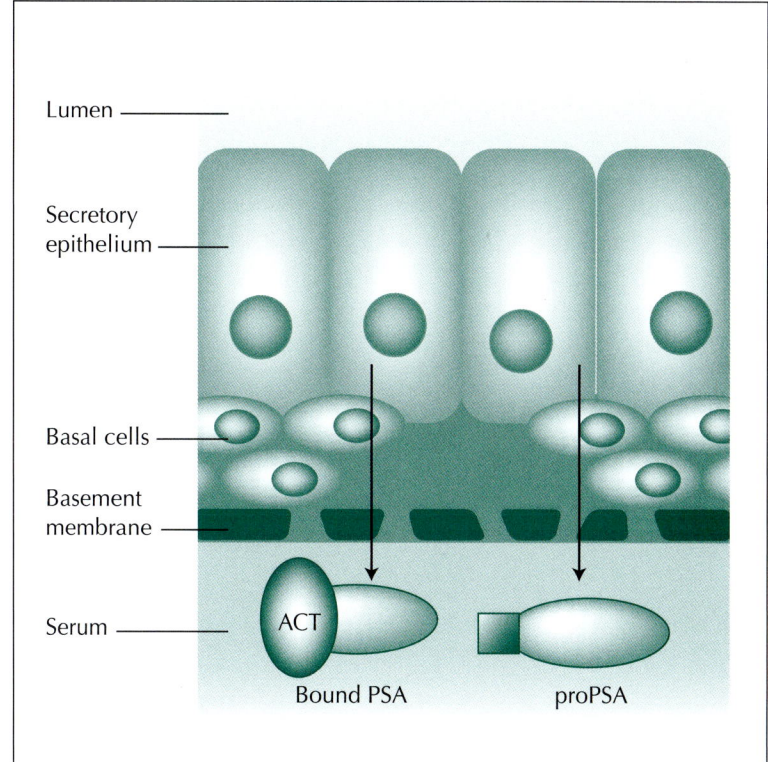

FIGURE 8-9. Prostate-specific antigen (PSA) synthesis and secretion in prostatic adenocarcinoma. In prostate cancer, loss of basal cells, basement membrane, and normal lumen architecture results in a decrease in the luminal processing of proPSA to active PSA, and active PSA to inactive PSA, with relative increases in bound PSA and proPSA in the serum [2].

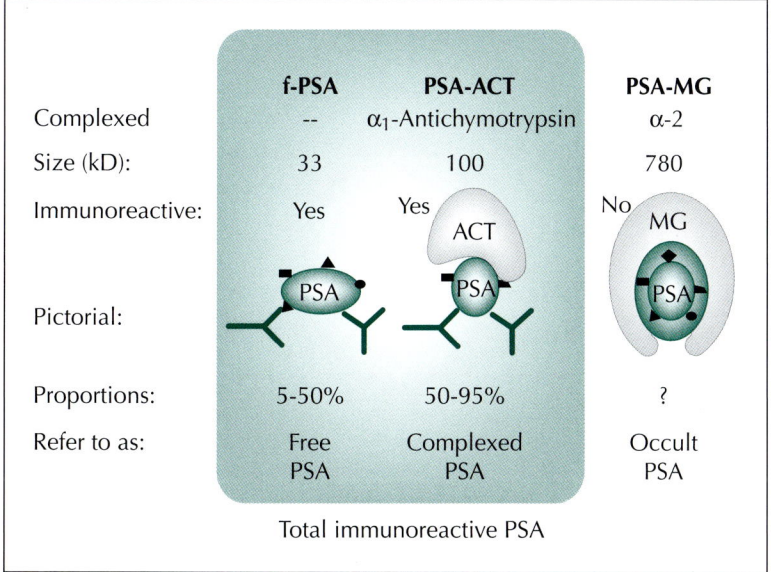

FIGURE 8-10. Major forms of prostate-specific antigen (PSA) in the serum. PSA is produced in the prostate columnar epithelial cells and secreted into the glandular lumen. The vast majority of kallikrein in the prostate is PSA that is initially expressed as precursor PSA (pPSA) but is found in its active form in the seminal fluid. More than 95% of the PSA in the seminal fluid is in its free form. In the serum, PSA complexes with α_1-antichymotrypsin (ACT) and α_2-macroglobulin (A2M) and is removed from the circulation by the liver serpin receptor and the A2M receptor on the reticuloendothelial cells, respectively. The smaller amounts of uncomplexed PSA forms are removed from the circulation through the renal system [14,15]. f-PSA—free PSA; PSA-MG—PSA-macroglobulin.

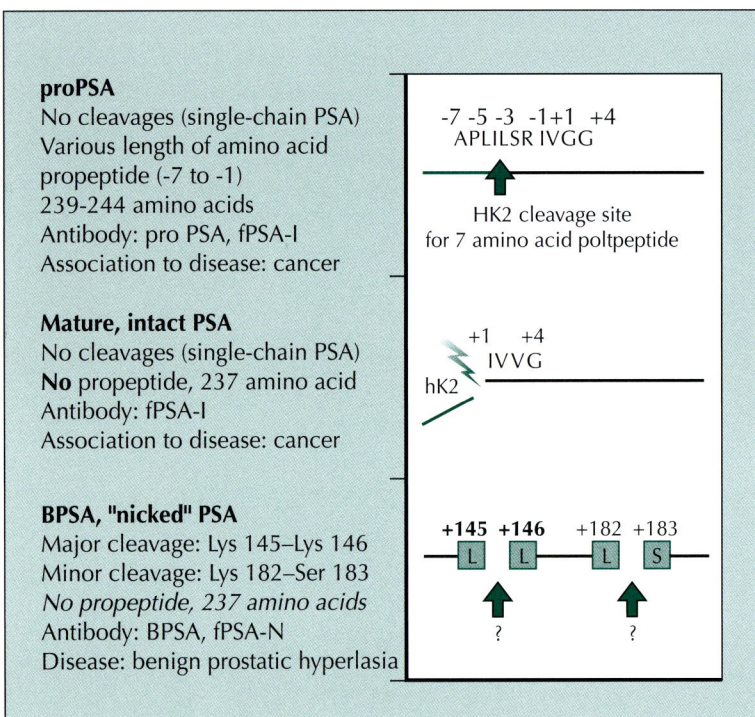

proPSA
No cleavages (single-chain PSA)
Various length of amino acid propeptide (-7 to -1)
239-244 amino acids
Antibody: pro PSA, fPSA-I
Association to disease: cancer

-7 -5 -3 -1+1 +4
APLILSR IVGG

HK2 cleavage site for 7 amino acid poltpeptide

Mature, intact PSA
No cleavages (single-chain PSA)
No propeptide, 237 amino acid
Antibody: fPSA-I
Association to disease: cancer

+1 +4
IVVG
hK2

BPSA, "nicked" PSA
Major cleavage: Lys 145–Lys 146
Minor cleavage: Lys 182–Ser 183
No propeptide, 237 amino acids
Antibody: BPSA, fPSA-N
Disease: benign prostatic hyperlasia

+145 +146 +182 +183
L L   L S
?   ?

▶ **FIGURE 8-11.** Free prostate-specific antigen (PSA) isoforms in the circulation. The detailed molecular nature of free PSA (fPSA) in the circulation has not yet been fully clarified, but free PSA has been concluded to be inactive because it is essentially nonreactive with the very large excess of inhibitors in the blood, mainly α_1-antichymotrypsin and α_2-macroglobulin. The two commonly proposed explanations for the presence of free PSA in the circulation are the proforms of the protein, which have been shown to possess little or no enzymatic activity, and internal cleavage at Lys145 to Lys146, which has been shown to inactivate PSA [16]. BPSA—baseline PSA; fPSA-N—nicked fPSA.

Molecular Forms of PSA and hK2: Literature Survey

| Molecular Form | Prostatic Tissue | | Seminal Plasma | Serum | |
	Carcinoma	Normal/BPH		PCa Patients	BPH Patients
tPSA	7.25 µg/mg protein	20.2 µg/mg protein	0.2–5 g/L, 30%–50% enzymatically active	>2 µg/L	1–20 µg/L
fPSA	5.58 µg/mg protein	15.1 µg/mg protein	>95% of tPSA	5%–30% of tPSA	10%–50% of tPSA
ACT-PSA	0.019 µg/mg protein	0.008 µg/mg protein	Not detectable	70%–95% of tPSA	50%–90% of tPSA
cPSA	0.068 µg/mg protein	0.099 µg/mg protein		70%–95% of tPSA	50%–90% of tPSA
API-PSA				3.2% of tPSA	4.1% of tPSA
ITI-PSA				<1% of tPSA	<1% of tPSA
A2M-PSA			Small amounts	12% of tPSA	17%
PCI-PSA			<5% of tPSA	Not detectable	
Nicked PSA	Smaller proportion	Higher proportion	~ 30% of tPSA	Small amounts	
proPSA	3.0% of tPSA	Small amounts	Not detectable	25% of fPSA	
bPSA	4.33% of tPSA	11.4% of tPSA 2.0 µg/mg protein			
thK2	0.12 µg/mg protein	0.19 µg/mg protein	2–12 mg/L	58 (0–235) ng/L 81 (0–931) ng/L	56 (0–577) ng/L 81 (0–818) ng/L
fhK2			Major fraction until 10 min after ejaculation	81%–96% of thK2	
ACT-hK2	Detected in Western blot			4%–19% of thK2	
API-hK2				Not detectable	
A2M-hK2				Present, rapid binding	
PCI-hK2			Major fraction until 10 min after ejaculation	In vitro, rapid binding	
Nicked hK2	Detected in Western blot		Major fraction of fhK2		
prohK2	70% of maximal immunoreactivity	45.5%		0.21 µg/L	0.09 µg/L
PI-6-hk2	~ 10% of thK2		Not detectable		

▶ **FIGURE 8-12.** Molecular isoforms of prostate-specific antigen (PSA) and hK2. It has been shown that PSA in serum exists in different molecular forms and that the measurement of these forms offers new possibilities to improve the diagnostic discrimination between prostate cancer and benign disease. The table lists the various isoforms of PSA and hK2 and their association with benign and malignant diseases of the prostate [17]. A2M—α_2-macroglobulin; ACT—α_1-antichymotrypsin; API—α_1-protease inhibitor; BPH—benign prostatic hyperplasia; bPSA—BPH nodule-associated PSA; cPSA—complexed PSA; fhK2—free hK2; fPSA—free PSA; PCa—prostate cancer; PCI—protein C inhibitor; PI-6-hK2—protease inhibitor 6 hK2; thK2—total hK2; tPSA—total PSA; ITI—inter-alpha–trypsin inhibitor. (*Adapted from* Stephan *et al.* [17].)

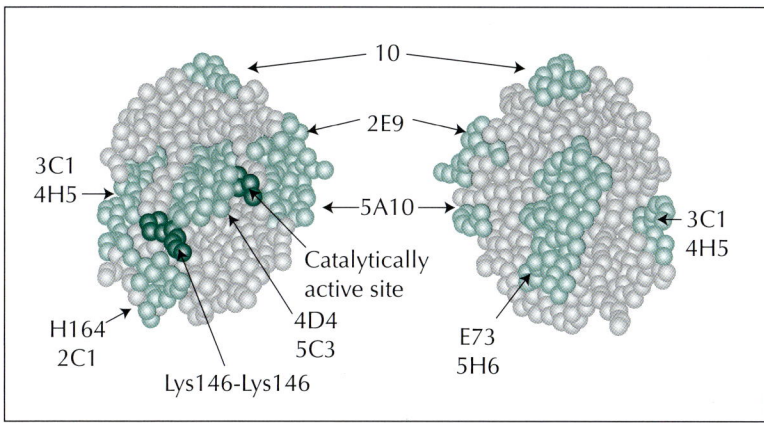

▶ **FIGURE 8-13.** Various prostate-specific antigen (PSA) antibody epitopes. Antibodies that bind to linear peptide sequences are mapped to this model of PSA. Seven independent antigenic domains are shown. Antibody 5A10 binds to the peptide sequence consisting of amino acids 84 to 91, 2E9 binds to amino acids 80 to 83, 10 binds to amino acids 150 to 164, 3C1 and 4H5 bind to amino acids 1 to 14, and H164 and 2C1 bind to amino acids 50 to 64, as presented by Nurmikko *et al.* [18]. E73 binds to the peptide sequence consisting of amino acids 215 to 229. Novel antibody 5H6 is mapped to the same epitope as E73 because it was bound to adjacent peptide sequence 225 to 237. The estimated binding site of 4D4 and 5C3, a novel epitope, is mapped to amino acids 135 to 144. The Lys145–Lys146 internal cleavage site and catalytically active sites are also shown [18]. (*Adapted from* Nurmikko *et al.* [18].)

Prostate Cancer Screening and PSA

Risk Classification	Age to Start Screening, y	Frequency of Screening
Low risk (*eg*, white, Asian male; no family history of prostate cancer)	50	Annually with serum PSA and DRE
High risk (African-American male or family history of prostate cancer)	40	Annually with serum PSA and DRE

▶ **FIGURE 8-14.** Prostate cancer screening and prostate-specific antigen (PSA). The topic of prostate cancer screening remains a controversial area. Current prostate cancer screening guidelines have been adopted by the American Cancer Society and the American Urological Association for men with a greater than 10-year life expectancy. In general, screening is recommended for men 50 years of age or older with an annual serum PSA and digital rectal examination (DRE).

Age-specific PSA Reference Values

Age Range, y	Normal Serum PSA Level, ng/mL
<40	<2.0
40–50	<2.5
51–60	<3.5
61–70	<4.5
>70	<6.5

▶ **FIGURE 8-15.** Age-specific prostate-specific antigen (PSA) reference values. In men who do not have prostate cancer, serum PSA levels correlate with age and total prostate volume. As men age, prostate volume increases an average of 0.7 to 1.5 mL per year, although men with benign prostatic hyperplasia appear to have higher prostate growth rates. However, independent of the effects of prostate volume, serum PSA levels increase with age in community populations. Oesterling *et al.* [19] proposed age-specific normal reference ranges based on these observations. (*Adapted from* Oesterling *et al.* [19].)

The Role of Percent Free PSA in Prostate Cancer Detection

PSA, ng/mL	Probability of Cancer, %	Free PSA, %	Probability of Cancer, %
0–2	1	N/A	N/A
2–4	15	N/A	N/A
4–10	25	0–10	56
		10–15	28
		15–20	20
		20–25	16
		>25	8
>10	>50	N/A	N/A

▶ **FIGURE 8-16.** The role of percent free prostate-specific antigen (PSA) in prostate cancer detection. In an attempt to improve the specificity of serum PSA testing, the role of percent free PSA was introduced. There is general agreement that the percent free PSA in serum provides additional benefit over total PSA alone in differentiating prostate cancer from benign disease. This has provided most benefit in patients with serum total PSA levels of 4 to 10 ng/mL. A higher percentage of free PSA is more likely associated with benign prostatic diseases. A free PSA cut point of 25% detected 95% of cancers while avoiding 20% of unnecessary prostate biopsies. For individual patients, a lower percentage of free PSA was associated with a higher risk of prostate cancer detection [20,21].

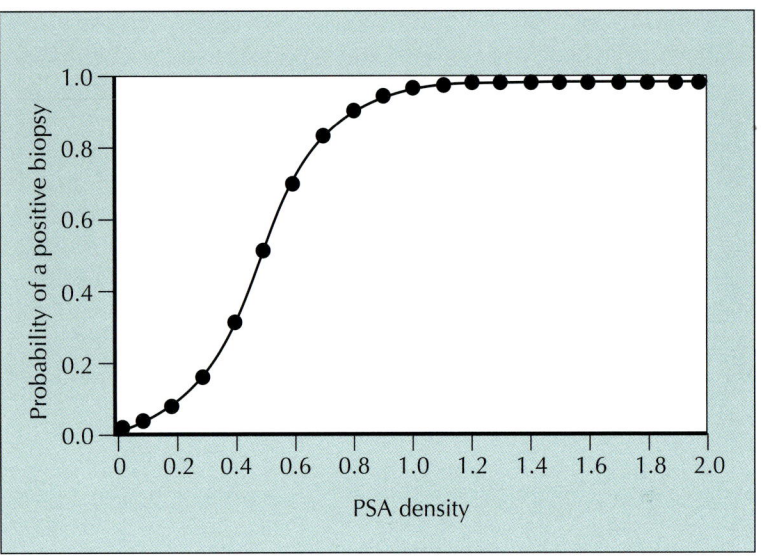

FIGURE 8-17. Prostate-specific antigen (PSA) density and prostate cancer detection. To further improve on the specificity of serum PSA testing, investigators have evaluated the role of PSA density (PSAD). PSAD is determined by dividing the serum PSA level by the transrectal ultrasound–determined prostate volume. Seaman *et al.* [22] evaluated men with serum PSA levels of 4 to 10 ng/mL and found that higher PSAD calculations were associated with a higher incidence of cancer detection. In men with prostate cancer, the mean PSAD was 0.29 compared with 0.19 in men without prostate cancer. Based on this, a cut point of 0.15 was chosen for PSAD [22,23].

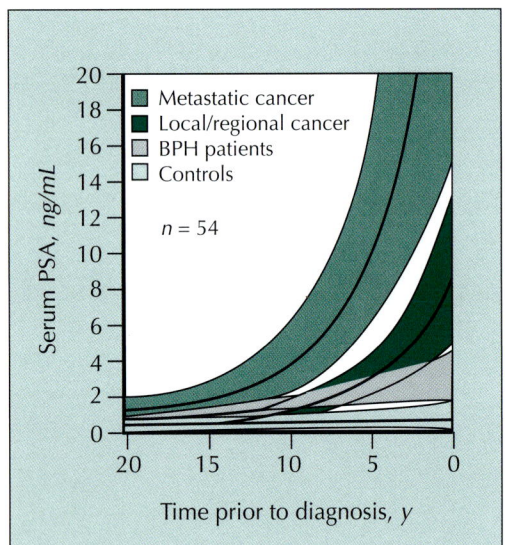

FIGURE 8-18. The role of prostate-specific antigen (PSA) velocity in prostate cancer detection. In general, prostate cancer increases serum PSA levels to a greater and more rapid extent than do benign prostatic diseases. Because serum PSA levels are directly related to the volume of prostate cancer and prostate cancer has a higher proliferative rate than benign diseases, it seems reasonable that men with prostate cancer should have a more rapid rise in serum PSA levels over time compared with men without prostate cancer. Previous studies have demonstrated a significant difference in PSA velocity in men without prostatic diseases (median PSA velocity of 0.03), men with benign prostatic hyperplasia (BPH; median PSA velocity of 0.12), and those with prostate cancer (median PSA velocity of 0.88). The most effective means of distinguishing between men with prostate cancer and men with BPH has been to use an average PSA velocity of more than 0.75 ng/mL per year, calculated based on three consecutive PSA measurements [24]. (*Adapted from* Carter *et al.* [24].)

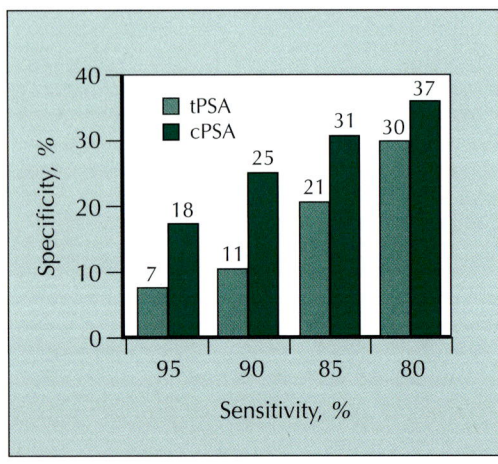

FIGURE 8-19. Sensitivity and specificity of complexed prostate-specific antigen (cPSA) compared with total PSA (tPSA). Brawer *et al.* [25] carried out a preliminary investigation with an assay specific for complexed PSA (PSA α_1-antichymotrypsin) and compared it with the total PSA assay. In this study, total and complexed PSA were measured in 300 men undergoing prostate biopsy, 75 with proven cancer and 225 with benign histologic findings. Generally, a trend was seen toward enhanced specificity for a complexed PSA compared with the total PSA assay at similar sensitivities. (*Adapted from* Brawer *et al.* [25].)

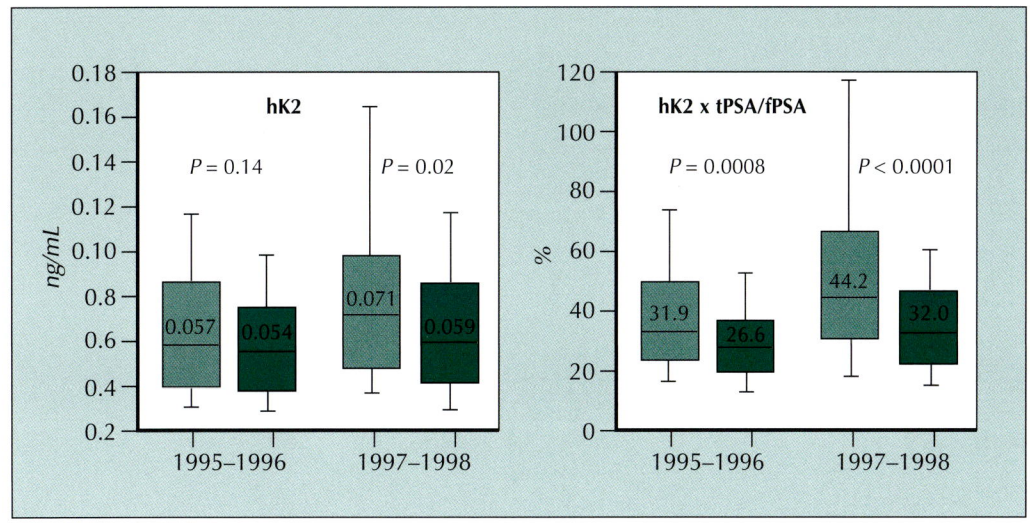

FIGURE 8-20. Role of hK2 in prostate cancer diagnosis. Based on a large biannual screening cohort from Sweden, Becker *et al.* [26] reported the value of hK2 in discriminating men with a diagnosis of cancer from those with benign disease. In the study, hK2 times the ratio of total (tPSA) to free PSA (fPSA) provided the best specificity. Shown are the two serum measurements (1995 to 1996 and 1997 to 1998) prior to the diagnosis of prostate cancer. The *shaded bars* represent the men subsequently diagnosed with cancer. (*Adapted from* Becker *et al.* [26].)

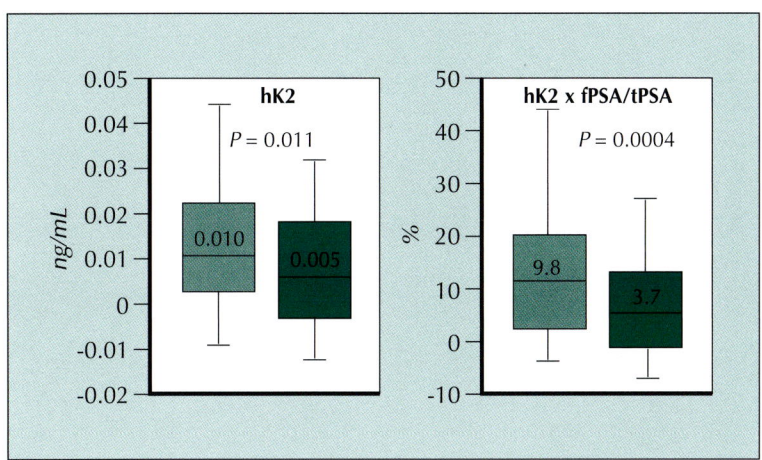

FIGURE 8-21. hK2 velocity and prostate cancer detection. In the same study, Becker *et al.* [26] evaluated the rate of change of hK2 and prostate-specific antigen (PSA) prior to the diagnosis of prostate cancer based on two serum measurements (1995 to 1996 and 1997 to 1998). A higher hK2 velocity was significantly associated with prostate cancer detection. The *shaded bars* represent men subsequently diagnosed with cancer. fPSA—free PSA; tPSA—total PSA. (*Adapted from* Becker *et al.* [26].)

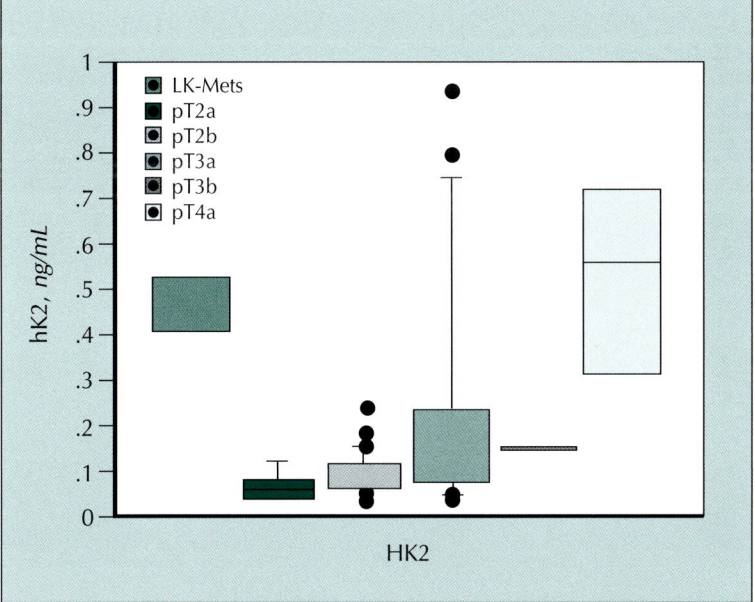

FIGURE 8-22. The role of hK2 in predicting the pathologic stage of prostate cancer. Higher levels of hK2 have been shown to be associated with an increasing incidence of non–organ-confined prostate cancer. Only one of 38 patients with a serum hK2 level greater than 0.2 ng/mL had organ-confined disease. Therefore, a high serum level of hK2 makes extraprostatic extension very likely [27].

A. The Partin Table Predicting for Pathologic Stage of Prostate Cancer

Gleason Score	PSA 0.0–4.0 Clinical Stage							PSA 4.1–10.0 Clinical Stage						
	T1a	T1b	T1c	T2a	T2b	T2c	T3a	T1a	T1b	T1c	T2a	T2b	T2c	T3a
Organ-Confined Disease														
2–4	90	80	89	81	72	77	—	84	70	83	71	61	66	43
5	82	66	81	68	57	62	40	72	53	71	55	43	49	27
6	78	61	78	64	52	57	35	67	47	67	51	38	43	23
7	—	43	63	47	34	38	19	49	29	49	33	22	25	11
8–10	—	31	52	36	24	27	—	35	18	37	23	14	15	6
Established Capsular Penetration														
2–4	9	19	10	18	25	21	—	14	27	15	26	35	29	44
5	17	32	18	30	40	34	51	25	42	27	41	50	43	57
6	19	35	21	34	43	37	53	27	44	30	44	52	46	57
7	—	44	31	45	51	45	52	36	48	40	52	64	48	48
8–10	—	43	34	47	48	42	—	34	42	40	49	46	40	34
Seminal Vesicle Involvement														
2–4	0	1	1	1	2	2	—	1	2	1	2	4	5	10
5	1	2	1	2	3	3	7	2	3	2	3	5	6	12
6	1	2	1	2	3	4	7	2	3	2	3	5	6	11
7	—	6	4	6	10	12	19	6	9	8	10	15	18	28
8–10	—	11	9	12	17	21	—	10	15	15	19	24	28	35
Lymph Node Involvement														
2–4	0	0	0	0	0	0	—	0	1	0	0	1	1	1
5	1	1	0	0	1	1	2	1	2	0	1	2	2	3
6	1	2	0	1	2	2	5	3	5	1	2	4	4	9
7	—	6	1	2	5	5	9	8	12	3	4	9	9	15
8–10	—	14	4	5	10	10	—	18	23	8	9	16	17	24

▶ **FIGURE 8-23. A** and **B,** The Partin table predicting for pathologic stage of prostate cancer. Several investigators have combined serum prostate-specific antigen (PSA) level, clinical stage, and biopsy Gleason score using multivariate analysis to improve the ability to predict pathologic stage. In 1997, Partin *et al.* [28] constructed a nomogram from 4133 untreated men with clinically localized prostate cancer undergoing radical prostatectomy at one of three major academic institutions. Patients were grouped into pathologic categories—*eg*, organ-confined disease, capsular penetration, seminal vesicle or lymph node involvement—assuming the worst pathologic outcome.

(*Continued on next page*)

B. The Partin Table Predicting for Pathologic Stage of Prostate Cancer

Gleason Score	PSA 10.1–20.0 Clinical Stage							PSA >20.0 Clinical Stage						
	T1a	T1b	T1c	T2a	T2b	T2c	T3a	T1a	T1b	T1c	T2a	T2b	T2c	T3a
Organ-Confined Disease														
2–4	76	58	75	60	48	53	—	—	38	58	41	29	—	—
5	61	40	60	43	32	36	18	—	23	40	26	17	19	8
6	—	33	55	38	26	31	14	—	17	35	22	13	15	6
7	33	17	35	22	13	15	6	—	—	18	10	5	6	2
8–10	—	9	23	14	7	8	3	—	3	10	5	3	3	1
Established Capsular Penetration														
2–4	20	36	22	35	43	37	—	—	47	34	48	52	—	—
5	33	50	35	50	57	51	59	—	57	48	60	61	55	54
6	—	49	38	52	57	50	54	—	51	49	60	57	51	46
7	38	46	45	55	51	45	40	—	—	46	51	43	37	2
8–10	—	38	40	46	38	33	26	—	24	34	37	28	23	17
Seminal Vesicle Involvement														
2–4	2	4	2	4	7	8	—	—	9	7	10	14	—	—
5	3	5	3	5	8	9	15	—	10	9	11	15	19	26
6	—	4	4	5	7	9	14	—	8	8	10	13	17	21
7	8	11	12	14	18	22	28	—	—	22	24	27	32	36
8–10	—	15	20	22	25	30	34	—	20	31	33	33	38	40
Lymph Node Involvement														
2–4	0	2	0	1	1	1	—	—	4	1	1	3	—	—
5	3	5	1	2	4	4	7	—	10	3	3	7	7	11
6	—	13	3	4	10	10	18	—	23	7	8	16	17	26
7	18	24	8	9	17	18	26	—	—	14	14	25	25	32
8–10	—	40	16	17	29	29	37	—	51	24	24	36	35	42

▶ **FIGURE 8-23.** (*Continued*) Using serum PSA, Gleason score of the prostate biopsy, and clinical stage, this nomogram can estimate with 95% confidence intervals the probability of a patient having one of these pathologic conditions. Validation of this study demonstrated that 72% of the time, these nomograms correctly predicted the probability of a pathologic stage to within 10%. (*Adapted from* Partin *et al.* [28].)

1. Lilja H: Biology of prostate-specific antigen. *Urology* 2003, 63(5 Suppl 1):27–33.

2. Balk SP, Ko YJ, Bubley GJ: Biology of prostate-specific antigen. *J Clin Oncol* 2003, 21:383–391.

3. Olsson AY, Lilja H, Lundwall A: Taxon-specific evolution of glandular kallikrein genes and identification of a progenitor of prostate-specific antigen. *Genomics* 2004, 84:147–156.

4. Olsson AY, Valtonen-Andre C, Lilja H, *et al.*: The evolution of the glandular kallikrein locus: identification of orthologs and pseudogenes in the cotton-top tamarin. *Gene* 2004, 343:347–355.

5. Diamandis EP, Yousef GM: Human tissue kallikreins: a new family of cancer biomarkers. *Clin Chem* 2002, 48:1198–1205.

6. Riegman PH, Vlietstra RJ, van der Korput JA, *et al.*: The promoter of the prostate-specific antigen gene contains a functional androgen responsive element. *Mol Endocrinol* 1991, 5:1921–1930.

7. Cleutjens KB, van Eekelen CC, van der Korput HA, *et al.*: Two androgen response regions cooperate in steroid hormone regulated activity of the prostate-specific antigen promoter. *J Biol Chem* 1996, 271:6379–6388.

8. Schuur ER, Henderson GA, Kmetec LA, *et al.*: Prostate-specific antigen expression is regulated by an upstream enhancer. *J Biol Chem* 1996, 271:7043–7051.

9. Kumar A, Mikolajczyk SD, Goel AS, *et al.*: Expression of pro form of prostate-specific antigen by mammalian cells and its conversion to mature, active form by human kallikrein 2. *Cancer Res* 1997, 57:3111–3114.

10. Takayama TK, McMullen BA, Nelson PS, *et al.*: Characterization of hK4 (prostase), a prostate-specific serine protease: activation of the precursor of prostate specific antigen (pro-PSA) and single-chain urokinase-type plasminogen activator and degradation of prostatic acid phosphatase. *Biochemistry* 2001, 40:15341–15348.

11. Lundwall A, Lilja H: Molecular cloning of human prostate specific antigen cDNA. *FEBS Lett* 1987, 214:317–322.

12. Bridon DP, Dowell BL: Structural comparison of prostate-specific antigen and human glandular kallikrein using molecular modeling. *Urology* 1995, 45:801–806.

13. Rittenhouse HG, Finlay JA, Mikolajczyk SD, Partin AW: Human kallikrein 2 (hK2) and prostate-specific antigen (PSA): two closely related, but distinct, kallikreins in the prostate. *Crit Rev Clin Lab Sci* 1998, 35:275–368.

14. Lilja H, Christensson A, Dahlen U, *et al.*: Prostate-specific antigen in serum occurs predominantly in complex with alpha 1-antichymotrypsin. *Clin Chem* 1991, 37:1618–1625.

15. Lilja H, Piironen TP, Rittenhouse HG, *et al.*: Value of molecular forms of prostate-specific antigen and related kallikrein, hK2, in diagnosis and staging of prostate cancer. In *Comprehensive Textbook of Genitourinary Oncology*, edn 2. Edited by Vogelzang NJ, Scardino PT, Shipley WU, Coffey DS. Philadelphia: Lippincott Williams & Wilkins; 2000:638.

16. Nurmikko P, Pettersson K, Piironen T, *et al.*: Discrimination of prostate cancer from benign disease by plasma measurement of intact, free prostate-specific antigen lacking an internal cleavage site at Lys145-Lys146. *Clin Chem* 2001, 47:1415–1423.

17. Stephan C, Jung K, Lein M, *et al.*: Molecular forms of prostate-specific antigen and human kallikrein 2 as promising tools for early diagnosis of prostate cancer. *Cancer Epidemiol Biomarkers Prev* 2000, 9:1133–1147.

18. Nurmikko P, Vaisanen V, Piironen T, *et al.*: Production and characterization of novel anti-prostate-specific antigen (PSA) monoclonal antibodies that do not detect internally cleaved Lys145-Lys146 inactive PSA. *Clin Chem* 2000, 46:1610–1618.

19. Oesterling JE: Age-specific reference ranges for serum PSA. *N Engl J Med* 1996, 335:345–346.

20. Catalona WJ, Richie JP, Ahmann FR, *et al.*: Comparison of digital rectal examination and serum prostate-specific antigen in the early detection of prostate cancer: results of a multicenter clinical trial of 6630 men. *J Urol* 1994, 151:1283–1290.

21. Keetch DW, Catalona WJ, Smith DS, *et al.*: Serial prostatic biopsies in men with persistently elevated serum prostate-specific antigen values. *J Urol* 1994, 151:1571–1574.

22. Seaman E, Whang M, Olsson CA, *et al.*: Prostate-specific antigen density (PSAD): role in patient evaluation and management. *Urol Clin North Am* 1993, 20:653–663.

23. Benson MC, Whang IS, Olsson CA, *et al.*: The use of prostate-specific antigen density to enhance the predictive value of intermediate levels of serum prostate-specific antigen. *J Urol* 1992, 147:817–821.

24. Carter HB, Pearson JD: PSA velocity: a new concept for the diagnosis of early prostate cancer. *Urol Clin North Am* 1993, 20:665–670.

25. Brawer MK, Meyer GE, Letran JL, *et al.*: Measurement of complexed PSA improves specificity for early detection of prostate cancer. *Urology* 1998, 52:372–378.

26. Becker C, Piironen T, Pettersson K, *et al.*: Testing in serum for human kallikrein 2, and free and total prostate specific antigen in biannual screening for prostate cancer. *J Urol* 2003, 170:1169–1174.

27. Haese A, Becker C, Noldus J, *et al.*: Human glandular kallikrein 2: a potential serum marker for predicting the organ confined versus nonorgan confined growth of prostate cancer. *J Urol* 2000, 163:1491–1497.

28. Partin AW, Kattan MW, Subong EN, *et al.*: Combination of prostate-specific antigen, clinical stage, and Gleason score to predict pathological stage of localized prostate cancer: a multi-institutional update. *JAMA* 1997, 277:1445–1451.

Clinical Evaluation of the Patient with Prostate Cancer

9

Andrew J. Stephenson & Peter T. Scardino

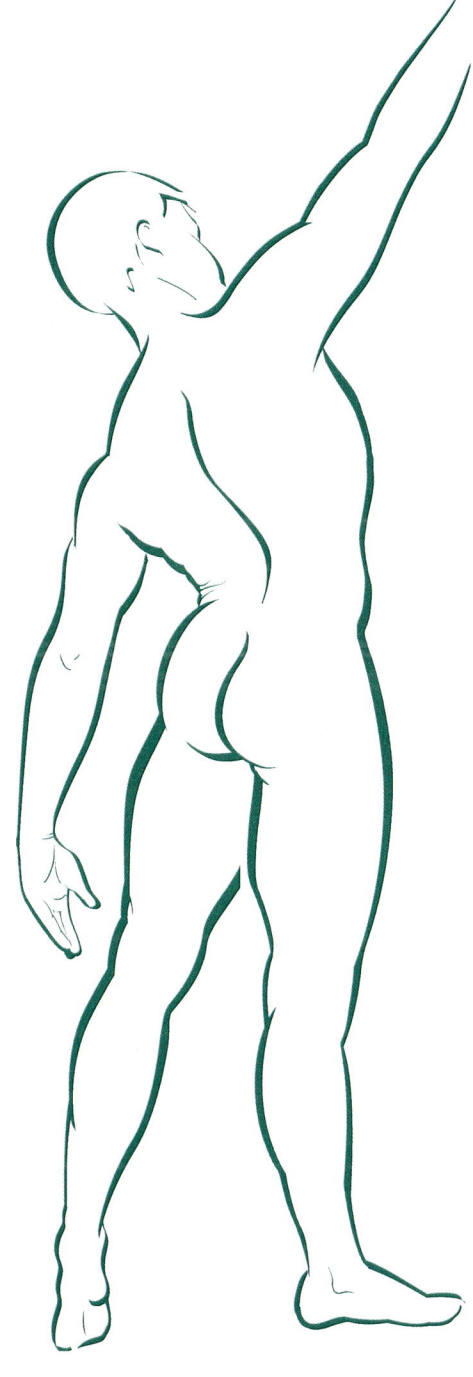

In 2005, an estimated 232,000 men in the United States will be diagnosed with prostate cancer and over 32,000 will die from this disease [1]. The mortality rate from prostate cancer has been declining over the last decade due, in large part, to early detection and effective local therapy [2]. Now we have definitive evidence that local therapy (specifically radical prostatectomy) decreases the chance of metastases and increases overall survival over a median follow-up of 8.2 years compared to patients randomized to watchful waiting [3]. Published series of patients treated by external-beam radiotherapy and brachytherapy have reported 10-year cancer control rates, for properly selected patients, similar to those achieved with radical prostatectomy [4,5]. Each of these treatment modalities is associated with a unique set of short- and long-term side effects, including altered bowel, urinary and sexual function, that may adversely affect quality of life.

Patients diagnosed with clinically localized prostate cancer face a daunting variety of treatment choices, including watchful waiting, brachytherapy and/or external-beam radiotherapy with or without neoadjuvant androgen-deprivation therapy (ADT), as well as radical prostatectomy by an open retropubic, perineal, or a laparoscopic approach, the last with or without robotic assistance. The selection of each of these treatment modalities is based, to varying degrees, on the individual characteristics of a patient's cancer and the likelihood of success with each modality, the anticipated treatment-related morbidity, patient co-morbidities, and patient preference. To help patients and their families make the right choices for their own particular situation, we recently published a book for the general public that describes the risks and benefits of each treatment in detail [6].

The preoperative characterization of each individual's prostate cancer in terms of its location, size, extent, and prognosis is a prerequisite for treatment selection and for designing a successful treatment plan. For example, for a patient treated with radical prostatectomy, a side-specific prediction of extracapsular extension may influence the surgeon to choose a wider plane of dissection and to partially (or completely) resect the neurovascular bundle on one side to reduce the likelihood of a positive surgical margin, while preserving the nerves responsible for potency to the greatest extent possible. For patients treated by radiation therapy, knowledge of a patient's prognosis before therapy may influence the decision to administer neoadjuvant or adjuvant androgen-deprivation therapy. Likewise, patients with low-volume, low-grade disease may be considered for watchful waiting.

Numerous preoperative variables for prostate cancer staging and prognosis have been identified, including clinical stage, serum prostate-specific antigen (PSA) level, biopsy Gleason sum, the location and number of positive biopsy cores, the quantity of cancer in the biopsy specimen, and the results of prostate imaging studies. No single parameter is either sufficiently sensitive or specific to dictate therapy. The urologist must consider all of these factors when designing a treatment plan. Traditionally, clinical judgment has formed the basis of patient counseling and informed decision-making. However, this can introduce considerable bias at all stages of the prediction process. Several studies have demonstrated that mathematical models called nomograms, which are based on a constellation of prognostic information, perform as well as, or indeed better than, clinical judgment. Nomograms have been developed that predict with a high level of accuracy the pathologic stage of prostate cancer [7–10], the presence and laterality of extracapsular extension [9], the probability of having indolent prostate cancer [11], and the likelihood of long-term cancer control following radical prostatectomy [12,13], external-beam radiotherapy [14], and transperineal brachytherapy [15].

The management strategy for patients with clinically localized prostate cancer must be highly individualized, considering the characteristics of the patient's cancer, his preferences, and his concerns about potential treatment-related morbidity. At our institution, we use these predictive models and the results of prostate imaging studies to counsel patients regarding local therapy options for clinically localized prostate cancer and for treatment planning. Ultimately, decision analysis models that consider the anticipated success of local therapy, treatment-related and disease-related morbidity, and their subsequent impact on quality of life would assist physicians and patients greatly in the management of clinically localized prostate cancer. Such models would enable physicians to individualize the care of patients with respect to the characteristics of their disease while addressing their fears, concerns, and preferences.

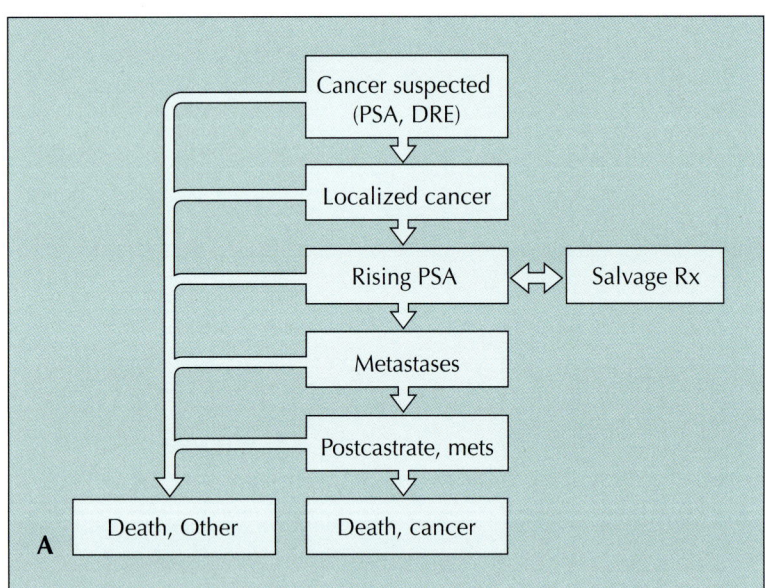

▶ FIGURE 9-1. A, Clinical states model. The treatment of patients with clinically localized prostate cancer is complicated by the protracted natural history of the disease and the late age at diagnosis. While the lifetime risk of developing prostate cancer is 16.7%, the lifetime risk of dying from prostate cancer is only 3.6% [16]. It is clear that definitive local therapy will not benefit many men with clinically localized prostate cancer, particularly those of advanced age or with significant co-morbidities. A clinical states model for prostate cancer considers both the natural (untreated) and treated history of the disease as a series of health states from diagnosis to death and illustrates the "race" between death from prostate cancer versus death from competing causes [17].

(Continued on next page)

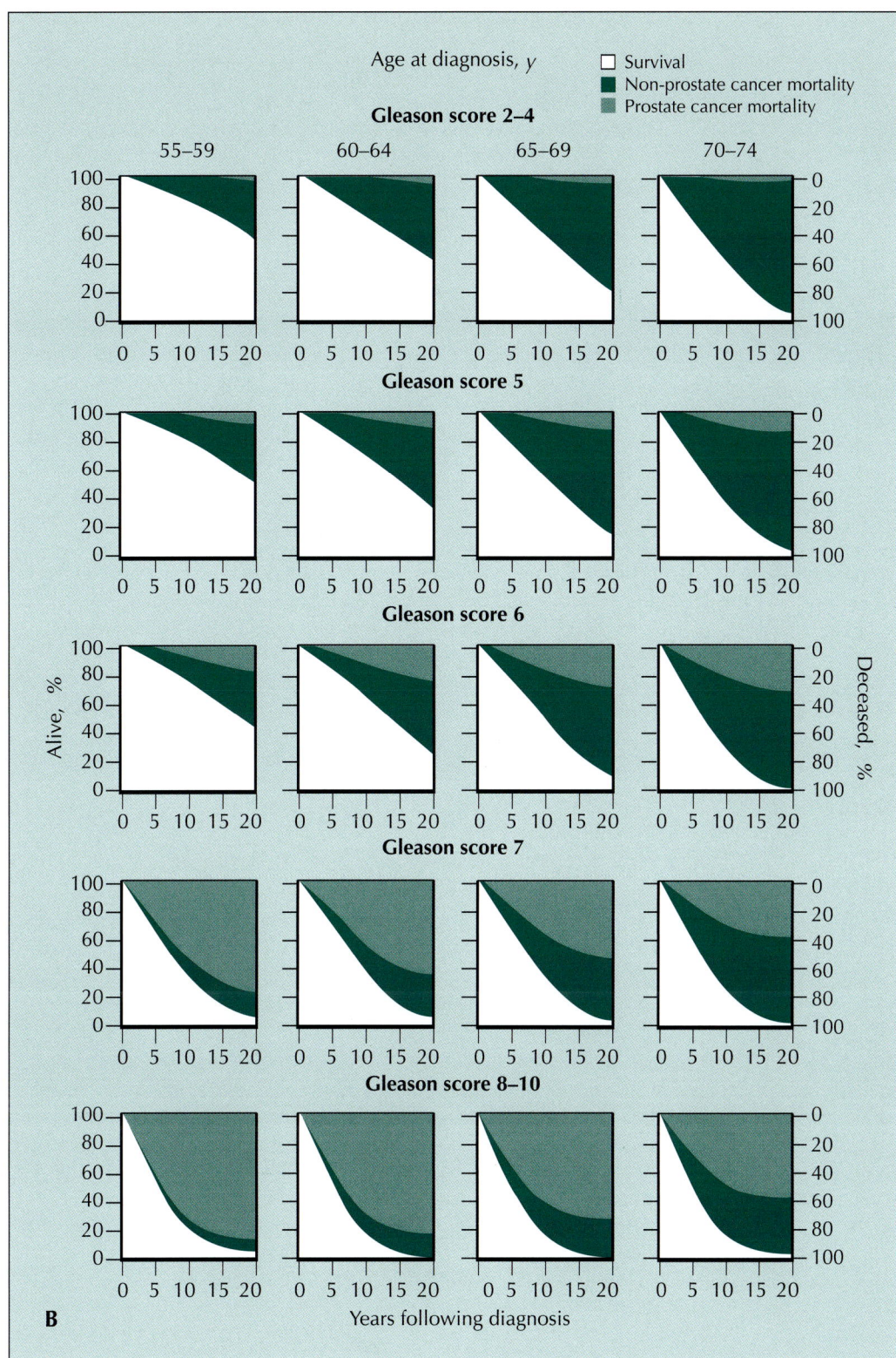

Age at diagnosis, y

☐ Survival
■ Non-prostate cancer mortality
■ Prostate cancer mortality

Gleason score 2–4

Gleason score 5

Gleason score 6

Gleason score 7

Gleason score 8–10

B   Years following diagnosis

▶ **FIGURE 9-1.** (*Continued*) **B,** For patients with clinically localized prostate cancer, the risk of death from competing causes generally exceeds the risk from prostate cancer. It is only after the development of metastatic disease that the risk of death from prostate cancer greatly exceeds that of competing causes. For men with clinically localized prostate cancer who do not receive definitive therapy, Albertsen *et al.* estimated the risk of death from prostate cancer and death from competing causes at 20 years after diagnosis, stratified by age and biopsy Gleason sum, as shown in Figure 9-1*B* [18]. The risk of dying from prostate cancer within 20 years of diagnosis is minimal for patients with Gleason 2–5 tumors, but high for those with Gleason 7–10 tumors. For men with intermediate grade (Gleason 6), deaths within 20 years of diagnosis are attributable to prostate cancer in 25% of men aged 55-64 and approximately one third of men aged 65–74. (Part A *adapted from* Scher and Heller [17]; Part B *adapted from* Albertsen *et al.* [18].)

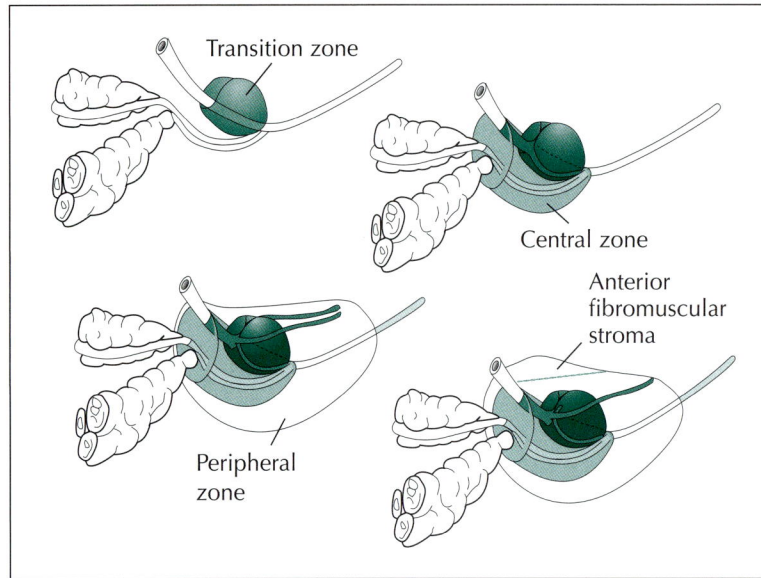

▶ **FIGURE 9-2.** Zonal anatomy. The prostate glandular structure can be divided into three zones, peripheral, transition, and central. More than 80% of prostate cancers arise in the peripheral zone (PZ), which contains 70% of the prostate glandular elements. The central zone surrounds the ejaculatory ducts and is the site of the primary lesion in fewer than 10% of cases. The transition zone (TZ), the site of development of benign prostatic hyperplasia (BPH), contains 10% of the glandular elements (although up to 80% in cases of BPH) and is the site of origin for less than 20% of prostate cancers. Due to their anterior location, TZ cancers frequently elude detection until they are of considerable size. Compared to

PZ tumors of similar size and grade, TZ cancers are associated with a favorable prognosis due to natural barriers to extension (*eg*, urethra, anterior fibromuscular stroma, fibrous plane between TZ and PZ) and inherent biologic differences.

The neurovascular bundles that contain the cavernous nerves, which are responsible for potency, travel in close proximity to the prostate gland on the posterolateral surface. Branches of the neurovascular bundles enter the prostate at the base (superior pedicle) and the apex (inferior pedicle) posterolaterally. The main route of extraprostatic spread of cancer is invasion along the conduits of the perineural spaces, which enables cancer cells to bypass the anatomical barrier of the prostate capsule. Extracapsular extension in the absence of perineural invasion is uncommon and is usually associated with large, high-grade tumors. Extracapsular extension most commonly occurs on the posterolateral surface of the prostate near the region of the neurovascular bundles. The distance from the prostate capsule to the neurovascular bundle is 2 to 5 mm at the inferior pedicle at the apex of the prostate, and 10 to 15 mm at the superior pedicle on the posterolateral surface of the prostate. Thus, among patients with extracapsular extension, the margin of safety to spare the neurovascular bundles completely and achieve a negative surgical margin may be only a few millimeters.

Successful radical prostatectomy is a surgical tour de tour that entails complete removal of the prostate and regional lymph nodes with negative surgical margins, whereas minimizing peri-operative complications and preserving urinary continence and erectile function. The operation is exquisitely sensitive to fine details in surgical technique, both in the risk of complications [19] and in long-term cancer control. In fact, the rate of positive surgical margins varies significantly among individual surgeons even when the cancers removed are corrected for all known prognostic factors [20]. (*Adapted from* Greene *et al.* [31].)

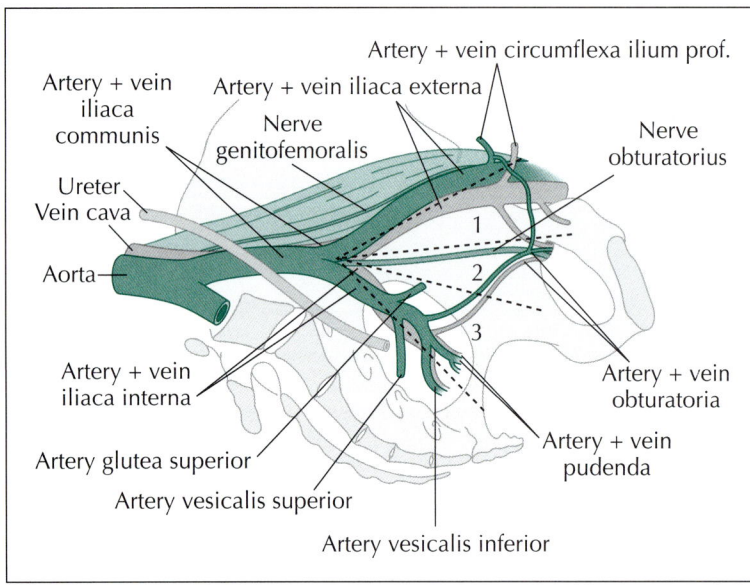

▶ **FIGURE 9-3.** Metastatic dissemination. The first echelon of lymph nodes draining the prostate are the external iliac (Zone 1), obturator (Zone 2), and internal iliac (Zone 3) nodes (*see* figure). If a pelvic lymph node dissection (PLND) is indicated, these nodes should all be removed. With complete PLND, 15% to 20% of patients with lymph node metastases are rendered free of biochemical recurrence of cancer 10 years after radical prostatectomy alone [21]. Whereas the incidence of lymph node involvement is less than 10% in most radical prostatectomy (RP) series, the overall rate of biochemical progression after RP ranges from 25% to 40%. Thus, hematogenous rather than lymphatic spread is the most common route for cancer dissemination. Prostate cancer has a propensity for metastatic spread to bone, typically the bony pelvis and axial spine. Visceral metastases to lung and liver are uncommon in the absence of extensive bone metastases and/or lymph node involvement. (*Adapted from* Bader *et al.* [32]).

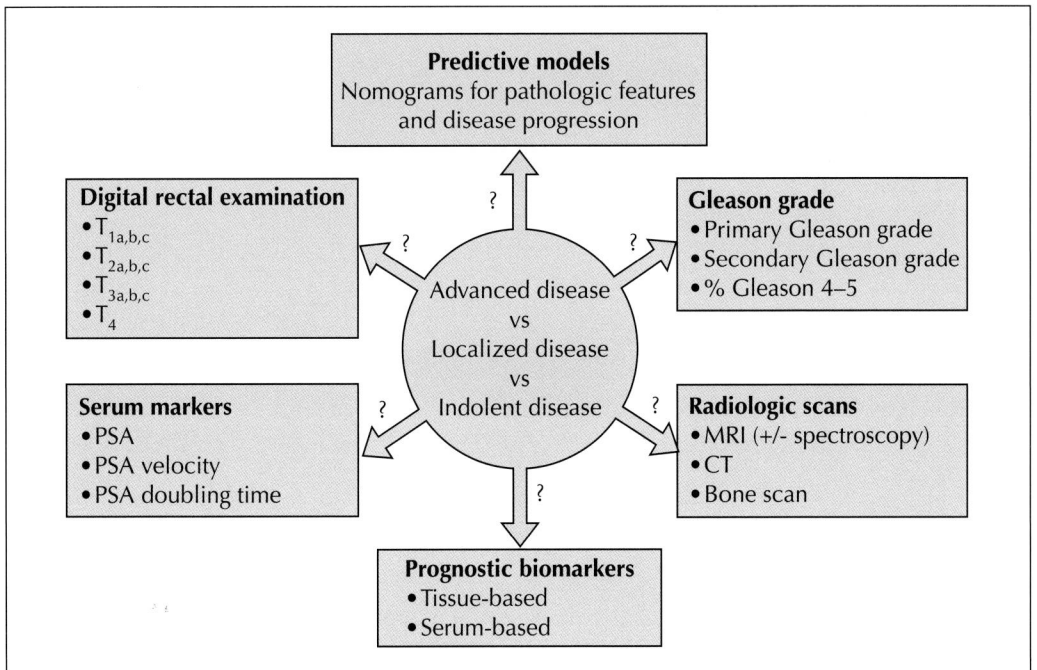

FIGURE 9-4. Risk Assessment. A fundamental tenant of the modern management of prostate cancer is that the choice and application of therapy should be tailored for each individual patient to the specific characteristics of his cancer. Making a decision when to treat and choosing a particular therapy should be based on the life expectancy of the patient, the risk of metastases and death posed by his particular cancer, the likelihood that the treatment will successfully interrupt the natural history of the cancer, the risks and complications of that therapy, and the patient's own utilities or values (is he more worried about living with an untreated cancer or suffering the side effects of therapy) [22]. Once a treatment is selected, optimizing the outcome requires accurate characterization the patient's tumor in terms of location, extent, biological activity, and prognosis. The key staging and prognostic parameters that assist the physician in assessing risk include the digital rectal examination, serum prostate-specific antigen (PSA) level, Gleason grade, systematic biopsy results, and appropriate imaging studies such as transrectal ultrasound (TRUS), endorectal coil magnetic resonance imaging (MRI) with or without spectroscopy, pelvic computed tomography (CT), and radionuclide bone scans. Prognostic models that accurately predict pathologic stage and estimate disease progression have been developed; these models are invaluable in developing a treatment plan based on the specific characteristics of an individual's prostate cancer. In the future, the identification of tissue or circulating biomarkers may enhance our ability to predict pathologic features and outcome as well as response to therapy. (*Adapted from* Partin [33–35].)

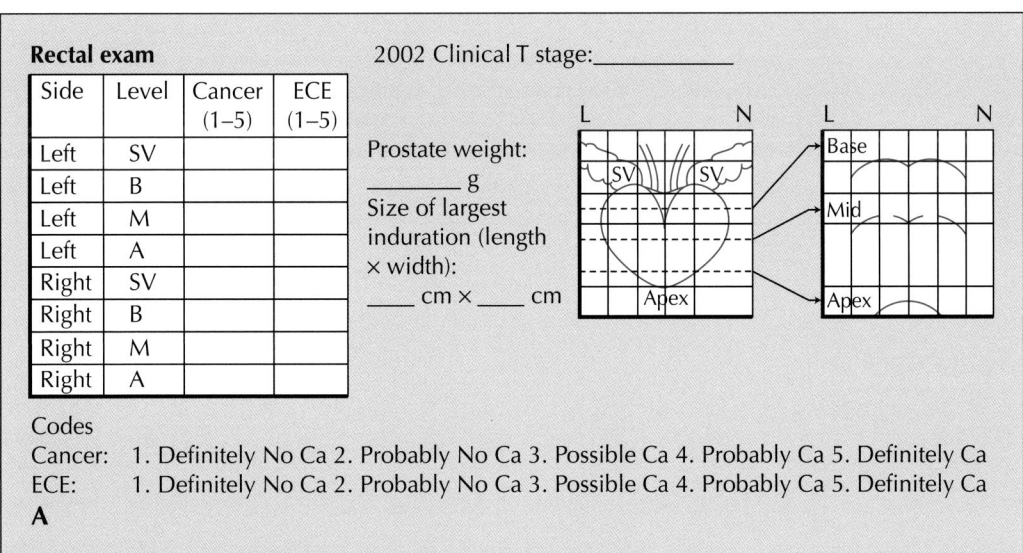

FIGURE 9-5. A, Touch diagram of the digital rectal examination (DRE). The results of a careful DRE should be recorded on a touch diagram in 3 dimensions (each line on the figure represents 1 cm), where the size, location, and extent of any suspicious induration or nodularity are noted. At our institution, we document on dorsoventral and cross-sectional view the site of DRE abnormalities, which are then graded on a scale from 1 to 5 to estimate the probability that abnormalities are related to cancer and the probability of extracapsular extension. The DRE results can provide important information about the resectability of a patient's cancer and the need for resection of the ipsilateral neurovascular bundle to achieve cancer control. Careful documentation of DRE findings is important for patients who elect to go on watchful waiting, as subsequent changes to the prostate exam can be interpreted more precisely.

(*Continued on next page*)

B. 2002 Clinical TNM Staging of Prostate Cancer

TNM stage	Description
T1	Clinical inapparent, not palpable or visible by imaging
T1a	Incidental histologic finding, ≤5% of resected tissue
T1b	Incidental histologic finding, >5% of resected tissue
T1c	Tumor indentified by needle biopsy, for any reason (*eg*, elevated PSA)
T2	Palpable or visible tumor, confined within the prostate
T2a	≤ 1/2 of one lobe
T2b	One lobe
T2c	Both lobes
T3	Tumor extends through the capsule
T3a	Extracapsular extension, unilateral or bilateral
T3b	Seminal vesicle involvement
T4	Tumor is fixed or invades adjacent structures
T4a	Invades bladder neck, external sphincter or rectum
T4b	Invades levator muscles or fixed to pelvic sidewalls

▶ **FIGURE 9-5.** (*Continued*) **B**, Clinical stage. The findings on DRE and pelvic imaging studies form the basis for the current tumor node metastasis (TNM) clinical staging system of prostate cancer. Prostate cancer clinical stage correlates with pathologic stage, but there are many exceptions. Some 20%–30% of patients without palpable abnormalities on DRE (clinical stage T1) and 40%–60% for patients with palpable nodules confined to the prostate on DRE (clinical stage T2) have extracapsular extension in the radical prostate-ctomy specimen. And 30% of patients with clinical stage T3 cancers prove to be organ-confined pathologically. A careful DRE is important to document the location, size, and extent of palpable abnormalities and to correlate these findings with the results of systematic biopsies and imaging studies of the prostate (TRUS and/or endorectal MRI). As a result of widespread PSA screening, 60%–70% of patients currently referred for radical prostatectomy at our institution have clinical stage T1c tumors. For these patients, the surgeon must rely on other information, such as the results of systematic biopsy and prostate imaging studies, for accurate clinical staging, and treatment planning.

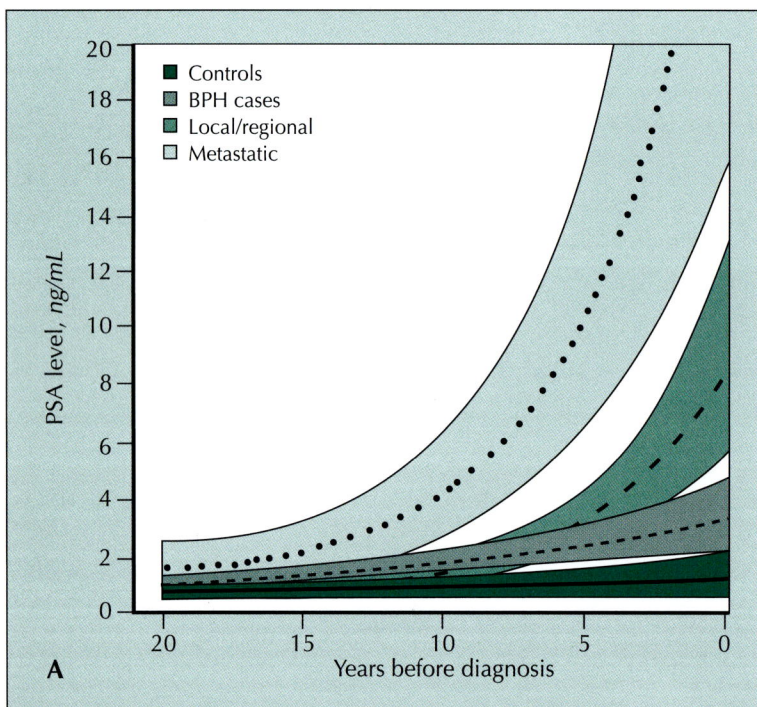

A

▶ **FIGURE 9-6.** **A**, PSA levels for men with and without prostate cancer. For every gram of tissue, prostate cancer increases the serum PSA level by 3 ng/mL compared to 0.3 ng/mL for benign prostate tissue. The absolute PSA level and the rate of rise over time have important prognostic significance for men with clinically localized prostate cancer. Higher absolute PSA levels are associated with greater tumor burden, more advanced pathologic features, and greater likelihood of disease progression after definitive local therapy [21]. However, an elevated PSA by itself is an inaccurate indicator of metastatic disease and should rarely be used to decide to forego definitive local therapy, as an estimated 50% of patients with PSA levels greater than 20 ng/mL at our institution were free of progression 15 years after radical prostatectomy alone. PSA measurably rises 10-15 years before the diagnosis of metastatic prostate cancer and 5 years or so before localized cancer would otherwise be detected. Carter *et al.* have documented that the rate of rise of PSA, referred to as PSA velocity, is much more rapid in men with prostate cancer and can be used to discriminate among patients with metastatic versus clinically localized cancer versus those without prostate cancer [23].

(*Continued on next page*)

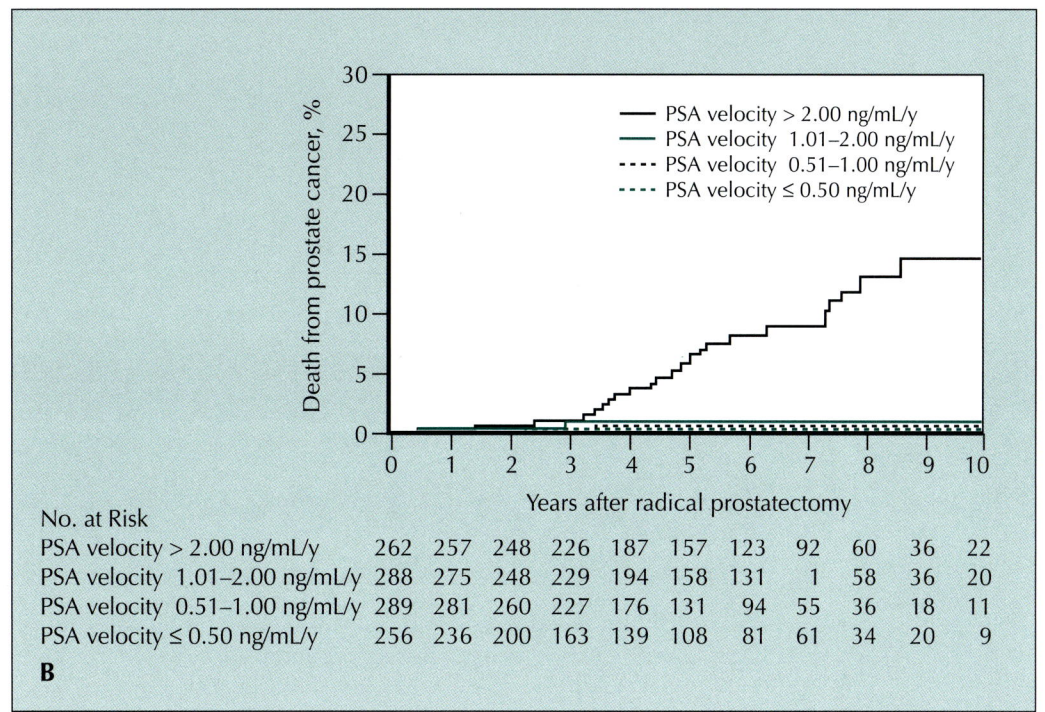

No. at Risk

PSA velocity > 2.00 ng/mL/y	262	257	248	226	187	157	123	92	60	36	22
PSA velocity 1.01–2.00 ng/mL/y	288	275	248	229	194	158	131	1	58	36	20
PSA velocity 0.51–1.00 ng/mL/y	289	281	260	227	176	131	94	55	36	18	11
PSA velocity ≤ 0.50 ng/mL/y	256	236	200	163	139	108	81	61	34	20	9

B

▶ **FIGURE 9-6.** (*Continued*) **B**, Recently, evidence that short-term PSA changes prior to radical prostatectomy predict for subsequent prostate cancer mortality was reported by D'Amico *et al.* [24]. In that study, men with a PSA velocity of 2 ng/mL/year or greater had a 10-fold increased risk of death from prostate cancer within 10 years relative to those with a PSA velocity less than 2 ng/mL/year, although this finding has not yet been confirmed in other series. PSA–prostate-specific antigen. (Part A *adapted from* Carter *et al.* [23] and Part B *adapted from* D'Amico *et al.*[24]).

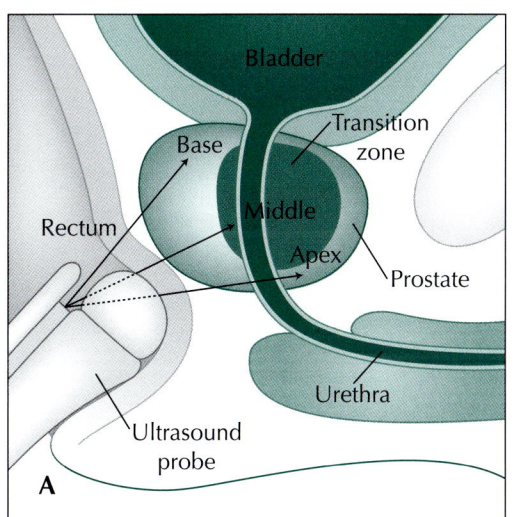

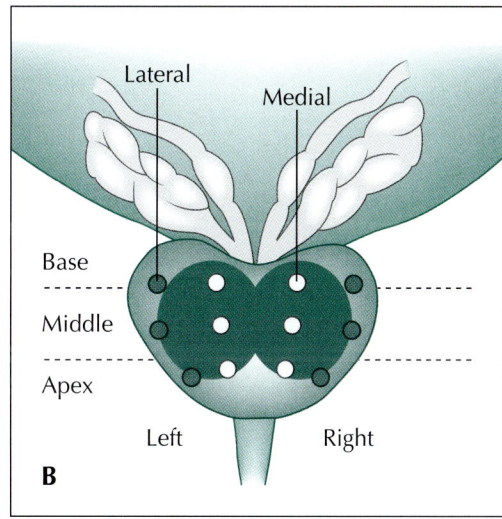

▶ **FIGURE 9-7.** **A** and **B**, Transrectal ultrasound-guided systematic needle biopsies of the prostate. Over 95% of prostate cancers are currently diagnosed by means of systematic TRUS-guided prostate biopsy with an 18-gauge needle. At our institution, we utilize an extended biopsy strategy. In addition to 2–3 directed biopsies of palpable lesions and lesions visible on transrectal ultrasound (or endorectal MRI), a total of 12 cores are taken systematically from the peripheral zone (medially and laterally from the apex, middle, and base of the prostate on each side) along with 2 cores from the transition zone. Each biopsy core is sent as a separate specimen rather than being bunched together as right- and left-sided cores. An extended biopsy strategy provides more information about the location and extent of prostate cancer (including Gleason pattern 4) than sextant biopsies. As a result of the increasing number of biopsy cores, the concordance rate between the biopsy Gleason sum and the prostatectomy Gleason sum has improved over the last decade from 28% to 56% (*see* Fig. 9-8). Information from prostate biopsy can be used for treatment planning (such as the decision to preserve or resect all or part of the neurovascular bundle to achieve a negative surgical margin) and for prostate cancer prognosis. Numerous studies have shown a correlation of the quantity of cancer in systematic biopsy specimens (expressed as the number of positive cores, percentage of positive cores, total percentage of cancer in cores, or ratio of cancer length to total core length) with extracapsular extension, seminal vesical invasion, positive surgical margins, lymph node metastases, and biochemical progression after radical prostatectomy. The percentage of positive biopsy cores is also reported to be a significant predictor of prostate cancer-specific mortality after 3 dimensional-conformal, external-beam radiotherapy. The presence of perineural invasion in biopsy specimens also predicts for the presence and laterality of extracapsular extension. TRUS–transrectal ultrasonography. (*Adapted from* Scardino and Kelman [6]; with permission.)

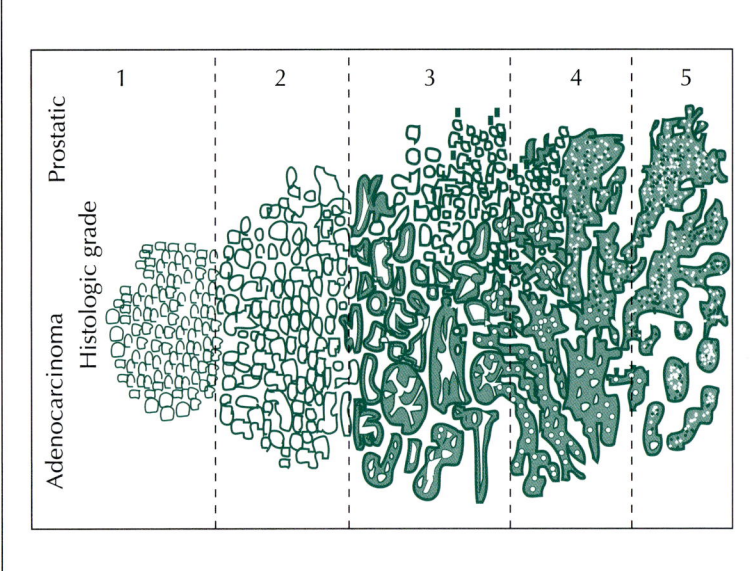

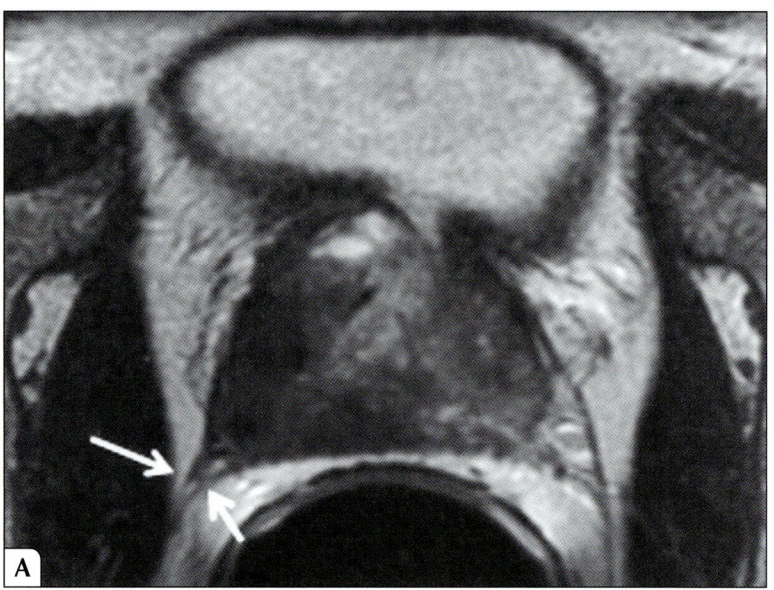

▶ **FIGURE 9-8.** Gleason grading system. The Gleason grading system is based on prostate cancer glandular architecture without respect to cytologic features. A Gleason grade from 1 to 5 is assigned to the primary tumor glandular pattern and also to the secondary tumor pattern based on the degree of disorder of the tissue. The Gleason score is obtained by combining these numbers; the score therefore ranges from 2 to 10. Because most prostate cancers are currently diagnosed by means of prostate core biopsy rather than transurethral resection, the majority of tumors are graded as Gleason score 6 to 10 as it is difficult to assign a Gleason pattern 1 or 2 on the basis of an 18-gauge needle biopsy. As is seen in Figure 9-1*B*, the biopsy Gleason score has important prognostic value for men with clinically localized prostate cancer. In general, patients with Gleason 8 to 10 tumors tend to present with advanced pathologic stage cancer (45% have seminal vesicle invasion and/or lymph node involvement) and their overall risk of progression is 60% at 10 years after radical prostatectomy alone. However, up to one-third of Gleason 8 to 10 cancers detected today are organ-confined, and 90% of these patients are free of disease at 10 years after radical prostatectomy. In contrast, 88% of Gleason 2 to 6 tumors are organ-confined and 98% of these remain free of cancer 10 years after radical prostatectomy. Within the Gleason 7 category, patients with primary Gleason pattern 4 tumors are more likely to have advanced pathologic features and to recur after radical prostatectomy than patients with primary Gleason pattern 3 tumors. The percentage of Gleason pattern 4 or 5 cancer in a biopsy or RP specimen correlates better with disease progression than the current Gleason grading system [25]. RP–radical prostatectomy. (*Adapted from* Gleason [36].)

▶ **FIGURE 9-9.** Local imaging studies. Given that most prostate cancers diagnosed today present without palpable abnormalities on digital rectal examination, the physician often must rely on the results of systematic prostate biopsy and imaging studies to determine the location and extent of disease. Transrectal ultrasonography (TRUS) has proven to be most useful for directing a biopsy needle during systematic biopsy. As a tool for the detection and staging of prostate cancer, however, TRUS has limited clinical utility. Relatively few cancers detected today are of sufficient size and echotexture to be visible by TRUS.

Magnetic resonance imaging (MRI) can be used to identify prostate cancer both locally and regionally. Endorectal MRI, which allows improved visualization of prostatic zonal anatomy and improved delineation of tumor location, volume, and extent, is performed by placing an inflatable, balloon-covered surface coil in the rectum. Patients are then imaged in a whole-body scanner. A full evaluation requires the use of both T1- and T2-weighted images. On T1 images, the prostate appears homogenous, and on T2 images, areas of cancer appear as zones of lower signal intensity surrounded by higher-intensity normal areas. To produce T2-weighted images of excellent resolution for local staging, thin slices (3 mm) and a small (14 cm) field of view are required. Post-biopsy hemorrhage can appear as high signal intensity areas on T1-weighted images, and this can make the distinction between normal and cancerous tissue more difficult. Hence, it is wise to wait at least 6 weeks after a biopsy to obtain an MRI of the prostate.

On endorectal coil MRI, extracapsular extension (*arrows*) can be identified by a contour deformity with a step-off or angulated margin, an irregular bulge or edge retraction, a breech of the capsule with evidence of direct tumor extension, obliteration of the recto-prostatic angle, or asymmetry of the neurovascular bundles, **(A)**.

(*Continued on next page*)

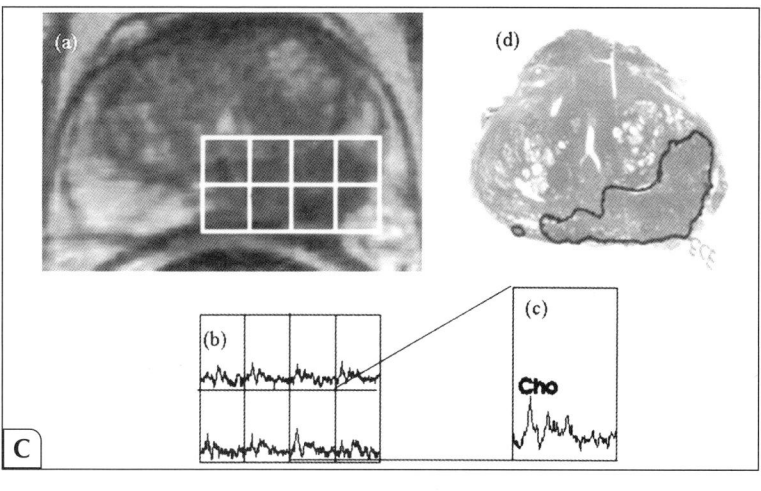

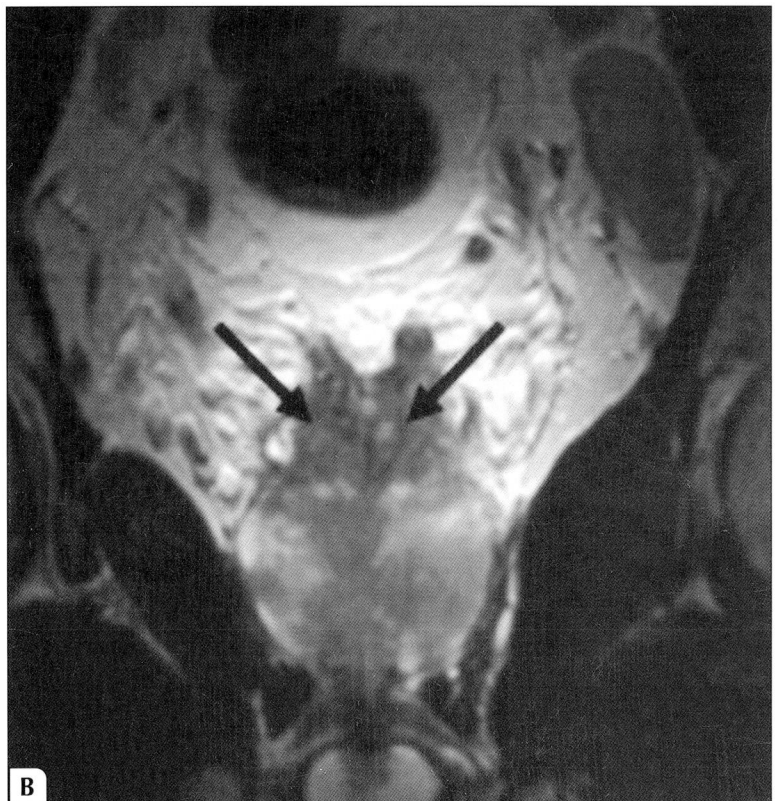

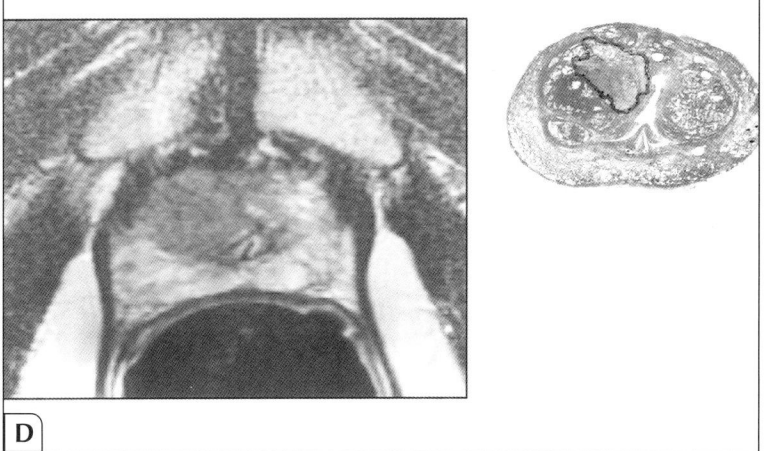

▶ **FIGURE 9-9.** (*Continued*) The criteria for seminal vesicle invasion include contiguous, low-signal—intensity tumor extension from the base of the gland into the seminal vesicles, tumor extension along the ejaculatory duct (nonvisualization of the ejaculatory duct), asymmetric decrease in the signal intensity of the seminal vesicles, and decreased conspicuity of the seminal vesicle wall on T2-weighted images, **(B).** Whereas transaxial planes of section are essential in the diagnosis of extracapsular invasion, the addition of coronal images facilitates the diagnosis. Combined axial, coronal, and sagittal planes of section facilitate the assessment of seminal vesical and bladder neck invasion. Endorectal MRI significantly improves the accuracy of predicting extracapsular extension when included in models along with PSA, clinical stage, Gleason score, and systematic biopsy results [26], and thus may significantly improve the surgeon's ability to modify the operation to avoid positive surgical margins during radical prostatectomy [27].

The reported accuracy of MRI in staging prostate cancer ranges from 54% to 90%, which has raised concerns about interobserver variability. Over the past few years, the diagnostic performance of experienced readers has improved, with reported accuracy reaching 75% to 93%, far exceeding that reported for either TRUS or CT. Magnetic resonance spectroscopic imaging (MRSI) has been used with MRI to increase specificity and reduce the interobserver variability. MRS detects metabolic activity of tissues and can differentiate cancerous from normal tissues based on ratios of creatine, choline, and citrate production and consumption. Cancerous tissue has been associated with lower levels of citrate and higher levels of choline and creatine when compared to tissue containing BPH or normal prostate, (*See Color Plate*) **(C).** The conjunctive use of MRI and MRSI may also help to predict for higher grade of cancer, with early image enhancement potentially being indicative of more aggressive, poorly differentiated tumors [28].

Whereas MRI has been most effective for detecting prostate cancer in the peripheral zone, it also has great potential for the evaluation of tumors located anterior to the urethra in the transition zone and/or peripheral zone, especially when it is combined with MRSI, (*See Color Plate*) **(D).** At our institution, approximately 20% of patients have the bulk of their cancers located anterior to the urethra. Systematic biopsy, TRUS, and DRE underestimate the extent of disease in anterior prostate cancers. Whereas these tumors tend to be of lower Gleason grade and less likely to have extracapsular extension compared to posterior tumors, they tend to be larger and are associated with a higher rate of positive surgical margins. The higher positive margin rate is likely a result of clinical understaging. Identifying anterior tumors with MRI aids in surgical planning, as a more distal transection of the dorsal venous complex over the urethra can be performed to minimize the chances of a positive surgical margin in that region. (*From* Mullerad *et al.* [37]; with permission.)

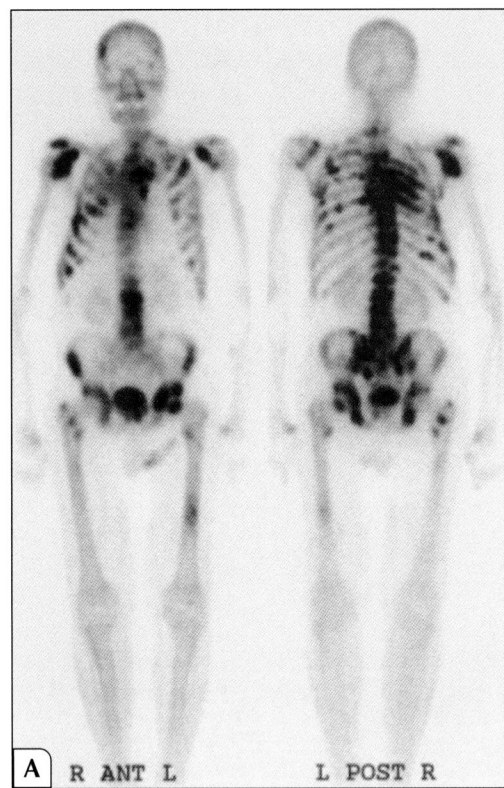

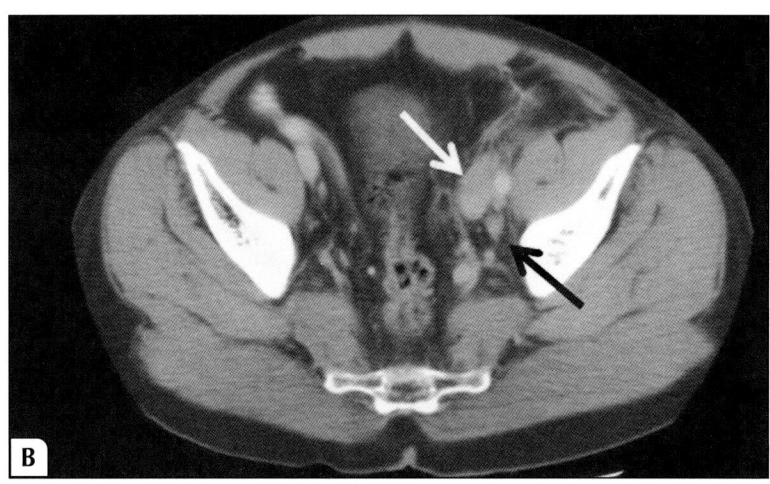

▶ **FIGURE 9-10.** Staging imaging studies for regional or distant metastatic disease. **A,** The radionuclide bone scan is widely used for detecting distant bony metastases in men with newly diagnosed prostate cancer. A policy of routine bone scans for all patients with clinically localized prostate cancer has been questioned due to the fact few such patients have a positive result, and positive findings are often related to benign causes which may delay cancer therapy unnecessarily. Computed tomography (CT) of the pelvis has proven to be of limited value in staging prostate cancer because most local extension is microscopic. **B**, CT is sensitive for detecting enlarged lymph nodes 10 mm or more in diameter, but the overall incidence of lymph node metastases (including microscopically positive nodes) is less than 5% (*arrows*). According to the National Comprehensive Cancer Network Clinical Practice Guidelines for prostate cancer, bone scans and pelvic CT imaging studies before definitive local therapy are recommended only in high-risk patients (pretreatment PSA >20 ng/mL, Gleason 8–10, clinical stage T3–T4, or the presence of symptoms). Although a baseline bone scan may be helpful to interpret subsequent bone scans in patients with progressive disease, we usually obtain a baseline study only after a patient's serum level of PSA begins to rise after radical prostatectomy. A rising PSA precedes the appearance of metastases visible on bone scan by 5 to 7 years. (*From* Mullerad *et al.* [37]; with permission.)

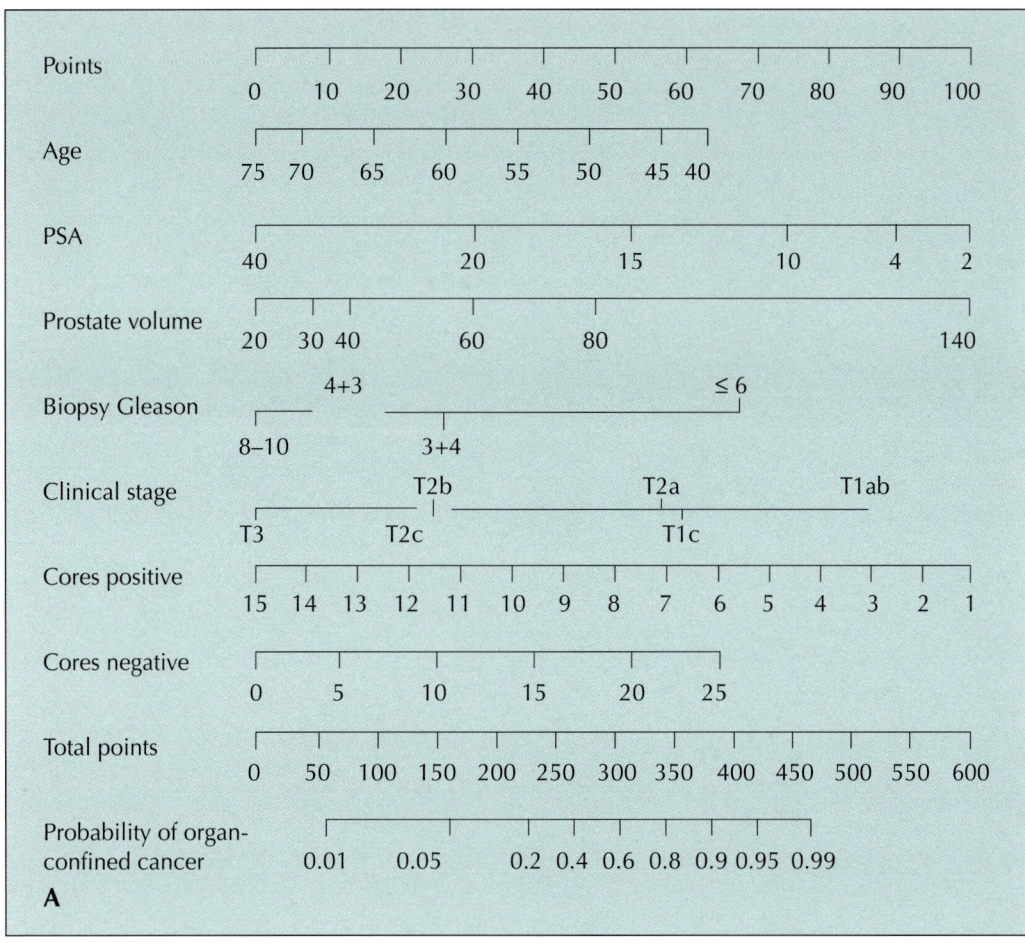

A

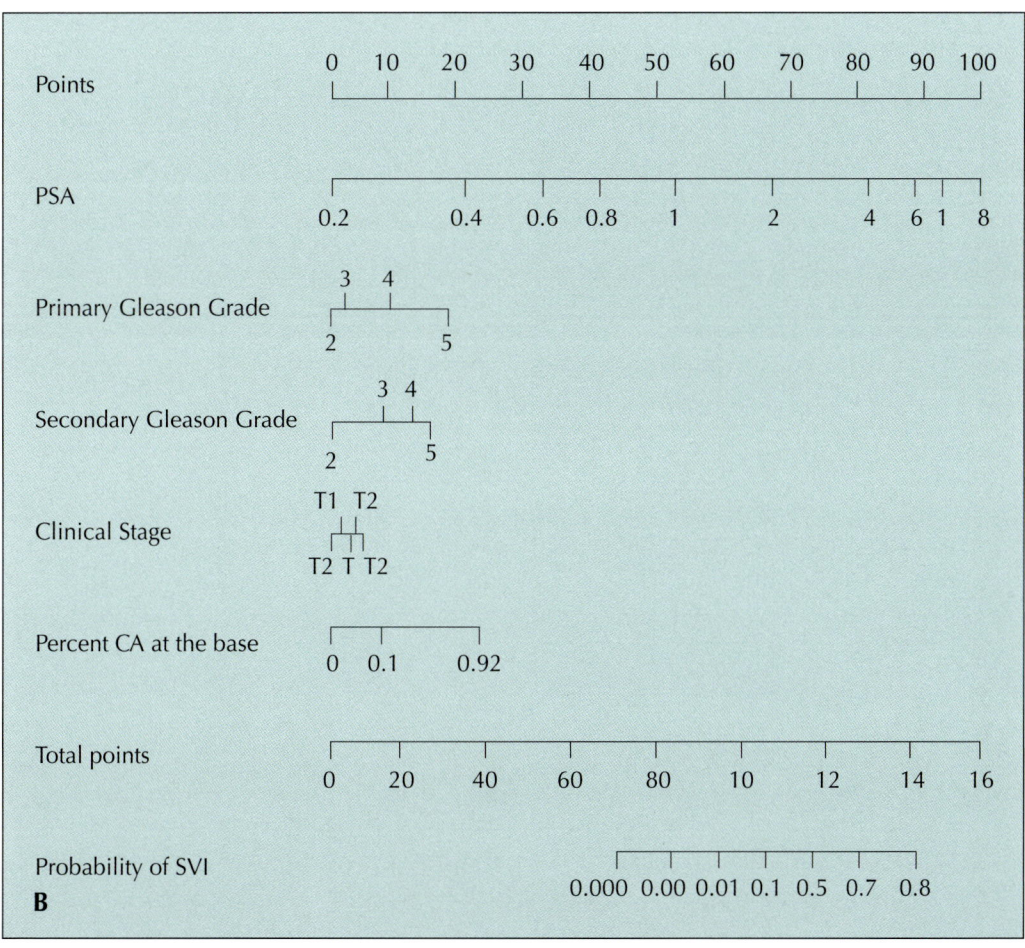

B

▶ **FIGURE 9-11.** Nomograms to predict
pathologic stage. Whereas numerous preoperative clinical and pathologic variables are associated with the presence of extracapsular extension,
seminal vesicle invasion, and lymph node
involvement, the value of any single parameter to
predict pathologic stage is limited. The ability to
accurately predict pathologic stage preoperatively
provides important information for surgical
planning. For example, determining the risk of
extracapsular extension on each side is important
if nerve-sparing radical prostatectomy is contem-
plated. Likewise, lymph node dissection may be
omitted in select patients at low risk for lymph
node metastases. It must be emphasized however,
that predicting pathologic stage does not necessarily predict prognosis. Patients with a low likelihood of organ-confined cancer are still candidates for definitive local therapy, as long-term
cancer control rates of 70% and 40% after
radical prostatectomy alone are reported for
patients with isolated extracapsular extension
and seminal vesicle invasion, respectively. The
"Partin" tables are a popular risk grouping system
used to predict pathologic stage as 1 of 4 mutually exclusive categories (organ-confined, isolated
extracapsular extension, seminal vesicle invasion,
lymph node involvement) based on preoperative
PSA, clinical stage and biopsy Gleason score
[10]. The Partin tables have limited clinical
utility in terms of determining the suitability of
nerve-sparing radical prostatectomy as they
predict the presence but not the laterality or location of extracapsular extension. We have recently
developed a series of continuous, multivariable
nomograms based on PSA, Gleason grade, clinical stage and the results of systematic biopsy to
predict the probability of organ-confined disease,
(**A**) [29], seminal vesicle invasion, (**B**) [8], and

(*Continued on next page*)

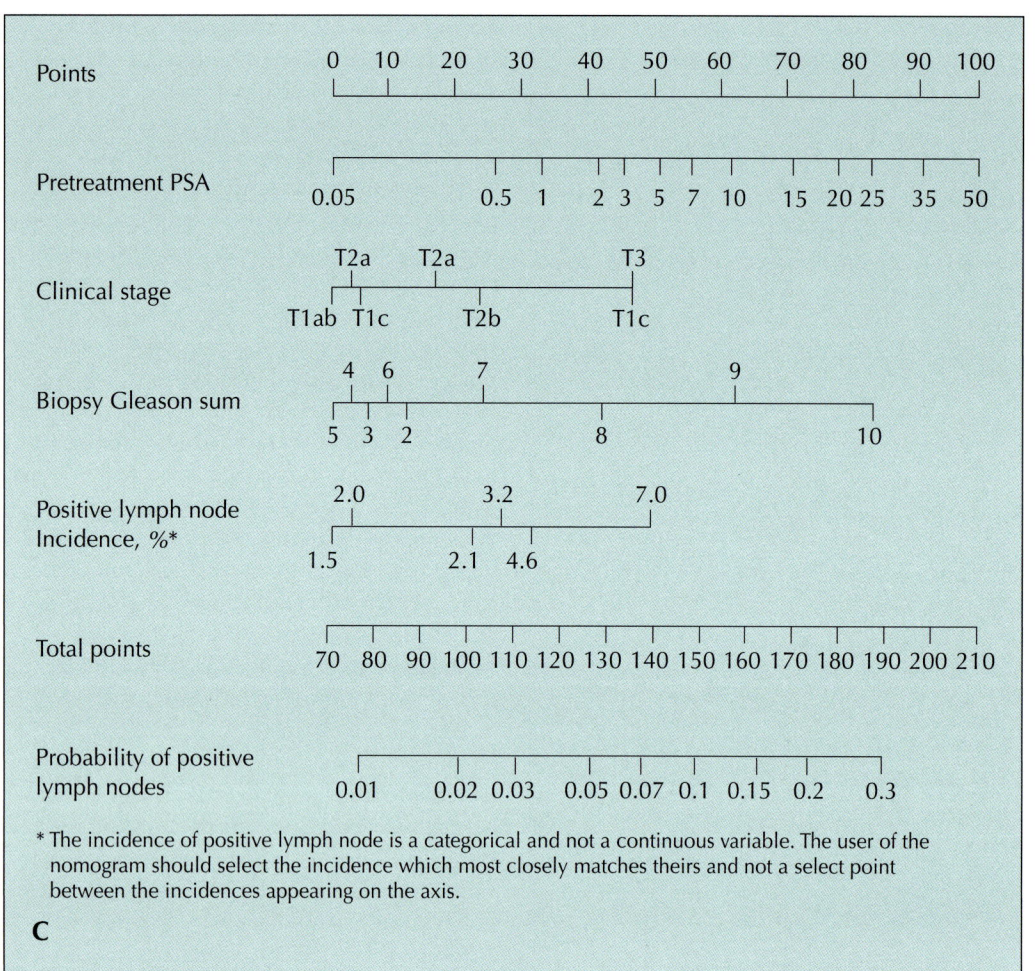

▶ **FIGURE 9-11.** (*Continued*) lymph node metastases, **(C)** [7]. In general, continuous, multi-variable models tend to have superior predictive accuracy compared to risk grouping systems, and each of these nomograms outperforms the Partin tables. We have also developed a nomogram to predict the side-specific probability of extracapsular extension, **(D)**, which has utility in decisions such as wide versus close dissection in the area of the cavernous nerves from the prostate [9]. (Part A *adapted from* Bianco *et al.* [29]; with permission; Part B *adapted from* Koh *et al.* [8]; with permission; Part C *adapted from* Cagiannos *et al.* [7]; with permission; Part D *adapted from* Ohori *et al.* [9]; with permission.)

* The incidence of positive lymph node is a categorical and not a continuous variable. The user of the nomogram should select the incidence which most closely matches theirs and not a select point between the incidences appearing on the axis.

C

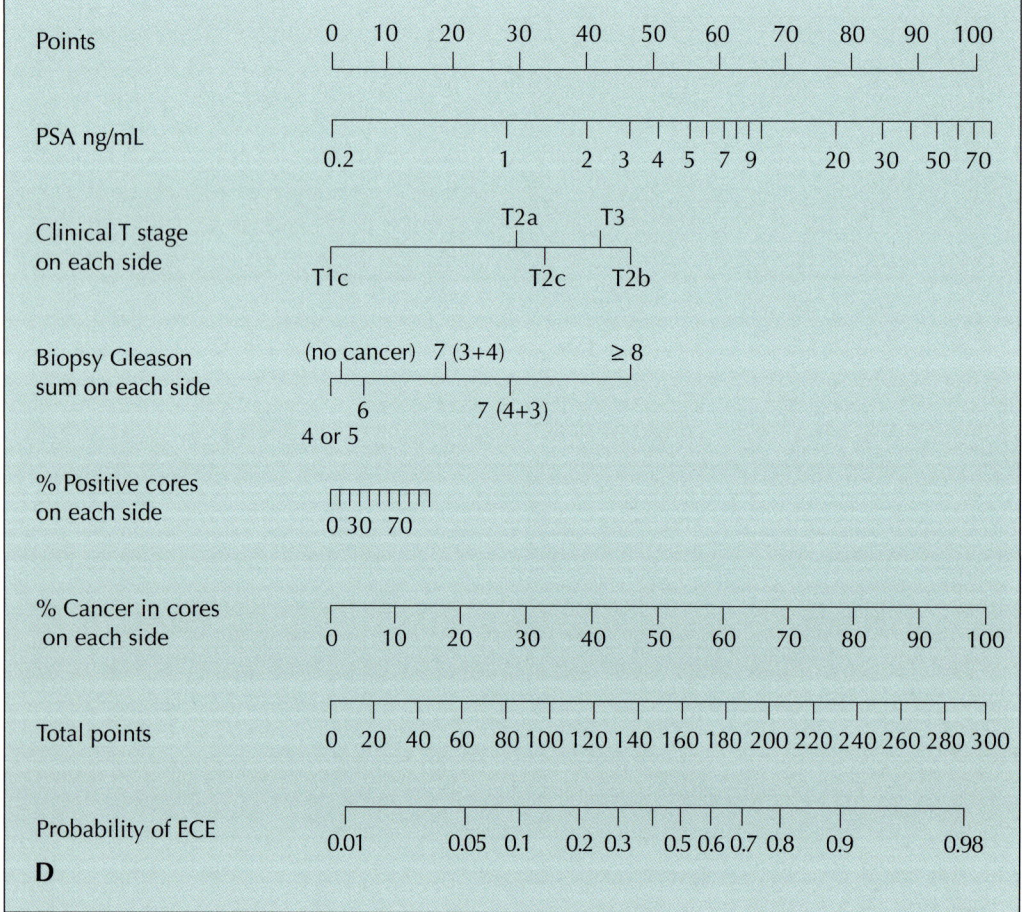

D

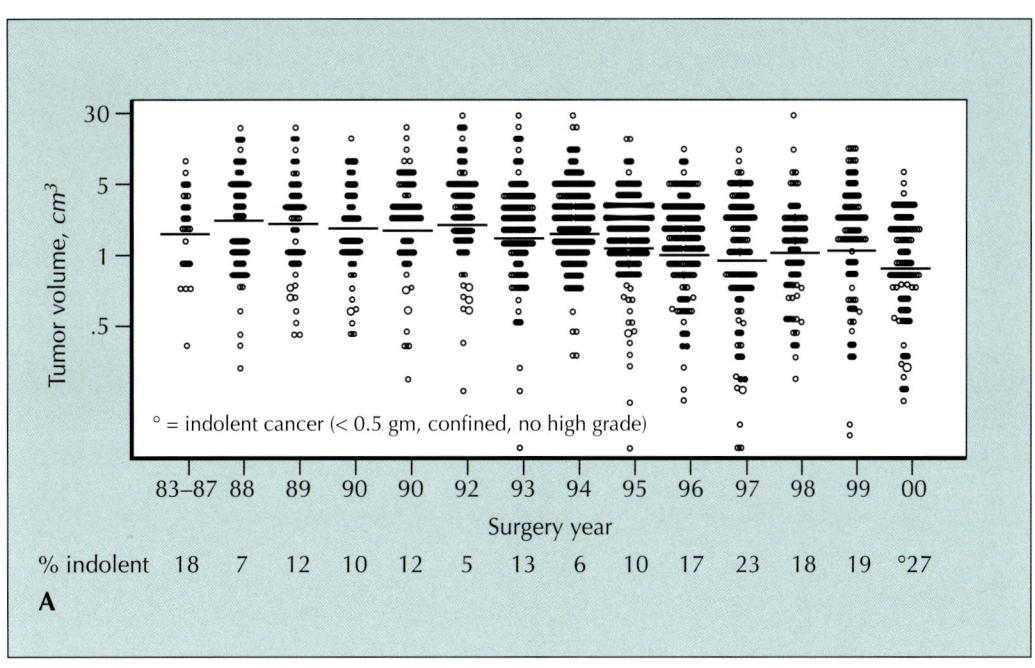

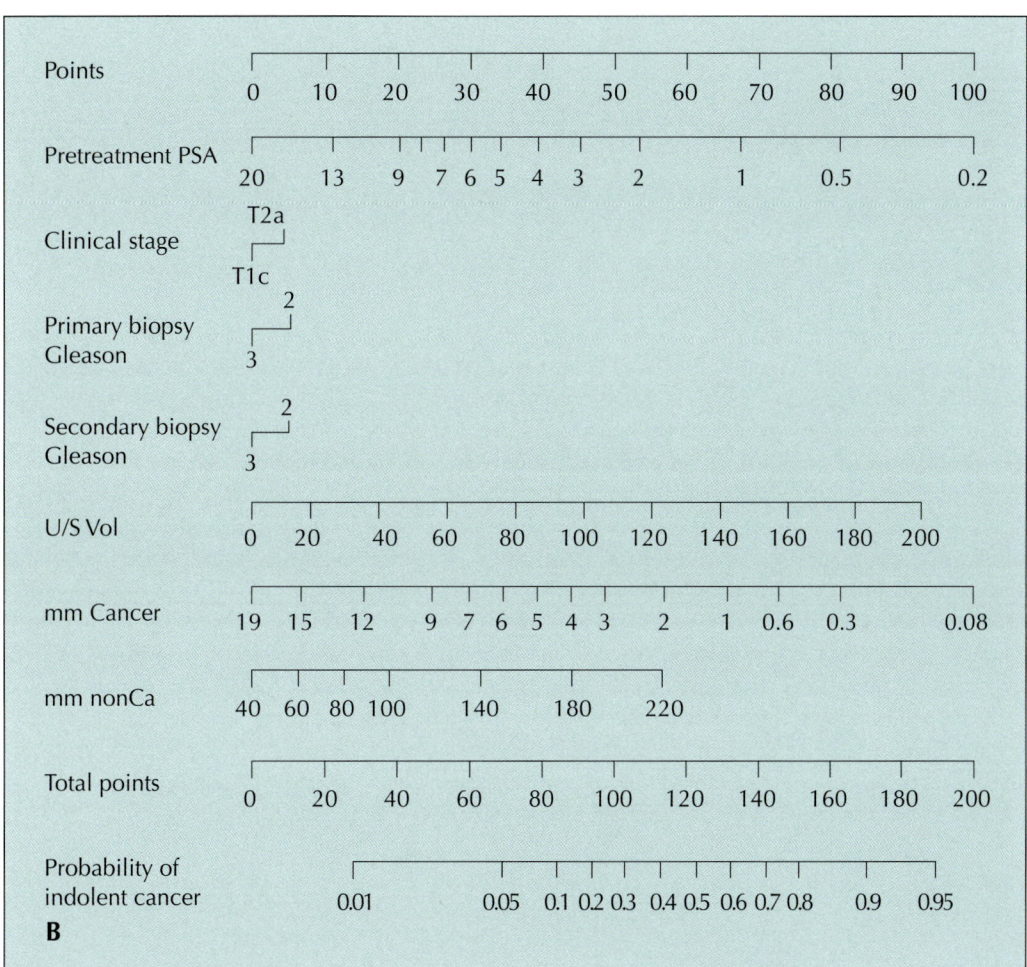

◗ **FIGURE 9-12.** Stage migration and frequency of indolent prostate cancer. As a result of widespread screening with serum PSA and the use of extended TRUS-guided prostate biopsy strategies, the majority of patients who are currently diagnosed with prostate cancer have low-volume disease confined to the prostate gland. Over the past 15 years, the median tumor volume in radical prostatectomy specimens at our institutions has decreased from approximately 2.5 cm³ in the 1980's and early 1990's to 0.6 cm³ in 2000. Moreover, the percentage of tumors considered to be indolent (confined to the prostate, less than 0.5 cm³ in volume, and without evidence of Gleason pattern 4 or 5) has increased from approximately 10% in the 1980's to 25%–30% today, **(A)**. The metastatic potential of tumors with these characteristics is considered to be negligible.

As a result of stage migration, an increasing proportion of patients are now apparently cured by definitive therapy, but there is also increasing danger that men with indolent tumors that pose little threat to their longevity will be subjected to the morbidity of radical therapy unnecessarily. Relatively few patients with newly diagnosed, clinically localized prostate cancer are considered for "watchful waiting" despite the realization that 25% or more of patients who undergo radical prostatectomy have indolent prostate cancer. This is due, in part, to patient anxiety about living with untreated "prostate cancer," the lack of reliable tools to identify progressive disease, and the difficulty in accurately identifying patients with indolent prostate cancer before prostatectomy. To better select patients for watchful waiting, we have developed a nomogram based on PSA, clinical stage, biopsy Gleason score, prostate volume by TRUS, length of cancer in the biopsy specimens, and length of noncancer in the biopsy specimens. This nomogram predicts, with approximately 90% accuracy, the probability of having indolent prostate cancer, **(B)** [11]. (Part B *adapted from* Kattan *et al.* [11]; with permission.)

A. System for Evaluating Progression in Patients Treated with Deferred Therapy

	1 Point	2 Points	3 Points
Gleason score increase	1	> 1	Any new Gleason pattern 4 or 5
PSA velocity (ng/mL/yr)	-	> 0.75 in 12 mo	> 0.75 in 24 mo
DRE/TRUS	Increasing old lesion*	New lesion not biopsy proven†	New biopsy proven lesion†
Biopsy specimens	-	Bilat or multifocal Ca	> 4 cores with Ca

*Greater than 25% increase in cross-sectional area (p/4 x perpendicular width).
†New nodule on DRE or hypoechoic lesion on TRUS separate from any previously recorded lesion.

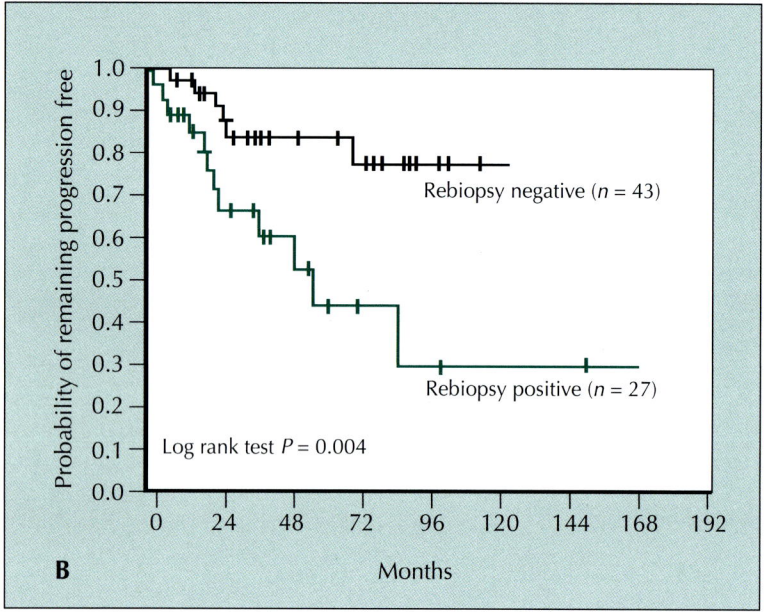

FIGURE 9-13. Watchful waiting as a treatment option for patients with low-grade, low-volume prostate cancer. Ideal characteristics of candidates for watchful waiting include a cancer with a low risk of metastatic progression and a short life expectancy due to advanced age or comorbidity. For the relatively few men with clinically localized prostate cancer who choose watchful waiting as a treatment option, most studies have reported that 50%–75% choose to receive definitive treatment with 4 to 5 years of diagnosis. The most common reasons for initiating treatment are patient anxiety and asymptomatic rises in the level of PSA without evidence of progression by repeat biopsy, digital rectal exam (DRE), or symptoms. We use the term "deferred therapy" rather than watchful waiting to designate patients with very low risk cancer who choose to defer therapy until there is clear evidence of progression. Patients who elect to go on a watchful waiting protocol at our institution are followed with regular PSA determinations, clinical assessment, periodic repeat TRUS biopsy, and endorectal MRI in select circumstances. A progression score was devised based on PSA velocity, changes in the prostate discernible by DRE, TRUS, or MRI, changes in the Gleason score, or an increase in the quantity or location of cancer in the biopsy specimen, **(A)**. Patients with 3 or more points by this system are considered to have progression and are recommended to receive definitive therapy. In our series, 67% of patients were free of progression at 5 years. None of the patients with progression who underwent radical prostatectomy have manifested evidence of recurrent disease [30]. The best predictor of those whose cancer will progress within 10 years, in our series, was the results of a repeat TRUS-guided biopsy; 11% of patients who had a first repeat biopsy that was negative for cancer had progression compared to 40% with a positive first repeat biopsy, **(B)**. Absent cancer on repeat needle biopsy therefore identifies cases highly unlikely to progress. These results demonstrate that deferred therapy is a feasible alternative to curative treatment in select patients with favorable, localized prostate cancer. DRE–digital rectal examination, TRUS–transrectal ultrasonography. (*Adapted from* Patel *et al.* [30]).

New Prognostic Markers Under Consideration

Circulating markers

Human glandular kallikrein 2 (hK2)
Plasma transforming growth factor β1
Plasma interlukin 6 soluble receptor
Circulating PSA, hK2, PSMA RNA by reverse transcription PCR assay
Circulating disseminated prostate cancer cells

Tissue-based markers

PTEN, Akt, p27^{KIP1} (CDKN1B)
Enhancer of zeste homolog 2 (EZH2)
Caveolin-1 (CAV1)
Bcl-2 (BAD)
E-cadherin (CDH1)
Tumor protein p53 (TP53)
Her-2/neu (ERBB2)

High-throughput, genomic-scale methodologies

Transcriptional profiling
Oligonucleotide microarrays
cDNA microarrays
Proteomics
MALDI-TOF (matrix-assisted laser desorption/ionization time-of-flight) mass spectrometry
SELDI-TOF (surface-enhanced laser desorption/ionization time-of-flight) mass spectrometry
Genomic profiling
Comparative genomic hybridization
High-density single nucleotide polymorphic allele (SNP) arrays

▶ **FIGURE 9-14.** New prognostic biomarkers in prostate cancer. In the context of prognostic models, the combination of PSA, Gleason grade, clinical stage, and systematic biopsy results performs well at predicting pathologic stage and probability of disease progression after definitive local therapy. However, the nomograms that predict these endpoints are far from perfect. In addition, stage, grade, and PSA are rather crude predictors of the response to systemic therapy. Tumorigenesis and metastatic progression occur as a result of molecular changes at the DNA, transcriptional, or translational level. Identifying the critical molecular events responsible for tumor progression may enhance our ability to predict outcome for the individual patient. Already, numerous tissue- and serum-based biomarkers have been shown to be independent predictors of prostate cancer progression; these include increased expression of enhancer of zeste homolog 2 (EZH2), caveolin-1 (CAV1), and Bcl-2 (BAD) and loss of expression of E-cadherin (CDH1), PTEN, p27kip1 (CDKN1B), and p53 (TP53). High-throughput, genomic-scale methodologies such as DNA microarrays and proteomics enable the identification of hundreds of prognostic molecular markers, including molecular pathways, simultaneously. In the future, molecular "fingerprints" of prostate cancer may be used to predict which patients will respond better to surgery versus radiation therapy, with or without (neo)adjuvant hormone therapy, chemotherapy, or other modalities. The identification of molecular pathways responsible for prostate cancer progression may lead to the development of targeted therapeutic strategies aimed at the specific molecular composition of an individual's cancer.

1. .Jemal A, Murray T, Ward E, *et al.*: Cancer statistics, 2005. *CA Cancer J Clin* 2005, 55:10–30.

2. Etzioni R, Legler JM, Feuer EJ, *et al.*: Cancer surveillance series: interpreting trends in prostate cancer—part III: Quantifying the link between population prostate-specific antigen testing and recent declines in prostate cancer mortality. *J Natl Cancer Inst* 1999,91:1033–1039.

3. Bill-Axelson A, Holmberg L, Ruutu M, *et al.*: Radical prostatectomy versus watchful waiting in early prostate cancer. *N Engl J Med* 2005, 352:1977–1984.

4. Kuban DA, Thames HD, Levy LB, *et al.*: Long-term multi-institutional analysis of stage T1-T2 prostate cancer treated with radiotherapy in the PSA era. *Int J Radiat Oncol Biol Phys* 2003, 57:915–928.

5. Ragde H, Elgamal AA, Snow PB, *et al.*: Ten-year disease free survival after transperineal sonography-guided iodine-125 brachytherapy with or without 45-gray external beam irradiation in the treatment of patients with clinically localized, low to high Gleason grade prostate carcinoma. *Cancer* 1998, 83:989–1001.

6. Scardino PT, Kelman J: In *Dr. Peter Scardino's Prostate Book: The Complete Guide to Overcoming Prostate Cancer, Prostatitis, and BPH.* New York, Avery Press; 2005.

7. Cagiannos I, Karakiewicz P, Eastham JA, *et al.*: A preoperative nomogram identifying decreased risk of positive pelvic lymph nodes in patients with prostate cancer. *J Urol* 2003, 170:1798–1803.

8. Koh H, Kattan MW, Scardino PT, *et al.*: A nomogram to predict seminal vesicle invasion by the extent and location of cancer in systematic biopsy results. *J Urol* 2003, 170:1203–1208.

9. Ohori M, Kattan MW, Koh H, *et al.*: Predicting the presence and side of extra-capsular extension: a nomogram for staging prostate cancer (discussion 1849). *J Urol* 2004, 171:1844–1849.

10. Partin AW, Kattan MW, Subong EN, *et al.*: Combination of prostate-specific antigen, clinical stage, and Gleason score to predict pathological stage of local-ized prostate cancer. A multi-institutional update. *JAMA* 1997, 277:1445–1451.

11. Kattan MW, Eastham JA, Wheeler TM, *et al.*: Counseling men with prostate cancer: a nomogram for predicting the presence of small, moderately differenti-ated, confined tumors. *J Urol* 2003;170:1792–1797.

12. Kattan MW, Eastham JA, Stapleton AM, *et al.*: A preoperative nomogram for disease recurrence following radical prostatectomy for prostate cancer. *J Natl Cancer Inst* 1998, 90:766–771.

13. D'Amico AV, Whittington R, Malkowicz SB, *et al.*: Biochemical outcome after radical prostatectomy, external beam radiation therapy, or interstitial radiation therapy for clinically localized prostate cancer. *JAMA* 1998, 280:969–974.

14. Kattan MW, Zelefsky MJ, Kupelian PA, *et al.*: Pretreatment nomogram for predicting the outcome of three-dimensional conformal radiotherapy in prostate cancer. *J Clin Oncol* 2000, 18:3352–3359.

15. Kattan MW, Potters L, Blasko JC, *et al.*: Pretreatment nomogram for predicting freedom from recurrence after permanent prostate brachytherapy in prostate cancer. *Urology* 2001, 58:393–399.

16. Scardino PT, Weaver R, Hudson MA: Early detection of prostate cancer. *Hum Pathol* 1992, 23:211–222.

17. Scher HI, Heller G: Clinical states in prostate cancer: toward a dynamic model of disease progression. *Urology* 2000, 55:323–327.

18. Albertsen PC, Hanley JA, Fine J: 20-year outcomes following conservative management of clinically localized prostate cancer. *JAMA* 2005, 293:2095–2101.

19. Begg CB, Riedel ER, Bach PB, *et al.*: Variations in morbidity after radical pro-statectomy. *N Engl J Med* 2002, 346:1138–1144.

20. Eastham JA, Kattan MW, Riedel E, *et al.*: Variations among individual surgeons in the rate of positive surgical margins in radical prostatectomy specimens. *J Urol* 2003, 170:2292–2295.

21. Hull GW, Rabbani F, Abbas F, *et al.*: Cancer control with radical prostatectomy alone in 1,000 consecutive patients. *J Urol* 2002,167:528–534.

22. Ohori M, Scardino PT: Localized prostate cancer. *Curr Probl Surg* 2002, 39:833–957.

23. Carter HB, Pearson JD, Metter EJ, *et al.*: Longitudinal evaluation of prostate-specific antigen levels in men with and without prostate disease. *JAMA* 1992, 267:2215–2220.

24. D'Amico AV, Chen MH, Roehl KA, *et al.*: Preoperative PSA velocity and the risk of death from prostate cancer after radical prostatectomy. *N Engl J Med* 2004, 351:125–135.

25. Stamey TA, McNeal JE, Yemoto CM, *et al.*: Biological determinants of cancer progression in men with prostate cancer. *JAMA* 1999, 281:1395–1400.

26. Wang L, Mullerad M, Chen HN, *et al.*: Prostate cancer: incremental value of endorectal MR imaging findings for prediction of extracapsular extension. *Radiology* 2004, 232:133–139.

27. Hricak H, Wang L, Wei DC, *et al.*: The role of preoperative endorectal magnetic resonance imaging in the decision regarding whether to preserve or resect neurovascular bundles during radical retropubic prostatectomy. *Cancer* 2004, 100:2655–2663.

28. Zakian KL, Sircar K, Hricak H, *et al.*: Correlation of proton MR spectroscopic imaging with Gleason score based on step-section pathologic analysis after radical prostatectomy. *Radiology* 2005, 234:804–814.

29. Bianco FJ, Scardino PT, Fearn PA, *et al.*: Prediction and natural history of organ-confined prostate cancer after radical prostatectomy. *J Urol* 2005, 173:271.

30. Patel MI, De CD, Lopez-Corona E, *et al.*: An analysis of men with clinically localized prostate cancer who deferred definitive therapy. *J Urol* 2004, 171:1520–1524.

31. Greene DR, Shabsigh R, Scardino PT: Urologic ultrasonography. In *Campbell's Urology*, edn 6. Edited by Walsh PC, Retik AB, Stamey TA, Vaughan ED JR. Philadelphia: WB Saunders; 1992:344–393.

32. Bader P, Burkhard FC, Markwalder R, *et al.*: Is a limited lymph node dissection an adequate staging procedure for prostate cancer? *J Urol* 2002, 168:514–518.

33. Partin AW: Issues in the Diagnosis and Prognosis of Prostate Cancer: A Slide Lecture Series. Oklahoma City: Cytodiagnostics (UROCOR); 1995.

34. Prostate Cancer: Management of Advanced Disease. Wilmington DE: ICI Pharmaceuticals;1995.

35. Jewett HJ: The present status of radical prostatectomy for stages A and B prostatic cancer. *Urol Clin North Am* 1975, 2:105–124.

36. Gleason D; Urologic Pathology: The Prostate. Edited by Tannenbaum M. Philadelphia: Lea & Febiger; 1997:171–198.

37. Mullerad M, Shukla-Dave A, Hricak H: Imaging in prostate cancer. In *Comprehensive Textbook of Genitourinary Oncology*, edn 3. Edited by Vogelzang NJ, Scardino PT, Shipley WU, Coffey DS. Philadelphia: Lippincott, Williams, and Wilkins; 2005.

Decision Making for Clinically Localized Prostate Cancer

10

Michael W. Kattan & Brian J. Miles

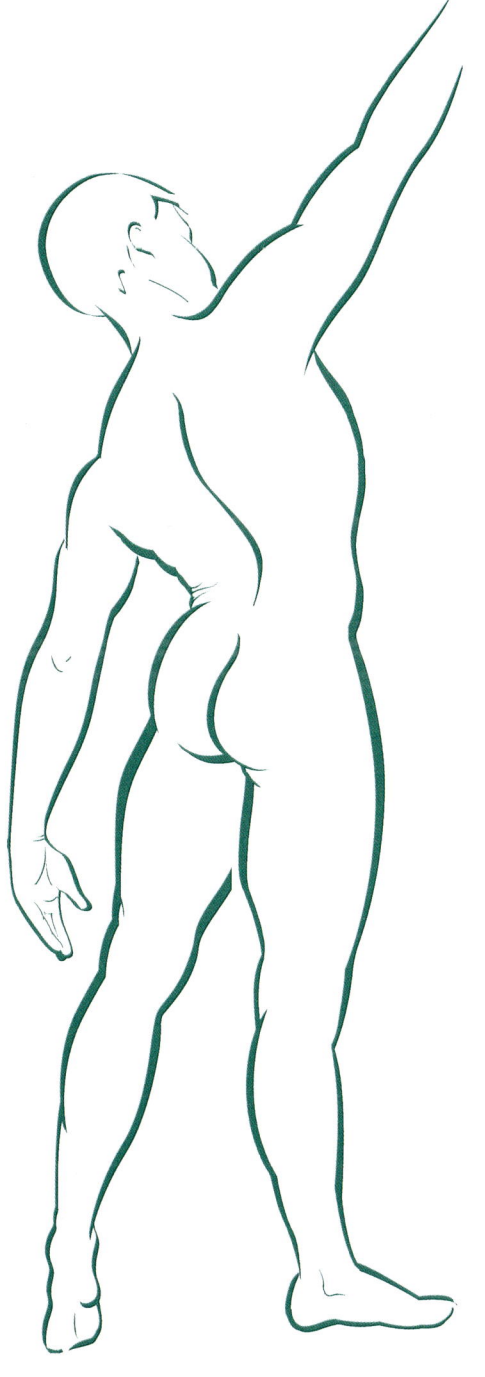

Treatment decision making for patients with clinically localized prostate cancer can be difficult. Because of the age of men at diagnosis, survival benefits associated with aggressive therapies such as surgery typically are estimated to be small, and patient preferences are very influential in determining the preferred treatment. This chapter reviews two different methods for assisting patients in choosing the treatment that is best for them. First, we consider the decision analytic approach, which directly incorporates patient preferences and survival estimates in suggesting the appropriate treatment. Because this approach is difficult to perform at the bedside, we also discuss a second method, nomograms, which are mathematical models that predict outcomes for the individual patient.

▶ **FIGURE 10-1.** The decision-making process for clinically localized prostate cancer. The patient with clinically localized prostate cancer faces a daunting decision. He has one of three mainstream paths from which to choose: surgery, external beam radiation therapy (EBRT), and brachytherapy. Alternatively, he may decide to "stay put" for a while (watchful waiting). For the most part, he is basing his decision on four issues: 1) whether his cancer will progress if left untreated, 2) how well an aggressive therapy would control his cancer, 3) the ability of a salvage therapy in the event that primary therapy fails, and 4) the side effects of each therapy. For the individual patient, each of these criteria is fundamentally a prediction; no outcomes, good or bad, are known with certainty. Further, each man places different values on side effects (*eg*, impotence). Because of all these issues, treatment recommendations for the individual patient must be tailored to his disease and preferences.

	Surgery	External beam	Brachytherapy	Watchful waiting
PSA progression				
Local progression				
Distant progression				
Survival				
Impotence				
Urinary frequency				
Urinary irritation/ obstruction				
Bowel problems				

▶ **FIGURE 10-2.** Using a spreadsheet to aid in making treatment decisions. Tailoring the treatment decision requires that each man construct his own "spreadsheet." The columns are the treatment options available to the patient, including watchful waiting. The rows are the possible outcomes, including disease progression, survival, and side effects. Each cell of the spreadsheet should contain a probability for the treatment/outcome combination. Once completed, this spreadsheet serves as a valuable decision aid for the patient. PSA—prostate-specific antigen.

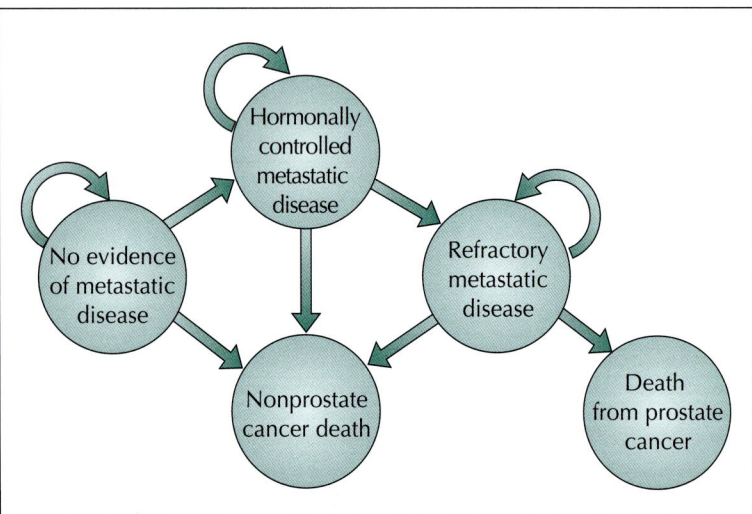

▶ **FIGURE 10-3.** Most decision analyses use computerized Markov models to represent treatment decisions. These models move patients through various health states (*eg*, healthy, sick, and dead). This figure represents a Markov model for clinically localized prostate cancer [1]. In this example, a theoretical cohort of patients begins in the health state ("no evidence of metastatic disease") (*left*). Every 6 months, a fraction of the cohort is allowed to progress in the direction of the arrows. The probabilities of progression are taken from the literature. *Circular arrows* indicate that it is possible for the patient to remain in that health state at the end of a 6-month period. The two death states are absorbing; they cannot be exited. Computerized Markov models such as this one allow survival estimation for various treatment strategies. If we assume that the patient will not prefer all health states equally, we may then be able to estimate quality-adjusted life expectancy by assigning different weights to the different health states. The quality-of-life adjustments, called *utilities*, can be estimated using several established techniques. (*Adapted from* Kattan *et al.* [1].)

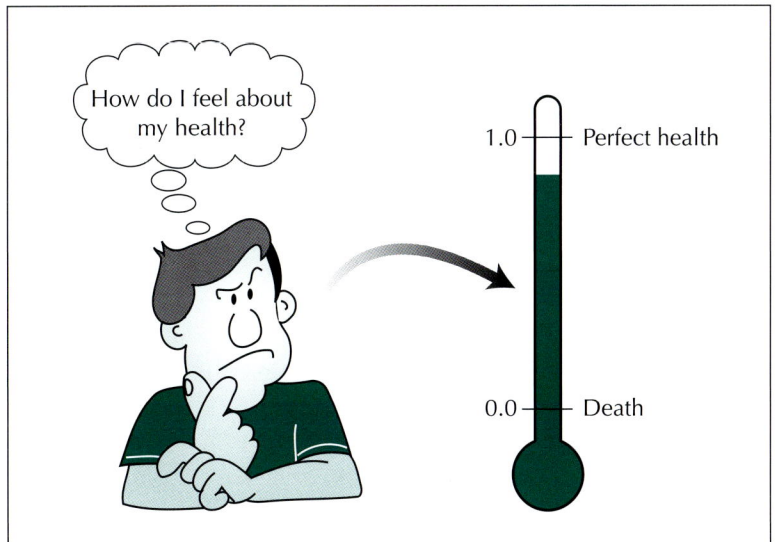

▶ **FIGURE 10-4.** Quality of life (QOL). There are numerous definitions of QOL, from the psychologic to the social; in general, QOL can be understood as a patient's ability to function in a manner commensurate with his needs, desires, and abilities. Although all traditional definitions help us approach a "sense" of QOL, none can globally capture what it is for all people. QOL can be defined only by each individual. Therefore, measuring QOL has been viewed as an inexact science fraught with misinterpretation, overinterpretation, and biased or inadequate questioning. However, the science of QOL evaluation has progressed to such an extent that dependable and reproducible results that allow investigators to estimate a patient's QOL are achievable. For the purposes of decision algorithms and models, QOL measurement must be reported numerically, on a scale from 0 to 1, in which 0 represents "death" and 1 represents "perfect health." The value of a utility is that all health states can be placed in this common scale.

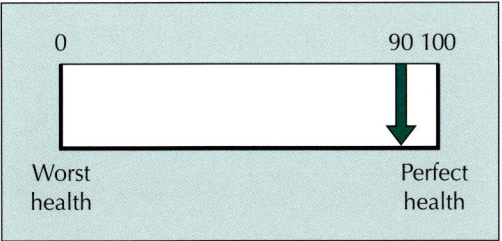

▶ **FIGURE 10-5.** Utility assessment with the rating scale. We can measure quality of life in several ways, but we need a numeric scale for use in computing a decision analysis. A simple approach is to ask clinicians to rate various health states (*eg*, impotence) and use their collective estimate for quality of life. However, such a strategy will not likely be sensitive to the preference of the individual patient. Instead, it is better to ask the patient himself how he would feel to have a particular complication. For example, we could ask the patient to place himself on a scale from 0 to 100. This is often called a "visual analog scale." It is easy to use, but it has an important limitation: the numeric score (*eg*, 90 of 100) does not have external meaning. What one patient considers a 90 may be very different from what another patient considers a 90.

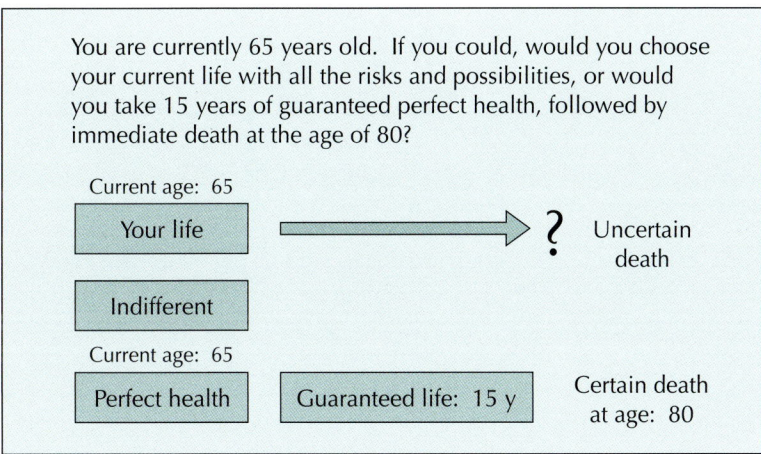

▶ **FIGURE 10-6.** The time-tradeoff technique. One way of measuring utilities (*ie*, health state preferences) is to use the time-tradeoff technique. This is one of the most common utility assessment techniques. With this method, the patient chooses between his current health/life expectancy and a guaranteed period of perfect health followed by immediate death.

The duration of guaranteed perfect health is varied until indifference is reached, and utility is calculated as the number of perfect health years divided by life expectancy. For example, patients might estimate the utility for impotence to be 0.8 and the utility for incontinence to be 0.7. This means that on average, patients would be willing to give up 10% of their life expectancy (0.8 − 0.7 = 0.1) to live with impotence rather than incontinence. Furthermore, a patient in this example would be willing to give up 20% of his life expectancy (1.0 − 0.8) to avoid impotence and remain in perfect health. As an example, the time-tradeoff technique works as follows for evaluating the utility for a person's current state of health. First, find the minimum amount of life in perfect health that the patient is willing to trade for his current life expectancy. Then divide the number of perfect health years by the life expectancy to obtain the utility for his current health state [2].

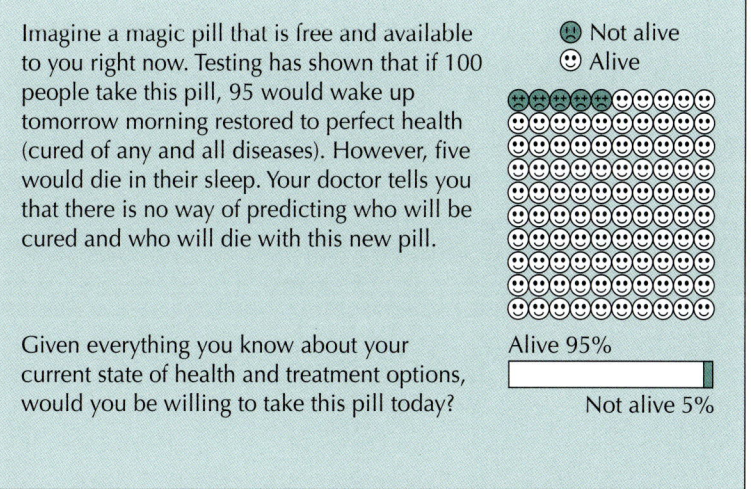

▶ **FIGURE 10-7.** Another method of utility assessment: the standard gamble. The patient is asked to consider taking a make-believe pill that will either cure him of his health problems or kill him. Conceptually, this method is very attractive because the patient is providing a probability: the maximum probability of death that the patient is willing to risk in order to eliminate his current health problems. This method has surprisingly high patient comprehension and test-retest reliability.

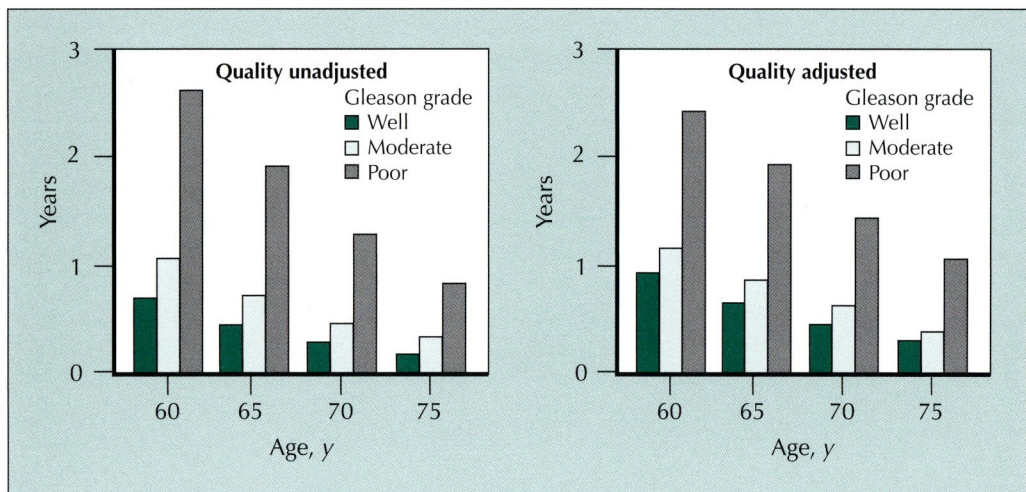

probability multiplied by quality of life (utility). This figure compares quality-adjusted survival with unadjusted survival. The values on the bars indicate how many years longer a radical prostatectomy patient is expected to live than is a watchful-waiting patient. For example, a 60-year-old man with poorly differentiated disease who chooses radical prostatectomy is expected to live 2.58 years longer than had he chosen watchful waiting. After adjusting for quality of life impact, that same man is expected to live an excess of 2.43 quality-adjusted years. Note that these estimates assume the patient has no comorbidity, and they do not specifically consider a particular patient's utilities. Instead, these estimates use group mean utilities. This is an important limitation because individuals of a group do not necessarily share the same utilities. (*Adapted from* Kattan *et al.* [3].)

▶ **FIGURE 10-8.** Quality-adjusted survival. Once we have developed the health states of interest in a Markov model, and reviewed the literature to obtain the probabilities of moving from one health state to another and the utilities of the health states, we can estimate survival and survival adjusted for quality of life under different treatment strategies. Quality-adjusted survival is survival

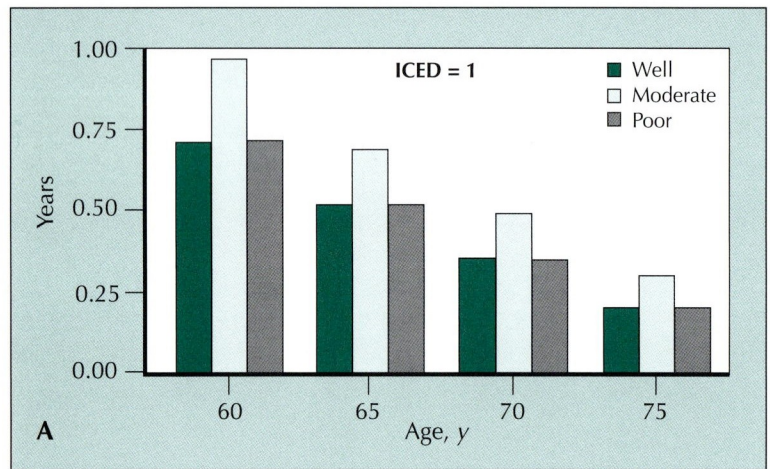

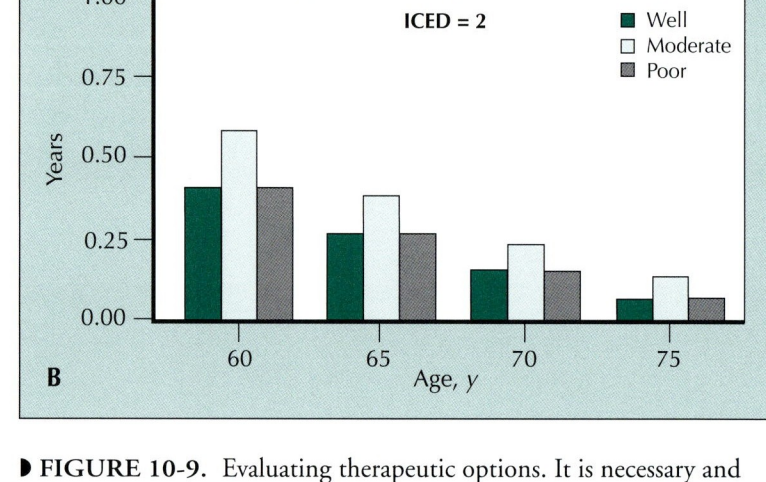

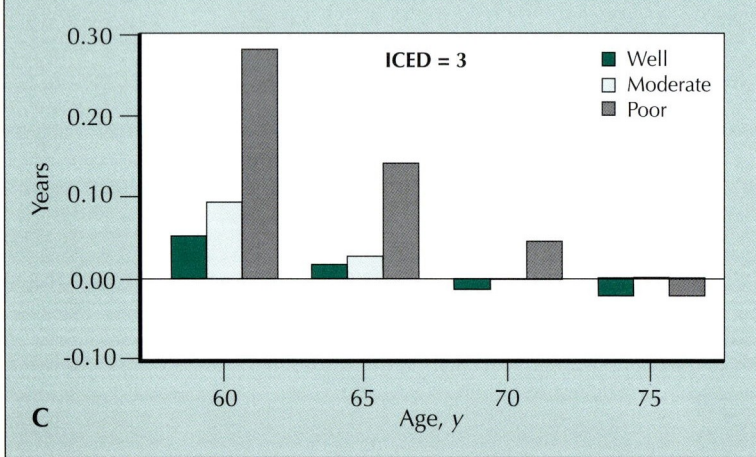

▶ **FIGURE 10-9.** Evaluating therapeutic options. It is necessary and important to consider the overall health of an individual when evaluating therapeutic options. In a very unhealthy patient (*eg*, with concomitant severe heart disease, diabetes, and Alzheimer's disease), aggressive surgical treatment of prostate cancer might be more immediately harmful than watchful waiting. This figure reflects the impact of comorbid conditions. As in Figure 10-8, the *vertical bars* indicate the additional quality-adjusted years of life that the patient is expected to derive from radical prostatectomy relative to watchful waiting.

The results of our model change when comorbidity is allowed to vary. The index of coexistent disease (ICED) is a measure from 0 (no comorbidity) to 3 (highest comorbidity). **A–C** show the results for ICED levels 1,2, and 3, respectively (based on data from Kattan *et al.* [1]). The vertical axes in these plots represent the additional years of life (quality-adjusted) that a radical prostatectomy patient is expected to live beyond the life expectancy of a watchful-waiting patient. Notice the decreasing benefit of radical prostatectomy as the comorbidity increases. Also, notice that when comorbidity is very high, watchful waiting is preferred in older men with low-grade disease. Still, individual preferences need to be measured. Measuring individual utilities on each patient is time consuming and expensive, however. For this reason, we are developing software that assesses utilities and allows the physician to enter clinical information and then compute the quality-adjusted survival estimates for that patient in a customized fashion (see our website: www.nomograms.org).

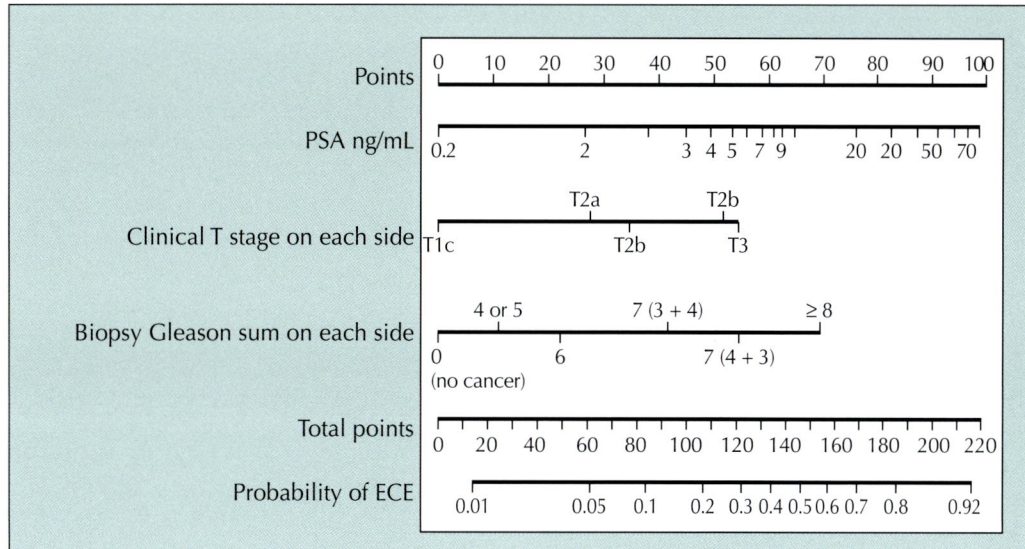

FIGURE 10-10. Nomograms. Markov modeling is difficult to perform on individual patients [4]. Furthermore, Markov models are designed for use in population and cohort studies. Because of this difficulty of use, many physicians prefer to use nomograms. These are mathematical devices (usually tables or charts) that predict the probability of an outcome for an individual patient. The main attraction of a nomogram is that it precisely predicts probabilities, which is something that humans have difficulty doing. Numerous studies have shown that nomograms predict more accurately than do human experts under most conditions [3–6].

This figure shows nomograms for predicting extracapsular extension (ECE). PSA—prostate-specific antigen. (*Adapted from* Ohori *et al.* [7].)

Predictive Value of Pathologic Stage

Pathologic Stage Grouping	Probability of PSA Recurrence at 5 Years, %
Organ confined	10
Nonorgan confined	50
Negative lymph nodes	20
Positive lymph nodes	88

FIGURE 10-11. Predictive value of pathologic stage. Although pathologic stage is an important endpoint to predict, it is difficult to interpret

for prognostic purposes. Many patients and physicians believe that organ-confined concerns are always cured with surgery, and that non–organ-confined cancers (extracapsular extension or seminal vesicle invasion or positive lymph nodes) are never cured. Neither statement is true. Although organ-confined cancers have a high cure rate, as shown in this figure, approximately 10% will fail. More importantly, nearly half of all non–organ-confined prostate cancers fail to progress by 5 years. In other words, the probability of organ confinement cannot be considered the progression-free probability. Final pathologic stage fails to provide a crisp breakpoint above which cancers always recur. For this reason, it would be more valuable to predict prostate-specific antigen (PSA) recurrence as an endpoint. (*Adapted from* Kattan *et al.* [8].)

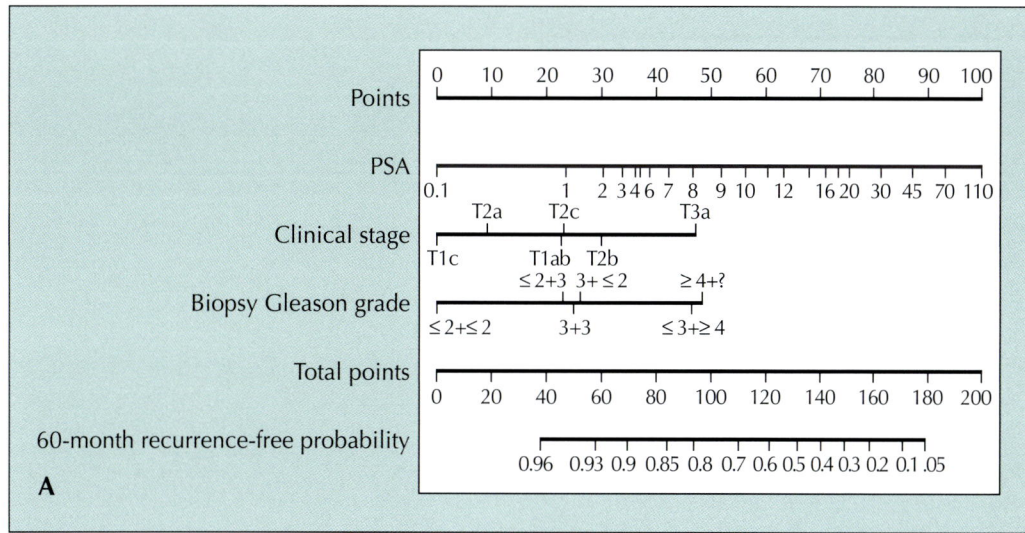

A

FIGURE 10-12. Nomograms for predicting prostate-specific antigen (PSA) recurrence within 5 years. Each of these tools predicts the probability that a man will experience PSA recurrence within 5 years of treatment, depending on whether or not he chooses surgery (**A**),

(*Continued on next page*)

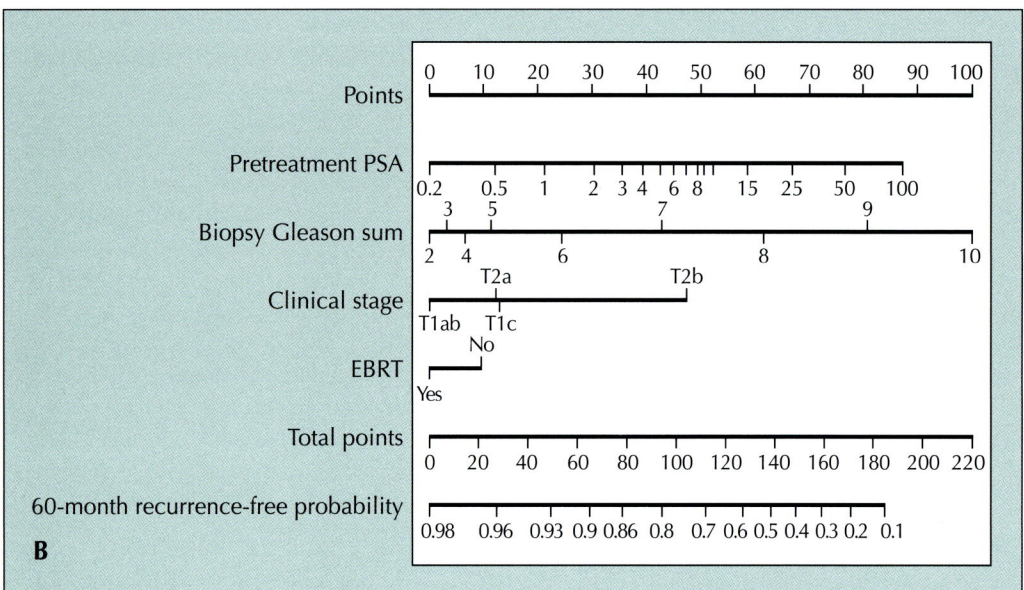

B

◗ **FIGURE 10-12.** (*Continued*) brachytherapy (**B**), or external-beam radiation therapy (EBRT) (**C**). They are available as downloadable software at http://www.nomograms.org or as a free web-enabled service at http://www.oncovance.com. (*Adapted from* Kattan *et al.* [9–11].)

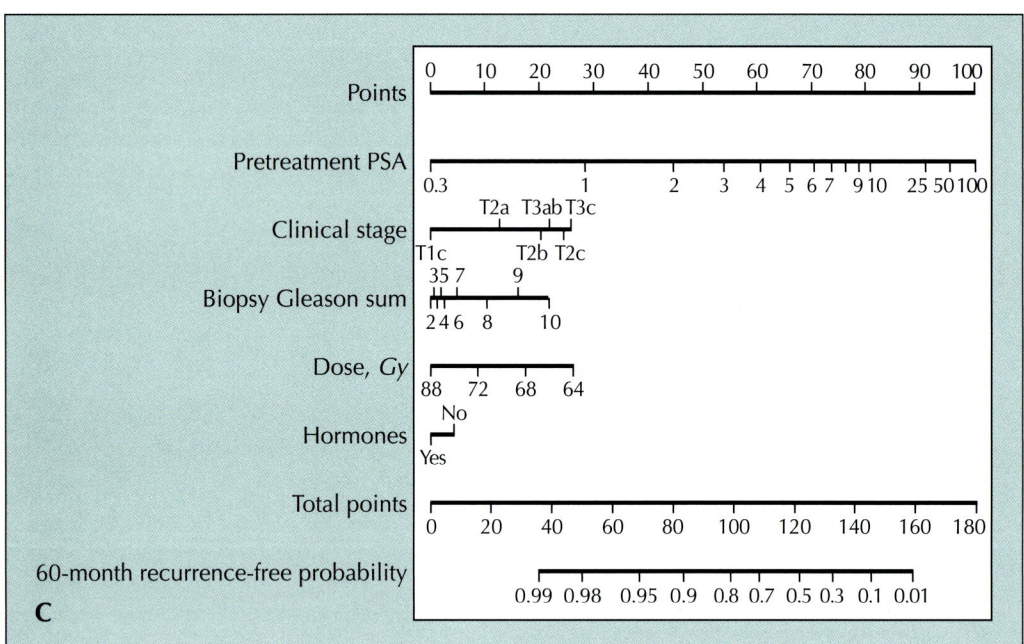

C

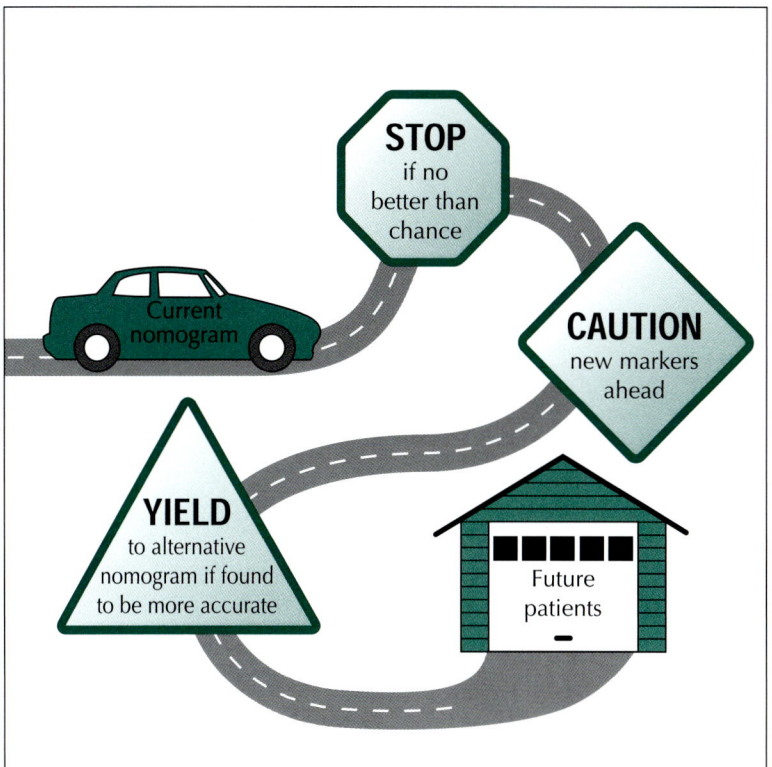

▶ **FIGURE 10-13.** Nomograms are not without limitations. Because they always predict probabilities of an event that will either occur or not, nomograms are always wrong! New markers may come along in the future that will improve our ability to predict, rendering some nomograms obsolete. Certainly, if a nomogram does not predict better than chance, it will not be useful. However, an imperfect prediction from a nomogram is still of value to the decision maker if it is the most accurate prediction currently available [12].

REFERENCES

1. Kattan MW, Cowen ME, Miles BJ: A decision analysis for treatment of clinically localized prostate cancer. *J Gen Intern Med* 1997, 12:299–305.

2. Kattan MW, Fearn PA, Miles BJ: Time trade-off utility modified to accommodate degenerative and life-threatening conditions. In *Proceedings of the 2001 AMIA Annual Symposium.* Bethesda: American Medical Informatics Association; 2001:304–308.

3. Kattan MW, Adams DA, Parko MS: A comparison of machine learning with human judgement. *J Manage Inf Surg* 1993, 9:37–57.

4. Cowen ME, Miles BJ, Cahill DF, *et al.*: The danger of applying group-level decision analyses for the treatment of localized prostate cancer to the individual. *Medical Decision Making* 1998, 18:376–380.

5. Ross PL, Gerigk C, Gonen M, *et al.*: Comparisons of nomograms and urologists' predictions in prostate cancer. *Sem Urol Oncol* 2002, 20:82–88.

6. Partin AW, Yoo J, Carter HB, *et al.*: The use of prostate specific antigen, clinical stage and Gleason score to predict pathological stage in men with localized prostate cancer. *J Urol* 1993, 150:110–114.

7. Ohori M, Kattan MW, Koh H, *et al.*: Predicting the presence and side of extracapsular extension: a nomogram for staging prostate cancer. *J Urol* 2004, 171:1844–1849.

8. Kattan MW, Stapleton AMF, Wheeler TM, Scardino PT: Evaluation of a nomogram for predicting pathological stage of men with clinically localized prostate cancer. *Cancer* 1997, 79:528–537.

9. Kattan MW, Eastham JA, Stapleton AMF, *et al.*: A preoperative nomogram for disease recurrence following radical prostatectomy for prostate cancer. *J Natl Cancer Inst* 1998, 90:766–771.

10. Kattan MW, Potters L, Blasko JC, *et al.*: Pretreatment nomogram for predicting freedom from recurrence following permanent prostate brachytherapy in prostate cancer. *Urology* 2001, 58:393–399.

11. Kattan MW, Zelefsky MJ, Scardino PT, *et al.*: Pretreatment nomogram for predicting the outcome of three-dimensional conformal radiotherapy in prostate cancer. *J Clin Oncol* 2000, 18:3352–3359.

12. Kattan MW: Statistical prediction models, artificial neural networks, and the sophism "I am a patient, not a statistic." *J Clin Oncol* 2002, 20:885–887.

Nerve-sparing Radical Retropubic Prostatectomy

11

*James A. Eastham
& David F. Jarrard*

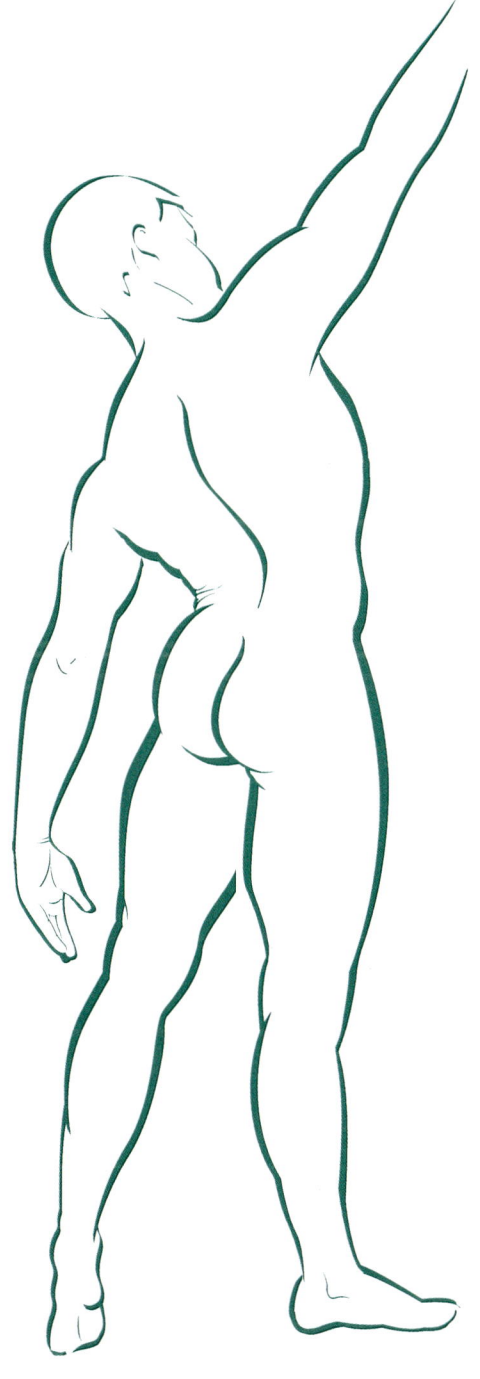

Radical retropubic prostatectomy (RRP) is among the most complex operations performed by urologists, challenging surgeons by results that are highly sensitive to fine details in surgical technique. Modern outcomes research has repeatedly documented how markedly the results and complications of this operation vary among surgeons, not only among those with less experience but also—even more so—among experienced surgeons. The elusive goals of modern RRP are to remove the cancer completely, with negative surgical margins, minimal blood loss, no serious perioperative complications, and complete recovery of continence and potency. No surgeon achieves such results uniformly. Various techniques work well in an attempt to accomplish these goals. The hope is that the reader will discern the important anatomic and surgical principles from this and other approaches that will allow him or her to improve his or her own technique.

For nearly a century, RRP has been an effective way to achieve long-term control of clinically localized prostate cancer. RRP offers several advantages over the perineal approach. The anatomy is more familiar to urologists, there are fewer rectal injuries, a staging pelvic lymphadenectomy can easily be performed, and the wide exposure offers greater flexibility to adapt the operation to each individual's anatomy, permitting more consistent preservation of the neurovascular bundles and a lower rate of positive surgical margins. RRP therefore has become the standard surgical procedure for removal of the prostate for treatment of localized prostate cancer.

Reports of long-term, cancer-specific survival rates after RRP have clearly shown that many such patients live out their lives free of cancer. Gibbons *et al.* [1] reported 82% cancer-specific survival at 15 to 35 years. Zincke *et al.* [2] reported 90% 10-year and 82% 15-year cancer-specific survival for 3170 patients with T1 to T2 NX M0 cancers treated with RRP. Han *et al.* [3], updating outcomes from Johns Hopkins, reported 96% 10-year and 90% 15-year actuarial cancer-specific survival for 2404 men undergoing RRP. Finally, Bianco *et al.* [4] reported 5-, 10-, and 15-year cancer-specific survival of 99%, 96%, and 93%, respectively, for 1700 men treated between 1983 and 2003, with a mean follow-up of 6 years (range 1 to 20 years). Clearly, RRP results in excellent long-term cancer-specific survival.

The efficacy of surgery, however, is based not only on cancer-specific survival, but also on the presence of a nondetectable serum prostate-specific antigen (PSA) level. Although rare cases of disease recurrence after RRP with an undetectable serum PSA level have been documented, in most men, a rising PSA level is the earliest indicator of persistent or recurrent cancer. From several major institutions, we now have remarkably similar 5-year, progression-free probabilities of 69% to 84% in more than 8700 patients treated between 1966 and 1998 [1–6]. Progression rates depend on the clinical stage, Gleason grade, and serum PSA level before RRP as well as on pathologic findings in the RRP specimen. Recently, Bianco *et al.* [4] calculated the risk of recurrence in 1700 consecutive patients with clinical stage T1 to T2 N0 or X, M0 prostate cancer scheduled for RRP and followed closely with serum PSA levels for 1 to 240 months (mean, 72 months). Progression, or treatment failure, was defined as a rising serum PSA greater than 0.2 ng/mL, clinical evidence of local or distant recurrence, or the initiation of adjuvant radiotherapy or hormonal treatment. At 5, 10, and 15 years, 84%, 78%, and 73%, respectively, were free of progression. Of particular interest are patients with high-grade cancers (Gleason sum, 7 to 10). Of patients with Gleason 3+4=7 cancers in the RRP specimen, 68% were free of progression at 15 years [4]. When the tumor was Gleason 4+3=7, in the RRP specimen, 51% were free of progression at 15 years [4]. Even patients with

Gleason sum 8 to 10 cancers fared well, with 27% free of progression at 10 years [4]. These progression rates are substantially lower than the 15-year cancer mortality rates reported in the watchful waiting series by Albertsen *et al.* [7] for patients with Gleason sum 7 to 10 cancers.

Since the late 1970s, clear definition of periprostatic anatomy has allowed the development of an operation more respectful of the intricate anatomy of the periprostatic tissues. Technical refinements have resulted in lower rates of urinary incontinence [8–10] and higher rates of recovery of erectile function [7,9,11,12], less blood loss and fewer transfusions [13–15], shorter hospital stays [16,17], and lower rates of positive surgical margins [18–21]. A thorough understanding of periprostatic anatomy that emphasizes vascular control permits the safe performance of an RRP with reduced morbidity. The purpose of this chapter is to provide surgeons with details about one approach to this operation, which has been modified frequently in a continual effort to improve the results.

PREOPERATIVE ASSESSMENT AND SURGICAL PLANNING

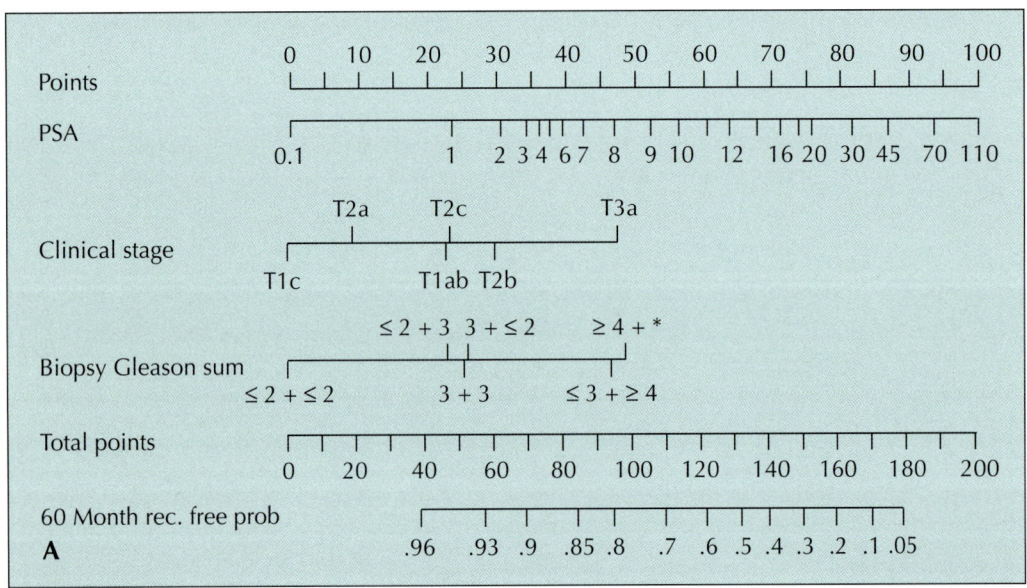

▶ **FIGURE 11-1.** Pretreatment nomograms. Radical retropubic prostatectomy (RRP) is recommended only for patients with clinically localized cancer (cT1 to T3a N0 or NX, M0, or MX) and a life expectancy of 10 or more years. Because of the risk inherent in major surgery, it should be reserved for patients with little or no systemic comorbidity. Although the risk of recurrence after RRP increases with higher clinical stage, Gleason grade, and serum prostate-specific antigen (PSA) levels, there are no absolute cutoff values that exclude a patient as a candidate. Accurate preoperative characterization of the cancer allows the surgeon to plan an operation tailored to the size, location, and extent of each patient's cancer, as well as the anatomy of each patient's prostate and periprostatic tissues. Today, the probability of successful treatment can be estimated from nomograms [22] that consider the important prognostic factors, such as clinical stage, Gleason grade, and serum PSA levels (**A**). Finally, the risk posed by the surgery (incontinence, erectile dysfunction, acute surgical morbidity) and the patient's own values must be brought into the decision-making process.

Bone and CT scans are generally not recommended for patients with a serum PSA level less than 20 ng/mL or a prostate biopsy (Bx) Gleason sum less than 6 because the positive yield is only 2% and 9%, respectively, in these groups [23]. The yield is higher in men with both a serum PSA level greater than 10 ng/mL and a Gleason sum greater than 7 cancer, or in individuals with Gleason sum greater than 8 cancers [23].

The results of systematic needle biopsy may indicate areas suspicious for extracapsular extension (ECE). Information about the location of positive biopsies, the length of cancer in each core, the grade of cancer, and the presence of perineural invasion can help characterize the location and extent of cancer within the prostate [24–27]. The presence of ECE is not a contraindication to RRP because long-term cancer control is possible in more than two thirds of patients with microscopic ECE [4]. However, knowledge of the presence and location of ECE will allow the surgeon performing RRP to modify the operation by performing a wider excision in the involved area so that the tumor can be removed with decreased risk of a positive surgical margin.

(Continued on next page)

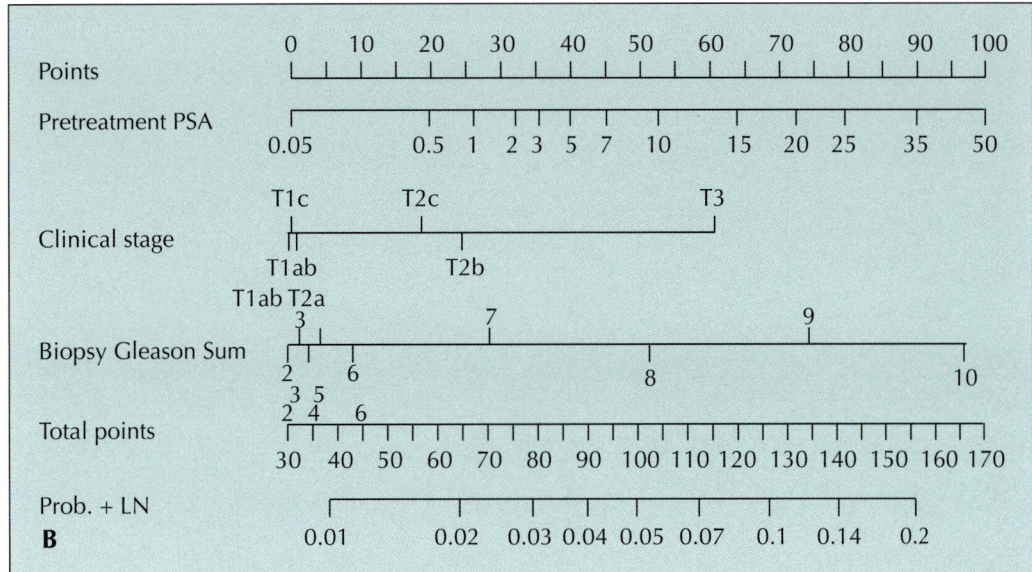

▶ **FIGURE 11-1.** (*Continued*) Improved imaging studies or other techniques that can detect ECE are urgently needed. With stage migration and improved patient selection, the rate of lymph node metastases in patients undergoing RRP has declined sharply over the last decade. As a result, the majority of patients gain no benefit from a pelvic lymph node dissection (PLND). Accurate preoperative prediction of lymph node status could eliminate the need for PLND for patients having the lowest risk of lymph node metastases. Radiographic imaging techniques, however, have low sensitivity for detecting microscopic lymphatic metastases. As a result, several investigators have created algorithms to predict lymph node status. Cagiannos *et al.* [28] examined preoperative predictors of lymph node metastases including pretreatment PSA, clinical stage (1992 TNM), and biopsy Gleason sum (**B**). These predictors were used in logistic regression analysis–based nomograms to predict the probability of lymph node metastases. Overall, 5510 patients were included and had complete clinical and pathological information. Lymph node metastases were present in 206 patients (3.7%). Pretreatment serum PSA (PreTxPSA), biopsy Gleason sum, and clinical stage represented predictors of lymph node status (*P* < 0.001). Bootstrap-corrected predictive accuracy of this three-variable nomogram (clinical stage, Gleason sum and PSA) was 0.76. The negative predictive value of the nomogram was 0.99 when it predicted a 3% or less chance of positive lymph nodes (+LN) [28]. This predictive tool can be used to select men for pelvic lymphadenectomy at the time of RRP.

The use of antibiotic prophylaxis is recommended for RRP, a clean-contaminated procedure. A broad-spectrum antibiotic (*eg*, a second- or third-generation cephalosporin) with activity against common skin and uropathogens should be given intravenously prior to the induction of anesthesia to achieve adequate serum concentrations at the time of the skin incision. (Part A *from* Kattan *et al.* [22], with permission and Part B from Cagiannos *et al.* [28], with permission.)

EARLY COMPLICATIONS: HEMORRHAGE, RECTAL INJURY, THROMBOEMBOLISM, AND BLADDER NECK CONTRACTURE

A. Estimated Blood Loss (EBL) in Patients Undergoing Radical Retropubic Prostatectomy

Series	Patients, n	Mean EBL, mL	Range
Rainwater *et al.* [29]	316	1020	100–4320
Zincke *et al.* [2]	1728	600	—
Eastham *et al.* [30]	954	800	150–5000
Coakley *et al.* [31]	143	1626	500–4400
Goldschlag *et al.* [32]	221	1073	—
Lepor *et al.* [33]	1000	819	—
Maffezzini *et al.* [34]	300	600	200–2200
Augustin *et al.* [35]	1243	1284	—

▶ **FIGURE 11-2.** Early complications in radical retropubic prostatectomy (RRP). Hemorrhage is the most common intraoperative complication during RRP (**A**). A more thorough understanding of the anatomy of the dorsal vascular complex and the periprostatic fascia has allowed development of techniques to control these vessels early in the course of the operation. By giving special attention to the major blood supply to the prostate and seminal vesicles, the surgeon can perform the RRP with reduced blood loss. The key steps in this surgical procedure are complete control of the dorsal vascular complex and anterior periprostatic veins, identification and control of the small branches from the neurovascular bundles to the prostate posterolaterally, and dissection of the seminal vesicles and vas with control of the many small vessels between the base of the bladder and the seminal vesicles. When bleeding is reduced, the surgeon can focus on complete excision of the cancer, selective preservation of the neurovascular bundles responsible for erection, and precise construction of the vesicourethral anastomosis.

(*Continued on next page*)

B. Perioperative Complications and Mortality of RRP in Contemporary Series*

Complications	Events, n (%)				
	Catalona et al. [36] (n = 1870)	Lerner et al. [37] (n = 1000)	Maffezzini et al. [34] (n = 300)	Augustin et al. [35] (n = 1243)	Overall (n = 4413)
Mortality	0 (0.0)	0 (0.0)	0 (0.0)	0 (0.0)	0/4413 (0.0)
Rectal injury	1 (0.1)	6 (0.6)	1 (0.3)	3 (0.2)	11/4413 (0.3)
Colostomy	—	0 (0.0)	0 (0.0)	0 (0.0)	0/4413 (0.0)
Ureteral injury	1 (0.1)	—	1 (0.3)	4 (0.3)	6/3413 (0.2)
Myocardial infarction	2 (0.1)	7 (0.7)	—	1 (0.1)	10/4113 (0.2)
Pulmonary embolism	39† (2.0)	6 (0.6)	1 (0.3)	2 (0.2)	48/4413 (1.1)
Thrombophlebitis/DVT	—	14 (1.4)	1 (0.3)	16 (1.3)	31/2543 (1.2)
Sepsis	—	2 (0.5)	—	3 (0.2)	5/2243 (0.2)
Wound infection or dehiscence	17 (0.9)	9 (0.9)	3 (1.0)	20 (1.6)	49/4413 (1.1)
Lymphocele	—	—	3 (1.0)	37 (3.0)	40/1543 (2.6)
Prolonged fluid leak	7 (0.4)	—	—	16 (1.3)	23/3113 (0.7)
Premature catheter loss	1 (0.1)	—	—	5 (0.4)	6/3113 (0.2)
Anastomotic stricture	71 (4.0)	87 (8.7)	2 (0.7)	—	160/2510 (5.0)

*Notice that complications are not mutually exclusive, that is, one patient may have had more than one complication.
†Includes all thromboembolic complications.

▶ **FIGURE 11-2.** (*Continued*) Other intraoperative complications occur much less frequently (**B**). Operative mortality, defined as death within 30 days of surgery, was not reported for the 4413 men summarized. Rectal injury was also uncommon, occurring in less than 1% of patients. Factors that predispose the patient to rectal injury include previous pelvic radiation therapy, rectal surgery, and/or transurethral resection of the prostate. Injury most often occurs during the apical dissection when the surgeon is unsure of the depth of incision. If a rectal injury occurs, it should not be repaired until after the prostatectomy has been completed. The injury is closed in two inverted layers. To reduce the potential of fistula formation, omentum may be placed between the rectum and vesicourethral anastomosis, although this is not generally found to be necessary. The omentum is mobilized by opening the peritoneum in the rectovesical cul-de-sac and delivering a segment of omentum through the opening. A colostomy is rarely necessary, unless the injury is extensive or there is evidence of proctitis from prior radiation treatment.

Deep venous thrombosis (DVT) and pulmonary embolism occur in approximately 2% of patients after RRP. Cisek and Walsh [38] reported thromboembolic complications in 2% of patients, which often occurred after discharge from the hospital. Patients are encouraged to ambulate soon after the operation and to perform dorsiflexion exercises while in bed to prevent venous stasis.

Bladder neck contracture is usually the result of poor mucosa-to-mucosa apposition at the time of the urethrovesical anastomosis. Eversion of the bladder neck mucosa and proper placement of the urethral sutures under direct vision will help reduce the incidence of this complication. Patients with a bladder neck contracture often note a dribbling urinary stream or symptoms of overflow incontinence. Assessment should include a urinary flow rate, determination of postvoid residual urine, and flexible cystoscopy to evaluate the anastomotic site. Most bladder neck contractures can be managed using a urethral dilating balloon. Severe bladder neck contractures may require cold-knife incision and, if recurrent, periodic dilatation to maintain an adequate urine flow.

LATE COMPLICATIONS: INCONTINENCE AND ERECTILE DYSFUNCTION

A. Incidence of Incontinence After Radical Prostatectomy

	Patients, n	% Incontinent	Definition of Incontinence
Series from investigator interviews			
Steiner *et al.* [39]	593	8	Leaks with moderate activity
Zincke *et al.* [2]	1728	5	Requires ≥ 3 pads/day
Kundu *et al.* [8]	2737	7	Any use of pads
Geary *et al.* [40]	458	20	Requires pads
Eastham *et al.* [9]	390	5	Leaks with moderate activity
Noh *et al.* [10]	244	23	Any use of pads
Series from patient surveys			
Litwin *et al.* [41]	98	25	"Bother" score
Murphy *et al.* [42]	1796	19	Requires pads
Walsh *et al.* [43]	62	5	Requires pads
Sebesta *et al.* [44]	674	32	Any pad use
Series from population surveys			
Stanford *et al.* [45]	1291	8.4	Severe incontinence
		21.6	Requires pads
Fowler *et al.* [46]	738	31	Pads or clamps

B. Results of Cox Proportional Hazards Analysis for Prediction of Spontaneous Recovery of Erections*

Preoperative parameters	Probability of Recovery of Potency by 24 mo, % (36 mo, %)		
Preoperative potency	Age < 60 y	Age 60.1–65 y	Age > 65 y
Full erection	63 (69)	44 (49)	37 (42)
Full erection, recently diminished	48 (54)	31 (36)	26 (30)
Partial erection	35 (40)	22 (25)	18 (21)
Preoperative and intraoperative parameters			
Bilateral nerve sparing			
Full erection	70 (76)	49 (55)	43 (49)
Full erection, recently diminished	53 (59)	34 (39)	30 (35)
Partial erection	43 (49)	27 (31)	23 (27)
Unilateral or bilateral neurovascular bundle damage			
Full erection	60 (67)	40 (46)	35 (41)
Full erection, recently diminished	44 (50)	28 (32)	24 (28)
Partial erection	35 (40)	21 (25)	18 (21)
Unilateral neurovascular bundle resection			
Full erection	26 (30)	15 (18)	13 (15)
Full erection, recently diminished	17 (20)	10 (12)	8.5 (10)
Partial erection	13 (15)	7.5 (8.8)	6.3 (7.5)

*For 314 patients undergoing radical prostatectomy since 1993 for cT1a to T3a prostate cancer based on preoperative and combination preoperative and intraoperative parameters. (Data from Rabbani et al. [12].)

▶ **FIGURE 11-3.** Late complications in radical retropubic prostatectomy (RRP). Urinary incontinence is still one of the most troubling side effects occurring after RRP. Although an anatomic approach to RRP has resulted in a diminished rate of incontinence, incontinence rates vary widely (**A**). Incontinence has been reported in 5% to 23% of postprostatectomy patients by surgeons from large medical centers and from 5% to 32% when reported by patients in response to quality-of-life questionnaires. These variations result from different definitions of continence, different patient populations, and different times of assessment after the operation. In a multivariate analysis, the factors independently associated with persistence of incontinence are increasing patient age ($P < 0.001$), surgical technique ($P < 0.001$), preservation of neurovascular bundles ($P < 0.01$), and development of an anastomotic stricture ($P < 0.01$) [9]. Over a 13-year period, the rate of urinary stress incontinence was 9% in a population of 581 patients who were continent before the operation [9]. Deliberate changes in surgical technique, introduced in 1990, however, resulted in a substantial improvement in the continence rate from 82% to 95% at 24 months [9]. These specific modifications include less manipulation of the urethra distal to the apex of the prostate, preservation of all periurethral tissue distal to the apex of the prostate, inclusion of a small amount of urethra and large amount of the oversewn lateral pelvic fascia covering the dorsal venous complex in the anastomotic sutures, and full-thickness eversion of the bladder neck to reduce the risk of an anastomotic stricture. The median time to recovery of complete urinary control in this series was 6 weeks, with 92% of patients continent at 12 months and 95% at 24 months [9]. Less than 1% of patients had leakage severe enough to require an artificial sphincter.

(Continued on next page)

Nerve-sparing Radical Retropubic Prostatectomy

149

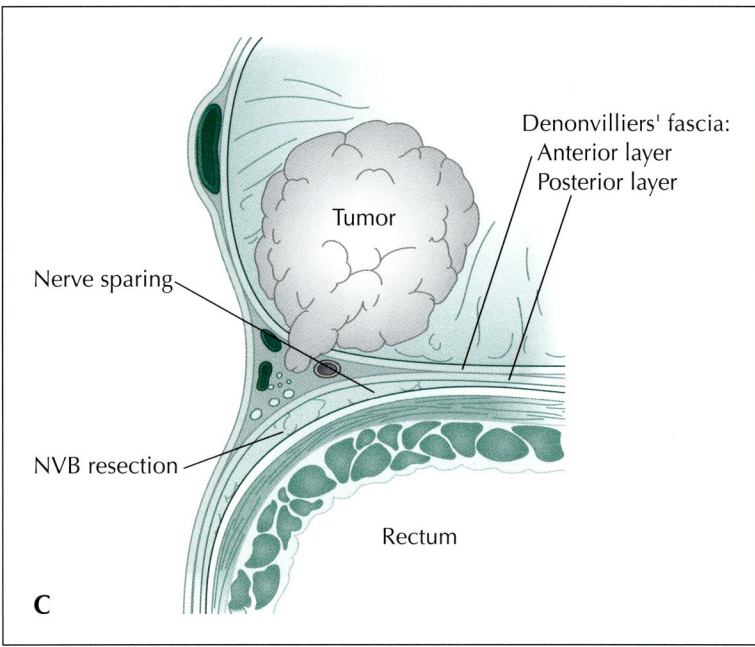

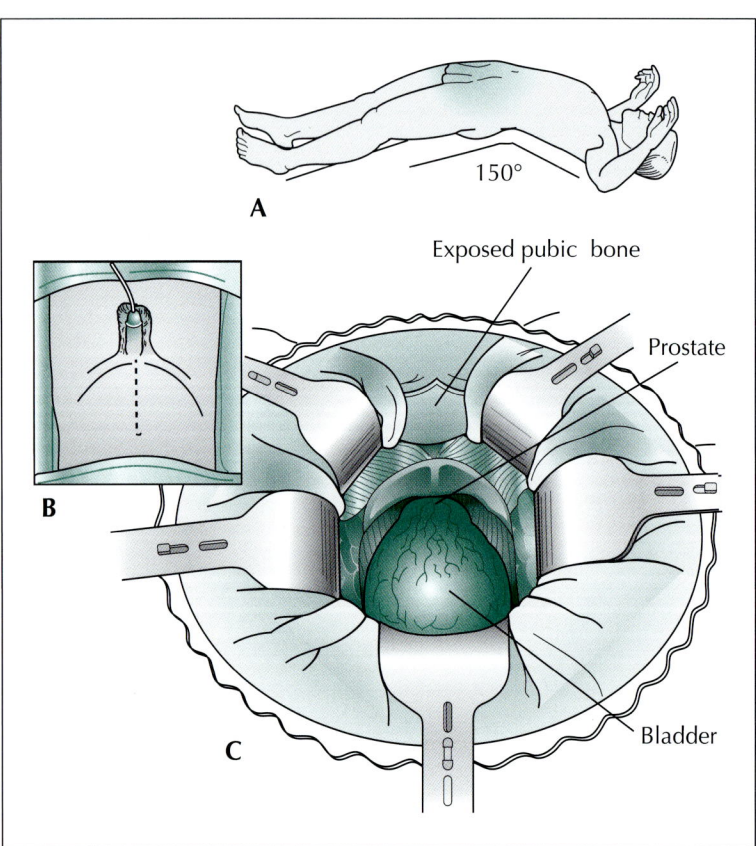

FIGURE 11-3. (*Continued*) Urodynamic studies of patients who are incontinent after RRP have not elucidated a predominant mechanism of incontinence. Most studies have suggested, however, that the functional length of the urethra is the most important factor in postprostatectomy incontinence. A "hands-off" approach to the external sphincter tissues beyond the apex of the prostate, fixation of the urethra within the pelvis, and preservation of the maximum amount of functional urethral length contribute significantly to the maintenance of continence after the procedure.

Potency is defined as the ability to obtain an erection that is sufficient for vaginal penetration and sexual intercourse. Current surgical techniques and a more precise understanding of the autonomic innervation of the corpora cavernosa allow preservation of sexual function in many men. Quinlan *et al.* [47] demonstrated that recovery of potency was quantitatively related to the preservation of nerves. They identified three factors associated with recovery of potency after RRP: age, clinical and pathologic stage, and preservation of the neurovascular bundles. Approximately 90% of men younger than 50 years were potent if either one or both neurovascular bundles were preserved. For men older than 50, return of potency was more likely if both neurovascular bundles were preserved rather than only one. Kundu *et al.* [8] reported potency in 76% of patients when both nerves were preserved and 53% when one nerve was spared. They also demonstrated a strong correlation of preservation of potency with age.

A nomogram is available to predict the return of potency based on a series of 314 previously potent patients treated since 1993 with RRP for clinically localized prostate cancer [12] (**B**). Factors significantly associated with recovery of spontaneous erections satisfactory for intercourse included the age of the patient, the quality of erections before the operation, and the degree of preservation of the neurovascular bundles. Time after surgery is also an important factor in the recovery of potency.

The anatomic approach to RRP has made it possible to completely remove the prostate, with reduced morbidity in the majority of patients with clinically localized prostate cancer. Removal of the cancer and preservation of the nerves responsible for erectile function are often competing goals (**C**). Cancers most often penetrate the prostatic capsule posterolaterally, directly over the neurovascular bundles (NVB). With deliberate attention to surgical planning, most patients can have both neurovascular bundles preserved with a low risk of a positive surgical margin.

OPERATIVE TECHNIQUE

FIGURE 11-4. Patient positioning. The patient is positioned supine. The table can be flexed as needed to gain access to the pelvis (**A**). The arms are abducted and externally rotated with the elbows flexed at 90°, with the wrists fixed to a frame that is positioned across the head of the patient. Through an 8- to 10-cm suprapubic midline incision extending toward the umbilicus (**B**), the transversalis fascia is incised sharply and the retropubic space entered. Care is taken not to sweep perivesical lymph nodes cephalad as the lateral pelvic sidewalls are exposed. A self-retaining Turner Warwick retractor (**C**) is effective in providing adequate pelvic exposure. Alternative retractors may be used according to the preference of the surgeon. Occasionally, a bony spur protruding from behind the symphysis pubis will compromise the view of the prostatic apex. The spur can be removed using an osteotome and mallet. An 18F Foley catheter is inserted, and the balloon is filled with 15 mL of sterile water.

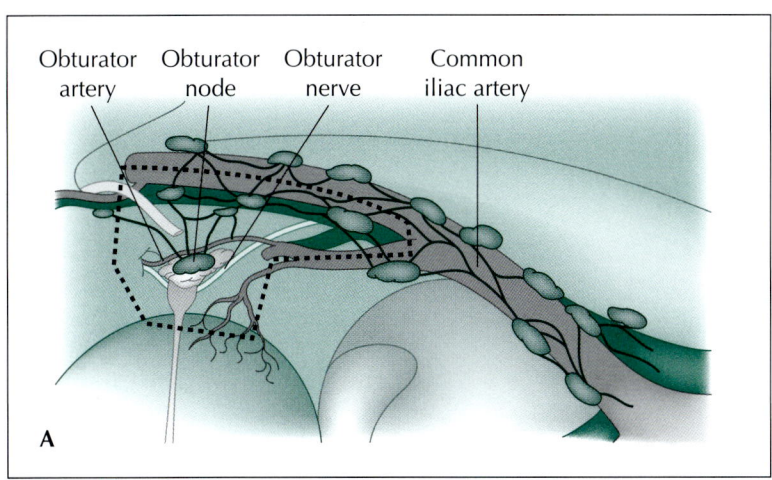

A

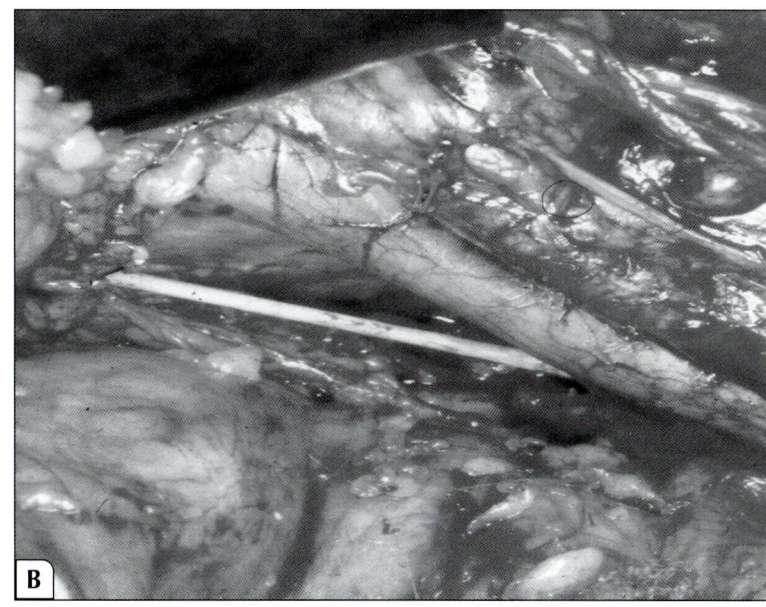

B

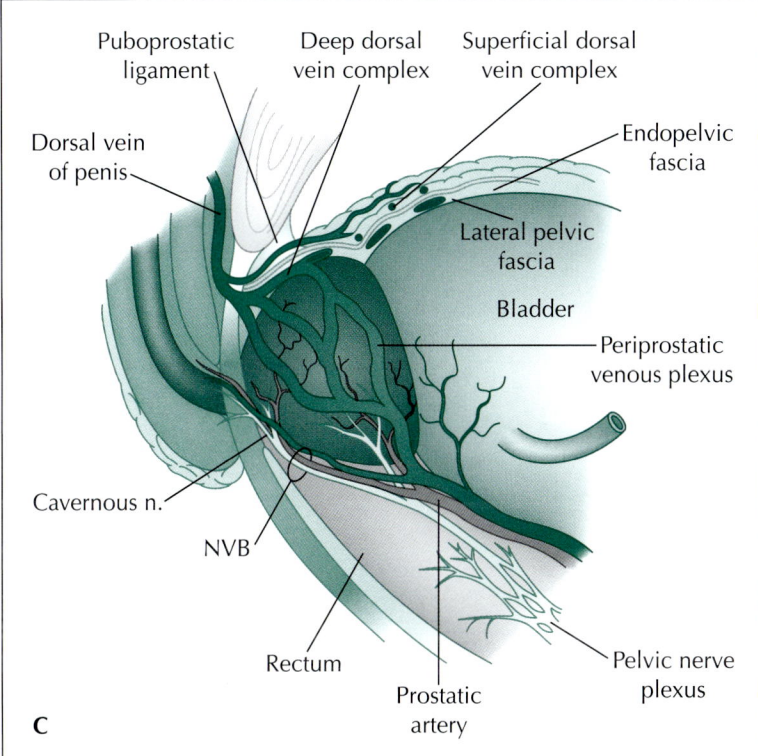

C

▶ **FIGURE 11-5.** (*See Color Plate*) A–C, The anatomic structures relevant to the pelvic lymph node dissection. A bilateral pelvic lymph node dissection is performed using the external iliac vein as the superior margin, the pelvic floor as the inferior margin, the obturator canal caudally, and the bifurcation of the common iliac vessels cranially. Lymphatic channels are carefully clipped to reduce the risk of lymphocele. NVB—neurovascular bundle.

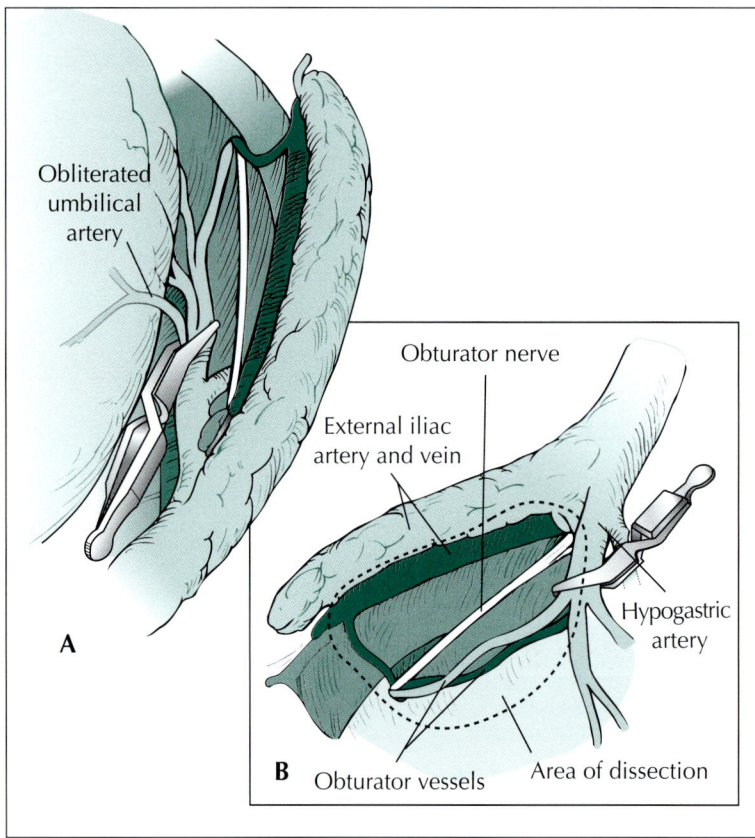

A

Obliterated
umbilical
artery

Obturator nerve

External iliac
artery and vein

Hypogastric
artery

B Obturator vessels   Area of dissection

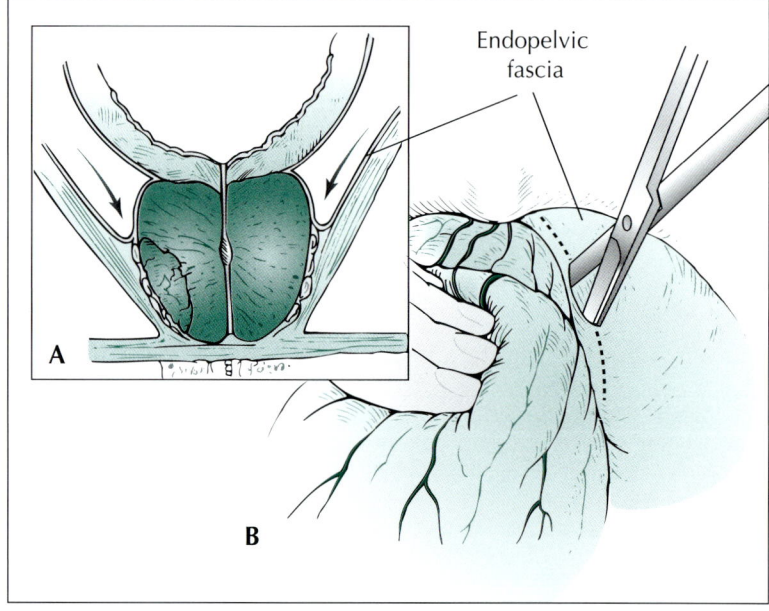

Endopelvic
fascia

A

B

▶ **FIGURE 11-6.** Periprostatic anatomy. A successful radical retropubic prostatectomy (RRP) requires a thorough knowledge of the periprostatic anatomy and a complete characterization of the individual's cancer. **A and B,** The anatomy of the dorsal vein complex and the periprostatic fascia has been defined, allowing the development of techniques to control these vessels early in the course of the operation. By giving special attention to the major blood supply to the prostate and seminal vesicles, the surgeon can perform the RRP with reduced blood loss, which facilitates complete removal of the prostate with preservation of continence and potency.

▶ **FIGURE 11-7.** Perforating the endopelvic fascia. Loose fatty tissue behind the symphysis pubis is gently teased out using nontoothed forceps to expose the superficial dorsal venous complex. The prostate is mobilized by incising the endopelvic fascia laterally (**A**), initially by puncturing the fascia with closed scissors into the deep natural groove between the prostate and the pelvic sidewall (**B**). This initial incision is extended in an anterior and posterior direction either bluntly or sharply. Care must be taken to avoid the venous plexus on the lateral aspect of the prostate. The fibers of the levator ani muscle can be swept off the lateral aspect of the prostate using a Kitner (peanut) dissector. Near the apex of the prostate, small branching vessels are often identified that can be controlled with hemoclips. The puboprostatic ligaments may either be incised sharply now at their insertion on the pubis or later during division of the dorsal vascular complex. The prostate is carefully palpated for induration. This information, together with preoperative information regarding the location of the cancer, will determine the feasibility and safety of a nerve-sparing procedure.

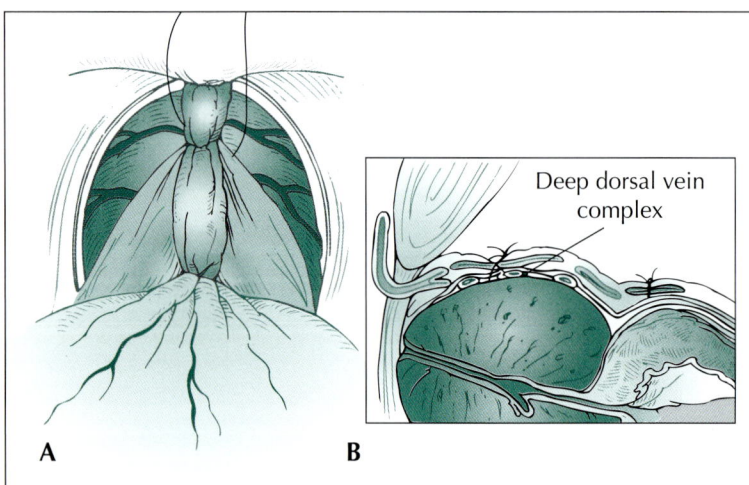

A   **B**

Deep dorsal vein
complex

▶ **FIGURE 11-8.** Control of the dorsal vascular complex. The superficial dorsal venous complex is controlled with a suture placed approximately 1 cm cephalad to the bladder neck, which is determined by its relationship to the catheter balloon. This suture limits back bleeding and also marks the anterior limit of the proximal dissection at the bladder neck during the final stages of the removal of the prostate (**A**). The incised endopelvic fascia and deep dorsal vascular complex are gathered in a figure-of-eight suture placed anteriorly over the midprostate (**B**). The suture is tagged with a hemostat for later use during the apical dissection. This suture should not be placed too close to the apex or too laterally as this may tether the neurovascular bundle, making it more susceptible to injury during its dissection later in the procedure.

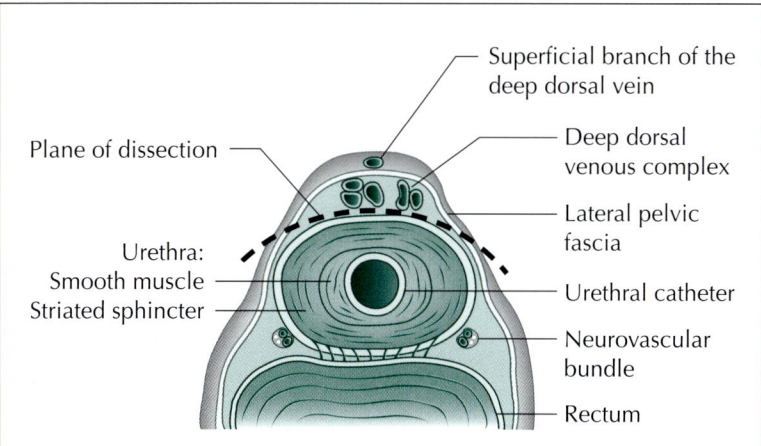

FIGURE 11-9. Anatomy of the dorsal vascular complex and urethra. Correct identification of the urethra and the avascular plane that runs below the dorsal vascular complex is critical to the initiation of the apical dissection. The Foley catheter serves as a guide. The apex and anterior surface of the prostate must be carefully avoided to prevent positive surgical margins in these areas.

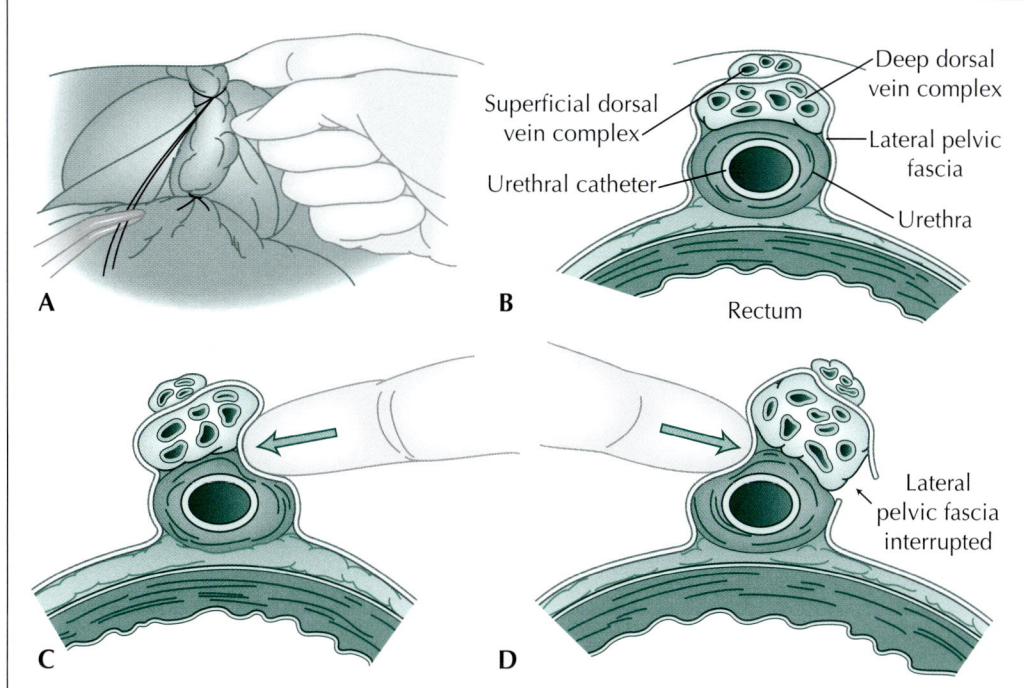

FIGURE 11-10. Isolation of the dorsal vascular complex from the urethra. Counter-traction placed on the hemostatic figure-of-eight suture around the deep dorsal vein complex at midprostate (Figure 11-8*B*) facilitates blunt finger dissection in the plane between the dorsal vein complex and the urethra (**A and B**). The lateral pelvic fascia is weakened with finger dissection applied from both sides (**C and D**). This must be done close to the apex of the prostate so as not to disturb the continence mechanism.

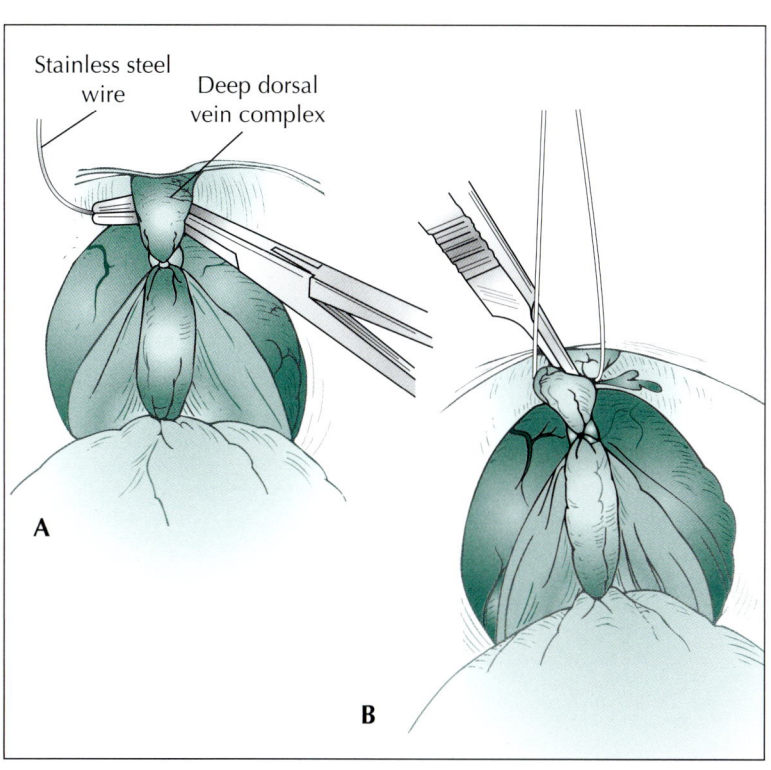

FIGURE 11-11. Division of the dorsal vascular complex. Once the plane of dissection has been identified, a long-tipped right-angled clamp is passed through the weakened fascia between the urethra and dorsal vascular complex and grasps a stainless steel wire that is looped on the end (**A**). The wire serves as a guide to allow a square transection of the dorsal vascular complex and its surrounding fascia using a no. 15 scalpel blade on a long handle (**B**). By this maneuver, the dorsal vascular complex can be divided close to or far from the apex of the prostate, as the surgeon chooses, with care taken to avoid a positive surgical margin.

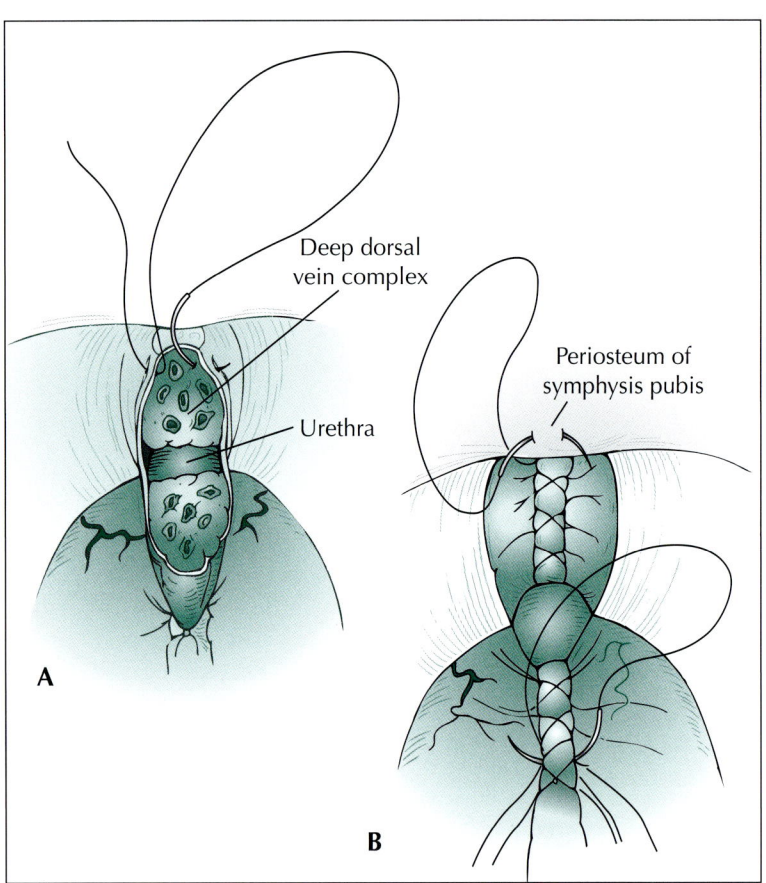

Deep dorsal
vein complex

Urethra

Periosteum of
symphysis pubis

A

B

▶ **FIGURE 11-12.** Control of bleeding from the transected dorsal vascular complex. Bleeding from the transected dorsal vascular complex is controlled by oversewing the cut edges of the lateral pelvic fascia vertically with a continuous suture (**A**), the last pass of which is brought through the periosteum of the pubis (**B**) to compress the superficial venous complex above the lateral pelvic fascia and to fix the fascia to the periosteum, simulating the function of the puboprostatic ligaments. Back bleeding from the ventral prostate is controlled with a continuous hemostatic suture. This suture is stopped short of the apex of the prostate, taking care not to draw the neurovascular bundles medially (**B**). With appropriate hemostasis, the surgeon should have a bloodless field to initiate the preservation of the neurovascular bundles.

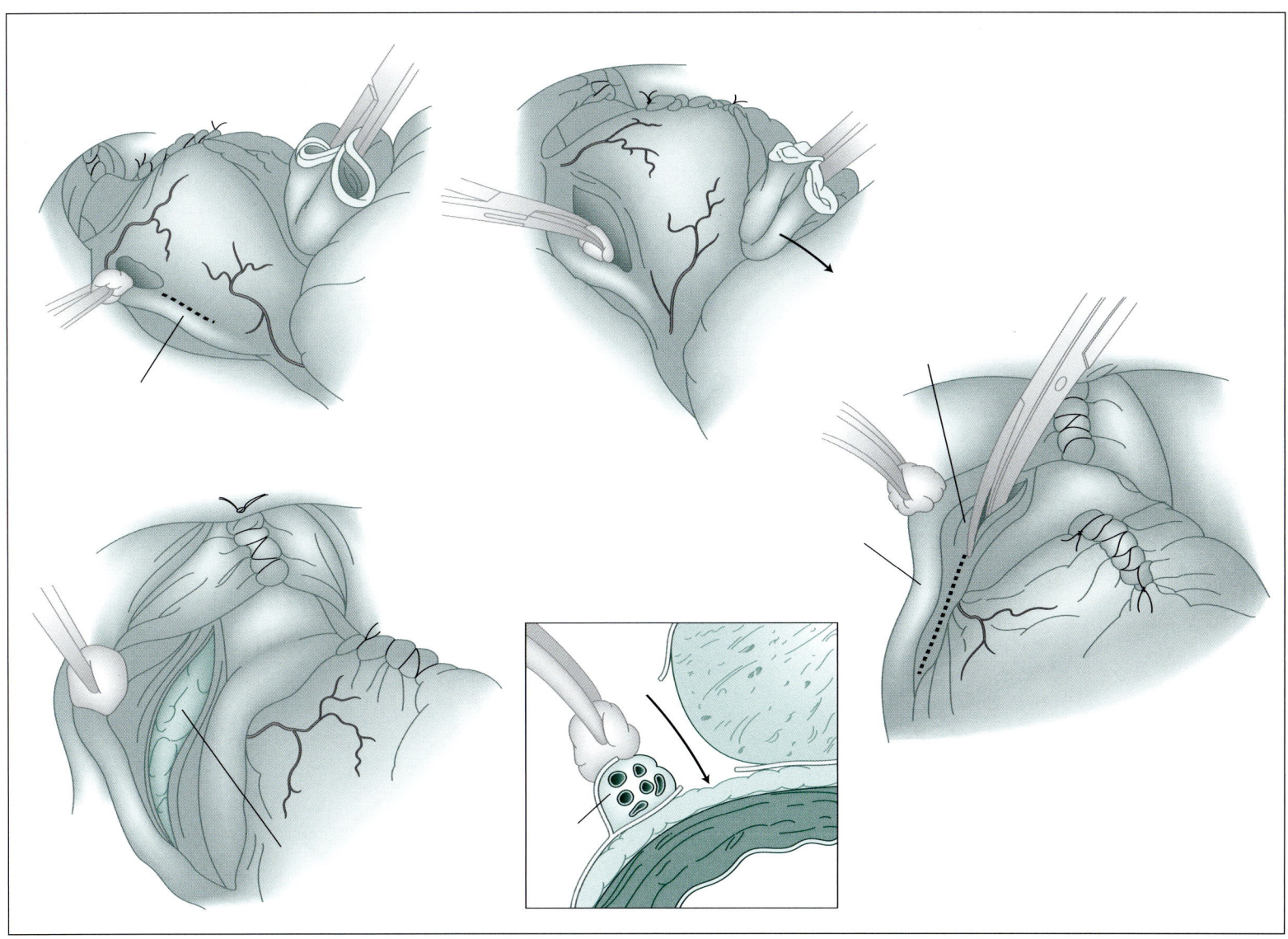

▶ **FIGURE 11-13.** Preservation of the left neurovascular bundle (NVB). After the dorsal vein complex has been divided and hemostasis attained, the prostate is rotated to the right with a sponge stick and any remaining levator ani muscle fibers are bluntly dissected away. The surgeon can examine the course of the NVB in relation to the prostate and any palpable tumor. Frequently, a shallow groove defines the superior margin of dissection for the preservation of the NVB. A plane of division of the lateral prostatic fascia is then chosen to assure a negative surgical margin while preserving as much of the NVB as possible. Once the plane of dissection has been selected, the lateral prostatic fascia is sharply incised in the groove between the prostate and the NVB. The NVB is most easily dissected away from the apical third of the prostate (**A and B**). The small branches of the vascular pedicle to the apex are clipped and divided. Care must be taken to avoid electrocautery near this neural tissue. The NVB is then gently dissected and displaced laterally, working from the apex toward the base. This should be done with a Kitner (peanut) dissector and/or a right-angled clamp. Finger dissection should be avoided on the NVB. Denonvilliers' fascia is then incised in the angle between the NVB and urethra at the apex of the prostate, releasing the NVB from the prostate and urethra (**C–E**). The appearance of perirectal fat will assure the surgeon that the layer has been incised completely. The plane of dissection is then developed sharply and/or bluntly. Special attention is paid to continuing the dissection of the NVB for a distance of almost 1 cm from the prostatourethral junction so that the nerves will not be tethered when the urethral anastomotic sutures are tied.

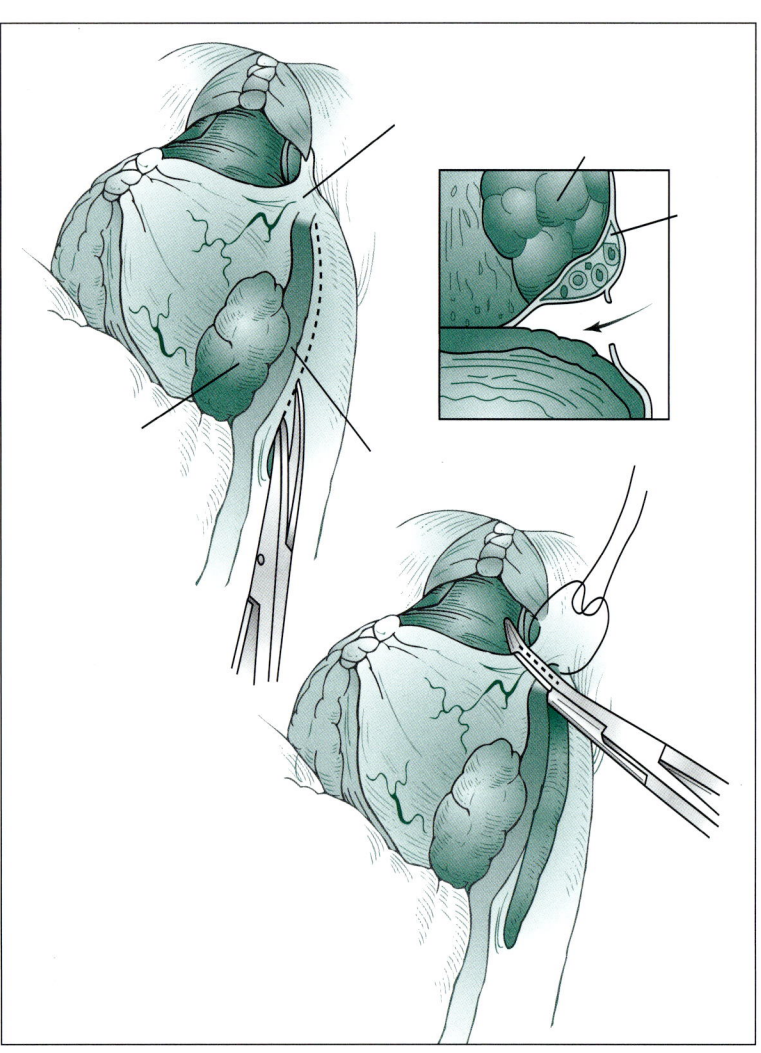

▶ **FIGURE 11-14.** Resection of the neurovascular bundle (NVB). If the cancer lies close to the NVB, all or part of the bundle should be resected to assure complete removal of the cancer. A plane of dissection is chosen laterally. If the entire bundle is to be resected, dissection begins over the lateral rectal wall in the fat beneath the NVB (**A and B**). The incision is extended distally, and the NVB is secured with clips or ties and divided distal to the apex of the prostate (**C**).

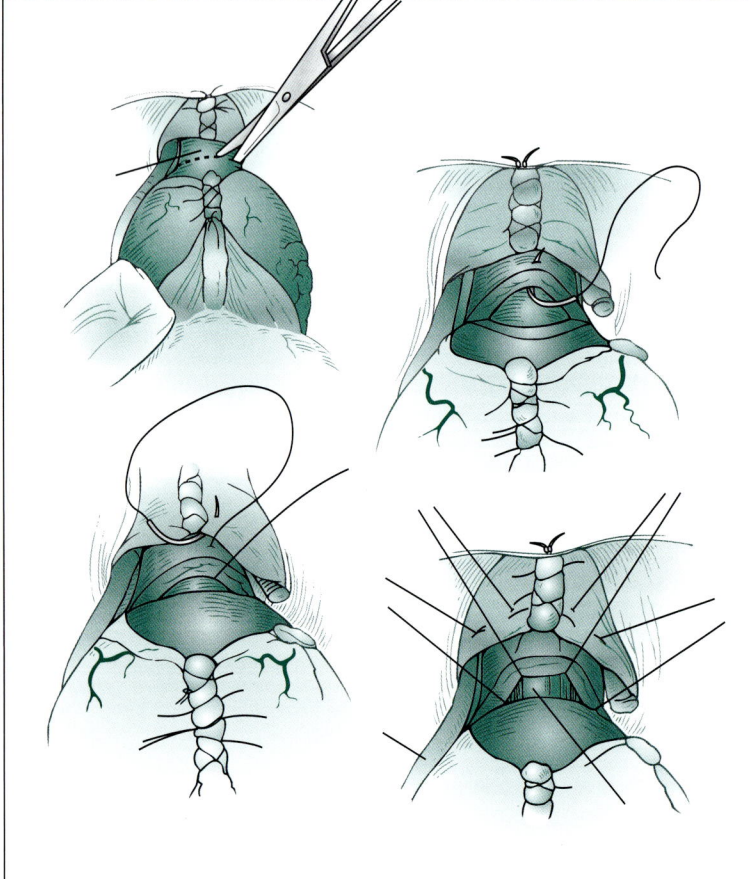

▶ **FIGURE 11-15.** Division of the anterolateral urethra and placement of the anterior anastomotic sutures. Close-up views of urethra at the prostatic apex, illustrating the site of anterior division. The urethra is divided 2 to 3 mm from the apex of the prostate (**A**), and four 2-0 Monocryl sutures are placed at regular intervals around the urethra (usually at 9, 11, 1, and 3 o'clock). Each suture includes the mucosa of the urethra (**B**) and then separately through the thick layer of lateral pelvic fascia (**C and D**) that was oversewn to control the dorsal vein complex. The catheter that was placed at the start of the procedure is withdrawn to expose the entire urethra. Care is taken to ensure that any posterior apical prostatic tissue is fully resected with the specimen by careful blunt dissection with a Kitner (peanut) dissector. NVB—neurovascular bundle.

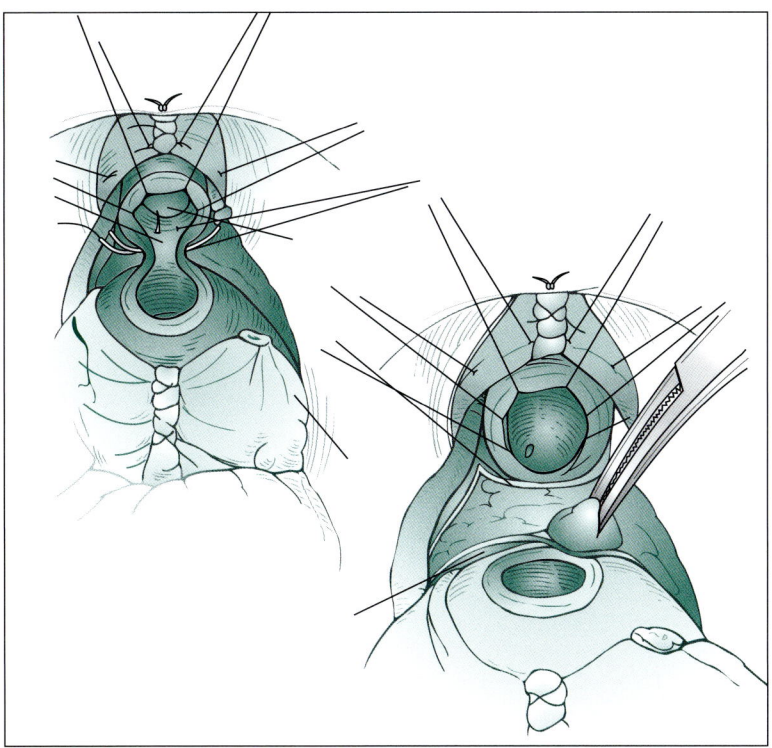

▶ **FIGURE 11-16.** Completion of the urethral division. Two posterior anastomotic sutures are placed at the 5 and 7 o'clock positions (**A**). After the surgeon ensures that the nerves have been dissected free (or divided), the remaining posterior urethra is divided. The previously made incisions in Denonvilliers' fascia are connected across the midline beneath the divided urethra (**B**). Sharp and blunt dissection is used to elevate the apex of the prostate together with Denonvilliers' fascia off the anterior rectal wall. The yellowish perirectal fat must be identified to assure the proper plane of dissection and to reduce the risk of a positive surgical margin. NVB—neurovascular bundle.

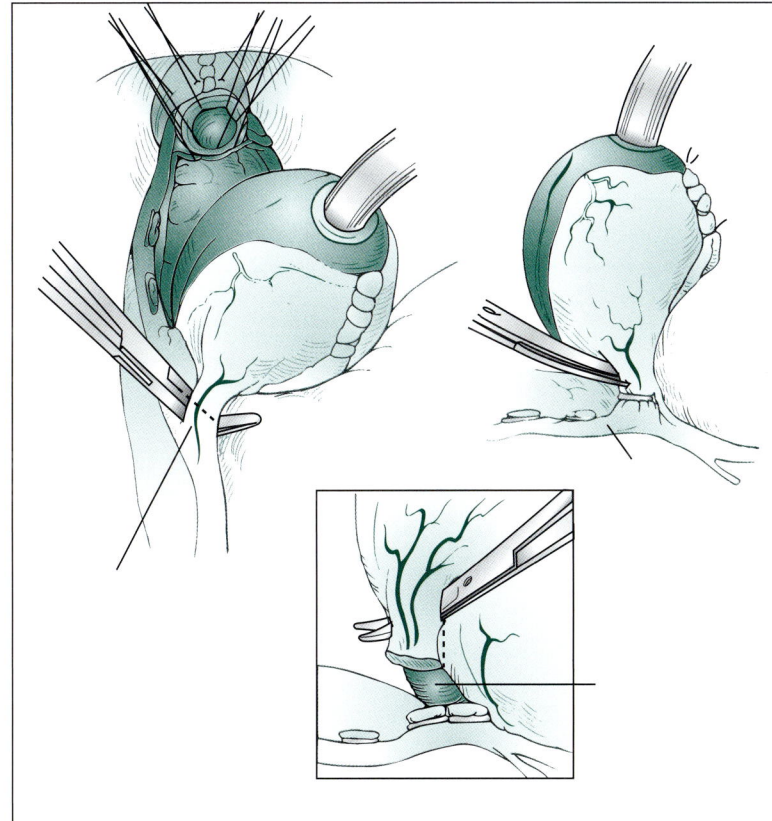

▶ **FIGURE 11-17.** Further mobilization of the prostate. A new catheter is placed through the prostate into the bladder to allow easier manipulation of the prostate, which is mobilized in a side-to-side fashion (**A**). Tension on the catheter should be avoided until the neurovascular bundles (NVB) have been completely released from the lateral aspect of the prostate. Small vessels between the NVB and prostate are controlled with small hemoclips placed parallel to the NVB. The lateral vascular pedicles of the prostate are identified and isolated with a right-angled clamp, working in an up-and-down motion to separate tissue appropriate for clip ligation (**B**) and division (**C**). This exposes the lateral aspect of the seminal vesicle. Further exposure is gained by division of the vascular bands between the bladder neck and the seminal vesicles and prostate (**C**). The surgeon needs to remain cognizant of the location of the NVB during this dissection because the NVB may be tented up and in the field of dissection secondary to ventral retraction of the prostate. In the posterior midline, Denonvilliers' fascia is divided transversely over the seminal vesicles.

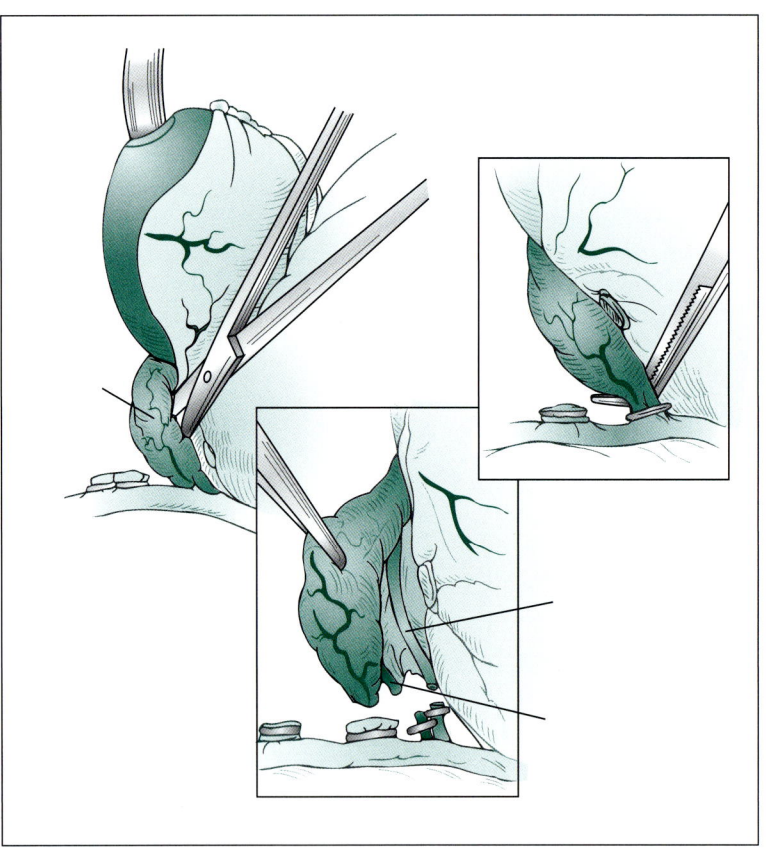

▶ **FIGURE 11-18.** Approach to the seminal vesicles. The seminal vesicles are typically approached laterally, and the plane between the seminal vesicles and the bladder is developed with scissors and finger dissection (**A**). The major vascular supply to the seminal vesicles lies anterior and lateral. When these vessels are clipped and divided close to the wall of the vesicle, it is easier to identify the large artery that enters at the apex of the seminal vesicle (**B**). The ampullae of the vas are clipped to include the vasal arteries and divided (**C**). The rectovesical fascia should be left covering the seminal vesicles.

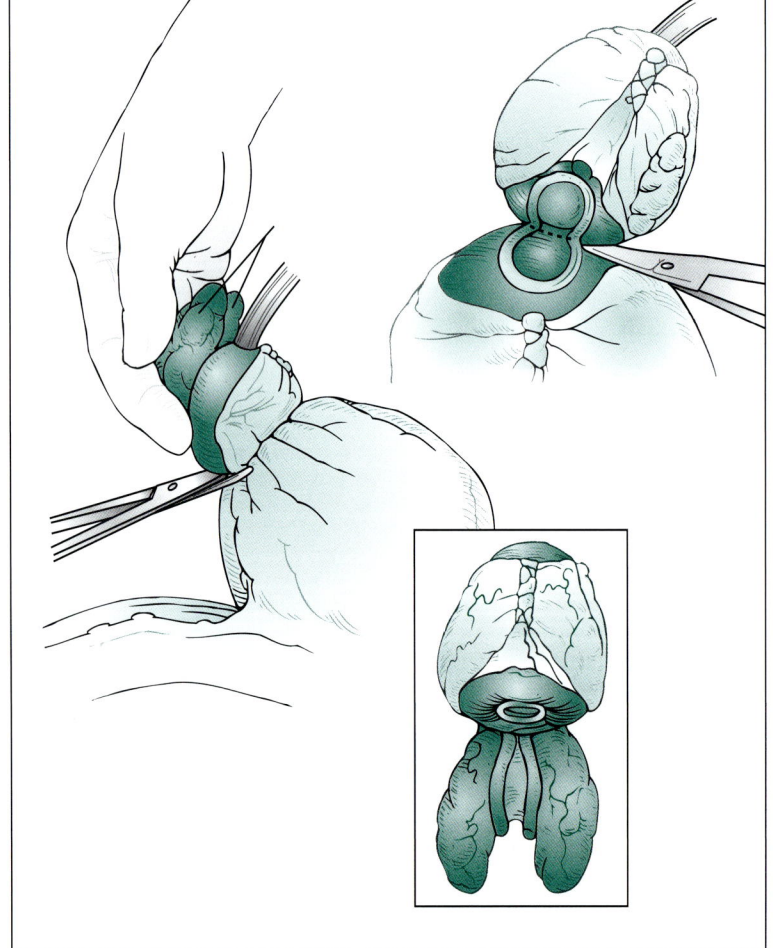

▶ **FIGURE 11-19.** Division of the bladder neck. The seminal vesicles and vasa are dissected off the posterior wall of the bladder (**A**). The bladder neck is divided anteriorly (**B**), and the Foley catheter balloon is withdrawn through this incision. No attempt is made to spare the bladder neck. Small vessels are controlled with the electrocautery. The ureteral orifices are identified prior to division of the posterior bladder neck. The resected specimen (**C**) is closely palpated and examined to determine the completeness of resection. Any margin suspicious for cancer may be tagged with a suture and the entire specimen sent to pathology for frozen section evaluation.

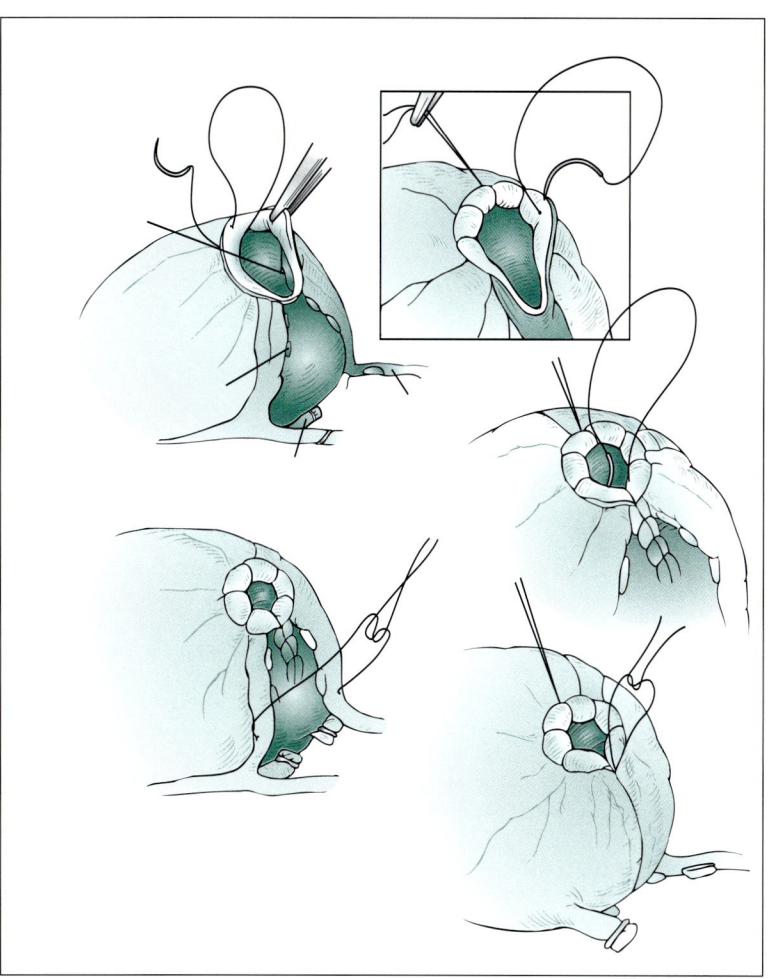

▶ **FIGURE 11-20.** Preparation of the bladder neck for anastomosis. The anterior bladder neck is reconstructed by fully everting the mucosa antero-laterally (**A and B**) with interrupted 4-0 Vicryl sutures. The posterior bladder neck is closed in a "tennis-racket" fashion with a continuous 2-0 Vicryl suture beginning at 6 o'clock and ending with a stitch that fully everts the bladder mucosa (**C**), providing an opening 24F to 30F in diameter. The suture closest to the trigone should include muscle but little mucosa to avoid tethering the ureteral orifices. In a separate layer, the lateral vascular pedicles of the bladder may be brought together in the midline to reinforce the closure and assure hemostasis (**D and E**).

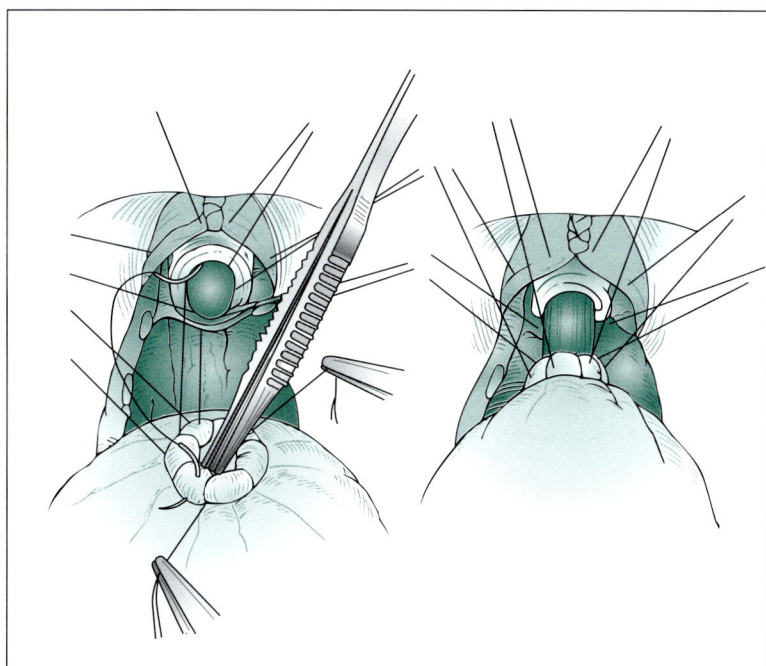

▶ **FIGURE 11-21.** The vesicourethral anastomosis. The anastomotic sutures previously placed through the urethra are now placed through their corresponding position in the bladder neck (**A**) to provide a mucosa-to-mucosa anastomosis (**B**). The sutures should be placed so that the knots are tied on the outside. The urethral catheter is placed into the bladder and the balloon inflated with 15 mL of sterile water. The operating table is taken out of the flex position to facilitate the advancement of the recon-structed bladder neck to the urethra. Two sponge sticks, one on each side of the Foley balloon, may facilitate apposition of the bladder neck and urethra. As the sutures are tied, care is taken to exclude the preserved neurovascular bundle by gentle downward displacement on it with a sponge stick.

The catheter is irrigated to provide a clear return and test the anasto-mosis for leakage. The catheter is secured to the patient's thigh without traction. Closed suction drains are placed in each obturator fossa. These are typically removed prior to discharge on the second postoperative day. Patients return to the office for catheter removal, without a prior cystogram, 10 to 14 days after the operation.

SUMMARY

Radical retropubic prostatectomy reliably eradicates the cancer in appropriately selected men with clinically localized prostate cancer. Although technically complex, this operation can generally be performed with a low level of acute and long-term morbidity, but the results are highly sensitive to fine details in surgical technique. Rates of blood loss, positive surgical margins, incontinence, and erectile dysfunction vary widely from surgeon to surgeon. With careful attention to surgical technique, cancer control rates should improve further, and the effect of the operation on quality of life should continue to decrease.

REFERENCES

1. Gibbons RP, Correa RJ Jr, Brannen GE, Weissman RM: Total prostatectomy for clinically localized prostate cancer: long-term results. *J Urol* 1989, 141: 564–566.

2. Zincke H, Oesterling JE, Blute ML, *et al.*: Long-term (15 years) results after radical prostatectomy for clinically localized (stage T2c or lower) prostate cancer. *J Urol* 1994, 152:1850–1857.

3. Han M, Partin AW, Zahurak M, *et al.*: Biochemical (prostate specific antigen) recurrence probability following radical prostatectomy for clinically localized prostate cancer. *J Urol* 2003, 169:517–523.

4. Bianco FJ, Dotan ZA, Kattan MW, *et al.*: 15-year cancer-specific and PSA-progression free rates after radical prostatectomy [abstract]. *J Urol* 2004, 171:313.

5. Trapasso JG, deKernion JB, Smith RB, Dorey F: The incidence and significance of detectable levels of serum prostate specific antigen after radical prostatectomy. *J Urol* 1994, 152:1821–1825.

6. Catalona WJ, Smith DS. Cancer recurrence and survival rates after anatomical radical retropubic prostatectomy for prostate cancer: intermediate results. *J Urol* 1998, 160:2428–2434.

7. Albertsen PC, Hanley JA, Gleason DF, Barry MJ: Competing risk analysis of men aged 55 to 74 years at diagnosis managed conservatively for clinically localized prostate cancer. *JAMA* 1998, 280:975–980.

8. Kundu SD, Roehl KA, Eggener SE, *et al.*: Potency, continence and complications in 3,477 consecutive radical prostatectomies. *J Urol* 2004, 172:2227–2231.

9. Eastham JA, Kattan MW, Rogers E, *et al.*: Risk factors for urinary incontinence after radical prostatectomy. *J Urol* 1996, 156:1707–1713.

10. Noh C, Kshirsagar A, Mohler JL: Outcomes after radical retropubic prostatectomy. *Urology* 2003, 61:412–416.

11. Walsh PC: Technique of vesicourethral anastomosis may influence recovery of sexual function following radical prostatectomy. *Urol Clin North Am* 1994, 2:59–65.

12. Rabbani F, Stapleton AM, Kattan MW, *et al.*: Factors predicting recovery of erections after radical prostatectomy. *J Urol* 2000, 164:1929–1934.

13. Goad JR, Scardino PT: Modifications in the technique of radical retropubic prostatectomy to minimize blood loss. *Urol Clin North Am* 1994, 20:65–74.

14. Maffezzini M, Seveso M, Taverna G, *et al.*: Evaluation of complications and results in a contemporary series of 300 consecutive radical retropubic prostatectomies with the anatomic approach at a single institution. *Urology* 2003, 61:982–986.

15. Lepor H, Nieder AM, Ferrandino MN: Intraoperative and postoperative complications of radical retropubic prostatectomy in a consecutive series of 1000 cases. *J Urol* 2001, 166:1729–1733.

16. Smith JA, Bray WL, Koch MO: Cost efficient management of the patient with localized prostate cancer. *AUA Update Series* 1997;16:122.

17. Leibman BD, Dillioglugil O, Abbas F, *et al.*: Impact of a clinical pathway for radical retropubic prostatectomy. *Urology* 1998, 52:94–99.

18. Eastham JA, Kattan MW, Riedel E, *et al.*: Variations among individual surgeons in the rate of positive surgical margins in radical prostatectomy specimens. *J Urol* 2003, 170:2292–2295.

19. Han M, Partin AW, Chan DY, Walsh PC: An evaluation of the decreasing incidence of positive surgical margins in a large retropubic prostatectomy series. *J Urol* 2004, 171:23–26.

20. Klein EA, Kupelian PA, Tuason L, Levin HS: Initial dissection of the lateral fascia reduces the positive margin rate in radical prostatectomy. *Urology* 1998, 51:766–773.

21. Wieder JA, Soloway MS: Incidence, etiology, location, prevention and treatment of positive surgical margins after radical prostatectomy for prostate cancer. *J Urol* 1998, 160:299–315.

22. Kattan MW, Eastham JA, Stapleton AMF, *et al.*: A preoperative nomogram for disease recurrence following radical prostatectomy for prostate cancer. *J Natl Cancer Inst* 1998, 90:766–771.

23. Albertsen PC, Hanley JA, Harlan LC, *et al.*: The positive yield of imaging studies in the evaluation of men with newly diagnosed prostate cancer: a population based analysis. *J Urol* 2000, 163:1138–1143.

24. Epstein JI, Walsh PC, Brendler CB: Radical prostatectomy for impalpable prostate cancer: the Johns Hopkins experience with tumors found on transurethral resection (stages T1A and T1B) and on needle biopsy (stage T1C). *J Urol* 1994, 152(Pt 2):1721–1729.

25. Canto EI, Slawin KM: Early management of prostate cancer: how to respond to an elevated PSA? *Annu Rev Med* 2002, 53:355–368.

26. Goto Y, Ohori M, Arakawa A, *et al.*: Distinguishing clinically important from unimportant prostate cancers before treatment: value of systematic biopsies. *J Urol* 1996, 156:1059–1063.

27. Bastacky SI, Walsh PC, Epstein JI: Relationship between perineural tumor invasion on needle biopsy and radical prostatectomy capsular penetration in clinical stage B adenocarcinoma of the prostate. *Am J Surg Pathol* 1993, 17:336–341.

28. Cagiannos I, Karakiewicz P, Eastham JA, *et al.*: A pre-operative nomogram identifying prostate cancer patients with decreased risk of positive pelvic lymph nodes. *J Urol* 2003, 170:1798–1803.

29. Rainwater LM, Segura JW: Technical consideration in radical retropubic prostatectomy: blood loss after ligation of dorsal venous complex. *J Urol* 1990, 143:1163–1165.

30. Eastham JA, Scardino PT, Yawn DH, *et al.*: Preoperative autologous blood donation in radical retropubic prostatectomy: a cost-effectiveness analysis. *Int J Technol Management* 2001, 3:322–326.

31. Coakley FV, Eberhardt S, Wei DC, *et al.*: Blood loss during radical retropubic prostatectomy: relationship to morphologic features on preoperative endorectal magnetic resonance imaging. *Urology* 2002, 59:884–888.

32. Goldschlag B, Afzal N, Carter HB, Fleisher LA: Is preoperative donation of autologous blood rational for radical retropubic prostatectomy? *J Urol* 2000, 164:1968–1972.

33. Lepor H, Nieder AM, Ferrandino MN: Intraoperative and postoperative complications of radical retropubic prostatectomy in a consecutive series of 1000 cases. *J Urol* 2001, 166:1729–1733.

34. Maffezzini M, Seveso M, Taverna G, *et al.*: Evaluation of complications and results in a contemporary series of 300 consecutive radical retropubic prostatectomies with the anatomic approach at a single institution. *Urology* 2003, 61:982–986.

35. Augustin H, Hammerer P, Graefen M, *et al.*: Intraoperative and perioperative morbidity of contemporary radical retropubic prostatectomy in a consecutive series of 1243 patients: results of a single center between 1999 and 2002. *Eur Urol* 2003, 43(2):113–118.

36. Catalona WJ, Carvalhal GF, Mager DE, Smith DS: Potency, continence and complication rates in 1870 consecutive radical retropubic prostatectomies. *J Urol* 1999, 162:433–438.

37. Lerner SE, Blute ML, Lieber MM, Zincke H: Morbidity of contemporary radical retropubic prostatectomy for localized prostate cancer. *Oncology* 1995, 9:379–382.

38. Cisek LJ, Walsh PC: Thromboembolic complications following radical retropubic prostatectomy. *Urology* 1993, 42:406–408.

39. Steiner MS, Morton RA, Walsh PC: Impact of anatomical radical prostatectomy on urinary continence. *J Urol* 1991, 145:512–514.

40. Geary ES, Dendinger TE, Freiha FS, Stamey TA: Incontinence and vesical neck strictures following radical retropubic prostatectomy. *Urology* 1995, 45:1000–1006.

41. Litwin MS, Hays RD, Fink A, *et al.*: Quality-of-life outcomes in men treated for localized prostate cancer. *JAMA* 1995, 273:129–135.

42. Murphy GP, Mettlin C, Menck H, *et al.*: National patterns of prostate cancer treatment by radical prostatectomy: results of a survey by the American College of Surgeons Committee on Cancer. *J Urol* 1994, 152:1817–1819.

43. Walsh PC, Marschke P, Ricker D, Burnett AL: Patient-reported urinary continence and sexual function after anatomic radical prostatectomy. *Urology* 2000, 55:58–61.

44. Sebesta M, Cespedes RD, Luhman E, *et al.*: Questionnaire-based outcomes of urinary incontinence and satisfaction rates after radical prostatectomy in a national study population. *Urology* 2002, 60:1055–1058.

45. Stanford JL, Feng Z, Hamilton AS, *et al.*: Urinary and sexual function after radical prostatectomy for clinically localized prostate cancer: The Prostate Cancer Outcomes Study. *JAMA* 2000, 283:354–360.

46. Fowler FJ Jr, Barry MJ, Lu-Yao G, *et al.*: Patient-reported complications and follow-up treatment after radical prostatectomy. The national Medicare experience: 1988–1990 (updated June 1993). *Urology* 1993, 42:622–629.

47. Quinlan DM, Epstein JI, Carter BS, Walsh PC: Sexual function following radical prostatectomy: influence of preservation of neurovascular bundles. *J Urol* 1991, 145:998–1002.

Laparoscopic Radical Prostatectomy

12

Karim Touijer
& Bertrand D. Guillonneau

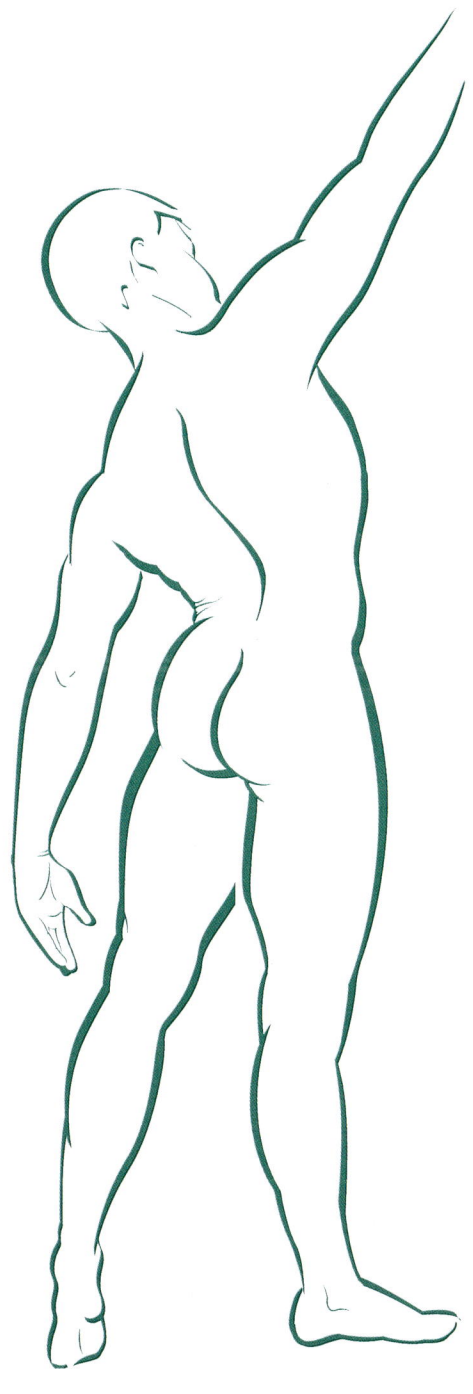

The integration of the laparoscopic approach into the surgical armamentarium has become a common practice in treating many urologic cancers. Its application to the treatment of clinically localized prostate cancer has gained increasing importance in the urologic oncology field. Although it is now safe, feasible, reproducible, and teachable, it remains technically challenging, and like that of any treatment for prostate cancer today, its success is tied to the accomplishment of a complete excision of the cancer with a preservation of quality of life to the greatest extent possible. Only then do a reduced morbidity and shorter convalescence become distinct advantages of the laparoscopic approach.

This chapter illustrates our technique of antegrade transperitoneal laparoscopic radical prostatectomy as currently performed at Memorial Sloan-Kettering Cancer Center and provides an overview of the oncologic and functional results.

There are no specific contraindications to the laparoscopic approach. However, certain conditions, such as extensive prior pelvic surgery, prior prostate surgery, pelvic radiation therapy, or morbid obesity, can raise the difficulty level of the procedure.

Preoperatively, patients receive an enema. Thromboprophylaxis is ensured with sequential compressive devices on both lower extremities and low molecular weight heparin, administered prior to surgery then daily afterward until discharge from the hospital. Thromboprophylaxis is essential given the presence of three risk factors: cancer surgery, pelvic surgery, and laparoscopy. Patients also receive antibiotic prophylaxis with a single preoperative dose of intravenous second-generation cephalosporin.

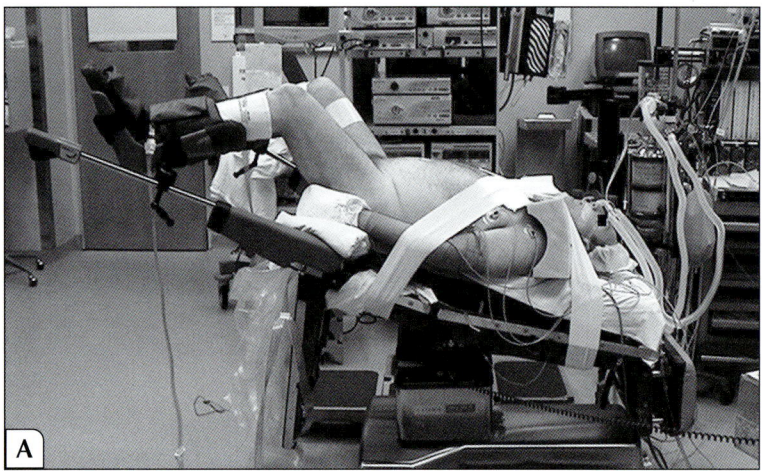

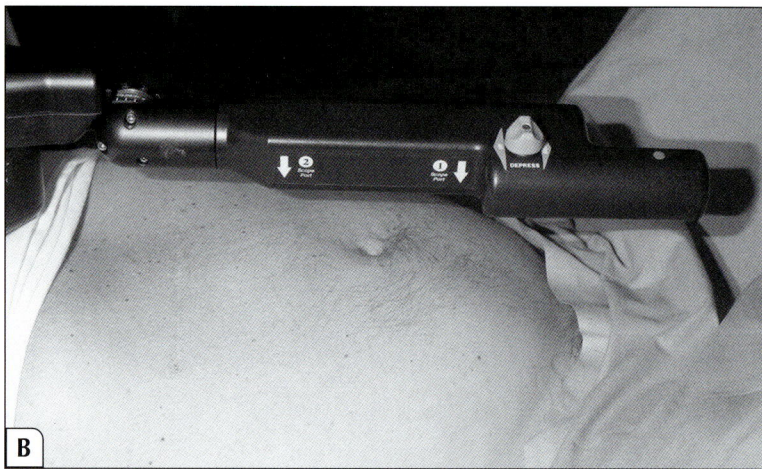

▶ **FIGURE 12-1.** Patient positioning. The operation is performed under general anesthesia. **A,** The patient is positioned in a low lithotomy position with both arms set along the body to avoid brachial plexus injuries. The shoulders are adequately padded, and the patient is secured to the operating table with surgical tape. We use a voice-controlled robotic camera holder, Automated Endoscopic System for Optimal Positioning (AESOP) 3000 (Computer Motion, Inc., Santa Barbara, CA). With both hands free, the assistant can concentrate and actively participate with total involvement in all the steps of the operation. **B,** The AESOP 3000 is mounted on the operating table, with the umbilicus placed between the two white arrows on the "forearm" of the robotic arm. This placement allows the robotic arm to easily reach the umbilicus. The patient and the AESOP are draped in a sterile fashion. A right-handed surgeon stands on the patient's left, with the assistant and the AESOP on the opposite side; the monitor is placed between the patient's legs, at the surgeon's eye level and as close as necessary.

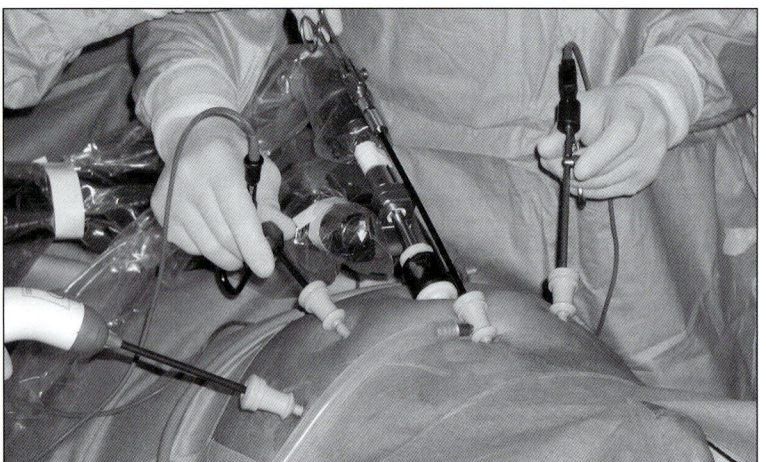

▶ **FIGURE 12-2.** Surgical ports placement. After a vertical and radial umbilical incision, a Veress needle is introduced into the peritoneal cavity and insufflation is started without exceeding a pressure of 12 mm Hg. A 10-mm trocar is inserted through the umbilicus for passage of the 0° laparoscope. The scope is mounted on the AESOP 3000 voice-controlled robotic camera holder (Computer Motion, Inc., Santa Barbara, CA). Four 5-mm working ports are inserted: one in the left iliac fossa, one in the right iliac fossa, one at McBurney's point, and one halfway between the umbilicus and the pubic symphysis. The patient is then placed in a steep Trendelenburg position, with careful attention paid to the patient's nose and the endotracheal tube as the lower limit of the AESOP is set. During the prostatectomy part of the operation, the surgeon uses the laparoscopic scissors and the bipolar cautery forceps; the assistant uses the laparoscopic suction device and the graspers.

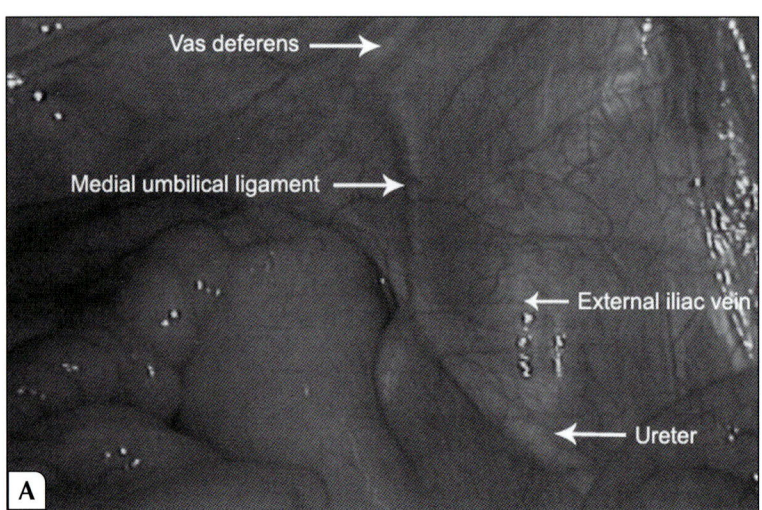

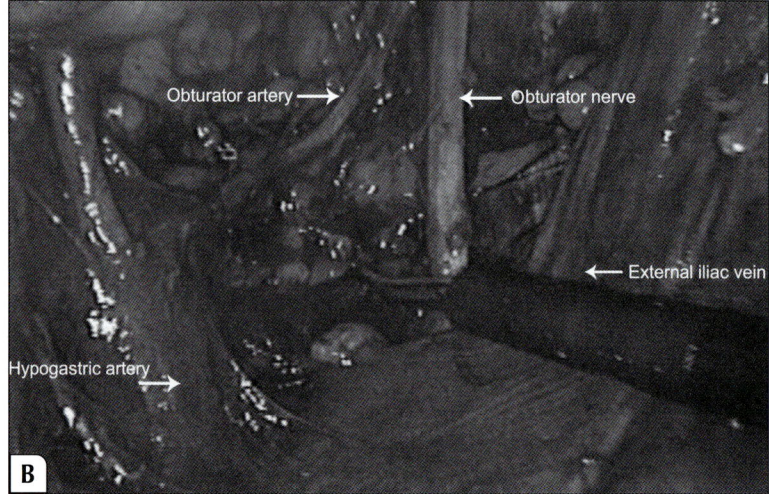

▶ **FIGURE 12-3.** Pelvic lymph node dissection. **A and B,** Bilateral pelvic lymph node dissection is performed. The peritoneum over the medial umbilical ligament is opened and all the lymphatic and fatty tissue lateral to the medial umbilical ligament, medial to the lateral pelvic side wall, distal to the iliac vessels bifurcation, proximal to Cooper's ligament, inferior to the external iliac vein, and superior to the hypogastric artery is removed.

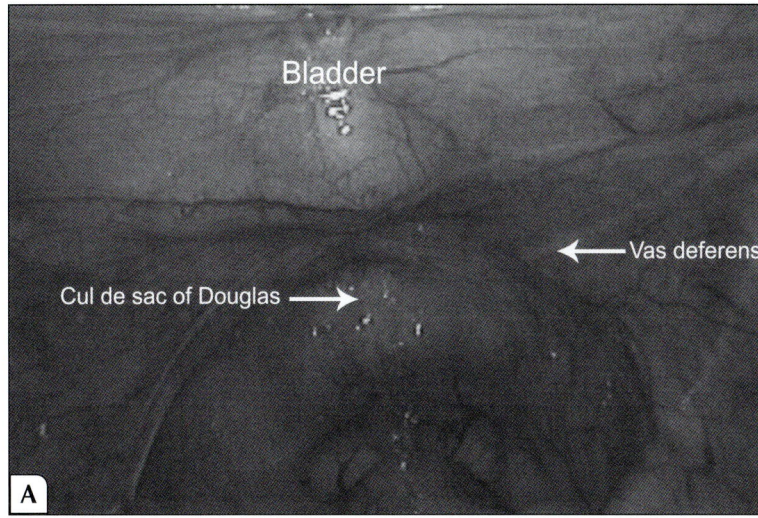

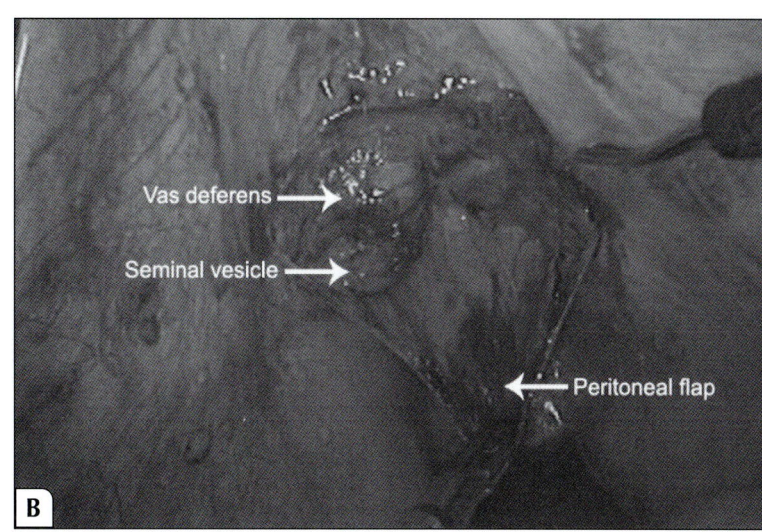

▶ **FIGURE 12-4.** Incising the cul-de-sac of Douglas. **A,** The sigmoid colon is held gently by the assistant, retracting the rectum cephalad. **B,** The surgeon incises the posterior vesical peritoneum transversally approximately 1 to 2 cm above the level of the cul-de-sac of Douglas. The dissection should then follow the inferior peritoneal flap. After coagulation of few subperitoneal vessels, the dissection enters into an avascular plane that should be developed. This exposes Denonvilliers' fascia. This step may be omitted if the patient's body habitus does not allow easy access to the cul-de-sac of Douglas; the seminal vesicles are then dissected at the time of bladder neck division.

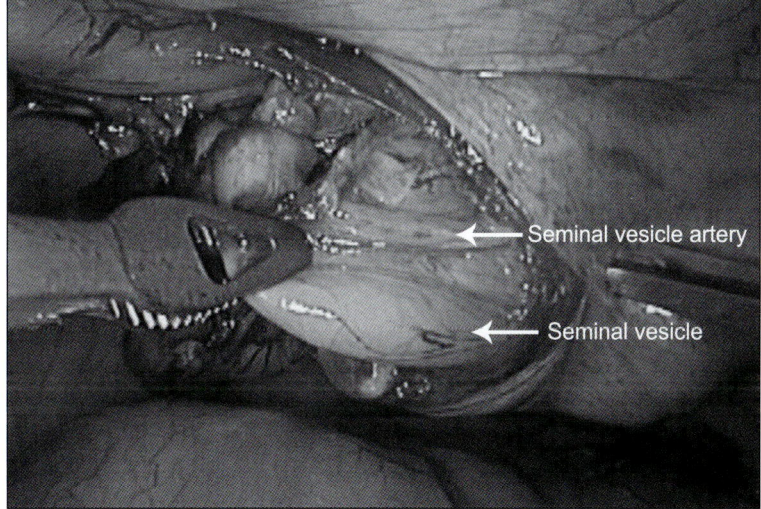

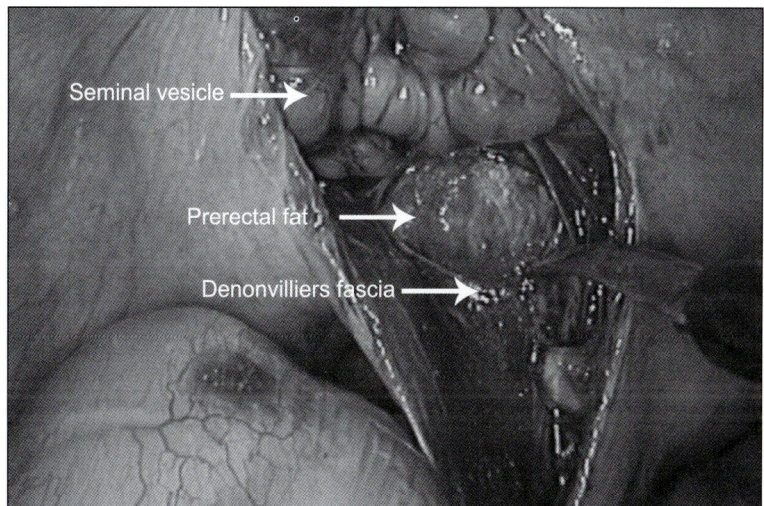

▶ **FIGURE 12-5.** Freeing the seminal vesicles. Once the peritoneum is opened, the outlines of the seminal vesicles and vasa deferentia are clearly visible. The vasa deferentia are dissected and coagulated with bipolar forceps then transected. One must be aware of and carefully coagulate the deferential artery running along the opposite side. Division of the vasa deferentia allows access to the seminal vesicles. The latter should be dissected along its surface to individualize its two vascular pedicles, one at the tip and the other at the base. These arteries are meticulously coagulated, with the bipolar forceps facing the seminal vesicles to avoid any thermal injury to the neural plexus in close proximity. The seminal vesicles are then completely mobilized, with the prostate as their sole attachment.

▶ **FIGURE 12-6.** Opening Denonvilliers' fascia. Incision of Denonvilliers' fascia allows an easier and safer dissection later in the operation by separating the rectum away from the prostatic pedicles. To facilitate the exposure, the assistant pulls the vasa deferentia upward and places Denonvilliers' fascia on tension. It will appear to have longitudinal striations under the magnification of the laparoscope. Denonvilliers' fascia is then incised medially and horizontally, bringing into view the prerectal fatty tissue. Further dissection toward the prostatic apex or laterally is not advised at this time.

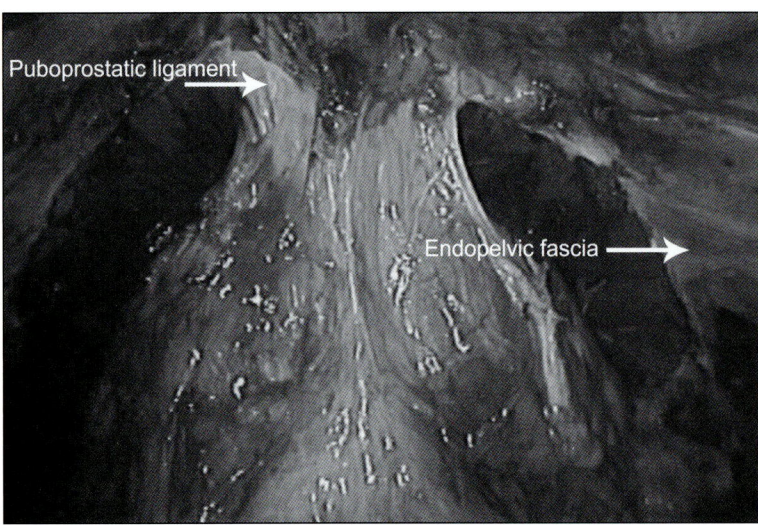

▶ **FIGURE 12-7.** Entering Retzius' space and exposing the endopelvic fascia. The bladder is filled with approximately 120 mL of saline to help identify the contours and pull it posteriorly. The anterior parietal peritoneum is incised from one umbilical ligament to the other. It is useless to divide the medial umbilical ligaments, but when a lymph node dissection has been previously performed, it is easier to follow the pubic bone that is already exposed to enter Retzius' space and then to transect the umbilical ligaments as high as necessary. Otherwise, by staying close to the medial aspect of the medial umbilical ligaments and heading laterally and caudally from there, the pubic arches are encountered. This dissection allows the clear identification of the urachus that is divided last, thus minimizing the risk of injury to the bladder. It is essential to free the bladder well from its anterior and lateral attachments in order to create a large working space and to allow a tension-free vesicourethral anastomosis at the end of the

operation. Once the bladder is freed anteriorly and laterally, it is then emptied with a syringe; because the patient is in Trendelenburg position, gravity drainage is never complete.

The fat over the fascia covering the prostate must be swept up laterally in order to expose clearly the intrapelvic fascia and the puboprostatic ligaments. The superficial dorsal vein is easily identified and coagulated with bipolar forceps. The endopelvic fascia is identified lateral to the prostate and incised on its line of reflection, uncovering the levator ani muscle fibers. Incision of the puboprostatic ligaments is done under visual control away from Santorini's venous plexus. The incision can be prolonged toward the fascia that covers the dorsal venous complex laterally. Although delicate, this step will delineate the anatomy and facilitate further dissection and exposure of the dorsal venous complex and the urethra later during the operation.

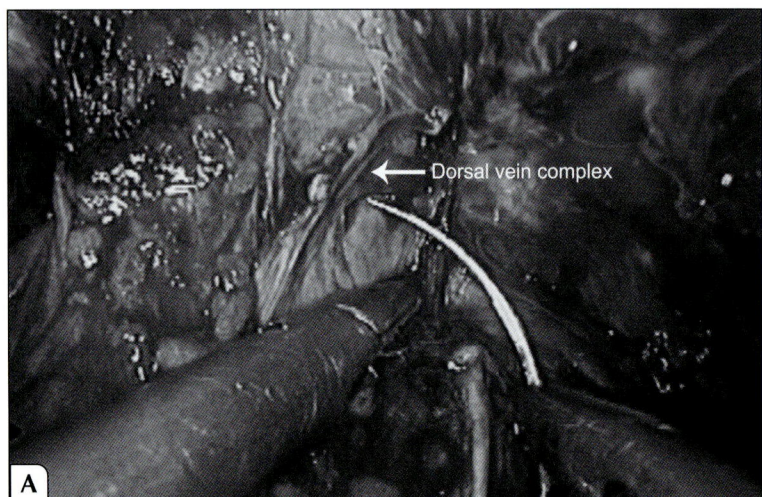

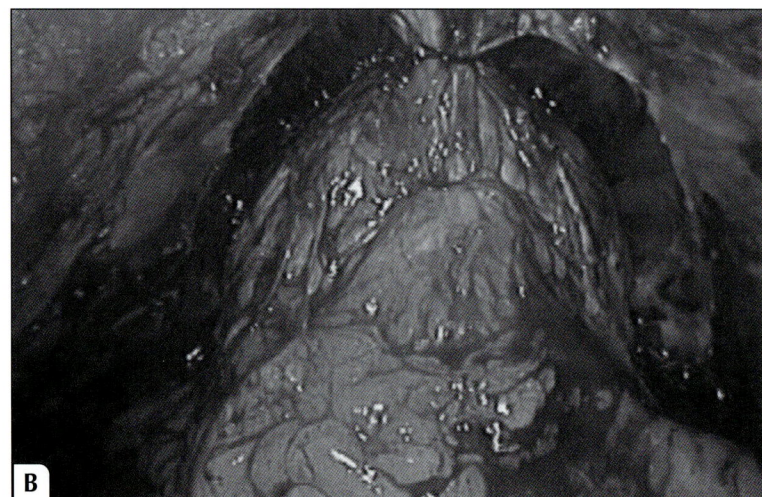

▶ **FIGURE 12-8.** Ligating the dorsal venous complex. **A,** The dorsal venous complex is ligated with a 2-0 resorbable suture on an SH needle passing underneath the venous plexus from one side to the other. For a right-handed surgeon, the needle is passed from the right side of the plexus to the left side, such that the curve of the needle follows the curve of the pubic symphysis. Transsection of the complex is unnecessary and will be done later, to avoid useless bleeding. **B,** A back-bleeding stitch ligating the preprostatic venous plexus is placed.

THIRD STEP: BLADDER NECK DISSECTION

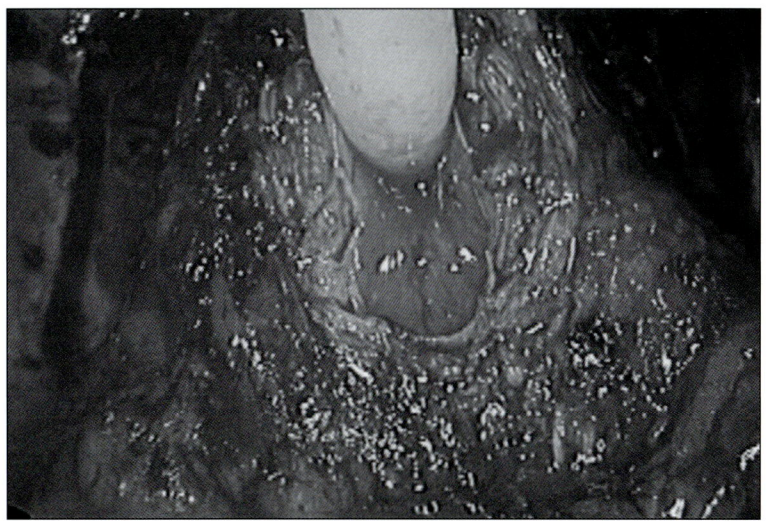

▶ **FIGURE 12-9.** Bladder neck dissection. The anatomic landmarks of this step are not as well defined. To identify the bladder neck area, the anterior preprostatic fat must be retracted cephalad, creating a faint outline of the anterior vesicoprostatic junction. The place where the bladder neck should be dissected is exactly where the fat becomes adherent. This step requires careful hemostasis anteriorly. The bladder neck is incised transversally, and the tip of the catheter is pulled up by a grasper via the suprapubic port to expose the posterior aspect of the bladder neck, allowing the surgeon to grasp the posterior bladder neck and separate the bladder from the prostate and reach the longitudinal muscular fibers between the prostate base and the bladder neck. This layer should be incised in order to gain access to the previously dissected retrovesical space. The vasa deferentia and the seminal vesicles are then simply brought into the operating field by the assistant. This maneuver exposes on both sides the lateral prostatic pedicles.

FOURTH STEP: LATERAL DISSECTION OF THE PROSTATE

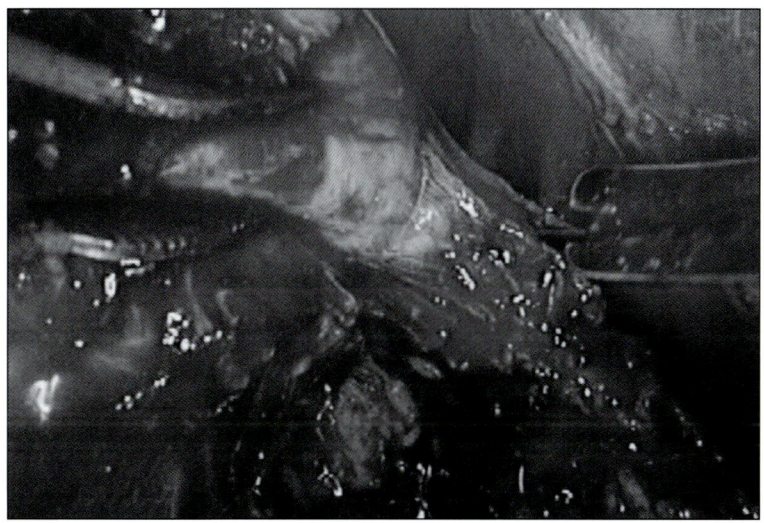

▶ **FIGURE 12-10.** (*See Color Plate*) Preserving the neurovascular bundles: interfascial technique. The assistant grasps the vas and the seminal vesicle and pulls them upward. The inferior and medial landmark is easily identified by the posterior layer of Denonvilliers' fascia, already dissected during the first step of the procedure; the superior and medial landmark is delineated by incising the periprostatic fascia along the prostate from the base to the apex. The lateral prostatic pedicle is controlled high on the base of the prostate, theoretically at a safe distance from the neurovascular elements of the bundle. The magnification allows a good visualization of the pedicles. However, because of the traction on the seminal vesicles, they appear to rise vertically, which facilitates their exposure but distorts their normal anatomic orientation. It is therefore important for the surgeon to reorient himself/herself constantly during the dissection of the pedicles and to be cognizant of the exact location of the neurovascular bundle.

Once the pedicle is controlled, the two fascial incisions (superior—periprostatic—and inferior—Denonvilliers' fascia) can be joined to develop, with careful and blunt dissection, an avascular interfascial plane, leaving laterally and posteriorly the neurovascular bundle partially recovered by a fascia, which reduces as much as possible the risk of mechanical injury to the bundle.

It is preferable to continue the apical dissection of the bundle after transecting the dorsal venous plexus, which gives mobility to the gland and facilitates the exposure of the apical and the distal third of the prostate.

If nerve sparing is not considered, the procedure is easier. The prostatic pedicles are transected far from the prostate, and the posterolateral attachments of the prostate are not dissected but simply controlled (using bipolar coagulation or clips) and divided. It is important to remember that although this step looks easier, the risk of rectal injury is higher because the dissection is performed close to the rectum, in the perirectal fat [1].

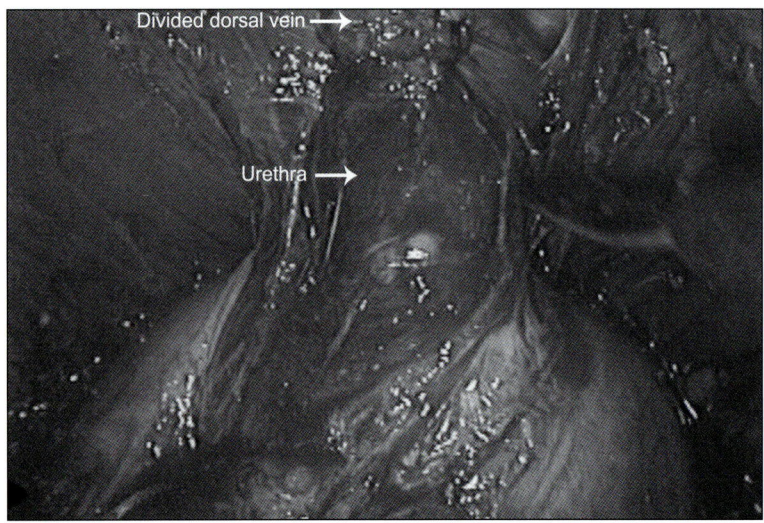

▶ **FIGURE 12-11.** Division of the dorsal venous complex. At this time, the only remaining prostatic attachments are the dorsal venous complex, the urethra, and the rectourethralis muscle. Because the dorsal vein has been ligated and the pedicles have been incised, there is little bleeding when the dorsal venous complex is incised. The incision is tangential to the prostate to avoid iatrogenic incision into the prostatic tissue at the apex. Gradually, an avascular plane of dissection situated between the dorsal venous complex and the urethra is developed to perfectly expose the anterior and lateral urethral walls.

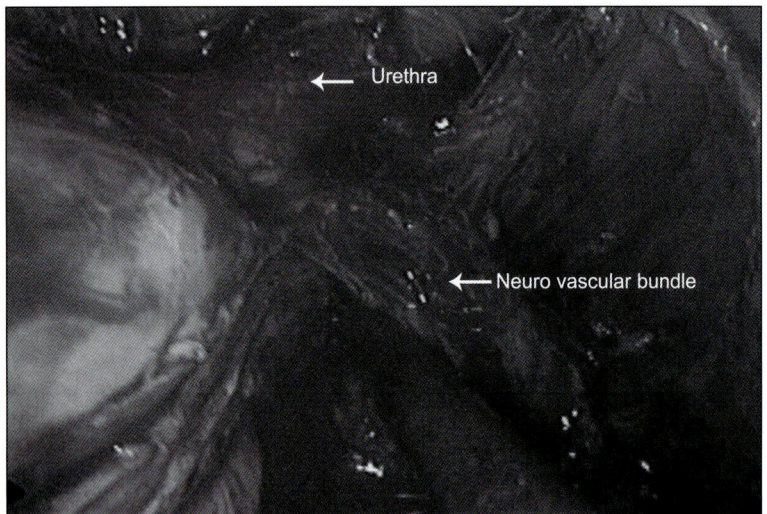

▶ **FIGURE 12-12.** Division of Denonvilliers' fascia. The remainder of Denonvilliers' fascia and the rectourethralis muscle fibers are divided. At the apex, the neurovascular bundles are divergent from the prostate but must be followed until their entrance into the pelvic floor, below and lateral to the urethra; the key element in this dissection is to follow the anatomic contours of the prostate. At the end of this step, the neurovascular bundles and the rectum are separated away from the prostate and the only attachment left is the urethra.

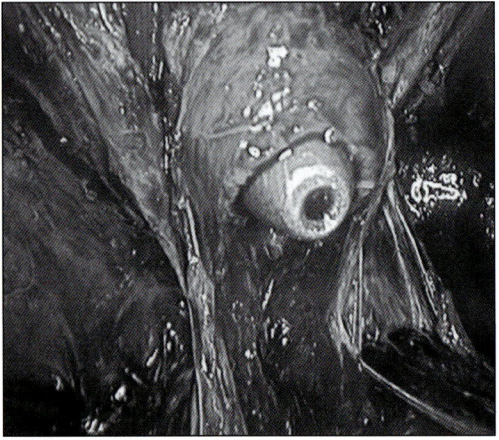

▶ **FIGURE 12-13.** (*See Color Plate*) Incising the urethra. The prostate is pulled cephalad, and the urethra is then sharply incised with laparoscopic scissors. The specimen is placed in a laparoscopic bag under the control of a 5-mm scope placed through a lateral port. An extension of the 10-mm umbilical incision is used to extract the specimen. The gland is macroscopically checked and sent to the pathologist for frozen section if necessary. The umbilical incision is carefully closed around a 10-mm trocar, and the abdomen is re-insufflated.

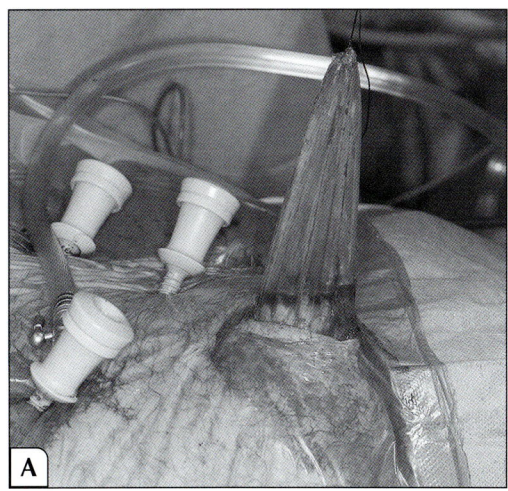
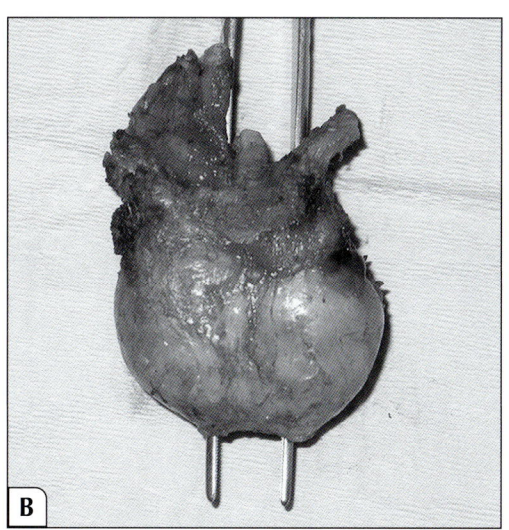
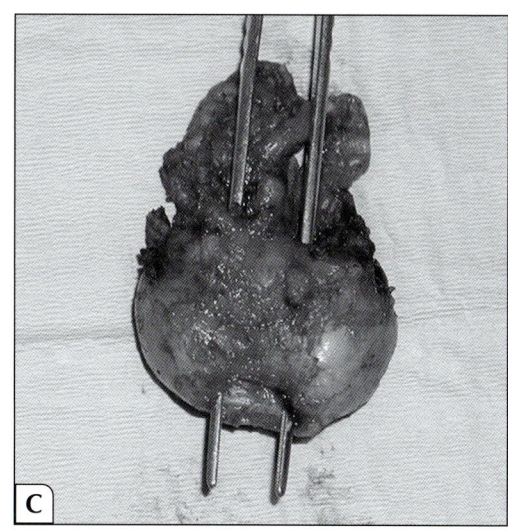

▶ **FIGURE 12-14.** Examination of the specimen. **A,** The specimen is retrieved prior to starting the anastomosis. **B and C,** The specimen is macroscopically examined and palpated to appreciate any suspicious areas for positive surgical margin and to obtain a frozen section for pathologic examination if needed [4].

It is not necessary to evert the bladder mucosa or to resize the bladder neck. However, in some cases with a large bladder neck, an anterior or posterior "tennis racket" reconstruction is required. Throughout this portion of the procedure, the surgeon works with two needle holders, using a 3-0 resorbable suture with an RB1 needle. All the sutures are tied intracorporeally. A Béniqué dilator helps guide the needle into the urethra. The first three sutures are posterior, placed at the 5, 6, and 7 o'clock positions, going inside-out on the urethra and outside-in on the bladder neck. These sutures are therefore tied intraluminally. Four other sutures are symmetrically placed at the 4 and 8, then the 2 and 10 o'clock positions, and tied outside the lumen. As a rule, for a right-handed surgeon, the right-sided stitches go outside-in on the bladder and inside-out on the urethra; the left-sided stitches go outside-in on the bladder and inside-out on the urethra.

Three final anterior stitches are placed at the 11, 12, and 1 o'clock positions, symmetric to the posterior stitches. The 11 and 12 o'clock stitches go outside-in on the urethra and inside-out on the bladder, whereas the 1 o'clock stitch goes outside-in on the bladder and inside-out on the urethra.

Once the sutures are tied, a Foley catheter is inserted [2,3]. The bladder is filled with 180 mL of saline to ascertain a watertight anastomosis and confirm the correct position of the catheter. Finally, the balloon is inflated with 10 mL of sterile water.

The abdominal pressure is lowered to 5 mm Hg to check for venous bleeding. One or two suction drains are placed, one anteriorly in Retzius' space and the other posterior, through the incision of the cul-de-sac of Douglas. The 5-mm trocars are removed under visual control, and the port sites are checked once more to exclude vascular injury, particularly of the epigastric vessels. At the end, the incisions are conventionally closed and dressed.

In a recent analysis of 400 laparoscopic radical prostatectomies performed at Memorial Sloan-Kettering Cancer Center, the positive surgical margin rate was 11%: 6.4% in pathologically organ-confined cancers (pT2) and 20.5% in cases with extracapsular extension (pT3). According to a validated quality-of-life questionnaire, at 6 months, 61% of the patients had no urine leak or had leakage of only a few drops and 74% were pad-free or wore one pad per day. Regarding potency, according to the same questionnaire, 45.5% of preoperatively potent patients who underwent a bilateral nerve-sparing procedure were potent at 6 months postoperatively. The mean operating time was 205 minutes (90 to 336 minutes), mean blood loss was 315 mL (100 to 1100 mL), and transfusion rate was 2.6%; patients stayed an average 1.8 nights (1 to 11 nights) in the hospital (Touijer K, Guillonneau B, unpublished data).

REFERENCES

1. Guillonneau B, Vallancien G: Laparoscopic radical prostatectomy: the Montsouris experience. *J Urol* 2000, 163:418–422.

2. Guillonneau B, Cathelineau X, Doublet JD, *et al.*: Laparoscopic radical prostatectomy: assessment after 550 procedures. *Crit Rev Oncol Hematol* 2002, 43:123–133.

3. Guillonneau B, Vallancien G: Laparoscopic radical prostatectomy: the Montsouris technique. *J Urol* 2000, 163:1643–1649.

4. Touijer AK, Guillonneau B: Laparoscopic radical prostatectomy. *Urol Oncol* 2004, 22:133–138.

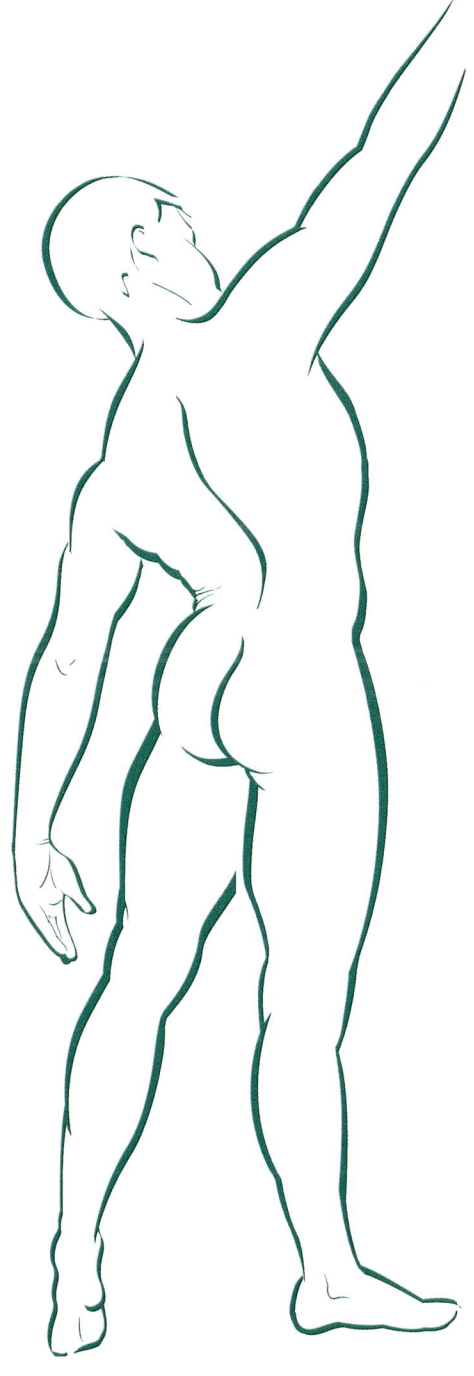

Robotic Radical Prostatectomy

13

Kevin M. Slawin & Naveen Kella

Over the past 5 years, the areas of debate regarding the treatment of localized prostate cancer have shifted dramatically. Prior to this period, there were many strong advocates resisting PSA-based screening for prostate cancer and questioning the role of treatment for localized disease in the absence of randomized trials proving a survival benefit. However, with the striking declines in advanced disease associated with screening programs, most dramatically in Tyrol, Austria, together with the unequivocal randomized data from Sweden proving a survival benefit from radical prostatectomy for clinically localized prostate cancer, the value of surgery for these patients is less frequently challenged. Key efforts now are focused on determining the appropriate PSA cutpoints for prostate cancer screening and on addressing the problem of overtreatment of patients with disease of lower grade and volume.

Variables often discussed now are the efficacy and morbidity of various treatment options for clinically localized prostate cancer. Treatment decisions require that patients and physicians weigh the risks and benefits of each option. Newer, minimally invasive options for the treatment of prostate cancer, such as robotic prostatectomy, impact this equation by offering high cancer control rates similar to those achieved with open, radical prostatectomy, but with a lower short-term, and potentially long-term, morbidity. The first great strides in addressing the morbidity of prostate cancer surgery were made through a better understanding of the surgical anatomy of the prostate, urinary sphincter, and neurovascular bundles, along with increased experience, as the number of radical prostatectomies performed ballooned in the late 1980s and 1990s [1]. These efforts led to a steady improvement in cancer control along with an improved quality of life for patients in the areas of urinary and sexual functions after surgery for prostate cancer.

More recently, technical advances in instrumentation, primarily in support of a laparoscopic approach to surgery, have supported a second revolution in radical prostatectomy surgery. Whereas laparoscopic approaches to the kidney gained acceptance by urologists, laparoscopic prostatectomy initially remained less popular because of the high degree of technical difficulty of this complex operation, and the long and steep "learning curve" associated with achieving its mastery. Challenges with laparoscopic prostate surgery include lack of depth perception, anti-intuitive "reverse motion" of the instruments, amplification of hand tremor, diminished dexterity in fine movements with the use of laparoscopic instruments due to the limited "degrees of freedom" (4 versus 6 for a surgeon's own hands), awkward ergonomics for the operating physician and a reduction in tactile feedback. Despite these challenges, a small cadre of talented surgeons, many of whom were expert laparoscopic surgeons but with limited training in oncology, became adept at laparoscopic prostatectomy, surging to the forefront of the field of surgical management of prostate cancer.

However, through the relentless drive of technology in the fields of computers and microelectronics, robotic techniques have emerged to provide a viable pathway for classically trained oncologic surgeons, skilled in open radical prostatectomy after years of practice and experience, to translate these skills into a minimally invasive approach to radical prostatectomy. This has leveled the field for all surgeons interested in pursuing minimally invasive approaches to prostate cancer surgery. The DaVinci robotic system (Intuitive Surgical, Inc., Mountain View, CA) allows surgeons to sit comfortably at a console and immerse themselves in a magnified (up to ten-fold) and 3-dimensional view of the surgical field. At the console, the surgeon controls instruments located on the surgical cart, which is the apparatus located patient-side. The surgeon has control of the stereoscopic camera as well as up to three robotic arms, which can wield various and interchangeable instruments. The instruments are able to articulate with wrist-like movements that allow six degrees of motion compared with four degrees possible with conventional laparoscopic instruments. Computer-filtration can eliminate surgeon tremor and finely scale a surgeon's motions up to 5:1, if desired. Moreover, instrument motions occur without perceptible delay to the surgeon. Because tactile feedback is limited, the surgeon is forced to rely on visual cues while dissecting and handling tissue.

The first robotic radical prostatectomies were performed by Binder and Kramer in Germany in May 2000 [2]. The advantages provided by robotic assistance for this highly complex and demanding surgical procedure have resulted in an increase in the number of surgeons performing the procedure. In 2004, robotic assistance was used in nearly 10% of all radical prostatectomies performed in the United States. However, the learning curve is still significant for performing a robotic-assisted laparoscopic prostatectomy. A study by Ahlering *et al.* [3] showed that 20 robotic cases were needed to achieve four-hour proficiency by a surgeon experienced in open procedures. For the initial 45 patients, the mean operating time was 3.45 hours (range 2.5–5.1 hours). Another requirement in laparoscopic surgery is a skilled assistant. Whereas many DaVinci robotic systems have an additional instrument arm, which allows the surgeon himself to help provide retraction, an experienced assistant is still invaluable for providing suction, irrigation, additional retraction, rapid instrument changes and occasional surgical cart troubleshooting.

GENERAL BENEFITS OF ROBOTIC SURGERY

Clear benefits of robotic surgery are the reduction in postoperative pain and length of hospitalization because of the minimally invasive nature of the procedure. Generally, our experience is that 90% of patients are ready for discharge the day after surgery. Reports in the literature corroborate our finding. Tewari *et al.* [8] noted that 93% of their patients are ready for discharge within 24 hours of surgery. Decreased blood loss associated with laparoscopic and robotic-assisted surgery is well documented in the literature. Blood loss in reported series has consistently been less than 200 cc and transfusion rates have been negligible. Narcotic usage is minimal, and many patients may not need patient-controlled analgesia with morphine. Many centers, including ours, find that a 24 hour course of ketorolac is sufficient for pain control during hospitalization followed by Tylenol and hydrocodone tablets afterwards. The Foley catheter remains in situ for one week. Earlier removal is possible but raises the risk of urinary retention.

Return to work or return to baseline activities seems anecdotally to occur earlier with robotic-operated patients. We allow patients to return to work and regular activities in as early as one to two weeks after surgery, especially those men who are not physical laborers.

URINARY CONTINENCE AND ROBOTIC SURGERY

Reports indicate that urinary continence returns earlier with a robotic prostatectomy. Tewari *et al.* [8] observed that 50% of patients achieved continence within 44 days after robotic surgery compared to 160 days with open surgery. In our experience, it is not unusual for patients to report wearing zero to one pad shortly after removal of the Foley catheter at one week, but we have not yet fully analyzed and reported our continence rates with validated questionnaires.

Further evaluation of continence rates is even more interesting when examining the rates of continence achieved by highly experienced open surgeons. For example, Ahlering *et al.* [9] compared a sequential series of 60 robotics patients (starting after his 45th robotic case) with the last 60 patients (out of hundreds) who had open surgery. From the robotics group, 76% of patients were completely continent 3 months after surgery, a proportion similar to that for his last group of 60 patients who underwent open radical prostatectomy [9].

With the robotic approach, excellent visualization at the prostatic apex results in maximal preservation of urethral length and minimizes inadvertent cautery damage to surrounding musculature and nerves. Whereas definite data are lacking, many consider preservation of urethral length as a contributor to return of continence [10]. Another aspect of the robotic approach is the ability to construct a watertight anastomosis. Again, whether urinary extravasation truly contributes to incontinence is an unanswered question. However, the ability to prevent urinary leaks does allow earlier removal of the catheter and perhaps reduces the incidence of bladder neck contracture due to urinary extravasation. Indeed, the reported incidence of bladder neck contracture in the robotic literature is extremely low.

In summary, promising data suggest an advantage in speed of return of continence and possibly total rate of return of continence with robotics. Additionally, as in open surgery, a surgeon's technique may ultimately be the driving factor in urinary continence. Robotics may better allow preservation of urethral length, construction of a watertight anastomosis, and bladder neck sparing, but surgeon skill and experience are still vital for consistent outcomes for urinary continence.

SEXUAL POTENCY AFTER ROBOTIC SURGERY

In laparoscopy, dissection of the prostate proceeds primarily in an antegrade fashion. The posterolateral neurovascular bundles are generally thickest proximally at the base of the prostate. As they are dissected under direct vision, they can be swept away towards the apex of the gland. Once at the apex, vision with robotics is superior to that with open surgery as long as the field is relatively bloodless. This visualization allows precise dissection of the neurovascular bundle away from the prostate at its apex. In total, these efforts likely contribute to preservation of sexual function. Of course, principles of nerve preservation during open surgery also apply to robotic surgery. Along with knowledge of the anatomy of the neurovascular bundles, minimal use of cautery and gentle handling of the neurovascular bundles are important.

Long-term data are available from some institutions that adopted robotics relatively early. For example, Tewari *et al.* [8] indicated that robotic surgery patients had an earlier return of erections than patients who had open surgery (50% return at a mean of 180 days versus 440 days for open radical prostatectomy patients). Undoubtedly, as with urinary continence, surgical technique and surgeon experience, rather than the use of the robot, will still be the primary factor determining the eventual success of nerve-sparing surgery.

COSTS OF ROBOTIC SURGERY

On a simplistic level, assessing the robotic prostatectomy from a cost-profit standpoint generally shows a poor financial return for the hospital. For example, in one report, a single center in the United States performed 174 procedures over a period of 18 months. The total hospital cost per radical prostatectomy was greater than the reimbursement per case by $148. In addition, this figure does not even account for the initial investment and annual maintenance for the robot, typically over 1 million dollars and 100,000 dollars, respectively [11].

At The Methodist Hospital in Houston, Texas, robotic prostatec-tomy produces net revenue, although over the past three years, open radical prostatectomy generated approximately $1000 more per case for the hospital. With growing experience and the currently decreasing time in the operating room achieved more recently, this differential in revenue will narrow. Further studies may also need to look beyond the hospital's finances and examine the cost of a radical prostatectomy from society's standpoint. Factors such as an earlier return to work, an earlier return of continence, and improved sexual function should be investigated to determine whether they are sufficient to justify the overall higher cost of robotic prostatectomy.

PREOPERATIVE CONSIDERATIONS

In general, radical prostatectomy is a treatment option for men with a life expectancy of 10 years or more. Any patient who is a candidate for open extirpation may also be a candidate for a laparoscopic robotic procedure. Conditions making laparoscopy more challenging include previous prostate surgery, whether open or endoscopic; abdominal surgeries, especially with usage of mesh; and adjuvant or salvage treatment, whether after radiation, hormonal therapy, or cryotherapy. The presence of a known median lobe calls for a surgeon who has achieved a higher level of expertise and comfort with this operation. Less experienced surgeons would be more likely to leave a portion of the median lobe behind, or have more difficulty in reconstructing the potentially wide bladder neck. Repair can be done posteriorly or anteriorly on the bladder neck depending on surgeon preference. The technique for performing the bladder neck reconstruction roboti-

cally is similar to the technique used in open surgery, but it can be difficult for the inexperienced robotic surgeon. Furthermore, a large prostate tends to lead to longer operating time because of the difficulty inherent in manipulating and placing traction on the prostate in a reduced space. However, we have successfully removed prostates over 130 grams in size. Removal of pelvic lymph nodes is recommended for patients with higher PSA or Gleason score. Surgeons can perform pelvic lymph node dissection laparoscopically with the DaVinci system, although a more complete node dissection can be achieved through the more standard, open procedure. The pneumoretroperitoneum can flatten the iliac veins, and dissection must be done delicately to avoid injury. Although a transperitoneal approach reduces the risk of a lymphocele, we exclusively utilize a retroperitoneal approach for robotic prostatectomy.

PREOPERATIVE PREPARATION

Surgeons need to discuss with their patients the risks of laparoscopy and traditional open surgery as well as the possibility of a robotic malfunction, which have been noted but are rare. Bowel preparations can be administered according to surgeon preference, although a simple enema on the morning of surgery is

the only preparation we recommend for both robotic and open prostatectomy. Especially during the transition period for "newly minted" robotic surgeons, patients should be keenly made aware that the surgeon may convert the case to an open approach if he for any reason, he feels the patient's interests favor conversion.

Positive Margin Rates of Multiple Published Series		
Series		**Positive margins, %**
Soloway (review of several centers)	(Open)	28
Lepor	(Open)	26
Scardino	(Open, 1154 cases)	pT2 7.8
	(498 cases)	pT3 20.8
Walsh	(Open, 4683 cases	All 9.2
	from 1997–2001)	pT3 22.7
Guillonneau	(Laparoscopic,	pT2 6.4
	400 cases at MSKCC)	pT3 20.5
Abbou	(Laparoscopic)	20
Rassweiler	(Laparoscopic)	24
Turk	(Laparoscopic)	26
Bollens	(Laparoscopic)	22
Sulser	(Laparoscopic)	18
Menon	(Robotic, >100 cases)	26, 17, 6
Ahlering	(Robotic, 140 cases)	24
Patel V	(Robotic, 450 cases)	10.5

▶ **FIGURE 13-1.** Positive margin rates of multiple published series. In oncology, a positive margin means an incomplete excision of the tumor. Whereas half or more of prostate cancer patients with a positive margin will remain cancer-free with long-term follow-up, efforts to reduce positive margins clearly lead to better biochemical progression-free rates [4]. In a study by Epstein *et al.* [5] patients with positive margins had 10-year biochemical progression-free rates of 55%, whereas patients with negative margins had progression-free rates of 80%. With open surgery, it has been shown that surgical technique is an independent predictor of positive margin status [6]. In robotics, the surgeon's technique also influences surgical margin rates. The improvement in visualization and precise movements during a robotic procedure come at the expense of tactile sensation, which some surgeons rely on to detect the presence of tumor extension [7]. Early series in robotics appear to show positive margin rates, which are at least comparable with many open and laparoscopic surgical series.

	First 50 cases	Second 50 cases	Last 17 cases
Baylor College of Medicine Single Surgeon Positive Margin Rate with Robotic Prostatectomy (*n*=117 cases) (Unpublished)			
pT2	42 (50)=84%	32 (50)=64%	16 (17)=94%
% + SM	3 (42)=7%	1 (32)=3%	0 (16)=0%
pT3	8 (50)=16%	13 (50)=26%	1 (17)=5.9%
% + SM	2 (8)=25%	3 (13)=23%	0 (1)=0%

▶ **FIGURE 13-2.** Baylor College of Medicine single surgeon positive margin rate with robotic prostatectomy. Positive margins typically are encountered at the prostatic apex or along the posterolateral aspect of the prostate where the neurovascular bundles are located. Interestingly, these are both locations where the robotic or laparoscopic approach can provide excellent visualization. With a straight (0 degree) or angled down (30 degree down) lens, surgical detail generally unappreciated in open surgery can be visualized to allow a more anatomical dissection, especially at the apex and alongside the neurovascular bundles. As surgeons experienced with radical prostatectomy migrate to the robotic platform, positive margin rates should improve. At Baylor College of Medicine, the single surgeon positive margin rate shows continuing improvement with experience, as shown in this table, and is comparable to those reported for open radical prostatectomy at our center, as well as at other centers of excellence. More importantly, data regarding long-term PSA PFS with robotic prostatectomy will require maturation of data to compare this more clinically significant outcome measure.

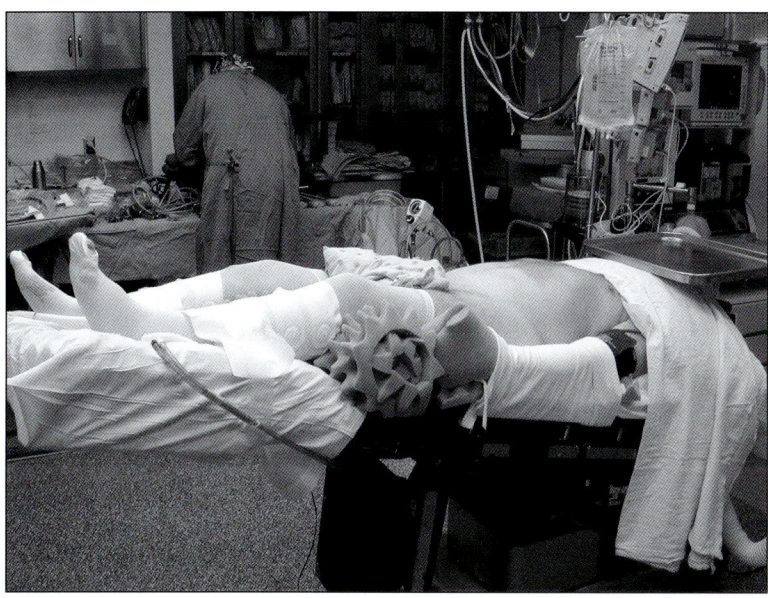

▶ **FIGURE 13-3.** Patient positioning. The patient is positioned supine in lithotomy position, or with split legs, to allow access for the robot between the legs of the patient. Arms are padded and tucked to the sides. This allows space for the assistant to work freely and also avoids possible interference with the optional fourth arm of the DaVinci robot. Depending on whether the approach is transperitoneal or extraperitoneal, the patient is placed maximally to moderately in Trendelenburg position. The surgical prep covers the genitalia to the xiphoid process and stretches laterally to just beyond the anterior superior iliac spines. For a four-arm system, the fourth arm is typically routed below the patient's left leg, or in some institutions, the right leg. The master-slave system of the DaVinci surgical system (Intuitive Surgical, Inc., Mountain View, CA) is comprised of the following: a surgeon's console with a 3-dimensional viewer, the surgical robot with either two or three working arms, and a camera arm. A patient-side assistant attaches instruments to the robotic arms and can change them throughout the course of the procedure. The assistant typically controls one or two laparoscopic ports for suctioning, retraction, suture passing, and eventual entrapment of the prostate in a specimen bag. At the console, the surgeon continually uses his hands and feet to move the instruments, to activate monopolar or bipolar electrocautery, and to position the camera.

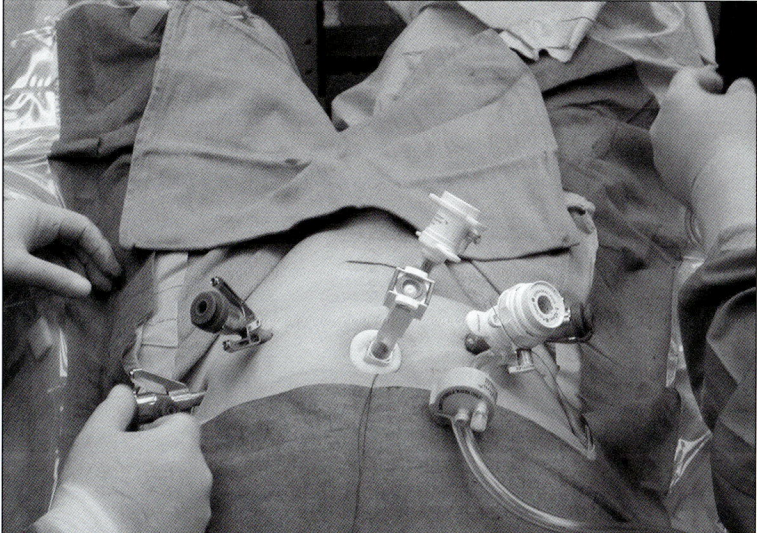

▶ **FIGURE 13-4.** Port placement. Two factors, the route of the procedure and the anatomy of the pubic bone, pubic rami, and anterior superior iliac spines primarily determine port placement. The decision to perform surgery transperitoneally or extraperitoneally dictates placement of the camera port 1 or 2 cm above the umbilicus if transperitoneal, or just below the umbilicus if extraperitoneal. The remaining ports are placed in a semicircular fashion, but the pubis should be used as the frame of reference, rather than the camera port [12]. The robotic arms have a finite length and positioning them further than 18 cm away from the pubis (measured when insufflated) risks making them unavailable for performance of the apical dissection or for the anastomosis. At the same time, the DaVinci arms need to be positioned sufficiently distant from the pubis to allow the anterior bladder takedown or a pelvic lymph node dissection. The robotic arms also need to be placed far enough apart to prevent instrument interaction. An 8 to 10 cm distance between each port (insufflated) appears ideal for avoiding interaction. In order to properly position the ports, we initially map out on the patient's skin the superior border of the pubic bone and the anterior superior iliac spines. After placement of the camera port, the primary right and left robotic arm positions are measured and marked on the lower abdomen. The position of the "fourth" arm is marked on the abdomen laterally to the left of the primary robotic trocar on the left side, all the way to the anterior iliac spine. Finally, a 5 mm assistant port in marked, two-finger breadths above the pubic bone, just to the right of the midline, and a 12 mm port between the camera port and the right sided robotic trocar are positioned. The 12 mm port is needed for passing needles, suctioning, and potentially for stapling the dorsal vein, as well as for entrapping the specimen.

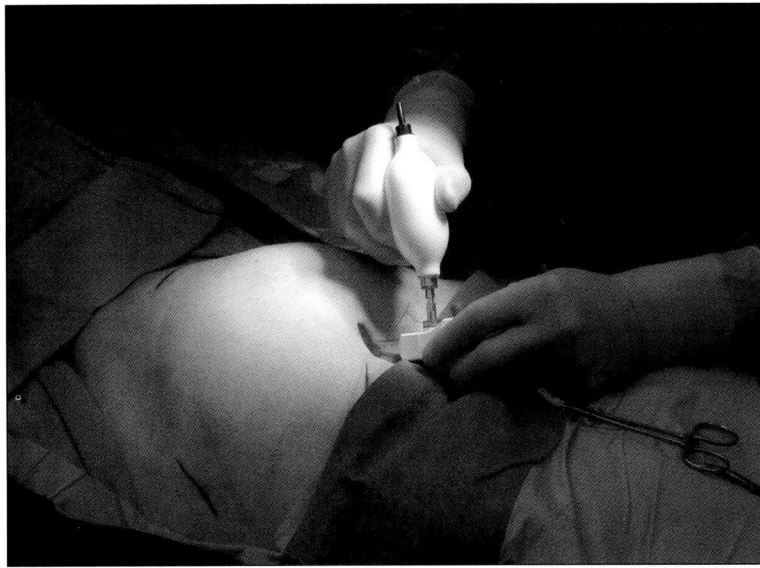

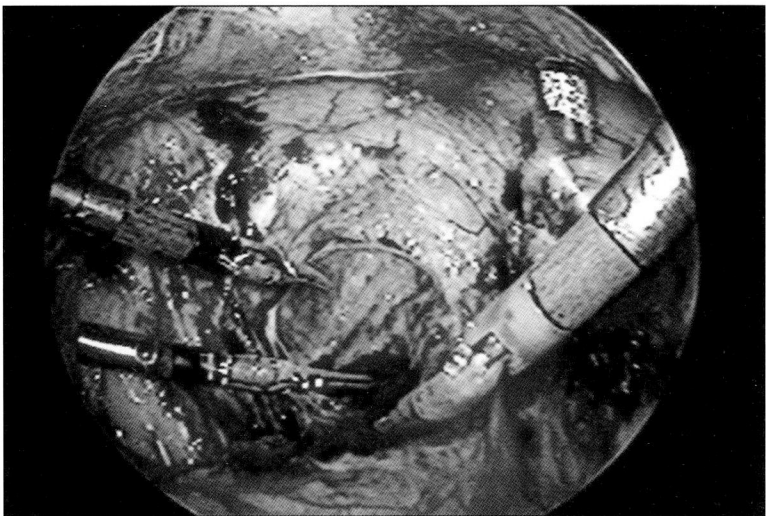

▶ **FIGURE 13-5.** Retroperitoneal insufflation. After making a 1–2 cm incision just below the umbilicus, the linea alba is exposed with an Army-Navy retractor, and the anterior rectus sheath is incised with an 11 blade, taking care to leave intact the posterior rectus fascia. Using finger dissection, the Space of Rhetzius is developed. A 2-0 prolene suture is place at the upper apex of the fascial incision and tagged. A "kidney-shaped" balloon dissection is then placed into the developed space and manually insufflated. After removing the deflated balloon dissector, the 10–12 mm camera port is inserted and a pneumoretroperitoneum of 13 mm Hg is established.

▶ **FIGURE 13-6.** (*See Color Plate*) Wide angle start. After approximately our first 50 cases, we have switched exclusively to the extraperitoneal approach, which we prefer because it requires less Trendelenburg, avoids the physiologic consequences of a pneumoperitoneum, takes advantage of the peritoneum to retract and protect the small bowel, and is less problematic in the rare event of a urine leak postoperatively. Using an extraperitoneal approach, the bladder is swept posteriorly by the pneumoretroperitoneum and the surgeon has immediate access to the prostate at the outset.

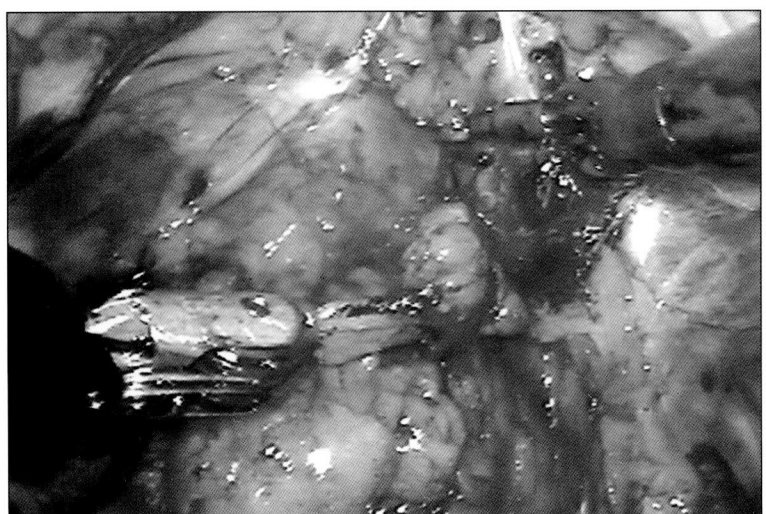

▶ **FIGURE 13-7.** Clearing of working space. As with conventional laparoscopy, clearing the working space allows improved visualization of surgical planes and diminished problems of clogging the suction device if there is bleeding. The fat is cleared from the endopelvic fascia and puboprostatics to the junction between the prostate and the bladder.

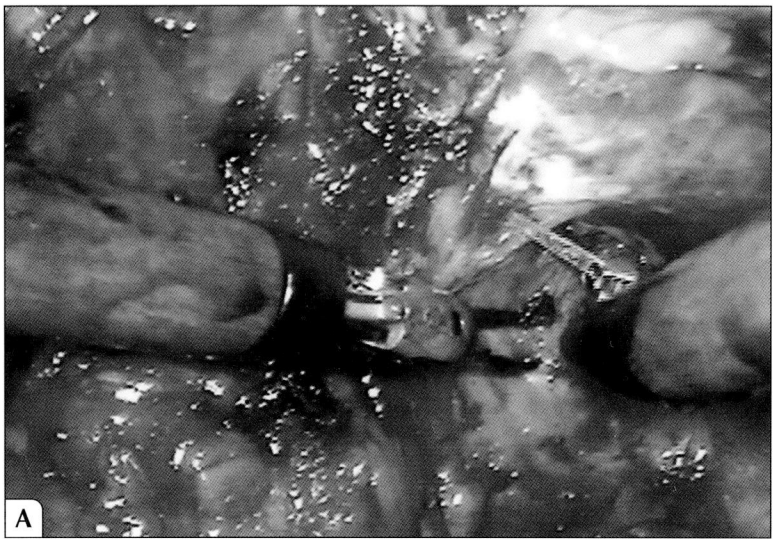

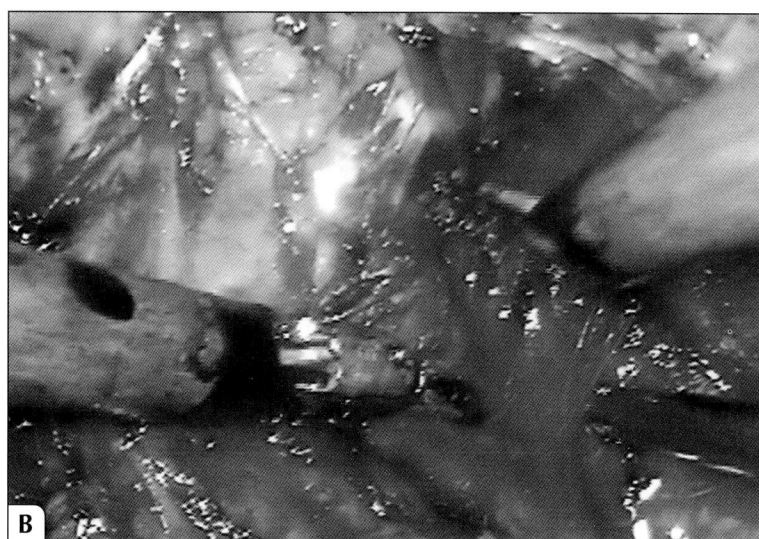

▶ FIGURE 13-8. (*See Color Plate*) **A**, Endopelvic fascia, and **B**, apical dissection. Sharp scissor dissection or electrocautery can start the endopelvic dissection lateral to the prostate. Work is carried proximally to the prostaticovesical junction, which is identifiable by a "V" shaped tongue of perirectal fat. As the condensations of the endopelvics move distally, they merge into the puboprostatic ligaments. Levator and pubourethral musculature appears to regularly insert into the visceral fascia of the prostate laterally, and forms a "sling" around the dorsal vein fascia distally. We spare as much musculature as possible by using blunt dissection primarily, and bipolar electrocautery only when necessary.

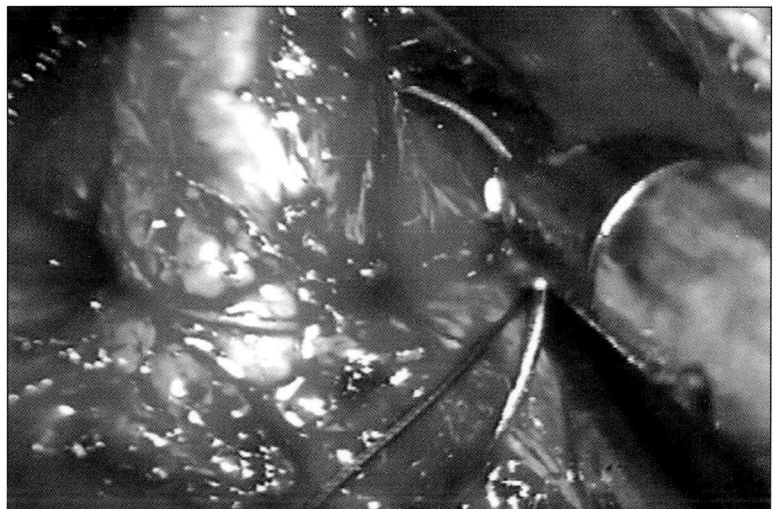

▶ FIGURE 13-9. Control of dorsal vein complex. The surgeon can decide whether to use a suture ligature or stapler at the apex. An EndoGIA stapler can nicely expose the urethra with minimal bleeding, but requires more dissection of the DVC and puboprostatics to allow placement of the device. Urethral transection theoretically is possible with the stapler. When distinguishing the urethra is difficult, gentle manipulation of the Foley catheter can help in identifying the demarcation between urethra and the dorsal venous complex. This same maneuver is useful when throwing a suture ligature to control the DVC. An advantage of using the stapler is the resulting clear visualization of the urethra. This will allow a precise urethral dissection and potentially reduce iatrogenic apical margins later in the operation [13]. Despite this, in our experience, a simple figure of eight suture using 0-Mersilene, which has a high coefficient of friction and thus resists slippage off of the DVC fascia, is all that is required to effectively control the DVC and is more cost efficient.

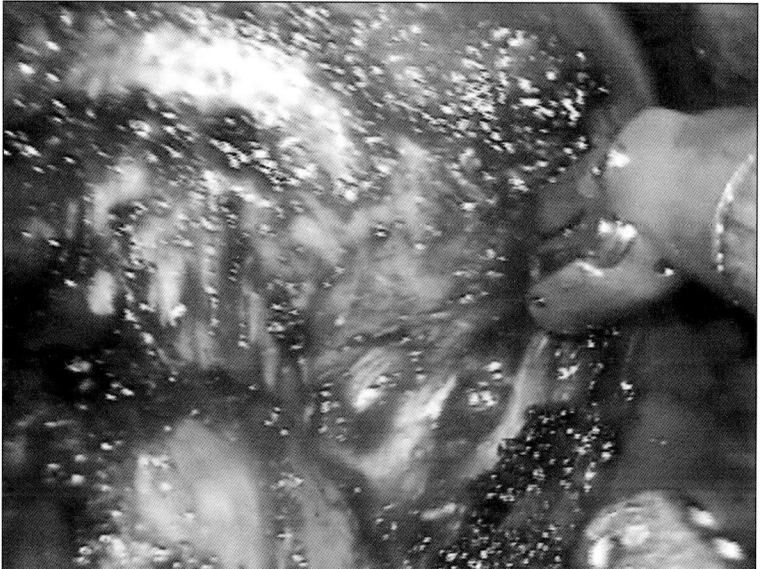

▶ FIGURE 13-10. Anterior bladder neck dissection. The successful dissection of the bladder neck is critical for creating the conditions for a simple urethrovesical anastomosis at the end of the procedure. The border between the prostate and bladder can be identified visually if the overlying prostatic fat is removed and is best identified at the lateral aspects. The 30 degree down lens provides a good view for this portion of the operation, and the surgeon can use it until the start of the urethral portion of the urethrovesical anastomosis. Moving the Foley catheter all the way into the bladder and then slowly pulling it back can also help identify the proper plane of dissection. An experienced assistant is invaluable for providing irrigation and counter-traction at this step. Our dissection proceeds close to the capsule of the prostate. Starting laterally on each side of prostaticovesicular junction, the surgeon uses the lateral aspect of the prostate as a landmark and starts the creation of a trough towards the midline. Bleeding can occur laterally with perivesicular veins and can occur if dissection occurs into the prostate or too far into the detrusor musculature. A combination of sharp and blunt dissection will identify the bladder neck in the midline, and the proper plan is maintained by staying in the layer of periprostatic fat, present between the bladder neck and prostate laterally. The lateral approach also nicely exposes any median lobe that might be present, thereby facilitating blunt dissection of this lobe off of the posterior aspect of the bladder neck.

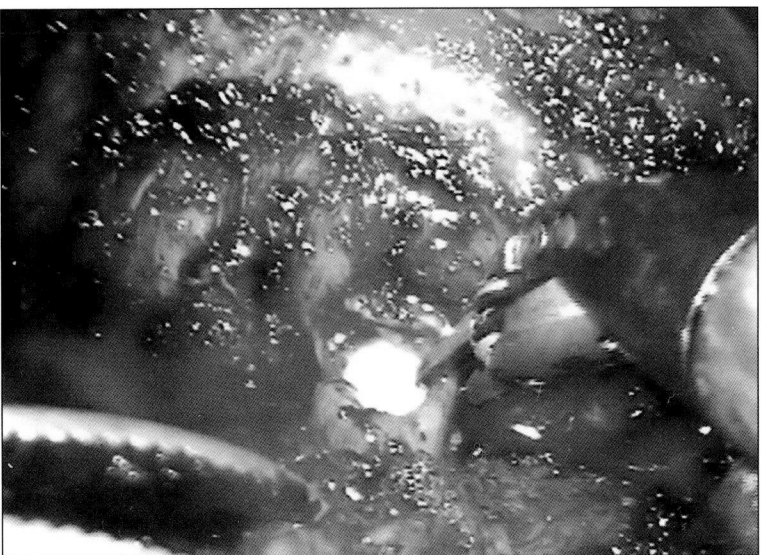

▶ FIGURE 13-11. Cut bladder neck. Cutting into the bladder will reveal the Foley catheter, which the fourth arm or the assistant can grasp to provide counter-traction for the posterior bladder neck dissection.

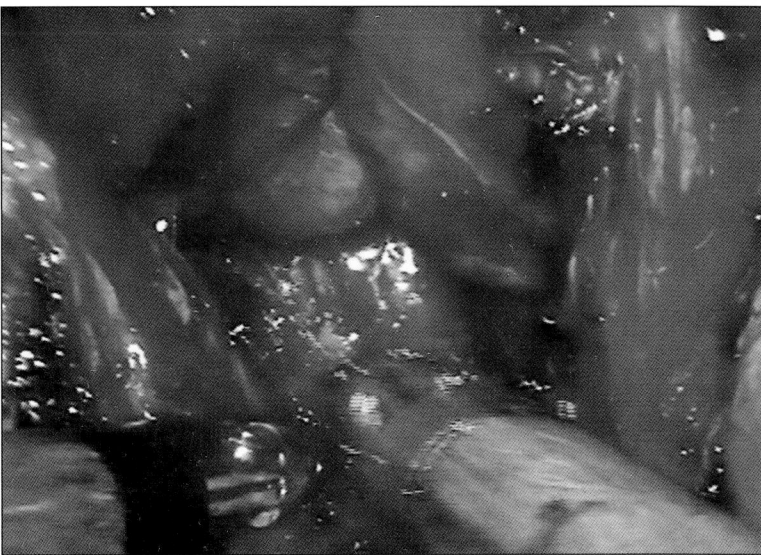

▶ FIGURE 13-12. Posterior bladder neck dissection. After the Foley catheter is elevated by the assistant, the bladder neck mucosa can be seen posteriorly following the contour of the base of the prostate into the urethra. This bladder neck is developed starting laterally with sharp and blunt dissection, sweeping the bladder neck off of the prostate. The detrusor fibers will give way to expose the anterior layer of Denonvillier's fascia. At this point, it is convenient to transect the posterior lip of mucosa forming the bladder neck. Dissection can quickly proceed to the anterior layer of Denonvillier's fascia, already established laterally. If a median lobe is present, the steps are similar except that the mucosa covering the median lobe should be transected at the neck of the median lobe and then bluntly dissected to reach Denonvillier's fascia. If the ureteral orifices are difficult to locate, the anesthesiologist can administer intravenous methylene blue.

An important point is to establish the thickness of the bladder neck wall. The thickness usually is the same circumferentially. This can help as a landmark during difficult dissections and can prevent a button-hole dissection into the posterior bladder.

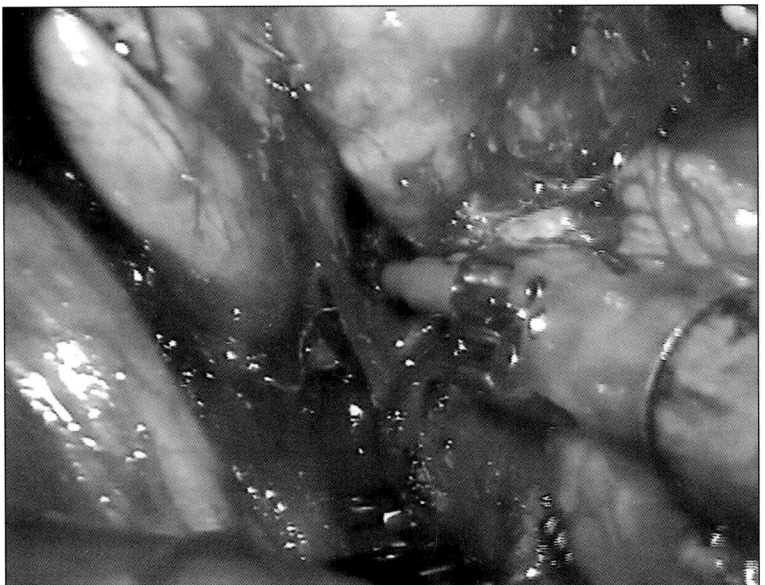

▶ FIGURE 13-13. Seminal vesicles and vasa. Cutting through the Denonvillier's fascia will reveal loose connective tissue encasing the seminal vesicles and vasa. This dissection can appear very deep, especially with a large prostate. To avoid dissecting into a hole, it is helpful to work laterally, as well as to continue to bring the bladder off the prostate. This will also help maintain orientation during this task.

We fully remove the seminal vesicles for oncologic purposes, but are careful to use scissor and bipolar dissection or clips to control the vessels to the vasa and the seminal vesicles to minimize injury to the neurovascular bundles.

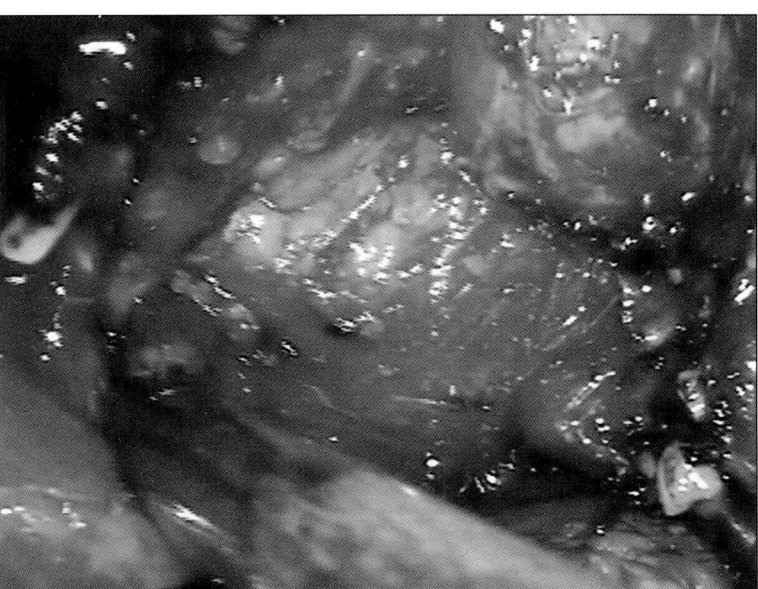

▶ FIGURE 13-14. Posterior dissection. To begin the posterior dissection, the seminal vesicles and vasa are grabbed and placed on upwards traction by the assistant. When posterior Denonvillier's fascia is transected close to the base of the prostate, the lobulated perirectal fat becomes apparent. Blunt and sharp dissection can establish the pedicles of the prostate. The plane of dissection should keep the posterior surface of the prostate apparent in order to avoid dissection too close or into the rectum. This posterior dissection can be carried all the way to the urethra if desired.

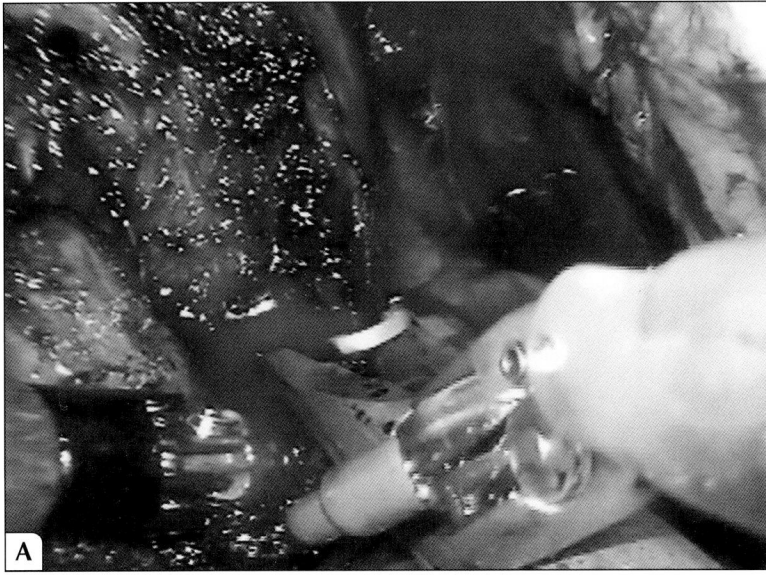

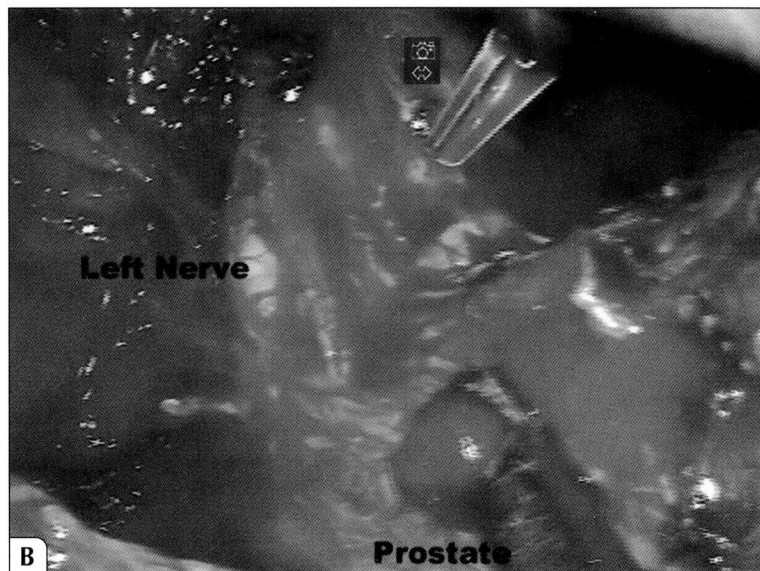

▶ **FIGURE 13-15.** (*See Color Plate*) **A,** Control of vascular pedicles and neurovascular bundle dissection. Anatomically, the vascular pedicles originate lateral to the seminal vesicles. Electrocautery or Weck clips are used to control the pedicles. With the increased magnification provided by the robot, the individual branches originating from the inferior vesicular artery can be coagulated precisely with bipolar cautery. As the pedi-

cles are dropped, the neurovascular bundles can be dissected away from the prostate. Moving in an antegrade fashion allows the bundles to be brought away from the prostate under direct vision. The bundles travel posterolaterally along the prostate and then are lateral and posterolateral to the urethra. **B** demonstrates a nerve-sparing approach, left.

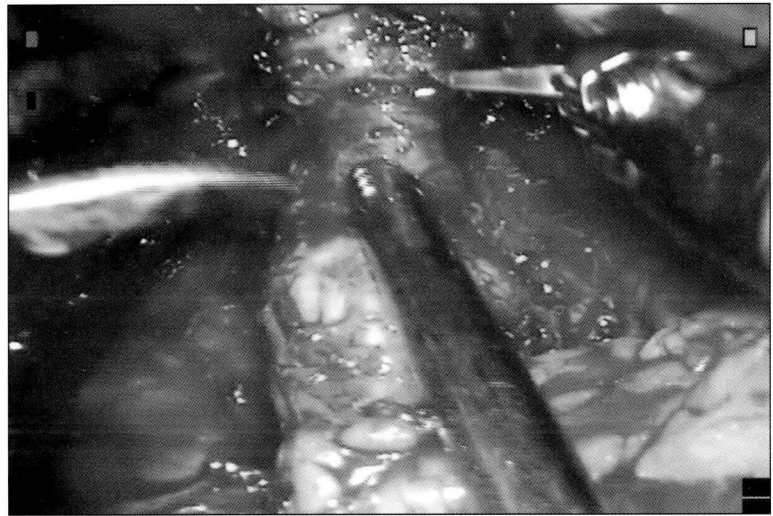

▶ **FIGURE 13-16.** (*See Color Plate*) Urethral transection and entrapment of prostate. Apical positive margins can be minimized and the urethral length can be maximized if the urethral transection is done under hemostatic conditions. The dorsal venous complex can occasionally start bleeding again due to slippage of the DVC suture, and a second hemostatic stitch should be placed in this circumstance to ensure bloodless visualization during this portion of the procedure. The fourth arm of the robot is useful at this stage to provide traction on the midprostatic suture anteriorly and cephalad. Transection through the uncut portion of the DVC staple line is done with a scissor, which is used to transect the urethra as well. Skilled open surgeons will find it comfortable to complete the distal portion of the neurovascular bundle dissection at this stage, in a retrograde fashion. A specimen sack is deployed to "bag" the prostate, which is then removed through the camera port incision. For larger prostates, this incision is extended slightly to allow specimen removal, and then shortened again with a 2-0 prolene suture to allow a tight seal when the camera port is replaced in order to complete the operation.

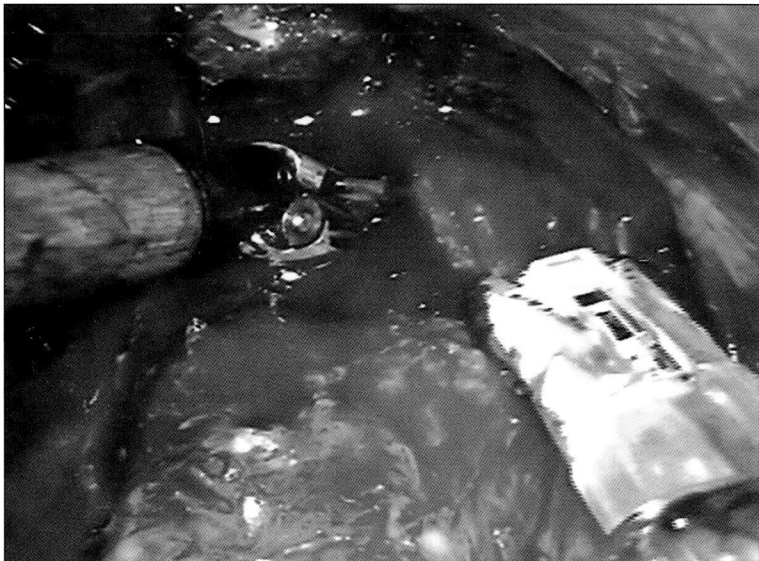

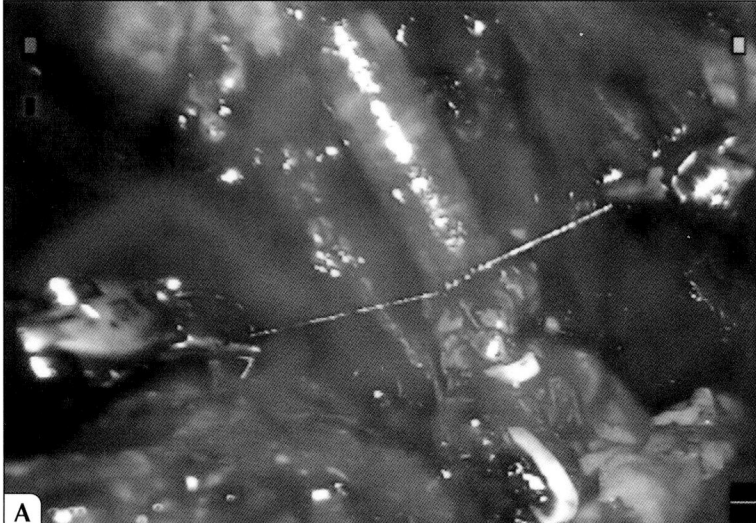

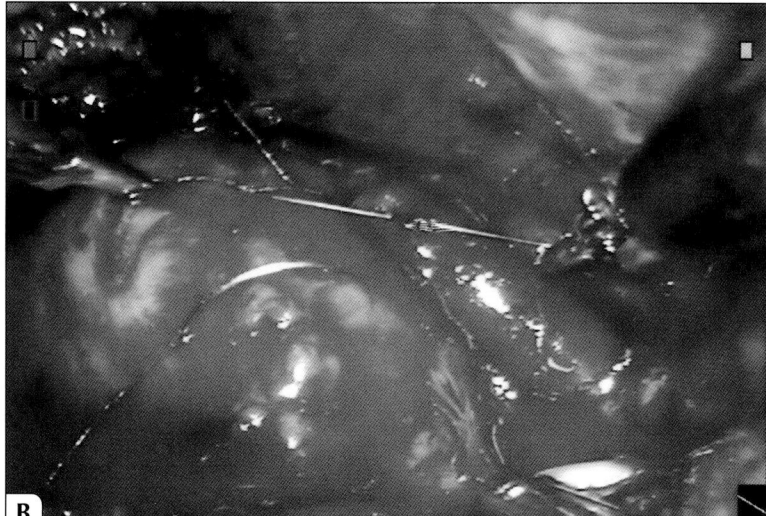

▶ FIGURE 13-17. Non–nerve sparing approach, right. In a small percentage of cases, the tumor grade and extent requires a non-nerve sparing approach unilaterally. The proximal and distal extent of the resected nerve is marked with clips.

▶ FIGURE 13-18. **A,** Proximal collagen graft, and **B,** distal collagen graft. For those patients requiring nerve grafting, the proximal and distal cut ends of the NVB are "stuffed" into the ends of a collagen tube allo-graft (Neuragen, OriginBiomedicinals, Inc., Nova Scotia, Canada) and secured with 5-0 prolene sutures.

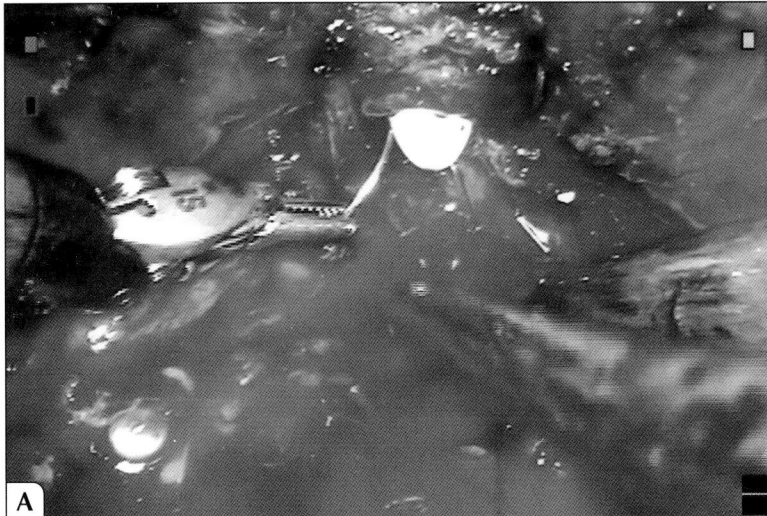

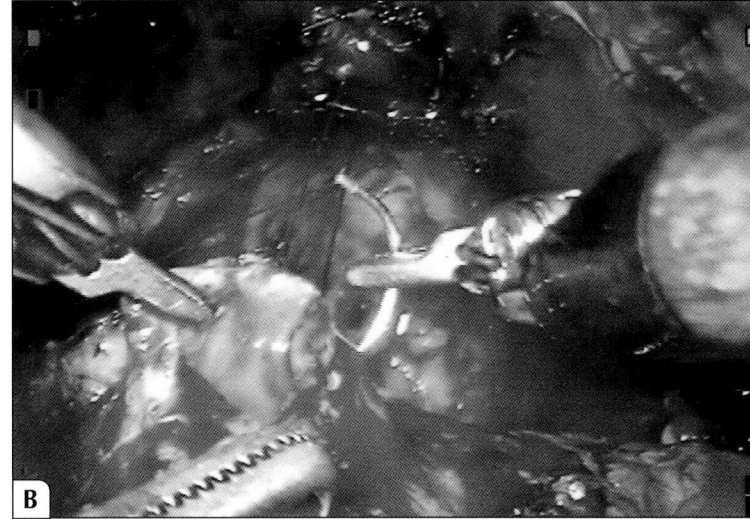

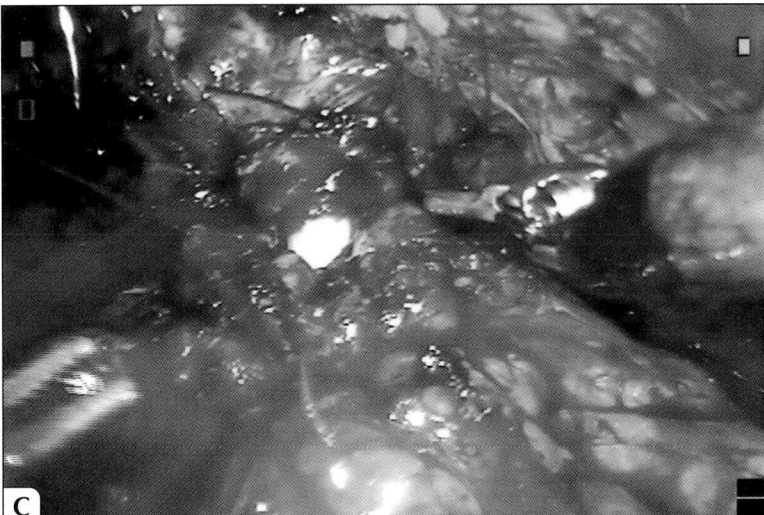

▶ **FIGURE 13-19. A–C.** Urethrovesical anastomosis. Perhaps the best example of the advantage of robotic surgery over conventional laparoscopy is in the performance of the anastomosis. The needle drivers can articulate at the wrist and thus allow sutures to be thrown precisely and with minimal trauma to surrounding tissues. A running, double-armed stitch popularized by Van Velthoven *et al.* [14] results in a watertight anastomosis. A few important points can make the anastomosis portion of the case move smoothly. Monocryl suture is useful because it can slide smoothly through tissue and thus accommodate the occasional tightening of the running anastomosis to prevent leaks. The fourth arm or the assistant can hold traction on the other arm of the stitch to prevent too much loosening of the anastomosis. If bladder neck reconstruction is needed, it can be done on the anterior or posterior portion of the bladder. If the tension required to bring the bladder down to the urethra seems to be too much, the best course of action is to place a few more throws before attempting to bring the anastomosis together. Multiple throws will dissipate the tension across the suture line and allow increased force to bring the anastomosis together.

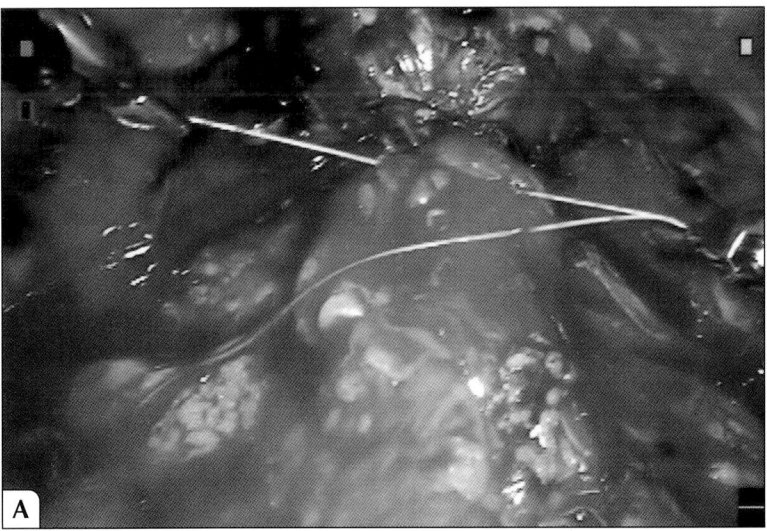

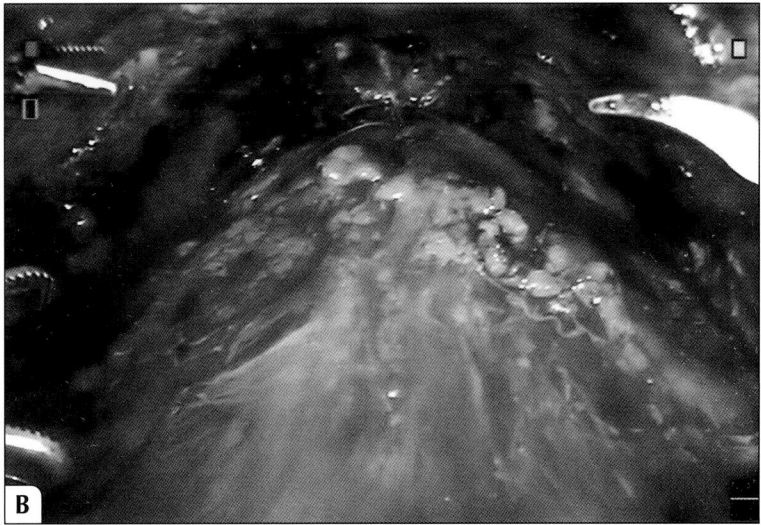

▶ **FIGURE 13-20. A,** Bladder neck suspension, and **B,** completion of procedure. Finally, a surgeon's knot is important to prevent the closure ties from coming apart. We typically approximate the DVC fascia to the anterior bladder neck with a final 2-0 Vicryl mattress suture to complete the procedure.

FUTURE

Almost 10% of all radical prostatectomy surgeries were performed robotically in 2004. As more surgeons surmount the learning curve, this percentage will increase. Implementation of training programs will be challenging but important to train the next generation of urologists to perform robotic surgery.

The benefits of robotic surgery include quicker recovery, diminished blood loss, and the faster recovery of continence. Data on sexual potency appear encouraging, but longer-term data from more robotic series are needed. Nerve-sparing is possible with robotics and will likely be technique dependent, just as in open surgery. Surgical positive margin rates appear to be comparable to or better than published rates from open series. However, most importantly, the use of the DaVinci system will not magically transform surgeons with limited knowledge or skill performing prostate cancer surgery into expert surgeons, or instantly improve their outcomes. Improved outcomes come only with experience and attention to the surgical anatomy of the prostate and an understanding of the biology of prostate cancer, regardless of the method used. Conversely, the DaVinci system can allow surgeons already adept at open radical prostatectomy after years of experience and hundreds or even thousands of cases to more readily translate this hard-won skill into minimally invasive surgery for prostate cancer.

REFERENCES

1. Walsh PC: Anatomic radical prostatectomy: evolution of the surgical technique. *J Urol* 1998, 160(6 Pt 2):2418–2424.

2. Binder J, Kramer W: Robotically-assisted laparoscopic radical prostatectomy. *BJU Int* 2001, 87(4):408–410.

3. Ahlering TE, Skarecky D, Lee D: Successful transfer of open surgical skills to a laparoscopic environment using a robotic interface: initial experience with laparoscopic radical prostatectomy. *J Urol* 2003, 170:1738–1741.

4. Grossfeld GD, Chang JJ, Broering JM, *et al.*: Impact of positive surgical margins on prostate cancer recurrence and the use of secondary cancer treatment: data from the CaPSURE database. *Urology* 2000, 163:1171–1177.

5. Epstein JI, Partin AW, Sauvageot J, *et al.*: Prediction of progression following radical prostatectomy. A multivariate analysis of 721 men with long-term follow-up. *Am J Surg Path 1996,* 20:286–292.

6. Eastham JA, Kattan MW, Riedel E, *et al.*: Variations among individual surgeons in the rate of positive surgical margins in radical prostatectomy specimens. *J Urol* 2003, 170:2292–2295.

7. Hernandez DJ, Epstein JI, Trock BJ, *et al.*: Radical retropubic prostatectomy. How often do experienced surgeons have positive surgical margins when there is extraprostatic extension in the region of the neurovascular bundle? *J Urol* 2005, 173:446–449.

8. Tewari A, Srivasatava A, Menon M; Members of the VIP Team: A prospective comparison of radical retropubic and robot-assisted prostatectomy: experience in one institution. *BJU Int* 2003 92:205–210.

9. Ahlering TE, Woo D, Eichel L, *et al.*: Robot-assisted versus open radical prostatectomy: a comparison of one surgeon's outcomes. *Urology* 2004, 63:819–822.

10. Coakley FV, Eberhardt S, Kattan MW, *et al.*: Urinary continence after radical retropubic prostatectomy: relationship with membranous urethral length on preoperative endorectal magnetic resonance imaging. *J Urol* 2002, 168:1032–1035.

11. Jean J: Cost-profit analysis of daVinci robotic surgery: Is it worth it? *J Urol* 2005, 173(4 suppl):7.

12. Pick DL, Lee DI, Skarecky DW, *et al.*: Anatomic guide for port placement for daVinci robotic radical prostatectomy. *J Endourol* 2004, 18:572–575.

13. Ahlering TE, Eichel L, Edwards RA, *et al.*: Robotic radical prostatectomy: a technique to reduce pT2 positive margins. *Urology* 2004, 64:1224–1228.

14. Van Velthoven RF, Ahlering TE, Peltier A, *et al.*: Technique for laparoscopic running urethrovesical anastomosis: the single knot method. *Urology* 2003, 61:699–702.

Brachytherapy for Prostate Cancer

14

Michael J. Zelefsky

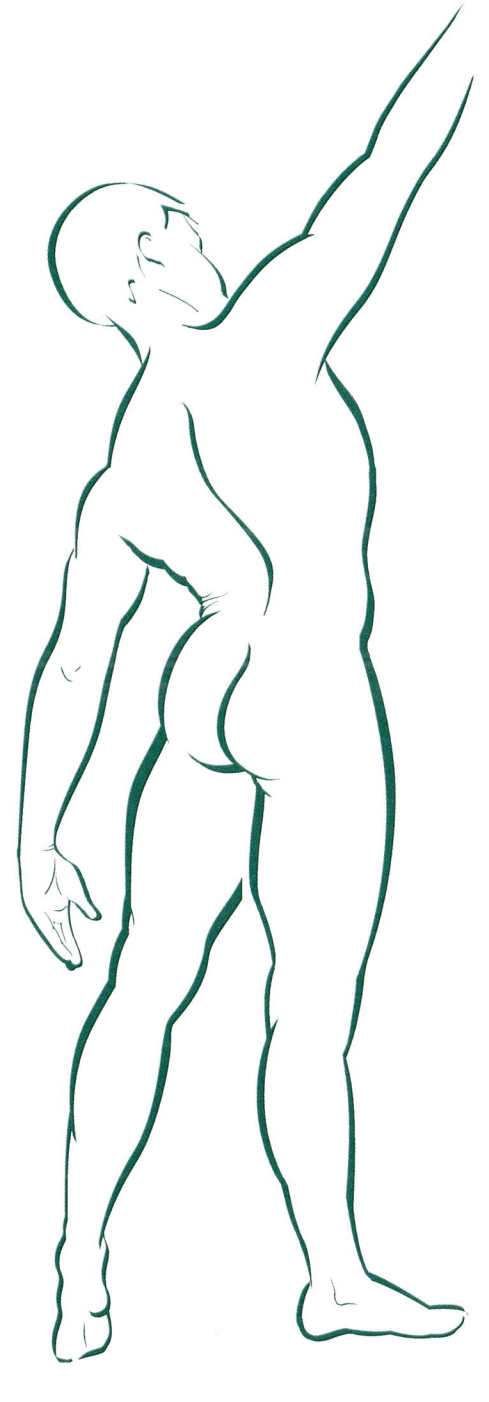

Brachytherapy has become an established and effective treatment intervention for patients with clinically localized prostate cancer. Fifteen year results have been reported using modern treatment techniques, and outcomes appear to be similar to what have been achieved with surgery or external beam radiotherapy. Newer approaches with brachytherapy have incorporated conformal treatment planning tools which more precisely tailor radiation doses to the target and more effectively minimize dose levels delivered to the urethra and rectum. Beams eye view, 3-dimensional target, and normal tissue reconstruction and intraoperative treatment planning are some of those tools now available to further enhance the conformality of the brachytherapy dose distribution. Combined approaches using permanent seed implantation with an abbreviated course of external beam radiotherapy is an effective form of dose escalation for patients with intermediate and selected high risk prostate cancer. High dose rate brachytherapy using temporary placement of Iridium-192 for several high dose fractions, in conjunction with a short course of external beam radiotherapy, is another effective technique to deliver concentrated doses to the prostate with a relatively low incidence of long-term complications. These newer techniques have effectively reduced acute and late toxicities of treatment and in turn have improved the quality of life of treated patients.

This chapter will summarize the appropriate selection criteria for considering brachytherapy for patients with low risk and more advanced stages of prostate cancer. The various forms of brachytherapy delivery and advantages of commonly used isotopes will be highlighted. Finally, the expected biochemical outcomes and treatment related side effects as well as potential complications of therapy will be reviewed.

Treatment Planning – Features of Preplanning and Intraoperative Planning Approaches

Preplanning

Highlights

Patient is planned several days to weeks before the procedure using the transrectal axial images of the prostate

Prostate and normal tissues are contoured on each of the images

Isodose distributions and dose volume histograms are obtained to determine in advance of the procedure the dose to prostate, urethra, and rectum

Advantages

Number of needles and seeds determined in advance and appropriate number of seeds can be ordered in advance which saves time during the procedure

Limitations

Necessary to recreate in the operating room the preplan geometry of the prostate and patient position in an attempt to simulate preplanning conditions

Need to account for intraoperative prostate edema secondary to needle placement which affects prostate size and shape

Intraoperative planning

Highlights

Patient is planned in the operating room using the transrectal axial images of the prostate. At Memorial Sloan-Kettering Cancer Center, needles are placed at the periphery of the prostate via ultrasound guidance. The images are then captured and downloaded into a treatment plan-ning system which calculates the ideal seed positions necessary to achieve optimal dose to the prostate with constrained dose levels delivered to the urethra and rectal wall [2,3]. Other commercially available systems can track position of deposited seeds and adjust the treatment plan, yet the exact location for the majority of the seed positions after placement within the gland is often difficult to see with ultrasound images due to hemorrhage, prostatic calcifica-tions, and image interference from other needles or other deposited seeds.

Isodose distributions and dose volume histograms are obtained in less than 1 minute after contouring and image downloading to intraoperative planning system. Computer-generated seed loading diagram obtained

Advantages

Real-time planning accommodates prostate edema and changes in geometry of the prostate which often occur during the actual procedure. Doses delivered to normal tissues can be appreciated real time and appropriate adjustments made to improve the dose distribution

Limitations

Need to approximate based on the prostate size, the number of seeds necessary to order before the case

Adds operating room time compared to preplanned implants; yet with updated available systems added, operating room time amounts to 10–20 minutes

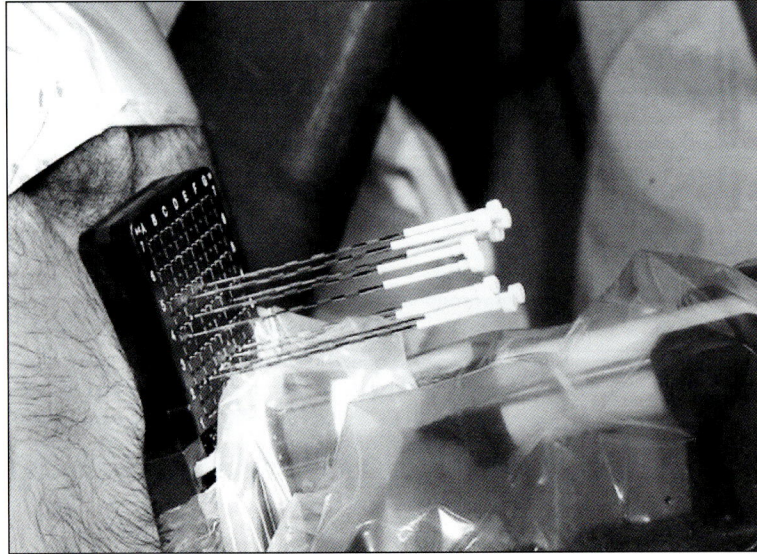

FIGURE 14-7. Figure 14-7 demonstrates peripheral needles in the process of being placed prior to image capture during intraoperative treat-ment planning.

Brachytherapy for Prostate Cancer

14

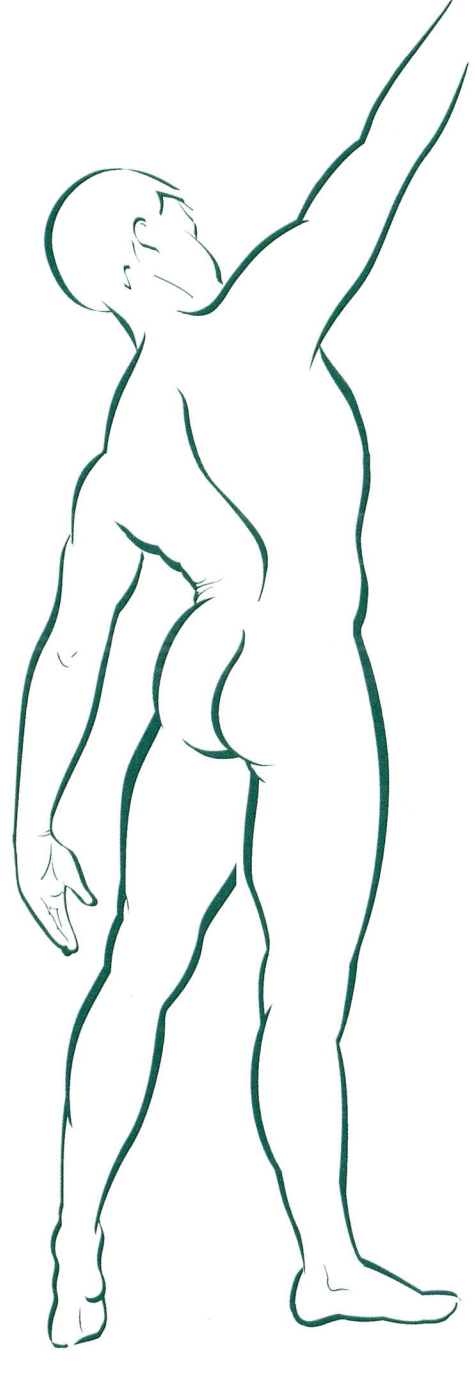

Michael J. Zelefsky

Brachytherapy has become an established and effective treatment intervention for patients with clinically localized prostate cancer. Fifteen year results have been reported using modern treatment techniques, and outcomes appear to be similar to what have been achieved with surgery or external beam radiotherapy. Newer approaches with brachytherapy have incorporated conformal treatment planning tools which more precisely tailor radiation doses to the target and more effectively minimize dose levels delivered to the urethra and rectum. Beams eye view, 3-dimensional target, and normal tissue reconstruction and intraoperative treatment planning are some of those tools now available to further enhance the conformality of the brachytherapy dose distribution. Combined approaches using permanent seed implantation with an abbreviated course of external beam radiotherapy is an effective form of dose escalation for patients with intermediate and selected high risk prostate cancer. High dose rate brachytherapy using temporary placement of Iridium-192 for several high dose fractions, in conjunction with a short course of external beam radiotherapy, is another effective technique to deliver concentrated doses to the prostate with a relatively low incidence of long-term complications. These newer techniques have effectively reduced acute and late toxicities of treatment and in turn have improved the quality of life of treated patients.

This chapter will summarize the appropriate selection criteria for considering brachytherapy for patients with low risk and more advanced stages of prostate cancer. The various forms of brachytherapy delivery and advantages of commonly used isotopes will be highlighted. Finally, the expected biochemical outcomes and treatment related side effects as well as potential complications of therapy will be reviewed.

B. Patients with Increased Likelihood for Acute and Late Symptoms after Prostate Brachytherapy
IPSS > 17 Patients with lower IPSS scores on concurrent α-blocker medications Prior urethral surgery or TURP Presence of prominent intravesical lobe (median lobe hypertrophy) Prior pelvic radiotherapy Active inflammatory bowel disease

▶ **FIGURE 14-1.** Selection criteria used for prostate brachytherapy. **A** and **B** summarize the selection criteria used for prostate brachytherapy. Ideal candidates for monotherapy are those with pretreatment characteristics associated with a low risk of extracapsular spread of disease (ECE) or seminal vesicle involvement (*ie*, PSA levels <10, low grade, low volume disease and early T stage). Those patients with higher risk of ECE are better suited for treatments which provide a biologically higher radiation dose to the prostate and extraprostatic tissues. The required escalation of dose can be accomplished with the delivery of brachytherapy in combination external beam radiotherapy. Other selection criteria listed in the tables attempt to identify patients with a lower likelihood of urinary morbidity after brachytherapy (lower IPSS scores, no prior urethral surgery). IPSS–International Prostate Symptom Score; PSA–prostate-specific antigen.

Characteristics of Commonly Used Isotopes for Brachytherapy			
	Iodine-125	**Palladium-103**	**Iridium-192**
Average energy (MeV)	0.028	0.021	0.318
Half-life	60 days	17 days	74 days
Dose rate	7 cGy/hour	21 cGy/hour	37.5 cGy/hour (45 Gy/5 days)
Utility	Permanent implants, low risk disease	Permanent implants, more often considered for higher Gleason tumors	High dose rate temporary implants
Advantages	Compared to Palladium-103, the radiation dose has a wider radial distance of exposure to provide broader dose coverage	Shorter half-life and decreased time period for radiation safety precaution compared to I-125	Ideal for temporary implants due to higher energy x-rays
Typical prescription dose	144 Gy	125 Gy	5.5–7 Gy fraction x 3 followed by 45–50 Gy of external beam radiotherapy

▶ **FIGURE 14-2.** Characteristics of commonly used isotopes for brachytherapy. This table describes the characteristics of the commonly used isotopes. Iodine-125 and Palladium-103 are most commonly employed for permanent interstitial implantation. A phase III randomized trial comparing the outcome of these two isotopes, when used for permanent interstitial implantation, has been performed and preliminary results of the study have not demonstrated significant differences in outcome.

Indications for Combining External Beam Radiotherapy with Permanent Seed Implantation

Gleason > 7 disease
PSA > 10
> 50% positive biopsy cores
 	
Contraindications for full dose external beam radiotherapy
  Dose to rectum, bladder determined by computer plan to exceed dose-volume tolerance constraints
  Bowel in close proximity to prostate precluding safe delivery of high dose external beam radiotherapy
  Bilateral hip replacements precluding adequate visualization of the prostate on treatment planning CT

▶ **FIGURE 14-3.** Indications for combining external beam radiotherapy with permanent seed implantation. The indications for using a combined regimen of brachytherapy and external beam radiotherapy are shown in this table. A typical regimen used at Memorial Sloan-Kettering Cancer Center (MSKCC) is I-125 permanent seed implant prescribing 110 Gy to the prostate target followed 60 days later with intensity modulated external beam radiotherapy (IMRT) delivering an additional 50.4 Gy. When Palladium-103 is selected as the isotope, the typical brachytherapy prescription dose is 100 Gy combined with IMRT. There are variations in practice patterns regarding the sequencing of external radiotherapy and seed implantation; other centers have initiated therapy with external radiotherapy followed by the implant boost. A phase III randomized trial 0232 conducted by the Radiation Therapy Oncology Group (RTOG) is currently underway testing the efficacy of combined regimens (external beam radiotherapy plus brachytherapy) versus seed implantation alone for intermediate risk disease. PSA–prostate-specific antigen.

Recommended Radiation Safety Precautions after Permanent Prostate Brachytherapy at MSKCC

	Implant radionuclide	
	I-125	Pd-103
Typical surface anterior dose rate on date of implant (mSv/hour)	Mean 40 Range 1–70	Mean 8 Range < 1–18
Typical 30 cm anterior (lap) dose rate on date of implant (mSv/hour)	Mean 6 Range < 1–15	Mean 3 Range < 1–8
Avoid close (ie, within 30 cm) contact or sleeping in the "spoon" position with infants, children, or pregnant women for extended periods of time (ie, >30 minutes per day)	6 months	3 months
Avoid sleeping in the "spoon" position (ie, in contact with the surface anterior area of the prostate) with a nonpregnant partner	6 months	No restriction
Security monitors – in case of alarms, carry card identifying the presence of implant	6 months	3 months
Strain urine to identify and catch potential lost seeds	1 week	
Sexual activity	1 week–1 month post implant	
Nonpregnant sexual partner	Use condom for first 5 ejaculates	
Pregnant sexual partner	Use condom until pregnancy completed	
Brief close contact (ie, hugging, kissing, shaking hands, etc)	No restrictions	

▶ **FIGURE 14-4.** Recommended radiation safety precautions after permanent prostate brachytherapy at Memorial Sloan-Kettering Cancer Center (MSKCC). In general, 5 half-lives of the isotope need to elapse before the implant is considered inactive or inert. Isotopes used for permanent interstitial implantation deliver low energy gamma x-rays which do not penetrate far beyond the seed. In fact, the radial distance of a radioactive iodine seed delivering its high dose is 1–1.5 cm circumferentially around the source. Nevertheless, with anywhere from 60–120 sources placed within the prostate gland, radioactivity can be detected during the first several months after a seed implant and appropriate precautions are prudent [1]. Recommended precautions are listed in this table.

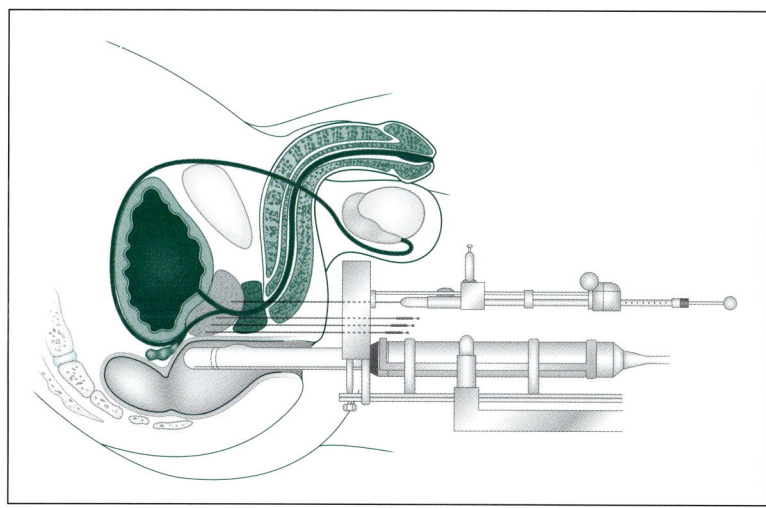

▶ **FIGURE 14-5.** Transperineal ultrasound guided approach. The patient is placed in an extended lithotomy position and needles are placed via ultrasound guidance. A stepping unit is fixed to the ultrasound unit so that axial images of the prostate can be obtained at 5 millimeter intervals. Sagittal or longitudinal images can also be obtained and are extremely helpful in guiding the needles to the base of the prostate and not through the bladder wall. The sagittal image is also useful for identification of the apex of the prostate gland. A 5–10 degree downward tilt of the tip of the ultrasound is recommended, as this better accommodates the probe to follow the posterior contour of the prostate. This would then reduce the risk of unnecessary needle positioning through the rectal wall. Visualization of the urethra is an important aspect of the procedure. A catheter is placed as shown in Figure 14-5 and/or a urethrogram can be performed with injection of aerated lubrication gel, which is well visualized on ultrasound images.

Treatment Planning – Features of Preplanning and Intraoperative Planning Approaches

FIGURE 14-6. Brachytherapy treatment planning and features of preplanning and intraoperative planning approaches.

Preplanning

Highlights

Patient is planned several days to weeks before the procedure using the transrectal axial images of the prostate

Prostate and normal tissues are contoured on each of the images

Isodose distributions and dose volume histograms are obtained to determine in advance of the procedure the dose to prostate, urethra, and rectum

Advantages

Number of needles and seeds determined in advance and appropriate number of seeds can be ordered in advance which saves time during the procedure

Limitations

Necessary to recreate in the operating room the preplan geometry of the prostate and patient position in an attempt to simulate preplanning conditions

Need to account for intraoperative prostate edema secondary to needle placement which affects prostate size and shape

Intraoperative planning

Highlights

Patient is planned in the operating room using the transrectal axial images of the prostate. At Memorial Sloan-Kettering Cancer Center, needles are placed at the periphery of the prostate via ultrasound guidance. The images are then captured and downloaded into a treatment planning system which calculates the ideal seed positions necessary to achieve optimal dose to the prostate with constrained dose levels delivered to the urethra and rectal wall [2,3]. Other commercially available systems can track position of deposited seeds and adjust the treatment plan, yet the exact location for the majority of the seed positions after placement within the gland is often difficult to see with ultrasound images due to hemorrhage, prostatic calcifications, and image interference from other needles or other deposited seeds.

Isodose distributions and dose volume histograms are obtained in less than 1 minute after contouring and image downloading to intraoperative planning system. Computer-generated seed loading diagram obtained

Advantages

Real-time planning accommodates prostate edema and changes in geometry of the prostate which often occur during the actual procedure. Doses delivered to normal tissues can be appreciated real time and appropriate adjustments made to improve the dose distribution

Limitations

Need to approximate based on the prostate size, the number of seeds necessary to order before the case

Adds operating room time compared to preplanned implants; yet with updated available systems added, operating room time amounts to 10–20 minutes

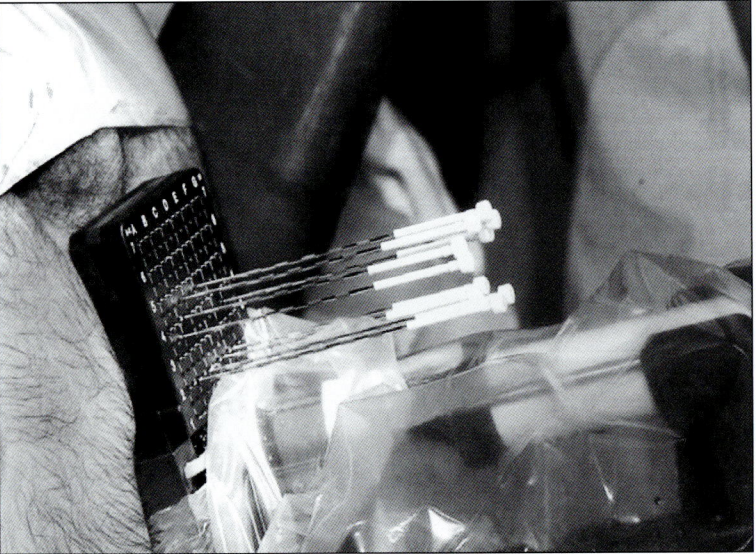

FIGURE 14-7. Figure 14-7 demonstrates peripheral needles in the process of being placed prior to image capture during intraoperative treatment planning.

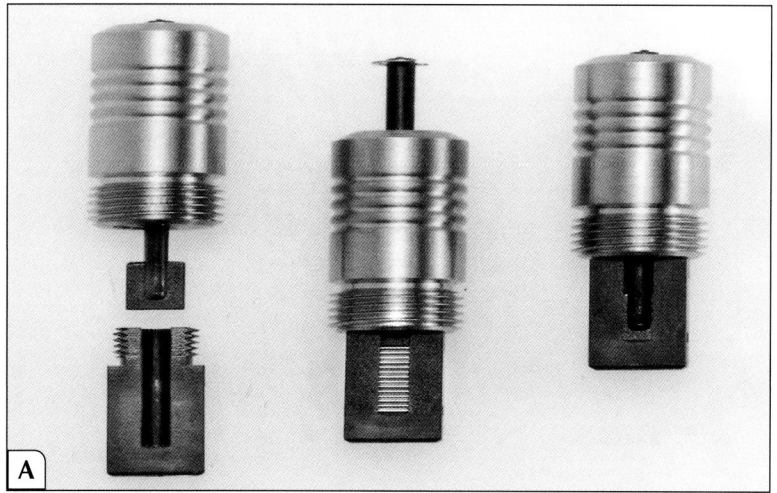

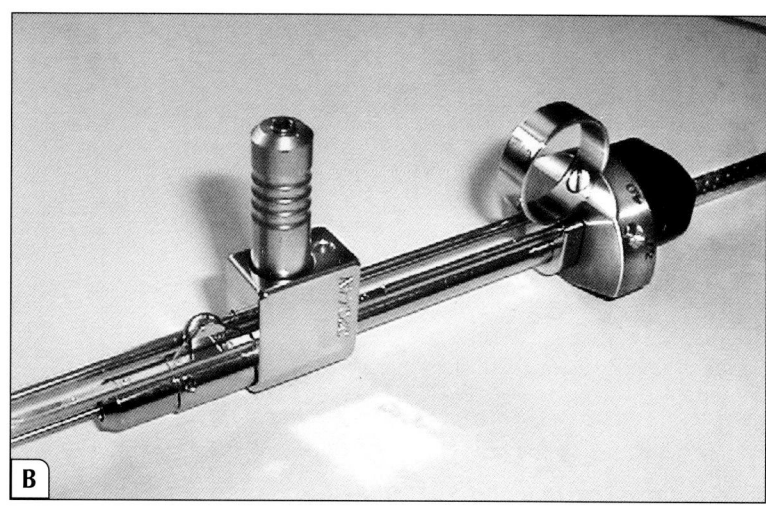

▶ **FIGURE 14-8.** Seed cartridges and applicator. **A** shows the shielded cartridge which houses the radioactive seeds and contains 15 seeds per cartridge. **B** demonstrates the Mick applicator (Mick Radio-Nuclear Instruments, Inc., New York) with the seed cartridge in place. In this case individual seeds are deposited within the gland, and the applicator retracts the needle at 5 millimeter (or other pre-determined) gradations to facilitate accurate seed placement. Another commonly used approach is placement of a strand of seeds within the gland, which may further reduce seed migration, –yet does not provide the flexibility of seed placement at customized spacing or intervals which can be required when using intraoperative conformal planning.

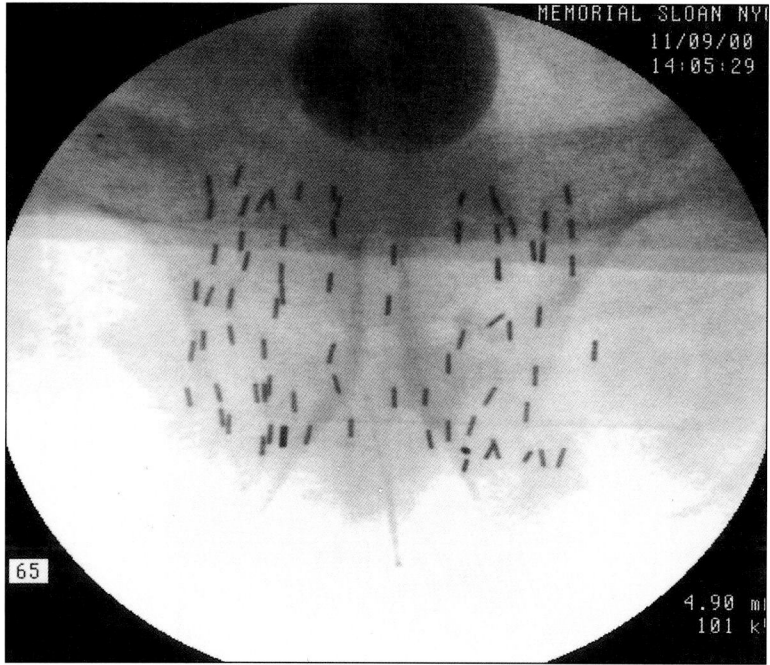

▶ **FIGURE 14-9.** Fluoroscopic image of I-125 seeds deposited within the prostate. Fluoroscopy is a useful intraoperative adjunct in addition to ultrasound to visualize seeds as they are being deposited and make immediate adjustments for enhanced seed positioning.

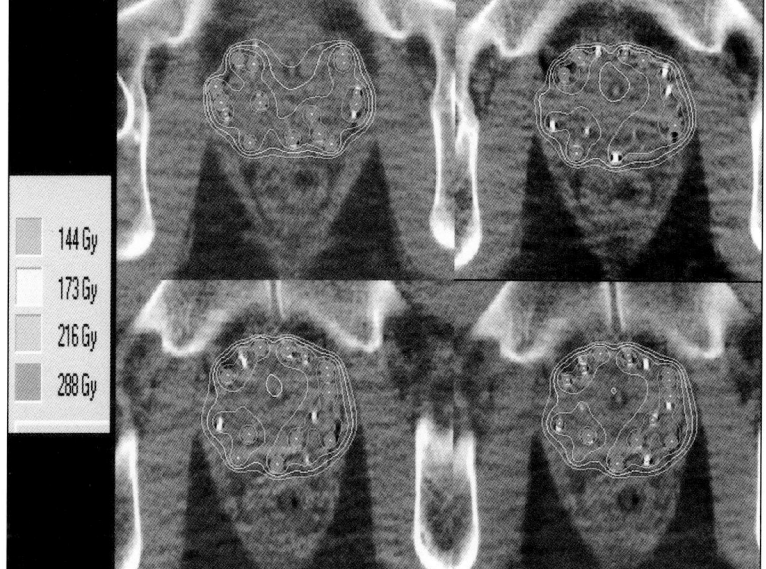

▶ **FIGURE 14-10.** (*See Color Plate*) Post-implantation evaluation. The American Brachytherapy Society [4] recommends that all patients should undergo postimplantation dosimetric evaluation. To accomplish this, CT scan is obtained on either the day of the implant procedure or 30 days after procedure (depending upon the institutional practice). Commercially available software is used to determine the actual 3-dimensional dose distributions for the prostate and normal tissues based upon the actual seed positions within the prostate and their proximity to the urethra and rectum. Dose volume histograms are then generated, which will display important dosimetric parameters of implant quality. The postimplant dosimetric evaluation represents a critical quality assurance tool after prostate implantation. It is helpful for the identification of suboptimal implants as well as providing feedback to the clinician as a guide for further technical improvements. Important dosimetric parameters for the target include V100 (volume of the prostate receiving 100% of the prescription dose) and the D90 (dose delivered to the 90% of the prostate gland). Several reports have documented that for I-125 implants, higher D90 levels have been associated with improved long-term biochemical outcomes [5,6]. Other parameters which are important to extract from the postimplantation evaluation include doses to the urethra and rectum. For these normal tissue structures, maximum, average doses and D30, *ie*, dose to 30% of the respective volumes for these structures have been reported.

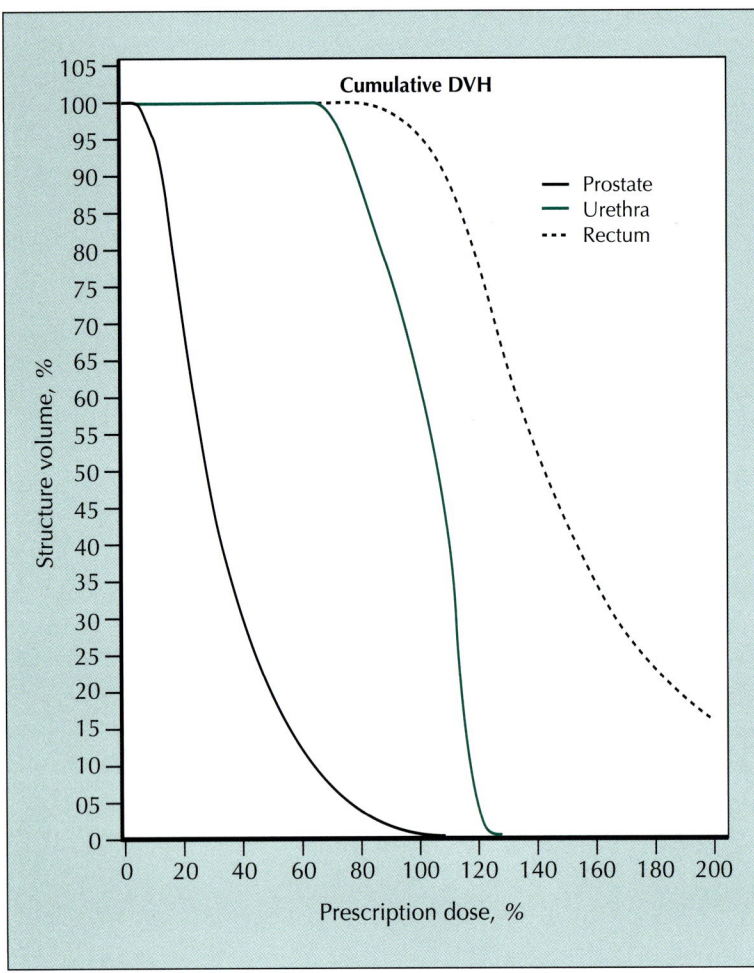

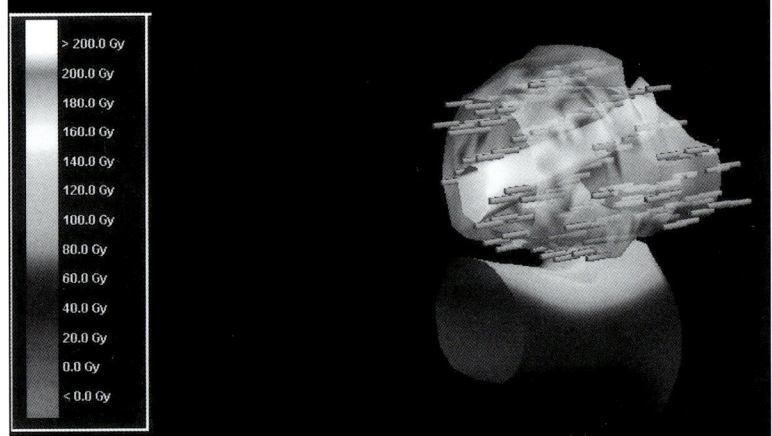

▶ **FIGURE 14-11.** A dose volume histogram (DVH) assessment based on a post-implantation CT scan. In the case illustrated, the v100 is above 95%, the D30 for the urethra is 110% of the prescription dose, and the D30 for the rectum is 40% of the prescription doses.

▶ **FIGURE 14-12.** (*See Color Plate*) Three-dimensional reconstruction of the dose clouds surrounding the target (*ie*, prostate) and the rectum (*blue*). The urethra traversing through the prostate is also shown.

A. Acute Symptoms after Permanent Prostate Brachytherapy

Acute Symptoms	Developing symptoms, %	Symptoms management
Acute urinary retention	3–7	Catheter placement for several days, α-blockers
Urinary obstructive symptoms	60–80	α-blockers, nonsteroidal anti-inflammatory medications
Rectal urgency	10–20	High fiber diet
Rectal bleeding	5	Sitz baths, cortisone suppositories, high fiber diet

B. Late Symptoms after Permanent Prostate Brachytherapy

Late symptoms	Developing symptoms, %	Median time to develop, mo	Recommended treatment approach
Impotence	20–80	12–24	Sildenafil citrate, vacuum pump devices, intracavernosal prostaglandin injections, penile implants
Urethral stricture	1–2	18–36	Urethral dilation, TURP
Chronic urinary obstructive symptoms	15–20	3–36	α-blockers
Rectal bleeding	4–6	10–12	Cortisone suppositories, sitz baths, high fiber diet
Rectal ulcer (grade 3–4)	≤ 1	12–24	Maintain conservative measures, argon laser treatments, formalin applications, avoid deep biopsies and cauterization procedures

▶ **FIGURE 14-13.** Summary of acute (**A**) and late (**B**) symptoms after permanent implantation. Brachytherapy for prostate cancer is associated with acute and potential late morbidity. Thus careful criteria need to be employed for treatment selection for the individual patient. In particular those patients with large glands, significant urinary obstructive symptoms, and prior urethral surgery are not optimal candidates for the procedure.

In general most acute symptoms resolve within the first year. Careful management of late symptoms is paramount. Aggressive strategies to address urethral and rectal complications such as overzealous biopsies and cauterization can lead to fistula development and should be avoided if possible. TURP–transurethral resection of the prostate.

Biochemical Relapse-free Survival Rates for Permanent Seed Implantation for Prostate Cancer

Series	Treatment	Patients, n	Median follow-up, mo	Low risk, %	Intermediate risk, %	High risk, %
Grimm et al. [7]	I-125	125	81	87	78	-
Blasko et al. [8]	Pd-103	230	42	94	82	65
Kollmeier et al. [9]	I-125	243	75	88	81	65
Merrick (Personal communication)	I-125	156	78	95	90	-
Zelefsky (Unpublished data) (using real time planning)	I-125	276	40	96	93	-
Beyer [10]	I-125/Pd-103	1266	50	85	78	58
Sharkey et al. [11]	Pd-103	1458	44	89	89	88
Potters et al. [12]	I-125/Pd-103	493	41	92	74	55

▶ **FIGURE 14-14.** Biochemical relapse-free survival rates for permanent seed implantation for prostate cancer.

Features of HDR Prostate Brachytherapy

Transperineal placement of afterloading catheters via ultrasound guidance in the prostate. After treatment planning, catheters are connected to an afterloading machine which houses the Iridum-192 source. The radioactive source is programmed to traverse through each of the catheters to deliver its high dose fraction

Permanent seeds not deposited

Less radiation safety considerations for the patient

Means of delivering several high dose fractions in a short period of time to the tumor which could serve as a radiobiologic advantage for improved tumor cell kill

Flexibility of computer planning to allow the Iridium-192 source to dwell for different lengths of time at various positions within the needles, which will in turn generate a highly conformal dose distribution of the radiation

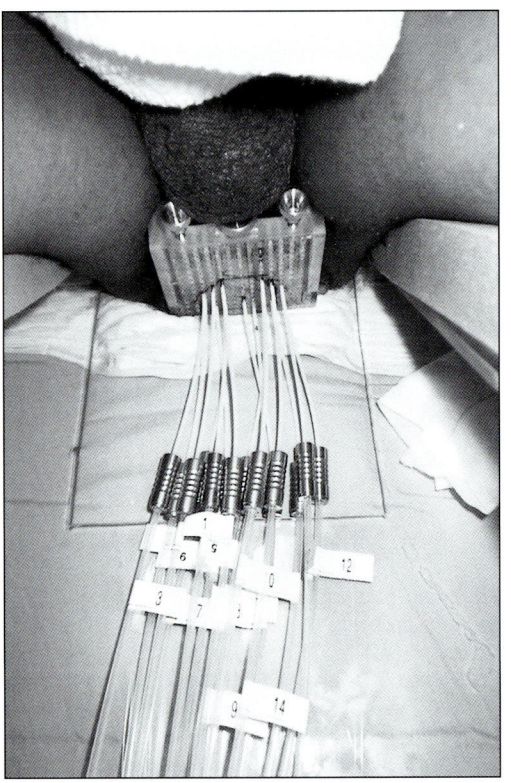

▶ **FIGURE 14-15.** Features and advantages for high dose rate (HDR) temporary implantation. High dose rate temporary prostate implants represent an excellent alternative for brachytherapy delivery to the prostate. In general the HDR treatment is used as a boost to deliver several high dose fractions (over a 24–36 hour time period) followed several weeks later with supplemental external beam radiotherapy to doses of 45–50.4 Gy. HDR fraction sizes have ranged from 4–9.5 Gy delivered with Iridium-192. The large fraction sizes (in comparison to the low dose implants and the conventional 1.8 Gy fraction sizes delivered with external beam radiotherapy) is a potential radiobiologic advantage of this form of therapy because of evidence that prostate cancer cells possess an enhanced capability to repair radiation damage between radiation fractions. It is therefore expected that such high dose fractions may be more effective in suppressing the repair of radiation injury to cancer cells resulting in improved tumor control. Ongoing Phase I-II single institution studies are testing HDR brachytherapy as a single modality treatment (without supplemental external beam radiotherapy) and preliminary results appear promising with low rates of treatment-related complications [13,14].

▶ **FIGURE 14-16.** Afterloading catheters transperineally inserted via ultrasound guidance. These catheters are in turn connected to cables of an afterloading machine which will serve as conduits for the radiation source to pass through.

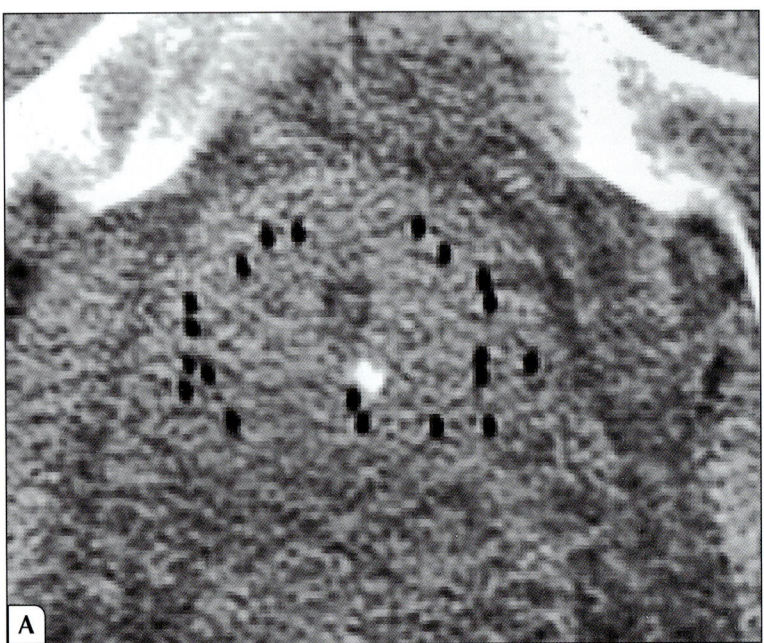

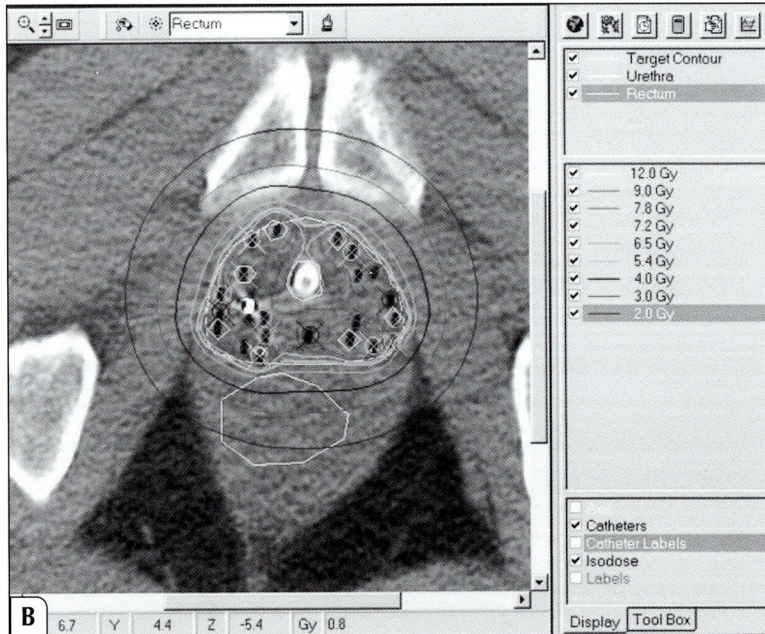

▶ **FIGURE 14-17.** (*See Color Plate*) Afterloading catheters. **A** shows the afterloading catheters in place and the dose distribution for an HDR fraction, **B**. For this patient, the dose per fraction was 6.5 Gy and the green 6.5 Gy isodose line demonstrates excellent coverage of the target volume with the prescribed dose.

Outcome of HDR Prostate Brachytherapy

Series	Patients, n	Median follow-up, y	Biochemical control according to risk group	Comments
Galalae et al. [15] (Multi-institutional study)	611	5	Favorable – 96% Intermediate – 88% Unfavorable – 69%	-
Demanes et al. [16] (Oakland, CA)	209	7.2	Favorable – 90% Intermediate – 87% Unfavorable – 69%	Grade 3 urinary toxicity was 6.7% most occurring in patients with prior TURP
Deger et al. [17] (Berlin)	442	5	Favorable – 81% Intermediate – 65% Unfavorable – 59%	-
Astrom et al. [18] (Sweden)	214	4	Favorable – 92% Intermediate – 88% Unfavorable – 61%	Urethra strictures in 13/214 patients

▶ **FIGURE 14-18.** Outcome of high dose rate (HDR) prostate brachytherapy.

REFERENCES

1. Dauer LT, Zelefsky MJ, Horan C, et al.: Assessment of radiation safety instruction to patients based on measured dose rates following prostate brachytherapy. Brachytherapy 2004, 3:1–6.

2. Zelefsky MJ: Three-dimensional conformal brachytherapy for prostate cancer. Curr Urol Rep 2004, 5:173–178.

3. Zelefsky MJ, Yamada Y, Marion C, et al.: Improved conformality and decreased toxicity with intraoperative computer–optimized transperineal ultrasound-guided prostate brachytherapy. Int J Radiat Oncol Biol Phys 2003, 55:956–963.

4. Nag S, Bice W, DeWyngaert K, et al.: The American Brachytherapy Society Recommendations for permanent prostate brachytherapy post implant dosimetric analysis. Int J Radiat Oncol Biol Phys 2000, 46:221–230.

5. Stock RG, Stone NN, Dahlal M, et al.: What is the optimal dose for 125-I prostate implants? A dose response analysis of biochemical control, posttreatment prostate biopsies and long-term urinary symptoms. Brachytherapy 2002, 1:83–89.

6. Potters L, Cao Y, Cauguru E, et al.: A comprehensive review of CT-based dosimetry parameters and biochemical control in patients treated with permanent prostate brachytherapy. Int J Radiat Oncol Biol Phys 2001, 50:605–614.

7. Grimm PD, Blasko JC, Sylvester JE, et al.: 10-year biochemical (prostate-specific antigen) control of prostate cancer with (125) I brachytherapy. Int J Radiat Oncol Biol Phys 2001, 51:31–40.

8. Blasko JC, Grimm PD, Sylvester JE, et al.: Palladium-103 brachytherapy for prostate carcinoma. Int J Radiat Oncol Biol Phys 2000, 46:839–850.

9. Kollmeier MA, Stock RG, Stone N: Biochemical outcomes after prostate brachytherapy with 5-year minimal follow-up: importance of patient selection and implant quality. Int J Radiat Oncol Biol Phys 2003, 57:645–653.

10. Beyer DC, Thomas T, Hilbe J, et al.: Relative influence of Gleason score and pre-treatment PSA in predicting survival following brachytherapy for prostate cancer. Brachytherapy 2003, 2:77–84.

11. Sharkey J, Cantor A, Solc Z, et al.: (103) Pd brachytherapy versus radical prostatectomy in patients with clinically localized prostate cancer: A 12-year experience from a single group practice. Brachytherapy 2005, 4:34–44.

12. Potters L, Cha C, Oshinsky G, et al.: Risk profiles to predict PSA relapse-free survival for patients undergoing permanent prostate brachytherapy. Cancer J Sci Am 1999, 5:301–306.

13. Martinez AA, Pataki I, Edmunson G, et al.: Phase II prospective study of the use of conformal high-dose rate brachytherapy as monotherapy for the treatment of favorable stage prostate cancer: a feasibility report. Int J Radiat Oncol Biol Phys 2001, 49:61–69.

14. Grills IS, Martinez AA, Hollander M, et al.: High dose rate brachytherapy as prostate cancer monotherapy reduces toxicity compared to low dose rate palladium seeds. J Urol 2004, 171:1098–1104.

15. Galalae RM, Martinez A, Mate T, et al.: Long-term outcome by risk factors using conformal high-dose rate brachytherapy (HDR-BT) with or without neoadjuvant androgen suppression for localized prostate cancer. Int J Radiat Oncol Biol Phys 2004, 58 :1048–1055.

16. Demanes DJ, Rodriguez RR, Schour L, et al.: High dose rate intensity modulated brachytherapy with external beam radiotherapy for prostate cancer: California endocurietherapy's 10-year results. Int J Radiat Oncol Biol Phys 2005, 61:1306–1316.

17. Deger S, Boehmer D, Roigas J, et al.: High dose rate (HDR) brachytherapy with conformal radiation therapy for localized prostate cancer. Eur Urol 2005, 47: 441–448.

18. Astrom L, Pedersen D, Mercke C, et al.: Long-term outcome of high dose rate brachytherapy in radiotherapy of localized prostate cancer. Radiother Oncol 2005, 74:157–161.

External Beam Radiotherapy for Prostate Cancer

15

*Mark K. Buyyounouski
& Alan Pollack*

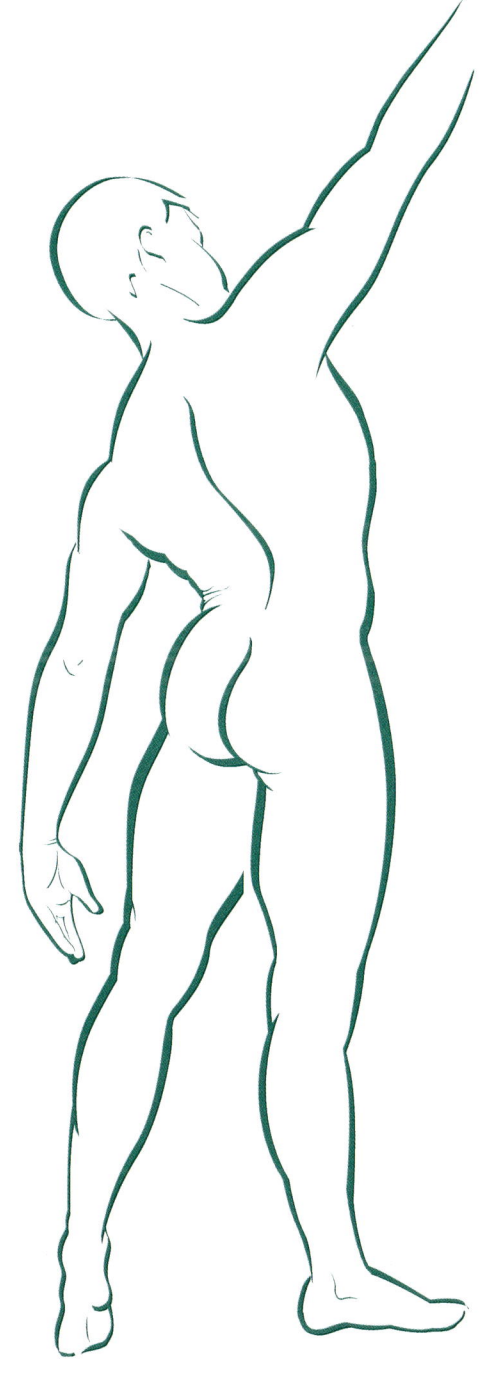

Prostate cancer is the most common nonskin cancer diagnosed in men across the United States. Contributing to the high rate is increasing patient awareness, screening with prostate-specific antigen (PSA), and ultrasound-guided biopsy methods. PSA is an extremely sensitive measure of prostate cancer that has changed the nature of the disease in terms of presentation and treatment outcome. As a consequence, there has been a shift in presentation to earlier stage, low-risk disease, and a recognition that we have not been curing as many men with radical prostatectomy or radiotherapy as once believed. These observations have been at the forefront of the impetus to develop more sophisticated methods of external beam radiotherapy (EBRT) delivery, such as three-dimensional treatment planning and conformal radiotherapy (3DCRT) and intensity-modulated radiotherapy (IMRT) and the combination of EBRT with androgen deprivation (AD). 3DCRT and IMRT are more precise at targeting the prostate and better spare the surrounding normal tissues, such that EBRT dose may be escalated. Dose escalation improves freedom from biochemical failure (FFBF). The combination of AD and EBRT improves FFBF and survival.

Prostate-specific antigen is also an outcome measure. Biochemical failure (BF) based on PSA is at times difficult to characterize in men treated with radiotherapy but is nonetheless an important correlate of clinical progression and the risk of dying from prostate cancer. Although there continues to be debate on the best definition of BF, biochemical parameters of relapse are foremost in decision making in men with prostate cancer who are treated with radiotherapy. The use of biochemical criteria has been instrumental in the development of clinical trials.

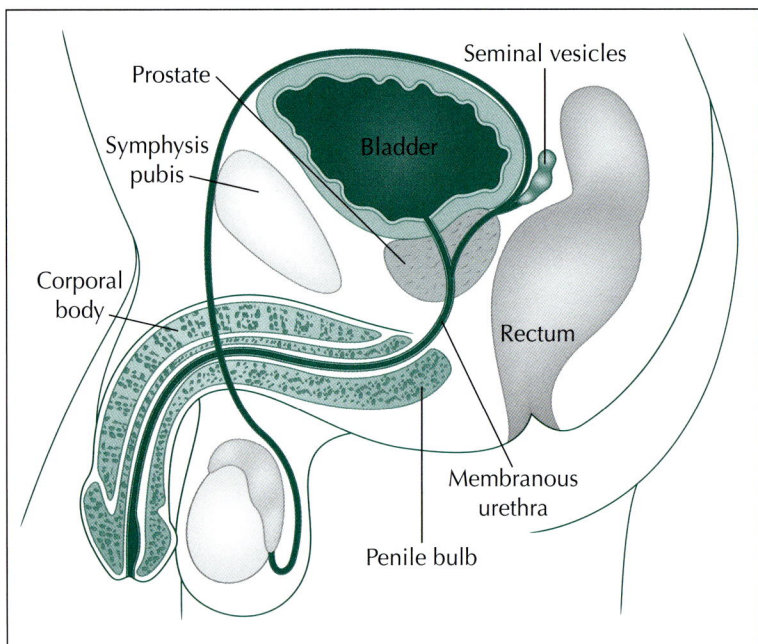

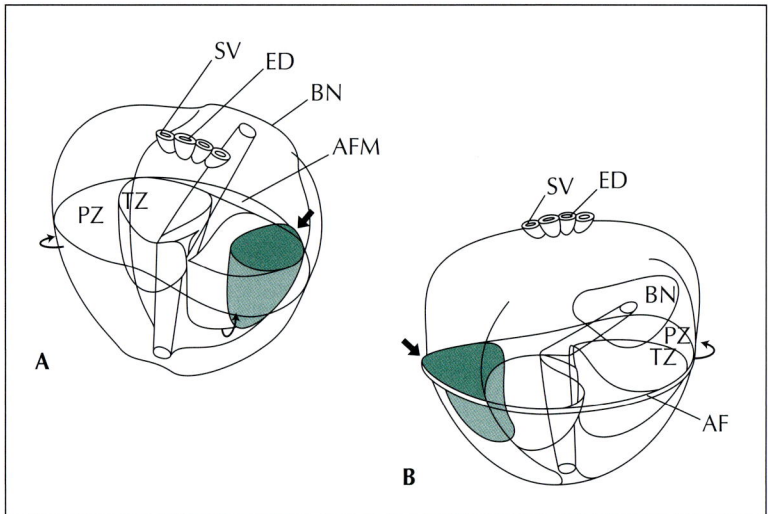

▶ **FIGURE 15-1.** Anatomy of the pelvis. The prostate is a glandular structure that is bounded superiorly by the bladder, inferiorly by the urogenital diaphragm that contains the membranous urethra, anteriorly by the pubic symphysis, laterally by the puborectalis muscle, and posteriorly by the rectum.

▶ **FIGURE 15-2.** Transparent perspectives of the zonal anatomy of the prostate and its relationship to surrounding structures. **A,** View from the rectal surface and above shows a transition zone (TZ) cancer (dark gray area) confined by the TZ boundary and penetrating the anterior fibromuscular (AFM) stroma (*arrow*). The TZ comprises approximately 5% of the prostate volume and consists of two pear-shaped lobes surrounding the proximal urethra. The TZ is a common site of nodular prostatic hyperplasia but is also the site of 10% of prostate cancer. **B,** View from the anterior surface and above shows a peripheral zone (PZ) cancer confined by the TZ boundary and penetrating capsule (*arrow*). *Curved arrows* indicate the place of cross section through the tumor. The PZ consists of 70% of the prostatic volume, which surrounds the transition and central zones and is the site of 80% of prostate cancers. AFM—anterior fibromuscular stroma; BN—bladder neck; ED—ejaculatory duct; SV—seminal vesicle. (*Adapted from* McNeal *et al.* [1], with permission.)

PATIENT EVALUATION AND RISK ASSESSMENT

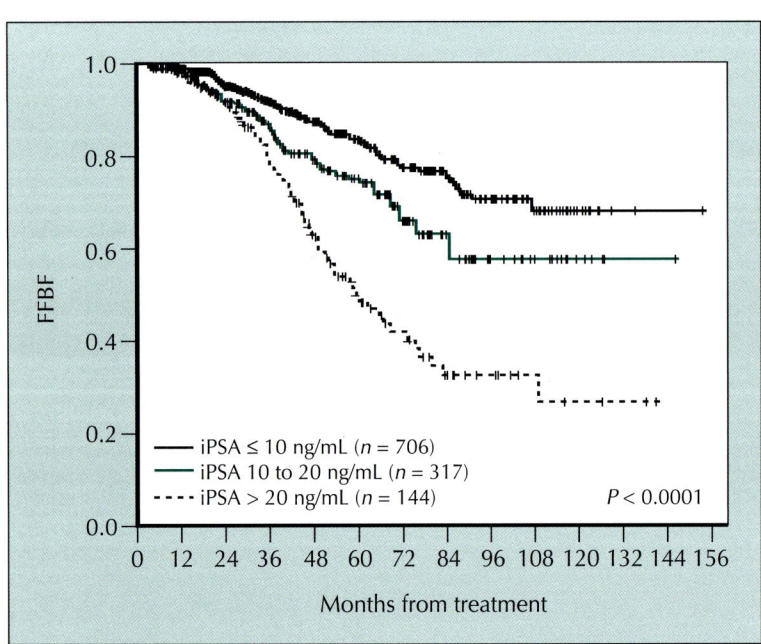

▶ **FIGURE 15-3.** Kaplan-Meier estimates of freedom from biochemical failure (FFBF) by initial pretreatment prostate-specific antigen (iPSA) level for 1167 men who received definitive three-dimensional conformal radiation therapy at Fox Chase Cancer Center between 1989 and 2001. Pretreatment prostate-specific antigen (PSA) is a strong predictor of patient outcome following radiation therapy but is not part of the American Joint Committee on Cancer staging system (*see* Fig. 15-4) because a relationship to survival has not been conclusively established. However, biochemical failure (BF), or a rising PSA profile following treatment, is a valid early end point for prostate cancer and has been standardized by the American Society of Therapeutic Radiation Oncology as three consecutive rises in PSA in 3- to 6-month intervals with backdating to the midpoint in time between the lowest post–external beam radiotherapy PSA (nadir PSA) and the first rise [2]. BF is a robust correlate of distant metastasis and disease-specific death [3]. *Vertical bars* represent censored events.

Clinical TNM Classification for Carcinoma of the Prostate Classification

Primary tumor (T)		Description
TX		Primary tumor cannot be assessed
T0		No evidence of primary tumor
T1		Clinically inapparent tumor neither palpable nor visible by imaging
	T1a	Tumor incidental histologic finding in 5% or less of resected tissue
	T1b	Tumor incidental histologic finding in more than 5% of resected tissue
	T1c	Tumor identified by needle biopsy (ie, elevated PSA)[*]
T2		Tumor confined within prostate[†]
	T2a	Tumor involves half of one lobe or less
	T2b	Tumor involves more than half of one lobe but not both lobes
	T2c	Tumor involves both lobes
T3		Tumor extends through the prostate capsule[‡]
	T3a	Extracapsular extension
	T3b	Tumor invades seminal vesicle(s)
T4		Tumor is fixed or invades adjacent structures other than seminal vesicles: bladder neck, external sphincter, rectum, levator muscles, and/or pelvic wall

Regional lymph nodes (N)

NX		Regional lymph nodes were not assessed
N1		No regional lymph node metastasis
N1		Metastasis in regional lymph node(s)

Distant metastasis (M)

MX		Distant metastasis cannot be assessed (not evaluated by any modality)
M0		No distant metastasis
M1		Distant metastasis

[*]Tumor found in one or both lobes by needle biopsy but not palpable or visible by imaging is classified as T1c.
[†]Tumor found in one or both lobes by needle biopsy but not palpable or reliably visible by imaging is classified as T1c.
[‡]Invasion into the prostatic apex or into (but not beyond) the prostatic capsule is classified not as T3, but as T2.

▶ **FIGURE 15-4.** Clinical TNM (tumor-nodes-metastasis) classification for carcinoma of the prostate. The rules for TNM classification according to the sixth edition of the American Joint Committee on Cancer staging handbook includes digital rectal examination (DRE) of the prostate and histologic or cytologic confirmation of prostate cancer [4]. In addition, it permits all information available before the first definitive treatment is used for clinical staging. For example, with the exception of T1c, imaging techniques such as transrectal ultrasound (TRUS) and endorectal coil magnetic resonance imaging (erMRI), as well as biopsy information such as tumor laterality (unilateral vs bilateral), may be used. The lack of definitive data concerning prediction of pathologic stage or patient outcome with TRUS [5,6], erMRI [7], and biopsy laterality information [8,9], together with the potential for significant stage migration as a consequence of using such imaging in staging, favors the use of DRE alone for the routine staging of prostate cancer.

The results with erMRI have the most potential for use in staging [10,11]. We use erMRI to confirm suspicion of extracapsular extension detected with DRE. For a patient with otherwise intermediate risk features and evidence of T3 disease on erMRI, we favor the addition of long-term androgen deprivation therapy [12,13].

Clinical pelvic lymph node staging with CT has a low detection rate for men with prostate-confined Gleason 2 to 7 disease [14]. Routine bone scans for the detection of distant metastasis may be reserved for patients with initial prostate-specific antigen (PSA) values greater than 10 ng/mL [15].

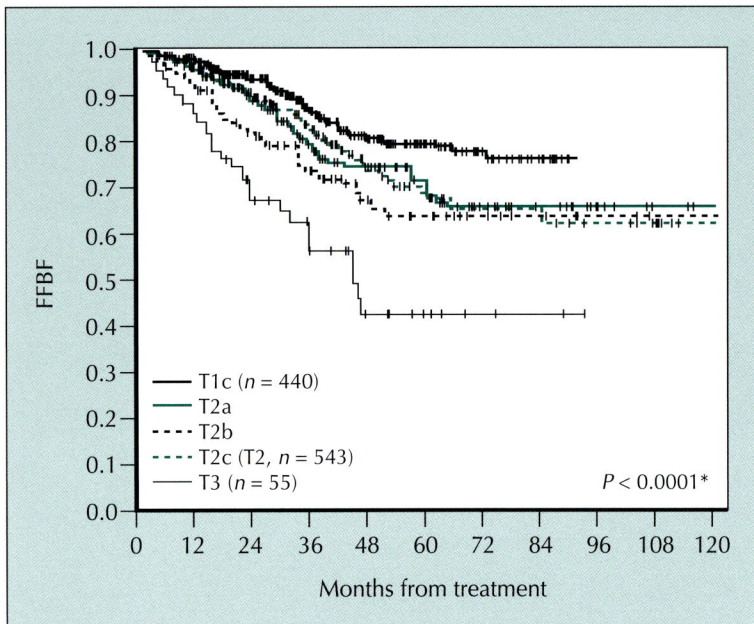

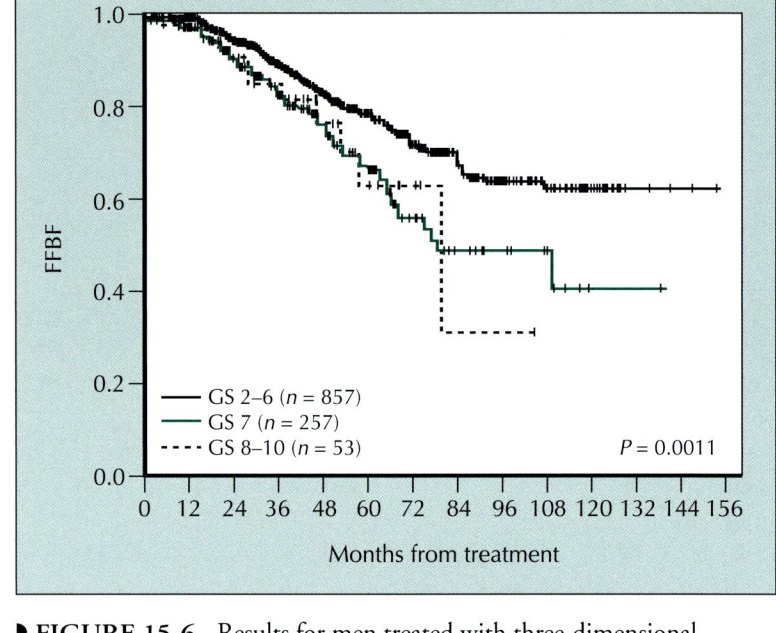

▶ **FIGURE 15-5.** Biochemical outcome by T category for men treated definitively with three-dimensional conformal radiotherapy alone at Fox Chase Cancer Center between 1989 and 1999. T2 subcategories were similar and intermediate between those with T1c and T3 disease. Five-year freedom from biochemical failure (FFBF) rates for the T2 subcategories were 70% for T2a, 72% for T2b, and 64% for T2c (*P* = 0.44). *Vertical bars* represent censored events. The *asterisk* represents the overall *P* value for T1c versus T2 versus T3. (*Adapted from* Buyyounouski *et al.* [8], with permission.)

▶ **FIGURE 15-6.** Results for men treated with three-dimensional conformal radiotherapy alone between 1989 and 2001 at Fox Chase Cancer Center by Gleason score (GS). The Gleason scoring system is the most commonly used grading system for prostate cancer [16]. The Gleason score consists of the sum of the major and minor glandular patterns, graded on a 1 to 5 scale. Gleason grade 1 denotes discrete glandular formation with slight disorganization, whereas Gleason grade 5 corresponds to an absence of glandular structures and anaplastic appearance. *Vertical bars* represent censored events. FFBF—freedom from biochemical failure. (*Adapted from* Chism *et al.* [20], with permission.)

The Single- and Double-Factor Risk Models

Risk	Single Factor	Double Factor
Low	iPSA ≤10 GS 2–6 T1–T2c*	iPSA ≤ 10 GS 2–6 T1–T2c
Intermediate	Presence of 1 or more:† iPSA > 10 and ≤ 20 GS 7	Presence of 1: iPSA > 10 GS ≥ 7 ≥ T3
High	Presence of 1 or more: iPSA > 20 GS 8–10 ≥ T3	Presence of 2 or 3: iPSA > 10 GS ≥ 7 ≥ T3

The single- and double-factor high-risk models are patterned after that described by D'Amico et al. [17] and Zelefsky et al. [18].
*T2b has sometimes been considered intermediate risk, and T2c has sometimes been considered intermediate or high risk [17,19]. In the Fox Chase database, these patients have about the same prognosis as patients with T2a disease in univariate and multivariate analysis, and so have been grouped in a favorable category here.
†No high-risk factors present. (Data from Chism et al. [20].)

▶ **FIGURE 15-7.** The single- and double-factor risk models. Two commonly used risk stratification schemes for clinically localized prostate cancer combine pretreatment initial PSA (iPSA), Gleason score (GS), and clinical T category (based on digital rectal examination) for assigning risk of biochemical failure after external beam radiotherapy (EBRT). The single-factor high-risk model used at Fox Chase Cancer Center (FCCC; modeled after D'Amico *et al.* [17]) classifies those with Gleason score 8 to 10, iPSA greater than 20 ng/mL, or T3/T4 disease as high risk. Included as intermediate risk are those with an iPSA of 10 to 20 ng/mL or Gleason 7 disease, as long as no high-risk factors are present. An alternative three-tier system used at Memorial Sloan-Kettering is the double-factor high-risk model [21]. In a comparison of these models by Chism *et al.* [20], the FCCC model resulted in more homogeneous groups. Low- and intermediate-risk patients are excellent candidates for EBRT alone, with 5-year biochemical failure–free survival. High-risk patients have been shown to benefit from long-term androgen deprivation in several randomized trials comparing EBRT with and without androgen deprivation therapy. (*Adapted from* Zelefsky *et al.* [18], with permission.)

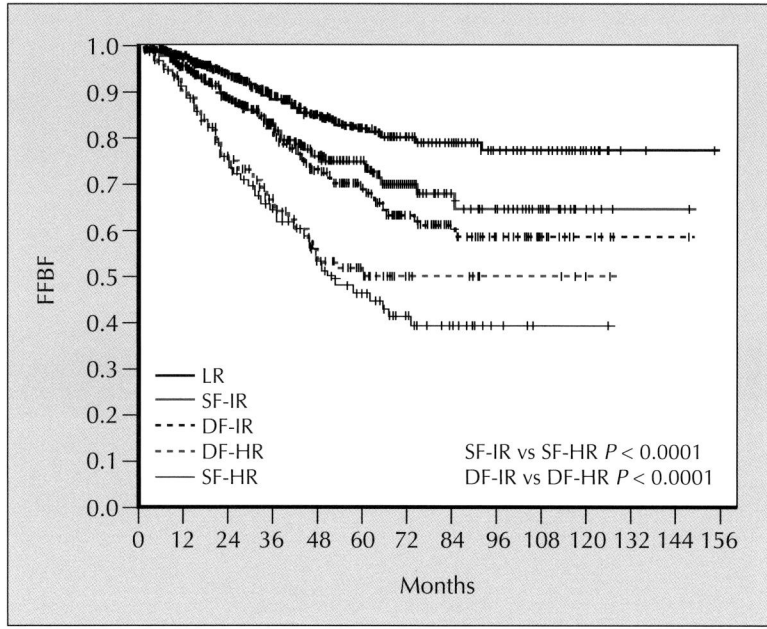

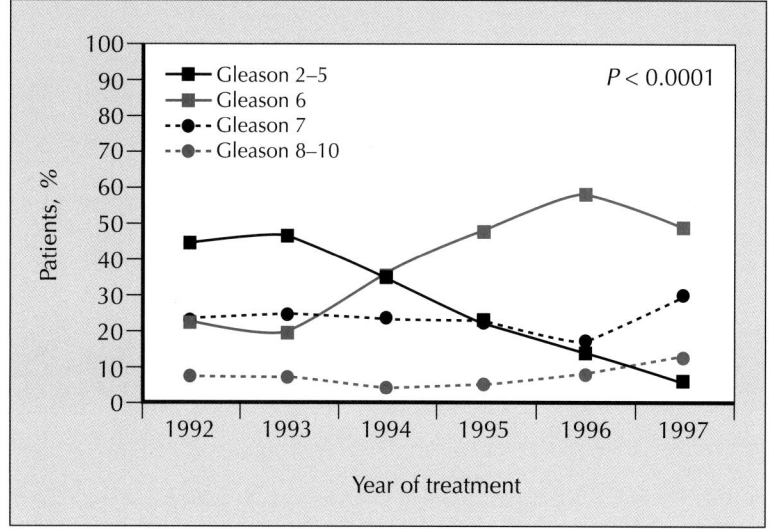

▶ **FIGURE 15-8.** Results for 1597 men treated with three-dimensional conformal radiotherapy alone for prostate cancer between 1989 and 2001 by the two risk groupings (single-factor [SF] and double-factor [DF]) shown in Figure 15-7. The selection of risk grouping can greatly influence freedom from biochemical failure (FFBF) results following external beam radiotherapy. Understanding the differences in risk stratification is central to the correct interpretation and comparison of outcomes between institutions, of dose escalation studies, and of studies testing additional therapies in combination with radiotherapy (*eg*, androgen deprivation therapy). Reserving the high-risk (HR) category for patients with the most ominous clinical features (Gleason score ≥ 8, prostate-specific antigen [PSA] > 20 ng/mL, or T3 disease) in the SF model translates to lower FFBF rates compared with the combination of PSA, Gleason, and T stage that denotes HR men in the DF model. This was explained by an "up-grouping" of DF-HR patients with more intermediate features compared with the SF method. Similarly, the presence of SF-HR men in the DF–intermediate risk (IR) group explains the slightly lower FFBF rate for the DF-IR group compared with the SF-IR group. The SF model is preferred over the DF model, given a preference to use a simple three-tier system. The nomograms of Kattan *et al.* [22] are more precise. *Vertical bars* represent censored events. LR—low risk for both SF and DF models. (*Adapted from* Chism *et al.* [20], with permission.)

▶ **FIGURE 15-9.** Percentage of patients with Gleason scores of 2 to 5, 6, 7, and 8 to 10 by year of treatment for 983 patients treated with conformal radiotherapy at Fox Chase Cancer Center between 1992 and 1997. A shift in Gleason score occurred during the 1990s, and by 1994, Gleason 2 to 5 disease was replaced by Gleason 6 disease as the most common grade found on biopsy. The shift to higher Gleason scores occurred in the setting of diagnosing patients with T1c disease more frequently and dropping pretreatment prostate-specific antigen. The Gleason score shift may be the result of replacing the secondary grade with the tertiary grade when the tertiary grade is higher [23] or less frequent diagnoses of Gleason 2 to 4 disease on prostate biopsy specimens at the recommendation of Dr. Epstein in 2000 [24]. In either case, the Gleason shift has occurred over time and has significant implications for the application of models incorporating Gleason score and nonrandomized analyses, such as sequential radiotherapy dose–escalation series. (*Adapted from* Chism *et al.* [25], with permission.)

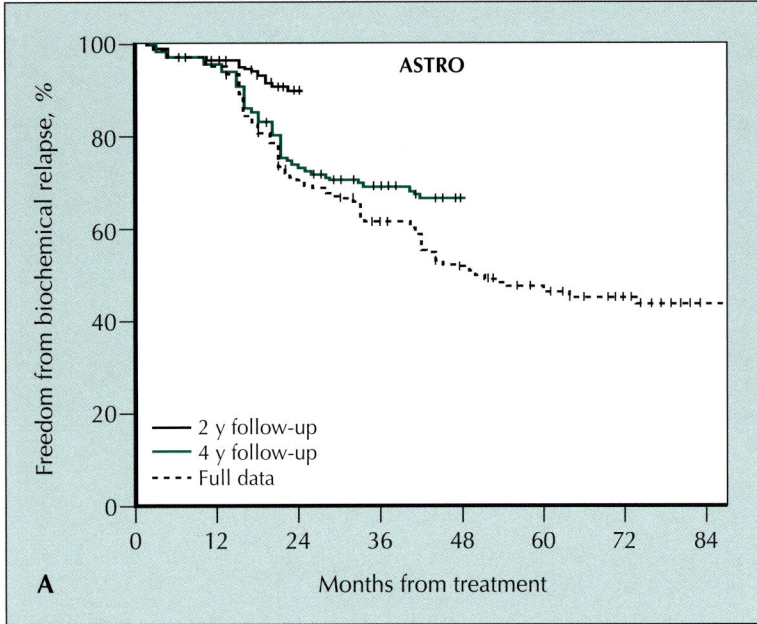

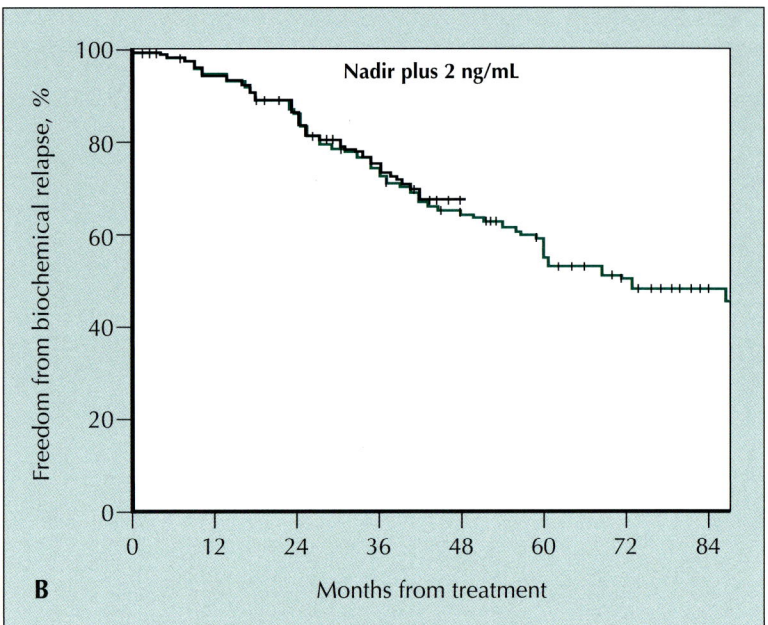

A — Months from treatment

B — Months from treatment

▶ **FIGURE 15-10.** The biochemical outcome for a cohort of patients at several follow-up intervals illustrating the effect of short follow-up bias on biochemical outcome with the American Society of Therapeutic Radiation Oncology (ASTRO) definition. Results with the (**A**) ASTRO and (**B**) nadir plus 2ng/mL definitions of biochemical failure (BF) are shown. The ASTRO definition is three consecutive rises with backdating of the time of failure to the midpoint between the lowest prostate-specific antigen (PSA) level (nadir PSA) after radiotherapy and the first PSA rise. The "Houston" definition [26–28] is the time at which the PSA rises 2 ng/mL above the nadir PSA; hence, there is no backdating in the nadir plus 2 ng/mL definition. The figure shows patients treated with curative intent with radiotherapy between July 1994 and June 1995 at the British Columbia Cancer Agency [27]. Follow-up data were selectively deleted from the dataset, resulting in the equivalence of 2, 4, or the full 8 years' maximal follow-up, with median follow-up times of 19, 41, and 72 months, respectively. Log rank–generated *P* values for differences between curves: *P* < 0.0001 (ASTRO) and *P* = 0.9 (nadir plus 2 ng/mL). The nadir plus 2 ng/mL definition is favored because it is less sensitive to variations in follow-up length, whereas the ASTRO definition is known to underestimate failure with short follow-up [29] because of backdating of failure. Furthermore, when androgen deprivation is added to radiotherapy, misclassifications using the ASTRO definition of BF occur in more than one fifth of men [30]. The nadir plus 2 ng/mL definition is much more accurate in classifying BF and predicting ultimate clinical failure (*eg*, distant metastasis). *Individual curves* for the nadir plus 2 ng/mL definition are not labeled because they overlie the full *data curve*. *Vertical bars* represent censored events. (*Adapted from* Pickles *et al*. [27], with permission.)

EXTERNAL BEAM RADIOTHERAPY TECHNIQUE

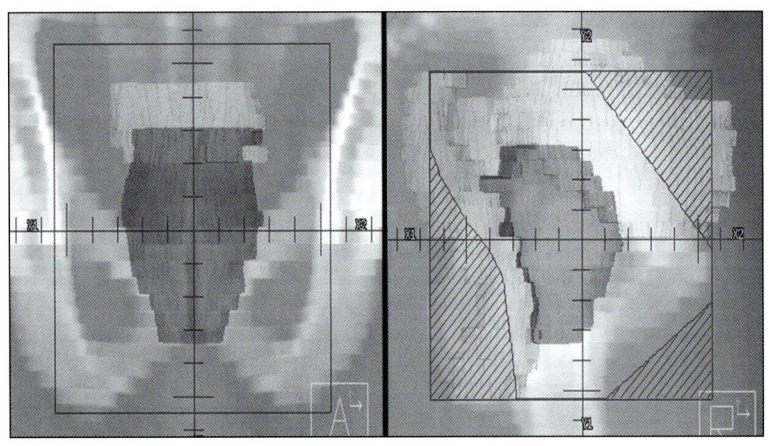

▶ **FIGURE 15-11.** *(See Color Plate)* Conventional radiotherapy fields. Digitally reconstructed radiographs of an anterior field (*left*; prostate and seminal vesicles shown) and a right lateral field (*right*; rectum, bladder, prostate, and seminal vesicles shown) are presented. On the right lateral field, the *hash marks* represent blocks over part of the rectum and bladder. A typical arrangement is a four-field box consisting of anterior, posterior, and right and left lateral fields. The maximum dose that can safely be delivered with these fields is 72 Gy. Above this dose, late bladder and bowel toxicity become more substantial. (*From* Pollack *et al*. [31]; with permission.)

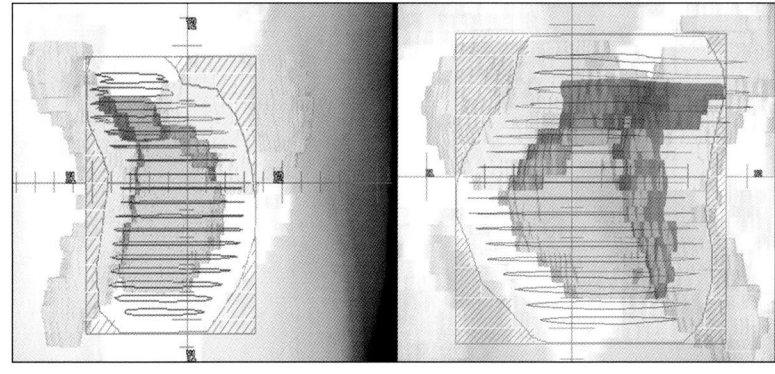

▶ **FIGURE 15-12.** *(See Color Plate)* Three-dimensional conformal radiotherapy (3DCRT) fields. In 3DCRT, the computer generates a three-dimensional reconstruction of the anatomy from a CT scan, allowing for the radiation fields to conform more precisely to the prostate and seminal vesicles. The target (prostate and seminal vesicles) may be viewed from any angle as a "beam's-eye view." Note how in the right lateral field (*left panel*), the blocks conform exactly to the shape of the blue wire frame margin (planning target volume) around the prostate and seminal vesicles. The planning target volume (PTV) accounts for uncertainties in target position and patient setup day to day. Note how on the oblique field (*right panel*), the block edge at the seminal vesicles superiorly is inside the PTV (wire frame); this was done as a compromise in coverage because too much rectum was being included. Such compromises are not needed with intensity-modulated radiotherapy, which is described later. An additional margin from the wire frame to the block edge allows for dose buildup or penumbra. A typical field arrangement is for five or more beam directions, such as laterals, right and left anterior obliques, and right and left posterior obliques (six fields).

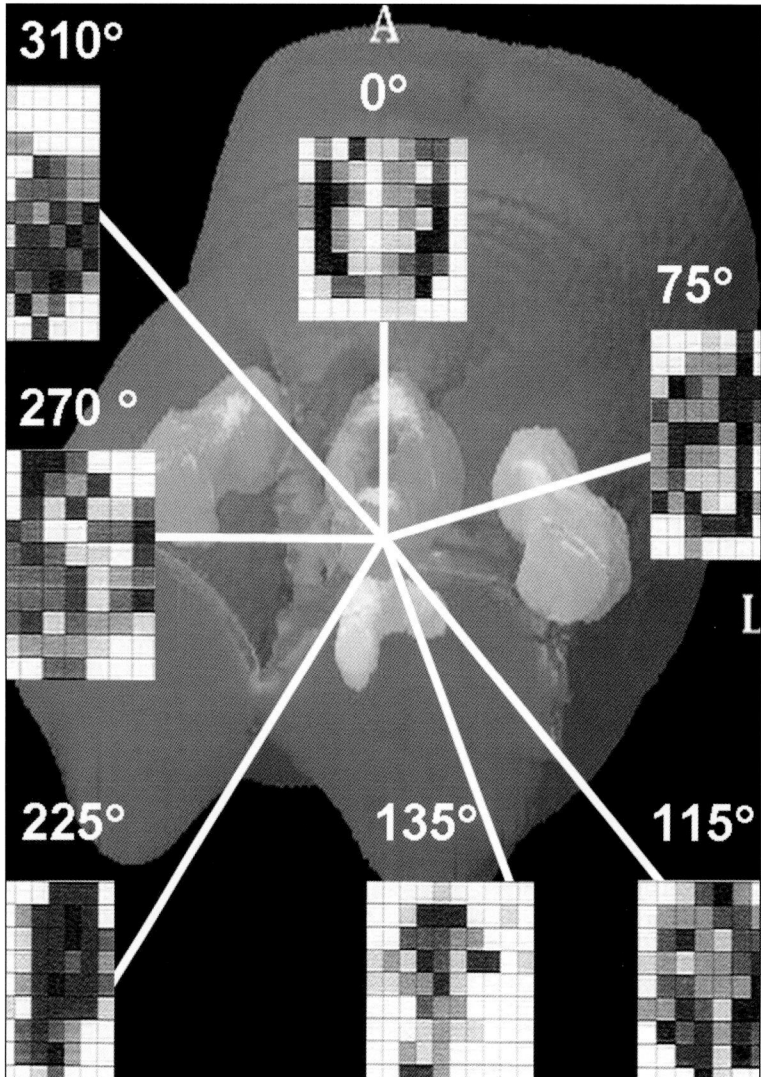

▶ **FIGURE 15-13.** *(See Color Plate)* Typical intensity-modulated radiotherapy (IMRT) field arrangement depicting the intensity maps for each beam angle. The treatment depicted consists of seven beam directions. In IMRT, the intensity for each beam may be varied by dividing each beam into multiple small squares or beamlets. The intensity of the dose in each beamlet is represented by different levels of gray; the darker the area, the more intense the radiation. The computer, using the method of inverse planning, iterates through a series of calculations to determine the ideal method of subdividing each beam into beamlets such that the normal tissues receive low doses relative to the prostate. (*Modified from* Price *et al.* [32]; with permission.)

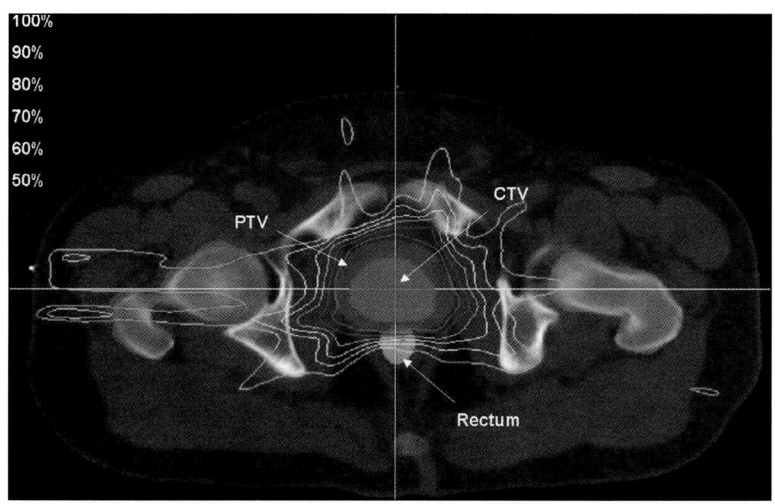

▶ **FIGURE 15-14.** *(See Color Plate)* An example of typical intensity-modulated radiotherapy dose distribution, seen on a transverse CT slice. There are a number of subjective and objective criteria that are used to determine whether the radiation treatment plan is acceptable. The treating physician will carefully assess the dose distribution on a CT slice–by–CT slice basis to ensure that the dose gradient across the normal tissues is abrupt, the coverage of the planning target volume (PTV) is satisfactory, and low doses in the target are not seen. CTV—clinical target volume.

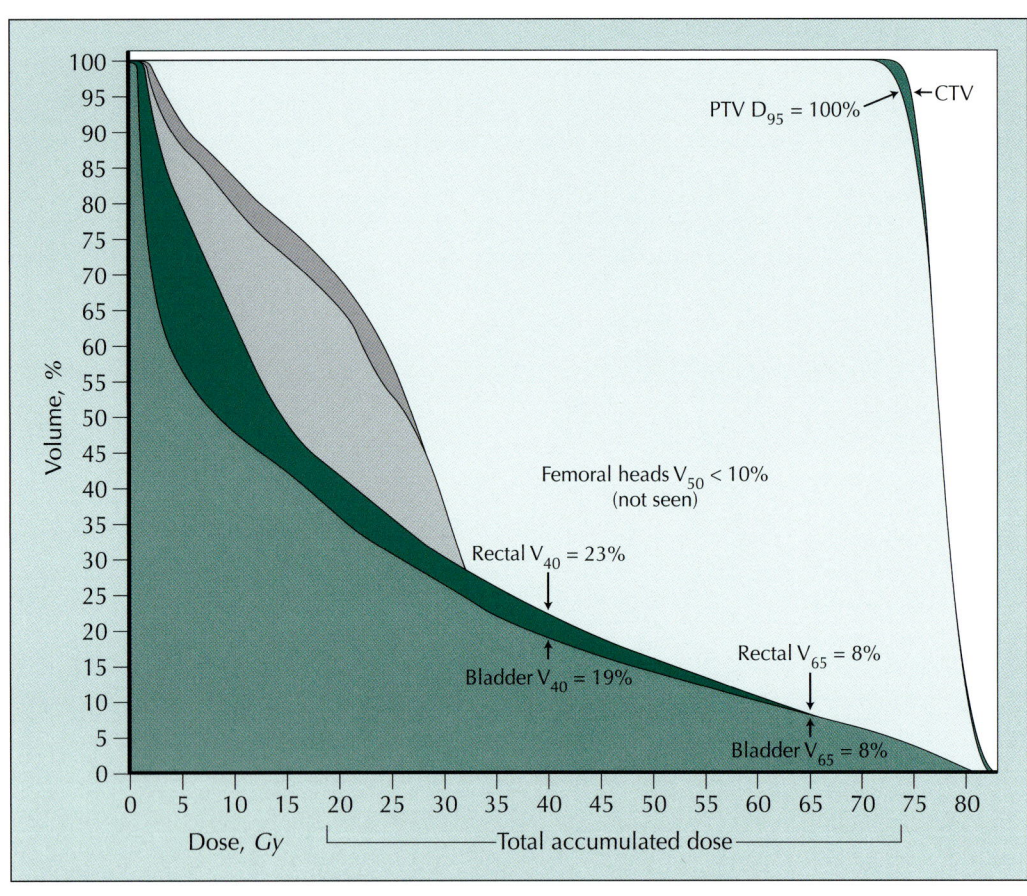

FIGURE 15-15. An example of a dose-volume histogram (DVH) analysis. Objective DVH criteria for the planning target volume (PTV), rectum, bladder, and femoral heads (*see* Fig. 15-16) have been adopted to evaluate intensity-modulated radiotherapy treatment plans. DVH criteria for normal tissue sparing are highly specific to the contouring method used. For example, the rectal DVH constraints outlined in Figure 15-17 are only applicable when the rectum is contoured from the ischial tuberosities to the sigmoid flexure encompassing the entire rectal volume (empty), similar to Radiation Therapy Oncology Group recommendations [33]. D_{95}—dose received by 95% of the volume; V_{40}, V_{50}, V_{65}—volume receiving 40%, 50%, and 65% of the prescribed dose volume, respectively.

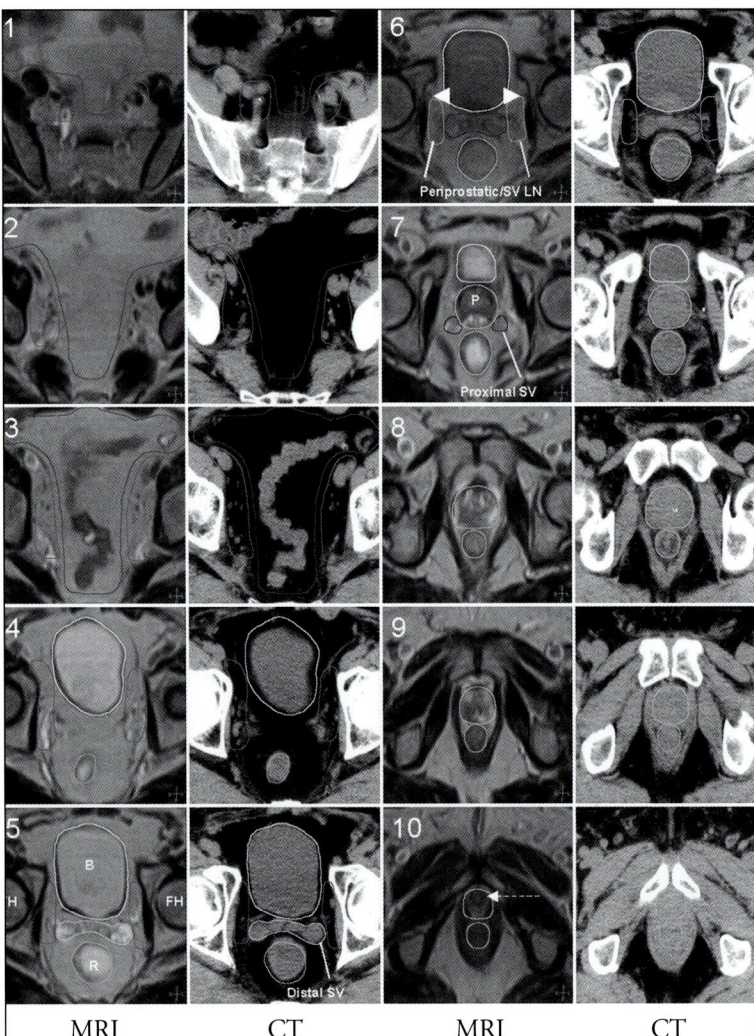

FIGURE 15-16. *(See Color Plate)* Target and normal volume definitions with MRI simulation used at Fox Chase Cancer Center, and corresponding fused CT images. MRI provides better images of the prostate boundaries, particularly at the base and apex. Based on the results of Radiation Therapy Oncology Group 94-13 [34], the pelvic lymph nodes are included for men with high-risk disease. As mentioned above, high-risk patients also receive extended androgen deprivation for 2 years or longer. The pelvic lymph node contours (red) begin at the level of the inferior aspect of the sacroiliac joint where the common iliac vessels bifurcate to the external iliac (*white arrow, panel 1*) and internal iliac vessels (*black arrow, panel 1*). The external iliacs are excluded from the pelvic lymph node volume as they exit the pelvis to enter the inguinal region. The obturator lymph node region is included bilaterally as the pelvic lymph volume continues inferiorly. The periprostatic/periseminal vesicle lymph node region (mustard) begins as the pelvic (obturator) lymph node (LN) region ends (*arrowheads, panel 6*).

A potential space that may contain the bowel (purple) is contoured in order to eliminate dose "dumping" into this region during the planning optimization. This method is used because 1) interfraction motion of the small bowel and sigmoid colon is unpredictable and not well understood and 2) a record of the dose received by this volume can be made and constrained appropriately. The rectal volume (dark green, R) begins at the rectosigmoid junction, where the rectum turns anteriorly at the superior aspect (between *panels 4 and 3*). The rectum ends inferiorly at the most inferior aspect of the ischial tuberosities. We have included the anus and rectum in one volume, but more recent evidence indicates that perhaps these structures should be separated [35]. The urinary bladder (yellow, B) is well visualized, without a need for contrast.

The prostate (rust, P) is well defined with MRI. The prostate–rectal interface and prostate apex (*dashed white arrow, panel 10*) are more clearly visualized on MRI, as compared with CT. The seminal vesicles (SVs) have a high signal intensity on T2-weighted MRI (*panel 7*, beginning of proximal SVs going superiorly) and are contoured separately into distal SVs (light blue) and proximal SVs (dark blue). The proximal SVs are typically defined as the first 0.9 cm. FH—femoral head.

Treatment Planning and Evaluation Scheme at Fox Chase Cancer Center

Volume	Target	Constraints Absolute (Hard)	Constraints Relative (Soft)	Comment
CTV1	Prostate Proximal seminal vesicles* Gross extracapsular extension	$D_{100} \geq 100\%$ prescription dose[†]	None	
PTV1	CTV1 + 8 mm, except 5 mm posteriorly	$D_{95} \geq 100\%$ prescription dose[†] $D_{max} < 17\%$ prescription dose[†] $V_{<65Gy} < 1\%$	Effective PTV: the slice-by-slice distance from the posterior edge of the prostate (CTV1) to the prescription isodose line is ~3 mm to 8 mm	The PTV is a 3D structure, and the distance between the CTV and prescription line varies
PTV2	Distal seminal vesicles (CTV2) + 8 mm, except 5 mm posteriorly	$D_{95} \geq 100\%$ prescription dose[‡]	None	The distal SVs are only treated in high-risk patients
PTV3	Lymph nodes (CTV3) + 8 mm, except 5 mm posteriorly	$D_{95} \geq 100\%$ prescription dose[‡]	None	If the bladder dose is too high, the lateral margins are brought down to 6 mm
Rectum	Entire rectal volume (empty) from the ischial tuberosities to the sigmoid flexure	$V_{65Gy} < 17\%$ $V_{40Gy} < 35\%$	The 90% dose line encompasses no more than the half-width of the rectum on any axial cut. The 50% dose line does not encompass the full rectum width.	The soft constraints are a way of ensuring a rapid dose gradient across the rectum
Bladder	Entire bladder volume (partially full)	$V_{65Gy} < 25\%$ $V_{40Gy} < 50\%$	None	Often times, bladder constraints are not met. These are not well defined and the least important.
Femoral heads	Right and left femoral heads to a level between the greater and lesser trochanters	$V_{50Gy} < 10\%$ for each	None	

*For T3b disease, most if not all of the seminal vesicles are treated to the full dose.
†Prescription dose: low risk = 76 Gy in 38 fractions; intermediate/high risk = 76–78 Gy.
‡Prescription dose: low/intermediate risk = N/A; high risk = 56 Gy delivered in 38 to 39 fractions.

▶ **FIGURE 15-17.** Treatment planning and evaluation scheme at Fox Chase Cancer Center (FCCC). The intensity-modulated radiotherapy (IMRT) planning volumes used at FCCC are shown. The clinical target volume (CTV) is constructed using a combination of subvolumes (ie, CTV1, CTV2, and so on) determined by the patient's respective risk group (low, intermediate, or high; see Fig. 15-7). In general, the CTV includes the prostate, any gross extracapsular extension, and proximal seminal vesicles (SVs; CTV1), including the distal seminal vesicles (CTV2) and lymph nodes (CTV3) in high-risk cases.

For low- and intermediate-risk patients at FCCC, the CTV includes the prostate and proximal SVs. Although the probability of proximal SV involvement is low, this region is included in the CTV1 because it is difficult to accurately identify the prostate-SV interface. Adequate coverage of the apex is of particular concern because it may be involved by tumor in more than 30% of men [36]. Lying in close proximity to the neurovascular bundles, the apex is a common site of perineural invasion, which provides a direct route of extracapsular/prostatic extension. Extracapsular extension, when seen, typically extends a maximum of 3 to 5 mm beyond the prostatic capsule [37–39]. For these reasons, we extend the CTV1 about 6 mm below where the prostate apex is believed to end. The planning target volume (PTV) is a margin around the CTV that takes into account the uncertainties of prostate location each day and patient setup. The PTV1 for the CTV1 incorporates 8 mm of margins in all directions, except posteriorly, where the margin is 5 mm to limit the dose received by the rectum. Although this margin is small, with daily correction of day-to-day (interfraction) prostate motion (see Fig. 15-18) the prostate falls within the PTV nearly all the time.

The coverage of lymph nodes outside the periprostatic and peri-SV regions is considered in CTV3 in men with high-risk disease, based on the recent results from Radiation Therapy Oncology Group 94-13 [34]. This adds considerable complexity to the construction of treatment volumes and dose calculations. At FCCC, the periprostatic, peri-SV and pelvic lymph node volumes used are slightly greater than a standard lymphadenectomy [40,41] and are included in the CTV3. They are contoured together, extending along the obturator, external iliac, and internal iliac vessels from the level of the prostate inferiorly to the bifurcation of the bifurcation of the common iliac vessels superiorly (see Fig. 15-16).

Volume expansion of the CTV3 to define a PTV3 to account for uncertainties is somewhat problematic because prostate motion is independent of the lymph nodes; prostate motion corrected using transabdominal ultrasound (see Fig. 15-18) could result in a shift of the PTV3 away from the lymph nodes, assuming the isocenter remains aligned with the bony anatomy. Because the standard deviation for prostate shifts is about 5 mm and the lymph nodes are considered a structure of secondary importance, we usually use the same PTV margins as those for the other structures (8 mm everywhere and 5 mm posteriorly), although we have sometimes limited the PTV3 to 6 mm lateral margins to limit bladder dose. Because lateral interfraction prostate displacement is typically small, this seems reasonable [42]. Presacral lymph nodes have not been treated at FCCC with IMRT. The goal is to treat as much of the lymph node regions as possible without compromising the delivery of high doses to the PTV1. Our results suggest that dose is of primary importance [43]. Risk groups: low risk = T1c to T2c, Gleason score 2 to 6, and pretreatment prostate-specific antigen (PSA) 10 ng/mL or lower; intermediate risk = Gleason score 7 or pretreatment PSA > 10 and less than or equal to 20 ng/mL; high risk = T3 to T4, Gleason score 8 to 10, or pretreatment PSA > 20 ng/mL. 3D—three-dimensional; D_{95}, D_{100}—dose received by 95% and 100% of the volume, respectively; D_{max}—maximum dose; V_{40Gy}, V_{50Gy}, V_{65Gy}, $V_{<65Gy}$—volume receiving 40, 50, 65, and less than 65 Gy, respectively.

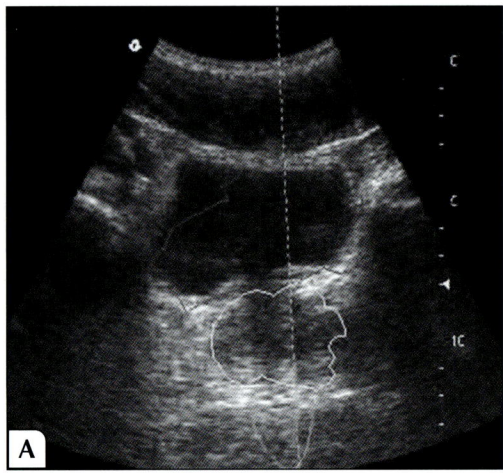 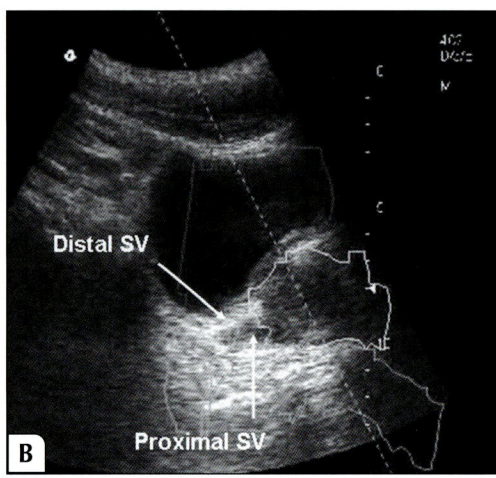

▶ **FIGURE 15-18.** *(See Color Plate)* Ultrasound (Sewickley, PA) alignment to correct for day-to-day (interfraction) prostate motion. There are a number of ways to correct for interfraction changes in prostate position, including the use of metallic seeds (fiducials), placement of a rectal balloon to immobilize the prostate, and daily CT scanning via a CT scanner in the treatment room or by acquiring a cone beam CT scan using a kilovoltage radiographic device attached to the gantry of the treatment machine. **A and B,** In the ultrasound example shown, the proximal (light blue) and distal (orange) seminal vesicles (SVs) have been outlined as separate structures [44].

RESULTS OF EXTERNAL BEAM RADIOTHERAPY ALONE

Sequential 3DCRT Dose Escalation Studies of External Beam Radiotherapy

| Study (Institution) | Year | Patients, n | Risk | 5-Year Results | | P Value |
				FFBF, % (Dose, Gy)	FFBF, % (Dose, Gy)	
Lyons *et al.* [45]	2000	738	Low	81 (< 72)	98 (≥ 72)	0.02
(Cleveland Clinic)			High	41 (< 72)	75 (≥ 2)	0.001
Hanks *et al.* [46]	2000	618	Low†	86 (< 70)	80 (≥ 70)	NS
(FCCC)			Int	29 (< 71.5)	66 (≥ 71.5)	< 0.05
			High	8 (< 71.5)	29 (≥ 71.5)	< 0.05
	2000	1213	Low	84 (< 67)	91 (> 67–70)	NS
Pollack *et al.* [47]			Low	91 (> 67–70)	100 (> 77)	NS
(MDACC)*			Int	55 (≤ 67)	79 (> 67–77)	0.0001
			Int	79 (> 67–66)	89 (> 77)	NS
			High	27 (≤ 67)	47 (> 67–77)	0.0001
			High	47 (> 67–77)	67 (> 77)	0.016
	2001	1100	Low	77 (≤ 70)	90 (≥ 75.6)	0.05
Zelefsky *et al.* [21]			Int	50 (≤ 70)	70 (≥ 75.6)	0.001
(MSKCC)			High	21 (≤ 70)	47 (≥ 75.6)	0.002
	2004	839	Low	81 (72–76)	78 (72–76)	NS
Pollack *et al.* [48]			Low	78 (72–76)	82 (> 76)	NS
(FCCC)			Int	24 (< 72)	65 (72–76)	0.0051
			Int	65 (72–76)	79 (> 76)	0.0096
			High	27 (72–76)	34 (> 76)	0.04

*Four-year results (published in a book chapter)
†Based on pretreatment prostate-specific antigen.
(Data from Hanks [49].)

▶ **FIGURE 15-19.** Sequential three-dimensional conformal radiotherapy (3DCRT) dose escalation studies of external beam radiotherapy (EBRT). The table presents a summary of the results of some of the retrospective 3DCRT dose escalation studies in which patients were subdivided by risk group. All risk groups display a gain in freedom from biochemical failure (FFBF) when EBRT doses are increased from less than 70 Gy to 70 Gy. In general, the greatest benefit is observed for intermediate-risk patients when doses are escalated above 70 Gy. However, some series revealed improvements in FFBF in low- and high-risk patients as well. Representative Kaplan-Meier curves from Fox Chase Cancer Center (FCCC) series are shown in Figure 15-20. Sequential dose escalation series such as these are confounded by changes in the patient population that occur over time, such as stage migration [50], the Gleason score shift [51,52], and the influence of length of follow-up on the calculation of biochemical failure using the American Society of Therapeutic Radiation Oncology definition [27,29]. Int—intermediate; NS—not significant; MSKCC—Memorial Sloan-Kettering Cancer Center; MDACC—MD Anderson Cancer Center. *(Adapted from Hanks [49], with permission.)*

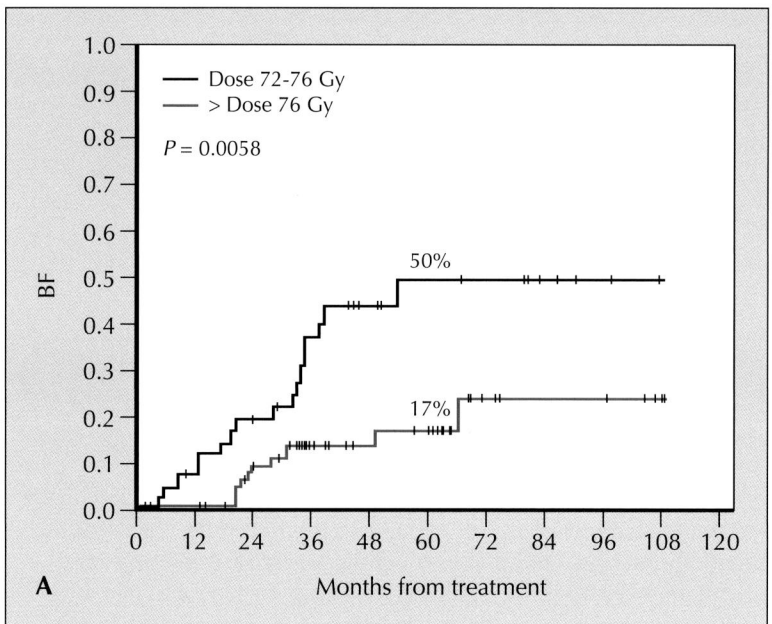

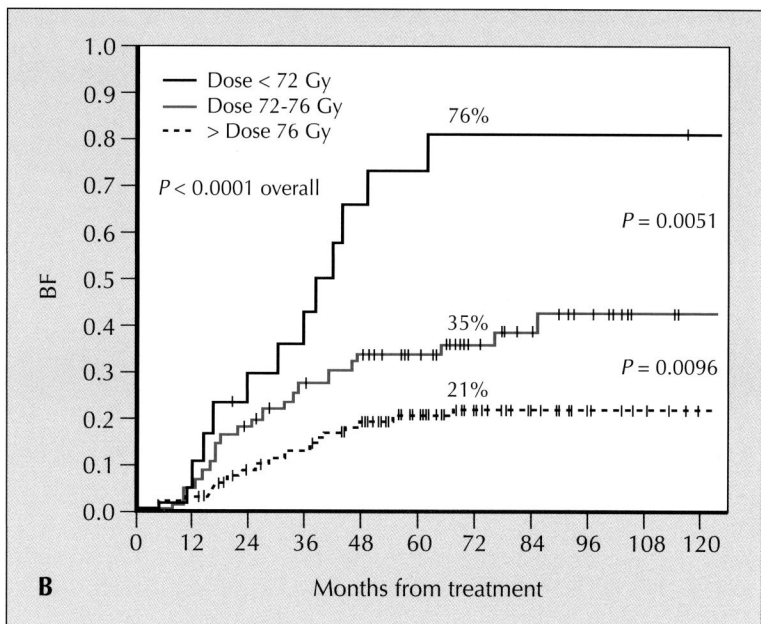

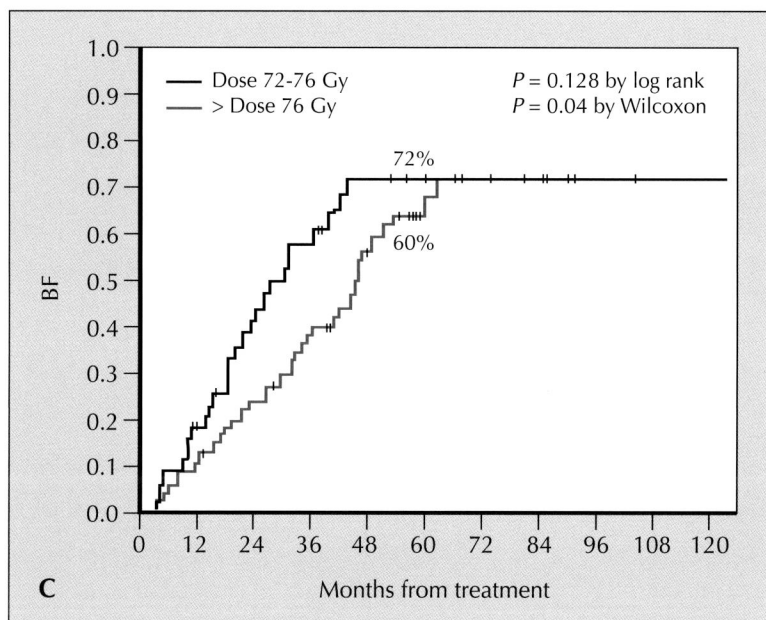

◗ **FIGURE 15-20.** Results for 839 patients who were treated with three-dimensional conformal radiotherapy alone at Fox Chase Cancer Center (FCCC) from 1989 to 1997 [48]. Shown here are the Kaplan-Meier curves from the FCCC dose escalation experience described in Figure 15-19 [31,53]. Log rank comparisons between dose groups are shown: (**A**) initial prostate-specific antigen (iPSA) less than 10 ng/mL and Gleason score 7 to 10, (**B**) iPSA 10 to 19.9 ng/mL, and (**C**) iPSA greater than 20 ng/mL. Comparisons between similar dose groups for iPSA less than 10 ng/mL and Gleason score 2 to 6 were not statistically different. *Vertical bars* represent censored events. BF—biochemical failure. (*Adapted from* Pollack *et al.* [48], with permission.)

Randomized Dose Escalation Studies of External Beam Radiotherapy in the PSA Era

Study (Institution)	Year	Patients, n	Risk	5-Year Results		P Value
				FFBF, % (Dose)	FFBF, % (Dose)	
Pollack *et al.* [53] (MDACC)	2002	305	Low	75 (70 Gy)	75 (78 Gy)	NS
			Int-High	43 (70 Gy)	62 (78 Gy)	0.012
Zietman *et al.* [54] (PROG 95-09)	2004	393	Low	65 (70.2 CGE)	83 (79.2 CGE)	0.002
			Int	60 (70.2 CGE)	79 (79.2 CGE)	0.01

▶ **FIGURE 15-21.** Randomized dose escalation studies of external beam radiotherapy (EBRT) in the prostate-specific antigen (PSA) era. Results from both the MD Anderson Cancer Center (MDACC) [53] and Proton Radiation Oncology Group (PROG) [54] randomized trials showed a statistically significant increase in freedom from biochemical failure (FFBF) when higher radiation doses were used. Dose escalation in the MDACC trial was accomplished using a three-dimensional conformal radiotherapy boost. In the PROG trial, the elevated dose was accomplished using a proton boost.

An early randomized dose escalation trial performed at Massachusetts General Hospital in the pre-PSA era did not show a disease-free survival or survival benefit when protons were used to boost the dose to the prostate to 75.6 CGE (cobalt-Gray equivalents), compared with 67.2 Gy using conventional techniques. A local control benefit, however, was demonstrated in men with poorly differentiated tumors [64].

The PSA-era trials from MDACC and PROG differ slightly in terms of which risk groups had the greatest gain from dose escalation. The MDACC group concluded that only the intermediate- to high-risk patients were affected. The PROG group concluded that both the favorable- and intermediate-risk patients were affected; they did not enter high-risk patients into their trial. The favorable-risk patients in the PROG trial did worse than described in retrospective series, casting some doubt about the extent of the gains observed in this risk group. Intermediate-risk patients consistently have exhibited a pronounced response to doses above 70 Gy. Int—intermediate; NS—not significant.

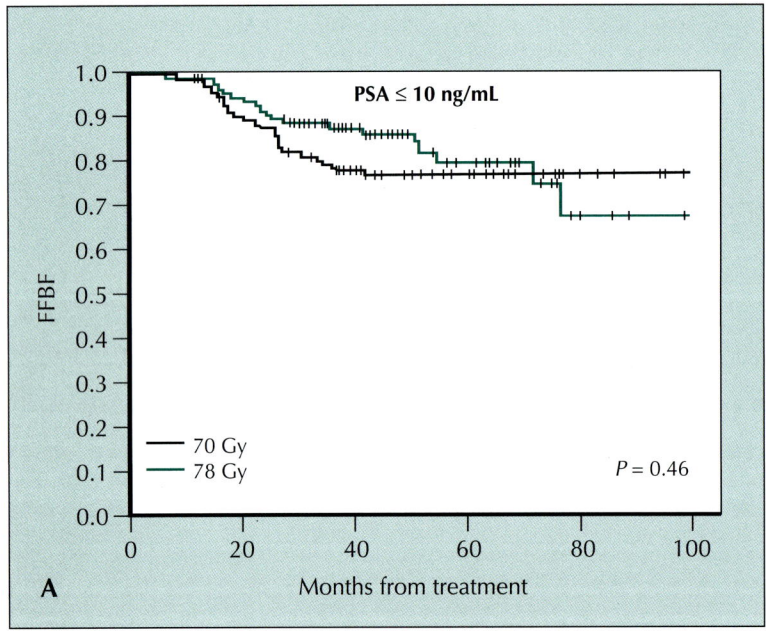

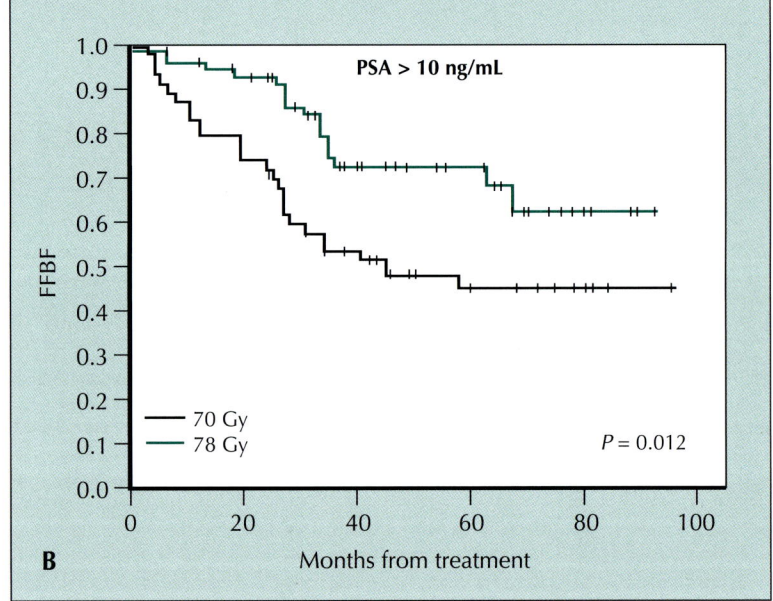

▶ **FIGURE 15-22.** Results of the MD Anderson Cancer Center (MDACC) trial. The results of the MDACC randomized trial illustrate the benefit of higher radiotherapy doses for the treatment of intermediate- and high-risk prostate cancer: (**A**) initial prostate-specific antigen (iPSA) 10 ng/mL or lower and (**B**) iPSA greater than 10 ng/mL. In this study, 301 assessable patients were randomized, with 150 receiving 70 Gy and 151 receiving 78 Gy (prescribed to isocenter). The clinical targeted volume (CTV) consisted of the prostate and seminal vesicles. The 70-Gy patients were treated with a conventional four-field box, with a field reduction after 46 Gy. The 78-Gy patients also received a four-field box to 46 Gy and then a six-field conformal boost to 78 Gy. The margins (CTV to block edge) on the conformal boost were 0.75 to 1.0 cm posteriorly and superiorly, and 1.25 to 1.5 cm anteriorly and inferiorly. The greatest benefit for dose escalation in the MDACC randomized trial was observed in men with a pretreatment prostate-specific antigen (PSA) greater than 10 ng/mL, who had a 19% absolute gain in freedom from biochemical failure (FFBF) at 6 years when treated to 78 Gy (*panel B*). The benefit in FFBF appeared to translate into a borderline reduction in distant metastasis (2% vs 12% at 6 years, *P* = 0.056); although there were only eight patients with distant metastasis at the time of the analysis. For the more favorable patients, with a pretreatment PSA of 10 ng/mL or less (*panel A*), no dose-related difference in FFBF or any other end point was observed. (*Adapted from* Pollack *et al.* [53].)

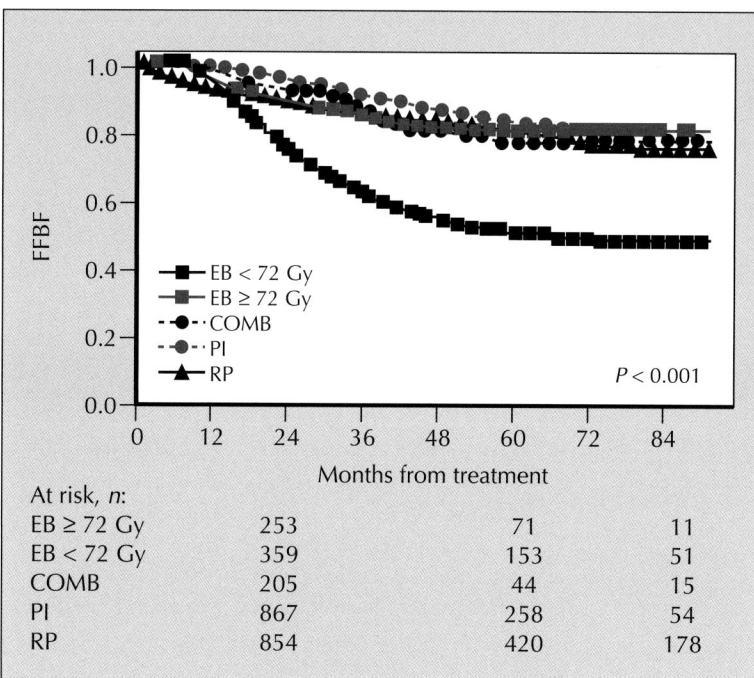

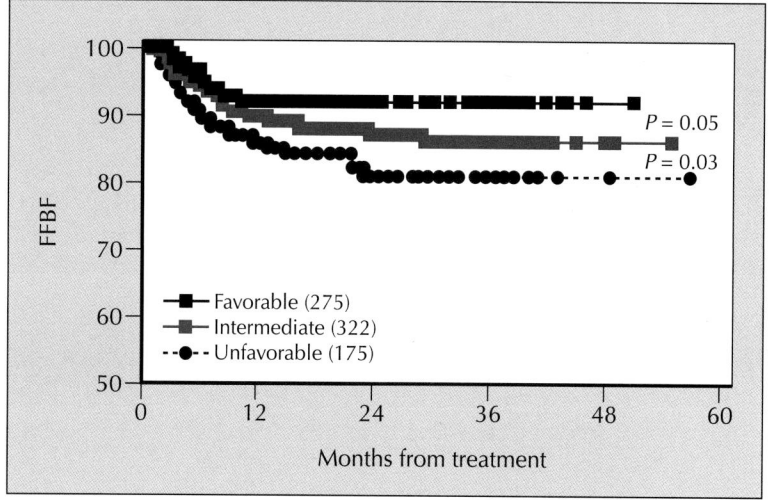

FIGURE 15-23. Freedom from biochemical failure (FFBF) by treatment modality for a study cohort including 2991 patients with clinical stage T1 and T2 prostate cancer consecutively treated at the Cleveland Clinic Foundation or Memorial Sloan-Kettering at Mercy Medical Center between 1990 and 1998 [55]. With the exception of men treated with external beam (EB) radiotherapy to a dose less than 72 Gy, biochemical outcome did not differ by treatment modality and no one technique proved superior. Biochemical failure was defined as three consecutive prostate-specific antigen (PSA) rises (3- to 6-month intervals) during follow-up for the radiotherapy-treated patients and a PSA greater than 0.2 ng/mL and two consecutive rises for the radical prostatectomy (RP)-treated patients. The results were similar when patients were subdivided into those with favorable and unfavorable prognostic features based on Gleason score, initial PSA, and stage. PI—prostate implant; COMB—combination external beam radiation therapy and prostate implant. Symbols represent censored events. (*Adapted from* Kupelian *et al.* [55], with permission.)

FIGURE 15-24. Results for 772 patients treated for clinically localized prostate cancer with intensity-modulated radiotherapy (IMRT) at Memorial Sloan-Kettering Cancer Center. IMRT reduces exposure of normal tissues to radiation by allowing for more precise dose conformality. As a result, doses may be increased. In the series displayed here, men were treated with IMRT to 81 to 86.4 Gy between April 1996 and January 2001. Freedom from biochemical failure by risk group (double-factor model) is shown. The results are very promising, although follow-up is still short. The number of patients at risk at 3 and 4 years for the favorable-risk group was 57 and six, respectively. The number of patients at risk at 3 and 4 years for the intermediate-risk group was 54 and eight, respectively. The number of patients at risk at 3 and 4 years for the unfavorable-risk group was 26 and three, respectively. PSA—prostate-specific antigen. (*Adapted from* Zelefsky *et al.* [56], with permission.)

Randomized Studies of External Beam Radiotherapy With or Without Androgen Deprivation Therapy

Institution	Risk	RT Dose	Length of AD	Result
RTOG 85-31 [57]	High	Standard	Permanent	LTAD + EBRT > RT*
Umea [58]	High	Standard	LTAD	LTAD + EBRT > RT*
EORTC [12]	High	Standard	LTAD	LTAD + EBRT > RT*
RTOG 86-10 [59]	High	Standard	STAD	STAD + EBRT > RT†
Harvard [60]	Int/high	Standard	STAD	STAD + EBRT > RT*
Quebec [61]	Int/high	Standard	STAD, ITAD	STAD/ITAD + EBRT > RT‡
PMH [62]	Int/high	Standard	STAD, ITAD	STAD + EBRT = ITAD + RT
RTOG 92-02 [13]	High	Standard	STAD, LTAD	LTAD + EBRT > STAD + RT†

*Overall survival improvement.
†Cause-specific survival improvement.
‡Improvement in positive biopsy rate at 12 and 24 months.

▶ **FIGURE 15-25.** Benefit of combination external beam radiotherapy (EBRT) and androgen deprivation (AD) in locally advanced prostate cancer. A number of randomized trials have shown that the combination of standard-dose EBRT and AD is superior to standard-dose EBRT alone. When reviewing these data, the length of AD should be considered. The criteria used at Fox Chase Cancer Center are that short-term AD (STAD) is for 6 months or less, intermediate-term AD (ITAD) is for more than 6 months and less than 2 years, and long-term AD (LTAD) is for 2 years or more. The figure shows that for those with high-risk disease who are treated with standard doses of

EBRT, the addition of LTAD consistently resulted in an overall survival improvement [12,57,58]. The combination of STAD and EBRT was also better than EBRT alone [59,60], but for high-risk patients, LTAD was better [13]. Because intermediate-risk patients have a substantial EBRT dose response, it is unclear what additional gains would result from the use of STAD to dose-escalated EBRT. Our policy is to use STAD in intermediate-risk patients with evidence of a high tumor volume on prostate biopsy (at least half the cores involved with cancer or an average tumor tissue content of > 20%). A formal phase III trial testing the effects of high-dose EBRT plus LTAD has not been tested in high-risk patients; however, this is our current policy, given the gains established for each method tested separately. EORTC—European Organisation for Research and Treatment of Cancer; Int—intermediate; PMH—Princess Margaret Hospital. RT—radiotherapy; RTOG—Radiation Therapy Oncology Group; Oncology Radiation Therapy Group; + —combination therapy; > —a benefit for the treatment to the left; = —equivalency.

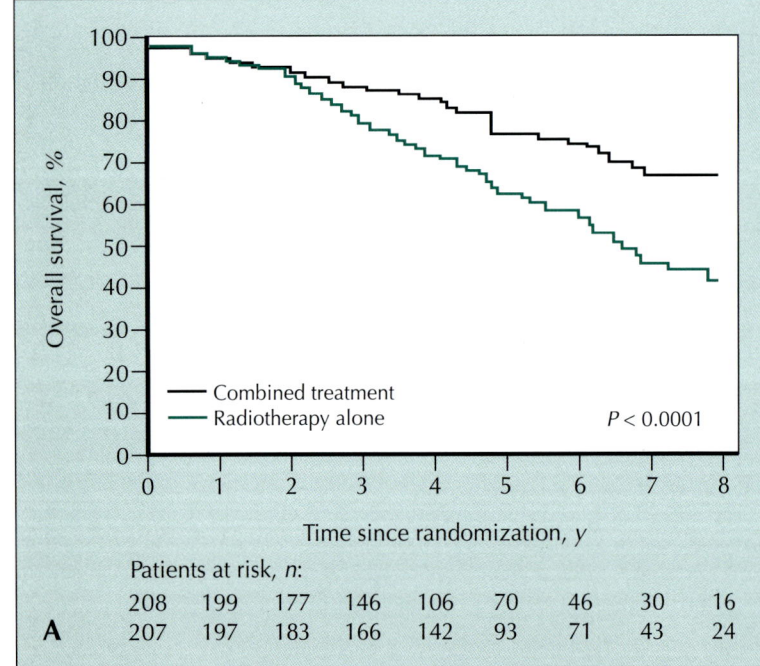
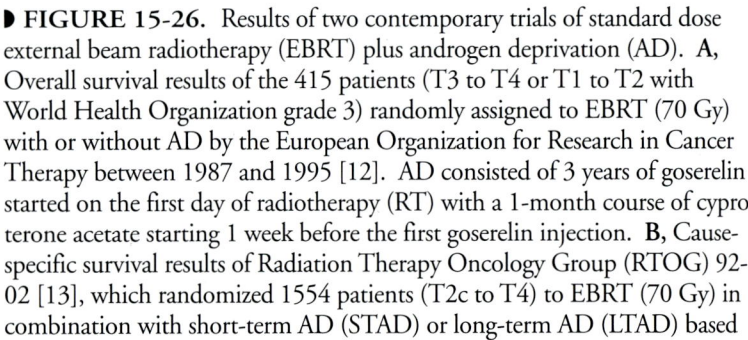
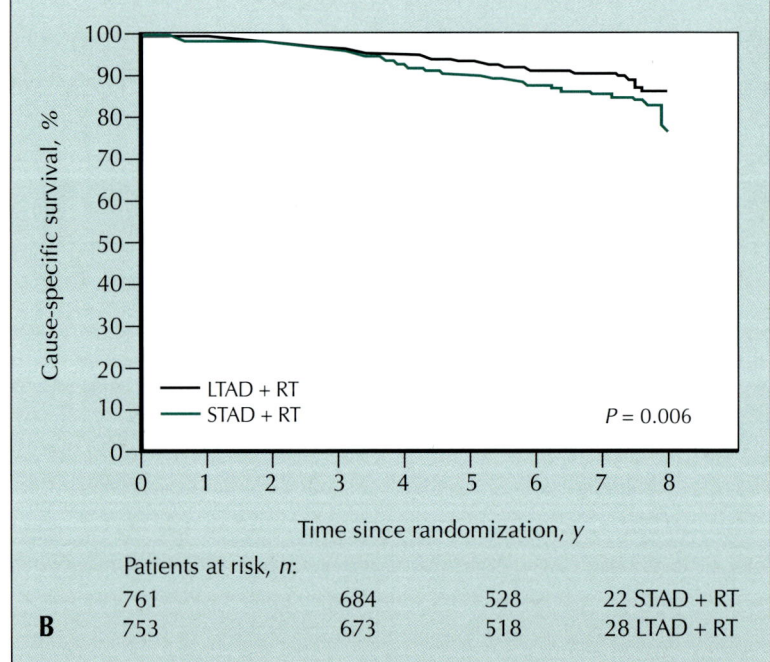

▶ **FIGURE 15-26.** Results of two contemporary trials of standard dose external beam radiotherapy (EBRT) plus androgen deprivation (AD). **A,** Overall survival results of the 415 patients (T3 to T4 or T1 to T2 with World Health Organization grade 3) randomly assigned to EBRT (70 Gy) with or without AD by the European Organization for Research in Cancer Therapy between 1987 and 1995 [12]. AD consisted of 3 years of goserelin started on the first day of radiotherapy (RT) with a 1-month course of cyproterone acetate starting 1 week before the first goserelin injection. **B,** Cause-specific survival results of Radiation Therapy Oncology Group (RTOG) 92-02 [13], which randomized 1554 patients (T2c to T4) to EBRT (70 Gy) in combination with short-term AD (STAD) or long-term AD (LTAD) based on results from two prior studies—RTOG 86-10 [59] and RTOG 85-31 [57]—which showed a dramatic reduction in both local and distant failures for the hormone-containing arm. All patients on RTOG 92-02 received a total of 4 months of goserelin and flutamide, 2 months before and 2 months during RT. Men randomized to LTAD received an additional 24 months of goserelin. The LTAD plus EBRT arm displayed significantly greater efficacy for all end points except overall survival (80.0% vs 78.5% at 5 years, P = 0.73), compared with the STAD plus EBRT arm. On subset analysis, a significant overall survival advantage was observed for the LTAD plus EBRT group among the patients with Gleason score 8 to 10 disease. (Panel A *adapted from* [12]; Panel B *adapted from* [13].)

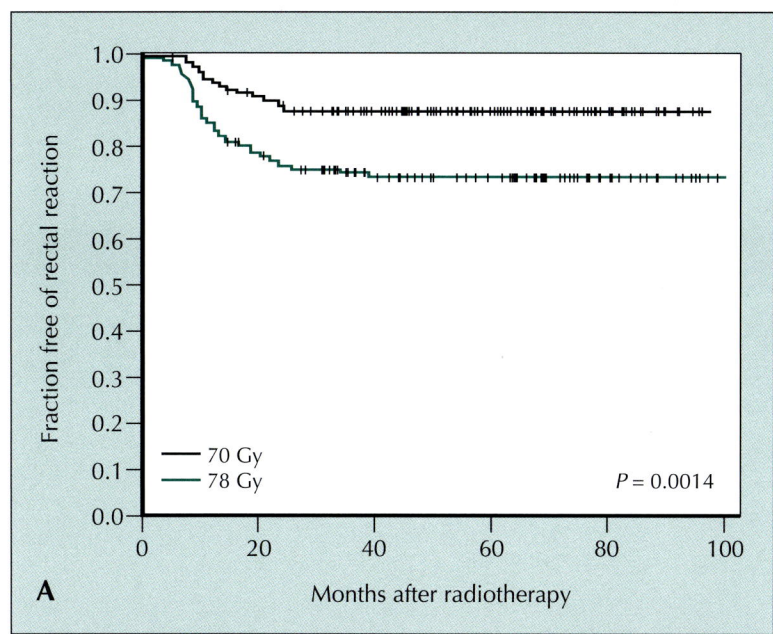

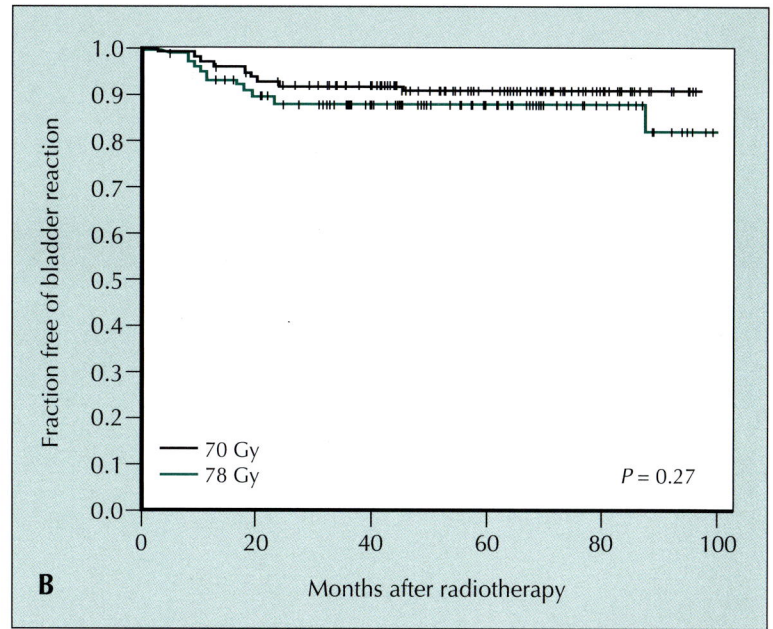

A

Months after radiotherapy

B

Months after radiotherapy

▶ **FIGURE 15-27.** The effect of radiotherapy dose on rectal (**A**) and bladder (**B**) toxicity illustrated by the results of the MD Anderson Cancer Center randomized dose-escalation trial. With a median follow-up of 5 years, there was a significantly higher rate of grade 2 or greater rectal toxicity in the high-dose arm. Treatment to 78 Gy was associated with a 6-year rate of rectal complications, which was 117% greater than that for 70 Gy (relative increase from 12% to 26%). No significant dose-related bladder complications were observed. (*Adapted from* Pollack *et al.* [53], with permission).

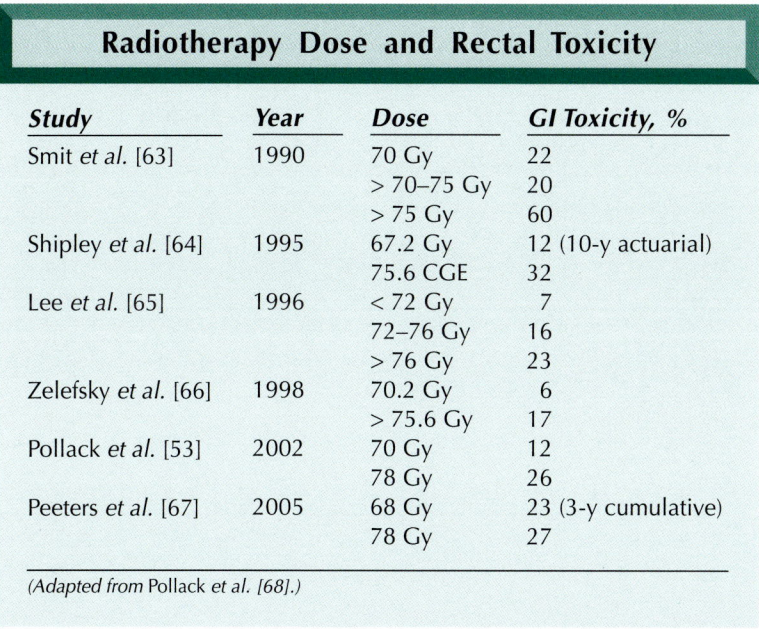

Radiotherapy Dose and Rectal Toxicity

Study	Year	Dose	GI Toxicity, %
Smit *et al.* [63]	1990	70 Gy	22
		> 70–75 Gy	20
		> 75 Gy	60
Shipley *et al.* [64]	1995	67.2 Gy	12 (10-y actuarial)
		75.6 CGE	32
Lee *et al.* [65]	1996	< 72 Gy	7
		72–76 Gy	16
		> 76 Gy	23
Zelefsky *et al.* [66]	1998	70.2 Gy	6
		> 75.6 Gy	17
Pollack *et al.* [53]	2002	70 Gy	12
		78 Gy	26
Peeters *et al.* [67]	2005	68 Gy	23 (3-y cumulative)
		78 Gy	27

(*Adapted from* Pollack et al. [68].)

▶ **FIGURE 15-28.** The association of radiation dose to rectal toxicity. Higher radiation dose is related to increased grade 2 or higher rectal reactions, with remarkable consistency among multiple groups. Only the recently described randomized trial results from Peeters *et al.* [67] have yet to show an effect of dose, because follow-up has been short. The significant increase in the rectal complication risk found in patients who received the higher dose in the MD Anderson Cancer Center randomized trial was not demonstrated until the median follow-up was 60 months [53] (*see* Fig. 15-22*A*). CGE—cobalt-Gray equivalents; GI—gastrointestinal. (*Adapted from* Pollack *et al.* [68], with permission.)

Rectal Volume and Rectal Toxicity

Study	Year	Dose	Rectum	GI Toxicity, %
Benk et al. [69]	1993	67–76 CGE	V76CGE < 40% ARW	19 (40-mo act.)[†]
		67–76 CGE	V76CGE 40% ARW	71
Lee et al. [65]	1996	74–76 Gy	Rectal block	10 (18-mo act.)
		74–76 Gy	No block	19
Dearnaley et al. [70]	1999	64 Gy	3DCRT	8 (5-y act.)
		64 Gy	Conventional RT	18
Boersma et al. [71]	1998	70 Gy	≤30%	0 (crude)
		70 Gy	> 30%	9
Pollack et al. [53]	2002	70–78 Gy	V70Gy 25%	16 (6-y act.)
		70–78 Gy	V70Gy > 25%	46
Kupelian et al. [72]	2002	78 Gy	≤15 mL	5 (2-y act)
		78 Gy	> 15 mL	22
Fiorino et al. [73]	2003	70–78 Gy	V50Gy ≤ 66%	8 (2-y act)
		70–78 Gy	V50Gy > 66%	32
		70–78 Gy	V70Gy ≤ 30%	8
		70–78 Gy	V70Gy > 30%	24
Cozzarini et al. [74]	2003	68–73 Gy	V50Gy ≤ 63%	7 (3-y act.)
		68–73 Gy	V50Gy > 63%	21
		68–73 Gy	V55Gy ≤ 57%	7
		68–73 Gy	V55Gy > 57%	21
		68–73 Gy	V60Gy ≤ 50%	7
		68–73 Gy	V60Gy > 50%	19
Koper et al. [35]	2004	66 Gy	V60Gy ≤ 70%	20 (3-y act.)
		66 Gy	V60Gy > 70%	52

[*]Severe rectal bleeding.
[†]Any rectal bleeding.
(Adapted from Pollack et al. [68].)

FIGURE 15-29. The association between rectal volume and rectal toxicity. The proportional increase in the volume of the rectum exposed to the same external beam radiotherapy dose is related to an increased risk of complications. These findings demonstrate that in addition to the dose prescribed (*see* Fig. 15-28), the volume of the rectum exposed to a specific radiation dose level is important. For any given dose, rectal complications are lower when a smaller volume is irradiated. Therefore, high prescription doses (≥ 75.6 Gy) can be used when specific dose-volume criteria are applied to limit the rectal exposure. The formulation of such criteria has been essential for prostate cancer dose escalation with intensity-modulated radiotherapy. 3DCRT—three-dimensional conformal radiotherapy; act.—actuarial; ARW—anterior rectal wall; CGE—cobalt-Gray equivalents; RT—radiotherapy; V_{50Gy}, V_{55Gy}, V_{60Gy}, V_{70Gy}, V_{76CGE}—volume receiving 50 Gy, 55 Gy, 60 Gy, 70 Gy, and 76 CGE, respectively. (*Adapted from* Pollack et al. [68], with permission.)

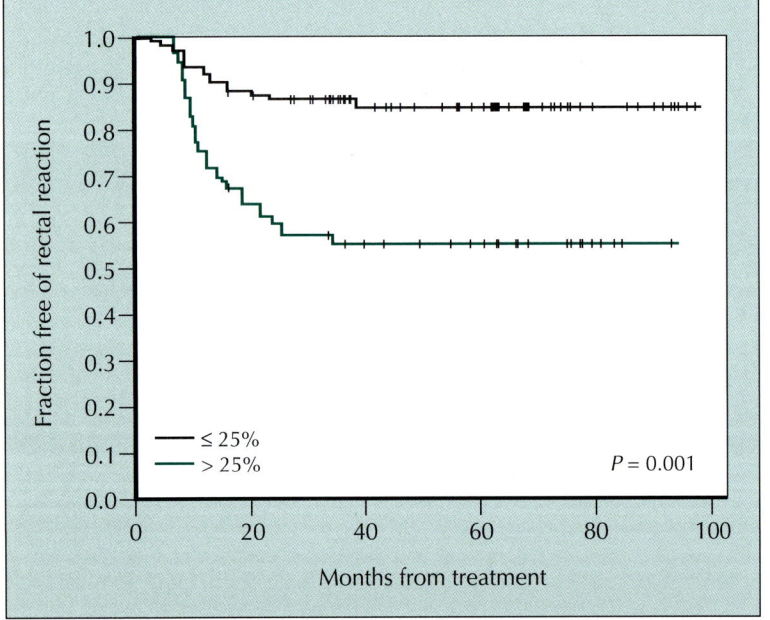

FIGURE 15-30. The dose-volume histogram relationship to grade 2 or higher rectal toxicity for the men participating in the high-dose arm of the MD Anderson Cancer Center randomized trial. When ≤ 25% of the rectum received ≥ 70 Gy , rectal toxicity was significantly reduced. (*Adapted from* Pollack et al. [53], with permission.)

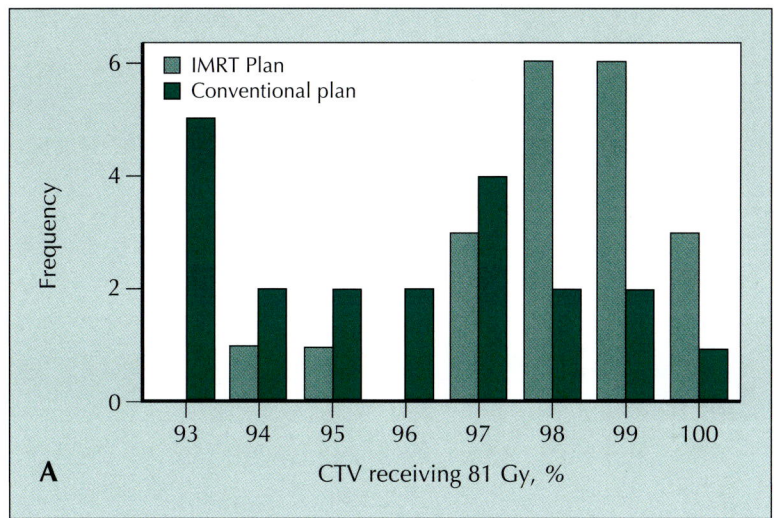

A CTV receiving 81 Gy, %

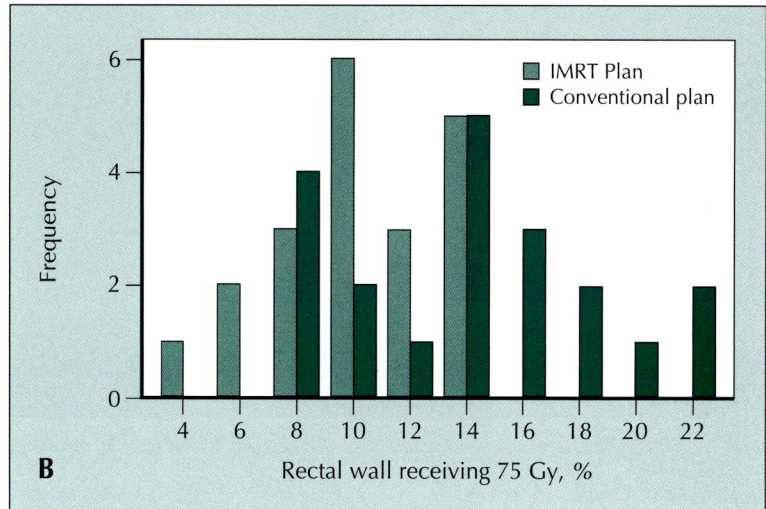

B Rectal wall receiving 75 Gy, %

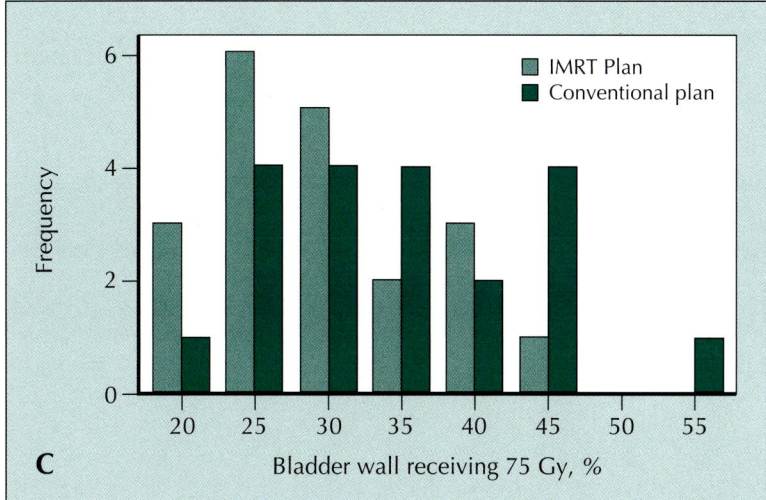

C Bladder wall receiving 75 Gy, %

▶ **FIGURE 15-31.** Intensity-modulated radiotherapy (IMRT) results in a lower percentage of normal tissue, and a higher percentage of the prostate, receiving high doses of radiation, as compared with three-dimensional conformal radiotherapy (3DCRT). The figure displays histograms of the percent clinical target volume (CTV) receiving 81 Gy (**A**), the percentages of the rectal wall carried to 75 Gy (**B**), and the percentages of the bladder wall receiving 75 Gy (**C**). Data were derived from dose-volume histograms generated from treatment plans of 20 randomly selected patients planned simultaneously from conventional 3DCRT and IMRT. Differences in the frequency distributions shown in *panels A, B, and C* are significant (*P* < 0.01). (*Adapted from* Zelefsky *et al.* [75].)

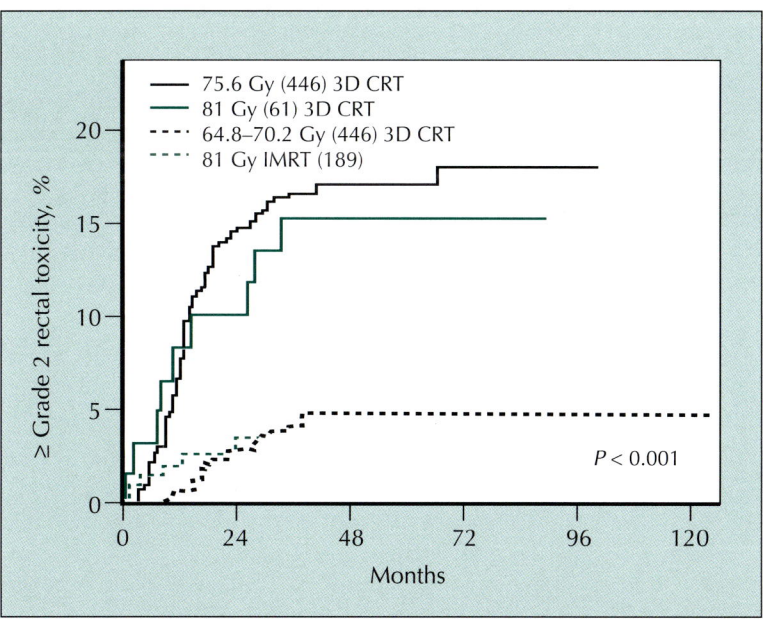

▶ **FIGURE 15-32.** The occurrence of grade 2 or higher rectal complications as a function of dose and external beam radiotherapy technique. These data are from the Memorial Sloan-Kettering Cancer Center's sequential prospective dose-escalation study [21]. The rates of grade 2 or higher rectal reactions are shown for patients treated with three-dimensional conformal radiotherapy (3DCRT) to 64.8 to 70.2 Gy, 75.6 Gy, and 81 Gy, and with intensity-modulated radiotherapy (IMRT) to 81 Gy. Escalating the 3DCRT dose to the prostate led to higher rates of rectal toxicity. IMRT was associated with a reduced rate of rectal toxicity by lowering the percentage receiving higher doses. This in turn has enabled further escalation of doses to the prostate [56]. (*Adapted from* Zelefsky *et al.* [21], with permission.)

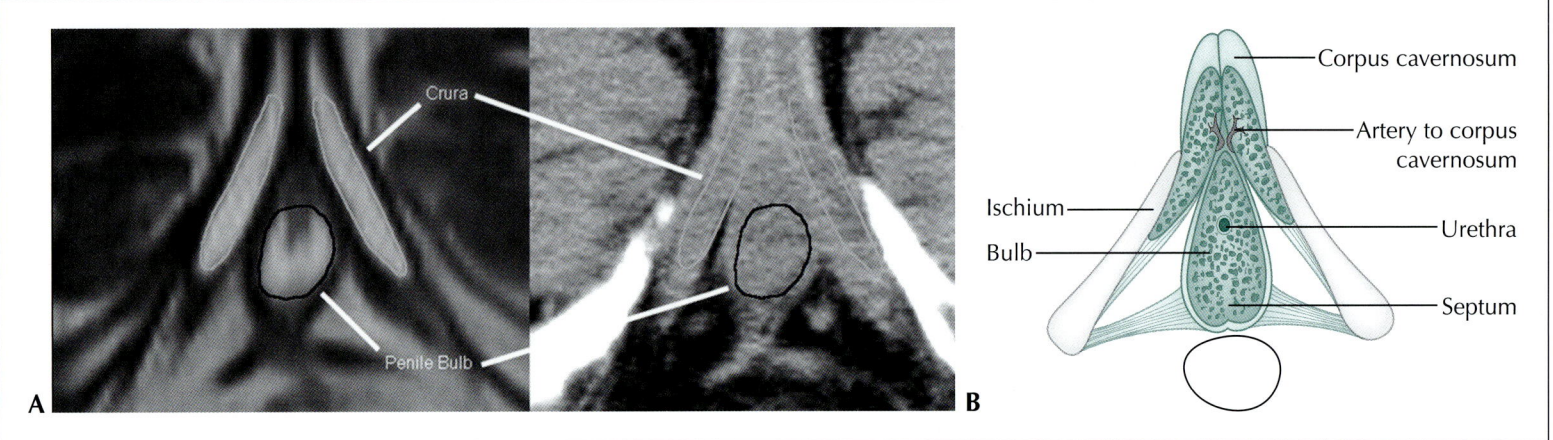

▶ **FIGURE 15-33.** Penile bulb and corporal body anatomy for external beam radiotherapy sparing and preservation of erectile function. **A,** MRI is superior to CT for defining these structures [76] as both appear as high signal intensity on T2-weighted images [76,77]. With respect to prostate delineation, MRI is also superior to CT and facilitates intensity-modulated radiotherapy planning to reduce the dose to these structures [78]. At Fox Chase Cancer Center, the penile bulb is defined as the bulbous, proximal portion of the corpora spongiosum and typically measures 1 to 2 cm in length. **B,** The corporal bodies are paired structures defined as the divergent, proximal portions of the corpora cavernosa and typically measure 2 to 3 cm in length before their departure from along the inner aspect of the ischial tuberosities. (*Adapted from* Buyyounouski *et al.* [79] and Hricak *et al.* [77], with permission.)

Penile Bulb Dose and Erectile Dysfunction After 3DCRT

Institution/Study	Year	Patients, n	Dose	Androgen Deprivation	Penile Bulb Dose	Potency
UCSF, Fisch *et al.* [80]	2001	21	76 Gy[*]	Yes[†]	14 Gy[‡]	No ED
					33 Gy[‡]	Slight ED
					51 Gy[‡] (P = 0.05)	Marked ED
RTOG, Roach *et al.* [81]	2004	158	31%, 68.4 Gy	Yes, 24%	49.8 Gy[§]	No ED
			69%, 73.8 Gy		60.3 Gy[§] (P = NR)	ED
Jefferson, Wernicke *et al.* [82]	2004	29	72 Gy	No	NR	No ED
					NR	ED

[*]Mean dose.
[†]The proportion of men who received androgen deprivation was not reported, but there was no difference observed in the proportion of patients remaining potent when comparing those who received hormonal therapy with those who did not.
[‡]Median dose to 95% of the penile bulb (D95).
[§]Median dose.

▶ **FIGURE 15-34.** The associations of radiation dose to erectile dysfunction (ED). Higher radiation dose appears to be associated with the incidence of ED, but the data are mixed and few. Fisch *et al.* [83] have demonstrated significantly higher penile bulb (PB) doses in men who developed ED. Roach *et al.* [81] also reported a higher median PB dose for men who developed ED following three-dimensional conformal radiotherapy (3DCRT) on dose levels I and II of Radiation Therapy Oncology Group (RTOG) 94-06, but statistical significance was not reported. Selek *et al.* [84] did not find a correlation in men treated in the MD Anderson Cancer Center prospective, randomized 3DCRT dose-escalation trial [53]; however, the definition of the PB used may have caused inaccuracies and/or inconsistencies in their PB dose determinations [85]. Wernicke *et al.* [82] did not compare PB doses between men with and without ED but instead demonstrated a volume effect (*see* Fig. 15-35). NR—not reported; UCSF—University of California, San Francisco.

Penile Bulb Volume and Erectile Dysfunction After 3DCRT

Institution/Study	Year	Patients, n	Dose	Androgen Deprivation	Penile Bulb Dose	ED Rate, %
UCSF, Fisch et al. [80]	2001	21	76 Gy*	Yes, NR[†]	D70 ≤ 40 Gy	0
					D70 > 40 Gy	82
RTOG, Roach et al. [81]	2004	15	31%, 68.4 Gy	Yes, 24%	DMedian < 52.5 Gy	25
		8	69%, 73.8 Gy		DMedian ≥ 52.5 Gy	50
Jefferson, Wernicke et al. [82]	2004	29	72 Gy	No	D30 ≤ 67 Gy	21
					D30 > 67 Gy	45
					D45 ≤ 63 Gy	21
					D45 > 63 Gy	45
					D60 ≤ 42 Gy	19
					D60 > 42 Gy	46
					D75 ≤ 20 Gy	21
					D75 > 20 Gy	45
MDACC, Selek et al. [84]	2004	28	78 Gy	No	NS	—

*Mean.
[†]There was no difference observed in the proportion of patients remaining potent when comparing those who received hormonal therapy with those who did not.

▶ **FIGURE 15-35.** The effect of penile bulb (PB) volume on the association of radiation dose to erectile dysfunction (ED). Three reports with three-dimensional conformal radiotherapy [81–83] have shown significant volume effects for the dose received by the PB and ED. These findings demonstrate that the volume of the PB exposed to a specific radiation dose is equally important as the dose itself. For any given dose, the ED rate is lower for smaller volumes irradiated. Comparison among studies is difficult because PB definitions may vary, but together they demonstrate that lower ED rates can be expected if smaller volumes of erectile tissue are irradiated. This is best seen in the study by Wernicke et al. [82], in which ED rates of 19% to 21% were observed when larger PB volumes received a low dose ($D_{75} \leq 20$ Gy) and high dose was limited to a smaller volume ($D_{30} \leq 67$ Gy). This dose–volume relationship is particularly important given the close relationship of the PB to the prostate apex. The distance from the PB to the prostate apex may range widely (5 to 33 mm) [86] in a region of very high dose fall-off. Therefore, small portions of the PB may receive high radiation doses [79]. D_{30}, D_{45}, D_{60}, D_{70}, D_{75}, D_{Median}—the dose received by 30%, 45%, 60%, 70%, 75%, and the median of the PB volume, respectively; MDACC—MD Anderson Cancer Center; NR—not reported; NS—not significant; RTOG—Radiation Therapy Oncology Group; UCSF—University of California, San Francisco.

EXTERNAL BEAM RADIOTHERAPY FOR NODE-POSITIVE DISEASE

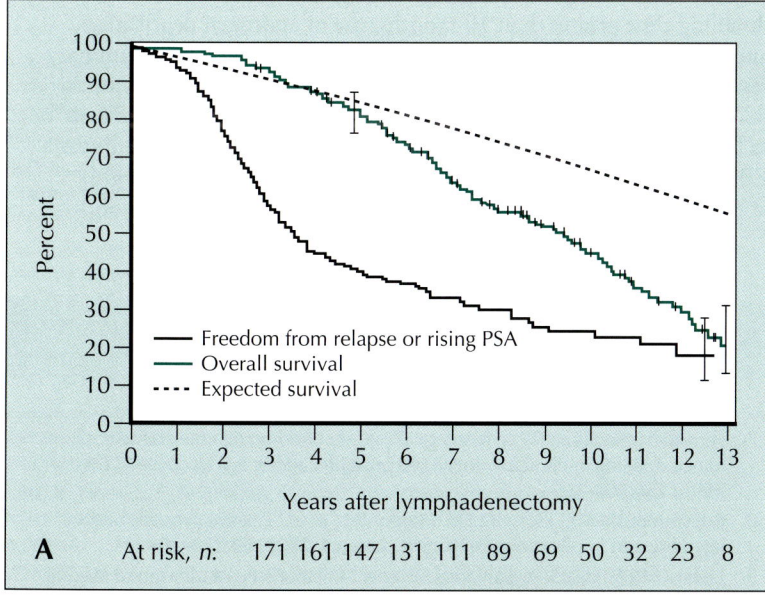
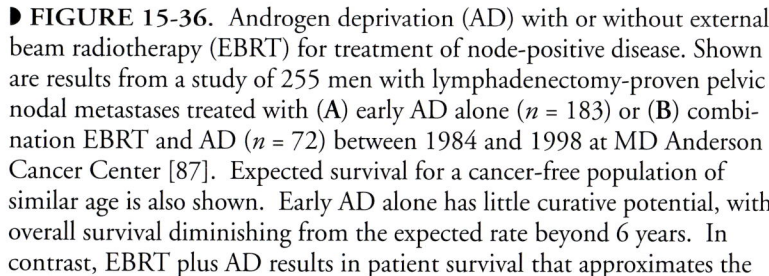

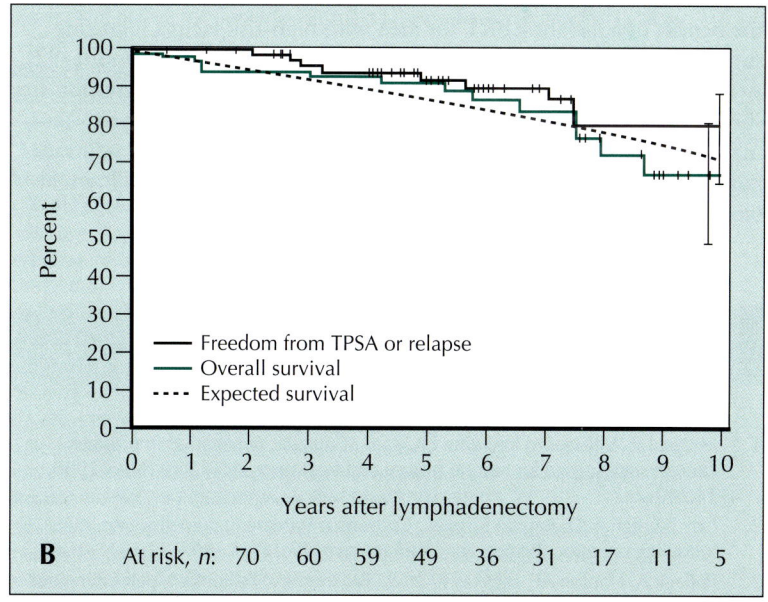

▶ **FIGURE 15-36.** Androgen deprivation (AD) with or without external beam radiotherapy (EBRT) for treatment of node-positive disease. Shown are results from a study of 255 men with lymphadenectomy-proven pelvic nodal metastases treated with (**A**) early AD alone (*n* = 183) or (**B**) combination EBRT and AD (*n* = 72) between 1984 and 1998 at MD Anderson Cancer Center [87]. Expected survival for a cancer-free population of similar age is also shown. Early AD alone has little curative potential, with overall survival diminishing from the expected rate beyond 6 years. In contrast, EBRT plus AD results in patient survival that approximates the age-matched expected survival and substantially improves biochemical control. Multivariate analysis for all patients identified the addition of EBRT as a significant determinant of outcome for all end points independent of Gleason score, T category, or initial prostate-specific antigen (PSA) [57,87,88]. Further support for the combination of local therapy in combination with AD comes from the surgical literature [89,90]. Men with node-positive prostate cancer should not be treated with AD alone or with local therapy alone if they have a 10-year life expectancy. (*Adapted from* Zagars et al. [87], with permission.)

58. Granfors T, Modig H, Damber JE, *et al*.: Combined orchiectomy and external radiotherapy versus radiotherapy alone for nonmetastatic prostate cancer with or without pelvic lymph node involvement: a prospective randomized study. *J Urol* 1998, 159:2030–2034.

59. Pilepich MV, Winter K, John MJ, *et al*.: Phase III radiation therapy oncology group (RTOG) trial 86-10 of androgen deprivation adjuvant to definitive radiotherapy in locally advanced carcinoma of the prostate. *Int J Radiat Oncol Biol Phys* 2001, 50:1243–1252.

60. D'Amico AV, Manola J, Loffredo M, *et al*.: 6-month androgen suppression plus radiation therapy vs radiation therapy alone for patients with clinically localized prostate cancer: a randomized controlled trial. *JAMA* 2004, 292:821–827.

61. Laverdiere J, Gomez JL, Cusan L, *et al*.: Beneficial effect of combination hormonal therapy administered prior and following external beam radiation therapy in localized prostate cancer. *Int J Radiat Oncol Biol Phys* 1997, 37:247–252.

62. Crook J, Ludgate C, Malone S, *et al*.: Report of a multicenter Canadian phase III randomized trial of 3 months vs. 8 months neoadjuvant androgen deprivation before standard-dose radiotherapy for clinically localized prostate cancer. *Int J Radiat Oncol Biol Phys* 2004, 60:15–23.

63. Smit WG, Helle PA, van Putten WL, *et al*.: Late radiation damage in prostate cancer patients treated by high dose external radiotherapy in relation to rectal dose. *Int J Radiat Oncol Biol Phys* 1990, 18:23–29.

64. Shipley WU, Verhey LJ, Munzenrider JE, *et al*.: Advanced prostate cancer: the results of a randomized comparative trial of high dose irradiation boosting with conformal protons compared with conventional dose irradiation using photons alone. *Int J Radiat Oncol Biol Phys* 1995, 32:3–12.

65. Lee WR, Hanks GE, Hanlon AL, *et al*.: Lateral rectal shielding reduces late rectal morbidity following high dose three-dimensional conformal radiation therapy for clinically localized prostate cancer: further evidence for a significant dose effect. *Int J Radiat Oncol Biol Phys* 1996, 35:251–257.

66. Zelefsky MJ, Fuks Z, Wolfe T, *et al*.: Locally advanced prostatic cancer: long-term toxicity outcome after three-dimensional conformal radiation therapy—a dose-escalation study. *Radiology* 1998, 209:169–174.

67. Peeters ST, Heemsbergen WD, van Putten WL, *et al*.: Acute and late complications after radiotherapy for prostate cancer: results of a multicenter randomized trial comparing 68 Gy to 78 Gy. *Int J Radiat Oncol Biol Phys* 2005, 61:1019–1034.

68. Pollack A, Price R, Dong L, *et al*.:IMRT for prostate cancer. In *Intensity Modulated Radiation Therapy: A Clinical Perspective*. Edited by Mundt AJ, Roeske JC. Hamilton, Ontario: BC Decker; in press.

69. Benk VA, Adams JA, Shipley WU, *et al*.: Late rectal bleeding following combined x-ray and proton high dose irradiation for patients with stages T3-T4 prostate carcinoma. *Int J Radiat Oncol Biol Phys* 1993, 26:551–557.

70. Dearnaley DP, Khoo VS, Norman AR, *et al*.: Comparison of radiation side-effects of conformal and conventional radiotherapy in prostate cancer: a randomised trial. *Lancet* 1999, 353:267–272.

71. Boersma LJ, van den Brink M, Bruce AM, *et al*.: Estimation of the incidence of late bladder and rectum complications after high-dose (70-78 GY) conformal radiotherapy for prostate cancer, using dose-volume histograms. *Int J Radiat Oncol Biol Phys* 1998, 41:83–92.

72. Kupelian PA, Reddy CA, Carlson TP, Willoughby TR: Dose/volume relationship of late rectal bleeding after external beam radiotherapy for localized prostate cancer: absolute or relative rectal volume? *Cancer J* 2002, 8:62–66.

73. Fiorino C, Sanguineti G, Cozzarini C, *et al*.: Rectal dose-volume constraints in high-dose radiotherapy of localized prostate cancer. *Int J Radiat Oncol Biol Phys* 2003, 57:953–962.

74. Cozzarini C, Fiorino C, Ceresoli GL, *et al*.: Significant correlation between rectal DVH and late bleeding in patients treated after radical prostatectomy with conformal or conventional radiotherapy (66.6-70.2 Gy). *Int J Radiat Oncol Biol Phys* 2003, 55:688–694.

75. Zelefsky MJ, Fuks Z, Happersett L, *et al*.: Clinical experience with intensity modulated radiation therapy (IMRT) in prostate cancer. *Radiother Oncol* 2000, 55:241–249.

76. Wallner KE, Merrick GS, Benson ML, *et al*.: Penile bulb imaging. *Int J Radiat Oncol Biol Phys* 2002, 53:928–933.

77. Hricak H, Marotti M, Gilbert TJ, *et al*.: Normal penile anatomy and abnormal penile conditions: evaluation with MR imaging. *Radiology* 1988, 169:683–690.

78. Steenbakkers RJ, Deurloo KE, Nowak PJ, *et al*.: Reduction of dose delivered to the rectum and bulb of the penis using MRI delineation for radiotherapy of the prostate. *Int J Radiat Oncol Biol Phys* 2003, 57:1269–1279.

79. Buyyounouski MK, Horwitz EM, Uzzo RG, *et al*.: The radiation doses to erectile tissues defined with magnetic resonance imaging after intensity-modulated radiation therapy or iodine-125 brachytherapy. *Int J Radiat Oncol Biol Phys* 2004, 59:1383–1391.

80. Fisch BM, Pickett B, Weinberg V, *et al*.: Dose of radiation received by the bulb of the penis correlates with risk of impotence after three-dimensional conformal radiotherapy for prostate cancer. *Urology* 2001, 57:955–959.

81. Roach M, Winter K, Michalski JM, *et al*.: Penile bulb dose and impotence after three-dimensional conformal radiotherapy for prostate cancer on RTOG 9406: findings from a prospective, multi-institutional, phase I/II dose-escalation study. *Int J Radiat Oncol Biol Phys* 2004, 60:1351–1356.

82. Wernicke AG, Valicenti R, Dieva K, *et al*.: Radiation dose delivered to the proximal penis as a predictor of the risk of erectile dysfunction after three-dimensional conformal radiotherapy for localized prostate cancer. *Int J Radiat Oncol Biol Phys* 2004, 60:1357–1363.

83. Fisch BM, Pickett B, Weinberg V, *et al*.: Dose of radiation received by the bulb of the penis correlates with risk of impotence after three-dimensional conformal radiotherapy for prostate cancer. *Urology* 2001, 57:955–959.

84. Selek U, Cheung R, Lii M, *et al*.: Erectile dysfunction and radiation dose to penile base structures: a lack of correlation. *Int J Radiat Oncol Biol Phys* 2004, 59:1039–1046.

85. Buyyounouski MK, Hanlon AL, Price RA Jr, *et al*.: In regard to Selek *et al*. erectile dysfunction and radiation dose to penile base structures: a lack of correlation. IJROBP 2004;59:1039–1046. *Int J Radiat Oncol Biol Phys* 2004, 60:1664–1665.

86. Taussky D, Haider M, McLean M, *et al*.: Factors predicting an increased dose to the penile bulb in permanent seed prostate brachytherapy. *Brachytherapy* 2004, 3:125–129.

87. Zagars GK, Pollack A, von Eschenbach AC: Addition of radiation therapy to androgen ablation improves outcome for subclinically node-positive prostate cancer. *Urology* 2001, 58:233–239.

88. Leibel SA, Fuks Z, Zelefsky MJ, *et al*.: The effects of local and regional treatment on the metastatic outcome in prostatic carcinoma with pelvic lymph node involvement. *Int J Radiat Oncol Biol Phys* 1994, 28:7–16.

89. Messing EM, Manola J, Sarosdy M, *et al*.: Immediate hormonal therapy compared with observation after radical prostatectomy and pelvic lymphadenectomy in men with node-positive prostate cancer. *N Engl J Med* 1999, 341:1781–1788.

90. Ghavamian R, Bergstralh EJ, Blute ML, *et al*.: Radical retropubic prostatectomy plus orchiectomy versus orchiectomy alone for pTxN+ prostate cancer: a matched comparison. *J Urol* 1999, 161:1223–1227; discussion 1227–1228.

91. Anscher MS, Clough R, Dodge R: Radiotherapy for a rising prostate-specific antigen after radical prostatectomy: the first 10 years. *Int J Radiat Oncol Biol Phys* 2000, 48:369–375.

92. Bolla M, Van Poppel H, Van Cangh P, *et al*.: Post-operative radiotherapy after radical prostatectomy improves progression-free survival in pT3N0 prostate cancer (EORTC 22911). *Int J Radiat Oncol Biol Phys* 2004, 60:S186.

93. Taylor N, Kelly JF, Kuban DA, *et al*.: Adjuvant and salvage radiotherapy after radical prostatectomy for prostate cancer. *Int J Radiat Oncol Biol Phys* 2003, 56:755–763.

94. Stephenson AJ, Shariat SF, Zelefsky MJ, *et al*.: Salvage radiotherapy for recurrent prostate cancer after radical prostatectomy. *JAMA* 2004, 291:1325–1332.

95. Pollack A, Hanlon AL, Pisansky TM, *et al*.: A multi-institutional analysis of adjuvant and salvage radiotherapy after radical prostatectomy. *Int J Radiat Oncol Biol Phys* 2004, 60:S186–S187.

Management of Erectile Dysfunction Following Radical Prostatectomy

16

Nelson E. Bennett & John P. Mulhall

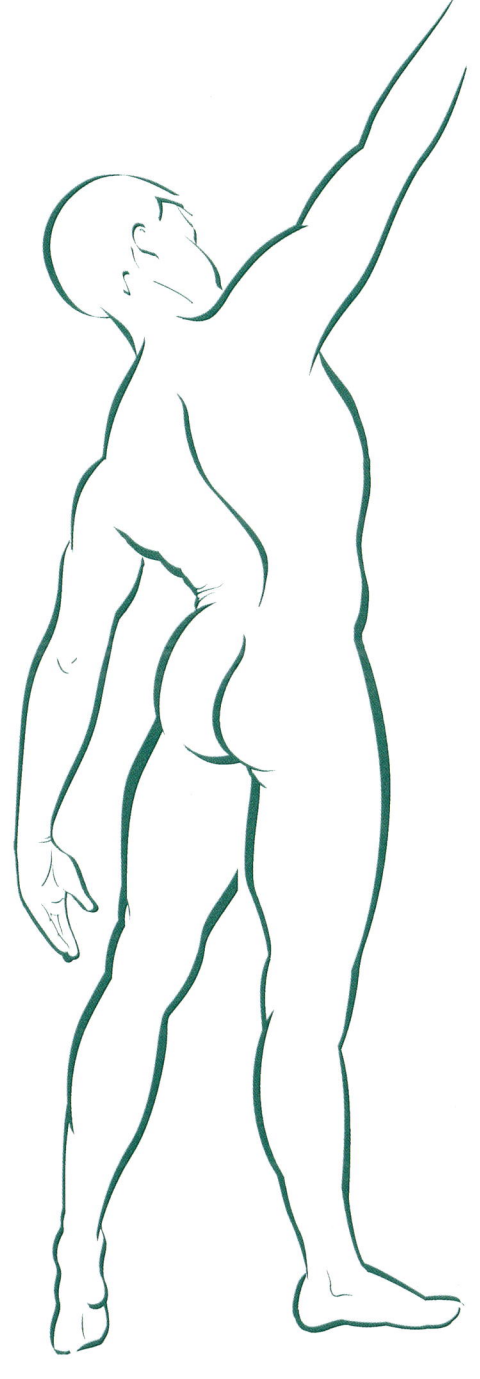

An estimated 200,000 men will be diagnosed with prostate cancer in 2005, and in more than 70% of these patients, the disease will be clinically localized [1]. Of these men, approximately half will undergo radical prostatectomy (RP) for definitive local therapy [2]. Although this procedure is technically successful in long-term disease control, the sexual dysfunction experienced by many men may be burdensome [3]. The consequences of sexual dysfunction, specifically reduction in self-esteem, impaired psychologic well-being, and relationship discord, are well established [4]. Prior to Walsh and Donker's [5] seminal description of the anatomic radical retropubic prostatectomy in 1982, erectile dysfunction was an invariable complication of RP. Since this description, potency preservation rates ranging from 20% to 90% have been reported [6].

It is irrefutable that the nerve-sparing status of the RP is predictive of the degree of recovery of erectile function, bilateral nerve sparing being associated with spontaneous and oral therapy–assisted erectile function results superior to those of unilateral nerve sparing, which in turn is more likely to lead to functional erections than is non–nerve-sparing surgery [7]. The term *nerve sparing* generally refers to the macroscopic preservation of the cavernous nerves. Although rarely reported in a quantitative fashion, at least to this point, there are clearly degrees of nerve sparing depending on the amount of nerve handling, stretching, and electrocautery use during RP, and preliminary reports suggest that such grading is predictive of erectile function outcomes [8].

Much attention is currently focused on strategies to minimize neural trauma or to correct it in a proactive fashion. Such strategies include preoperative, intraoperative, and postoperative maneuvers. Preoperative strategies potentially include the use of medications with neuroprotective properties to minimize cavernous neuropraxia [9]. Intraoperative approaches include optimization of surgical technique, cavernous nerve interposition grafting, and the use of intraoperative neurostimulation to aid in nerve identification prior to prostatectomy and following prostate removal to define cavernous nerve function prior to closure. Postoperative efforts are currently focused on the use of neuromodulatory drugs, which may have neuroregenerative properties.

Post–Radical Prostatectomy Sexual Dysfunctions

Erectile dysfunction
Anejaculation
Anorgasmia
Dysorgasmia (painful ejaculation)
Orgasm-associated urine leakage
Penile length alterations
Penile curvature

▶ **FIGURE 16-1.** Post–radical prostatectomy (RP) sexual dysfunctions. Although erectile dysfunction is recognized as a common post-RP occurrence, it is less well appreciated that other sexual dysfunctions may occur. In preoperative discussions with young men and men who have not completed their family, these patients need to be forewarned that they will be anejaculatory postoperatively. Although they remain candidates for sperm extraction (including vasal aspiration), they should be encouraged to bank semen specimens that can be cryopreserved for possible later use. This sperm will be usable only with in vitro fertilization (intracytoplasmic sperm injection). Many men observe the secretion of a clear, sticky fluid oozing from their urethral meatus; this emanates from the glands of Littre (urethral glands), which secrete this fluid in small quantities (< 0.5 mL) during high levels of arousal. There are data that indicate that a significant percentage of men have difficulty achieving orgasm following RP, and it is being increasingly appreciated that a proportion of men suffer from painful orgasm (dysorgasmia) after this operation [10]. The majority of men will leak urine at the time of orgasm on at least a few occasions after RP. The degree and persistency of this is usually correlated with diurnal continence level. Leakage of urine at orgasm is a significant barrier to satisfactory relations. Historically, condoms and the tricyclic antidepressant medication imipramine have been used with mixed success and acceptability for patients. More recently, we have been using the ACTIS band, the variable-tension band that has been used with the intraurethral suppository MUSE (Vivus, Menlo Park, CA). This band obstructs urine leakage at orgasm, with a high level of reliability and acceptance by patients. Morphologic changes in the penis are well documented in the literature (*see* Fig. 16-3).

Orgasmic Dysfunction Following Prostatectomy

Study	Year	Operation	Orgasmic Dysfunction
Barnas *et al.* [10]	2004	RP	74% had alterations in orgasm
			14% had orgasmic pain
Goriunov *et al.* [11]	1997	TURP	188/818 (23%) had orgasmic pain
Koeman *et al.* [12]	1996	RP	11% had orgasmic pain
			82% had diminished orgasmic intensity
Bergman *et al.* [13]	1979	RC	25% had anorgasmia
			17% had reduced intensity
Steg *et al.* [14]	1988	TURP	36% had alterations in orgasm

▶ **FIGURE 16-2.** Orgasmic dysfunction following prostatectomy. Barnas *et al.* [10] reported on 239 patients who had previously undergone a radical retropubic prostatectomy. Twenty-two percent of the patients had no change in orgasm intensity, 37% reported a complete absence of orgasm, 37% had decreased orgasm intensity, and 4% reported more-intense orgasms post prostatectomy compared with preoperatively. Dysorgasmia occurred in 14% of the patients, and the most common location was the penis. Pain was reported to occur always (with every orgasm) in 33%, frequently in 13%, occasionally in 35%, and rarely in 19%. Most patients (55%) experienced orgasm-associated pain of less than a minute's duration. Goriunov *et al.* [11] reported on orgasm alterations in surgically treated benign prostatic hyperplasia (BPH) patients. This group reported that 188 of 818 such patients (23%) suffered from dysorgasmia after their surgery.

Koeman *et al.* [12] reported pain during orgasm in 11% of post–radical prostatectomy (RP) patients, and 82% complained of diminished orgasmic intensity after surgery. The study by Bergman *et al.* [13] of 43 men who had undergone cystoprostatectomy for bladder cancer found 25% of postoperatively sexually active men unable to attain orgasm, and 17% of those able to achieve orgasm by masturbation found the sensation impaired. Steg *et al.* [14] reported that 36% of postprostatectomy patients who had BPH described their sensation of orgasm as "different" after surgery. Thus, it is well documented that following prostate and radical pelvic surgery, men have changes in orgasm. Currently, however, most clinicians spend little time discussing these changes prior to surgery or managing the problem effectively postoperatively. RC—radical cystoprostatectomy; TURP—transurethral resection of the prostate.

Penile Length Alterations Following Radical Prostatectomy

Study	Year	Patients, n	Timing of Length Measurements	Results
Fraiman et al. [15]	1999	100	Preoperatively and < 6 mo post RP	Mean reduction length of 9% Mean volume loss of 22%
Munding et al. [16]	2001	31	Preoperatively and 3 mo post RP	71% had objective length loss 48% had loss of > 1 cm Loss range: 0.5–4 cm
Savoie et al. [17]	2003	63	Preoperatively and 3 mo post RP	68% had objective length loss 19% had > 15% length loss Nerve sparing not predictive

▶ **FIGURE 16-3.** Penile length alterations following radical prostatectomy (RP). The literature supports the concept that men complain of penile length loss and that objective measures confirm this in the RP patient population [15–17]. Fraiman et al. [15] studied 100 men less than 6 months after RP, taking preoperative and postoperative flaccid and erect measurements and demonstrating an overall mean reduction in erect penile length of 9% but a mean reduction in volume of 22%. Munding et al. [16] studied 31 men, measuring penile length in the stretched flaccid state (accepted as equivalent to erect length) and showing that 71% had a decrease in penile length compared with preoperative length; 48% of the men demonstrated a greater than 1-cm loss, with a range of loss between 0.5 and 4 cm. Savoie et al. [17] studied 63 patients, taking preoperative measurements followed by repeat measurements at 3 months postoperatively, and demonstrated that 68% had some degree of length loss. The authors also showed that in this population, there was no difference between patients with erectile dysfunction and those without it postoperatively.

Although many patients have been told that removal of the prostate shortens the urethra by 2 to 3 cm, this concept has no scientific basis because the urethra is fixed at the urogenital diaphragm so that at the time of the vesicourethral anastomosis, the bladder is brought down to the urethra at this level. The reasons for penile volume changes can be explained by appreciating four concepts: 1) penile structural anatomy, 2) cavernous nerve injury–associated structural alterations in the penis, 3) cavernosal hypoxia-induced structural changes in the penis, and 4) sympathetic hyperinnervation.

The corpora cavernosa are composed of two distinct tissues, the corporal smooth muscle and the tunica albuginea. Penile smooth muscle is under contractile and relaxation forces. Relaxation is accomplished through the release of nitric oxide (NO) and the generation of the second messenger cyclic nucleotides, cyclic GMP and cyclic AMP [18]. Contractility of the smooth muscle is generally tonic and under the control of erectolytic neurotransmitters such as adrenaline. Any factors that result in reduced NO secretion (as occurs in patients with lower motor neuron lesions, such as patients with diabetes and those who have had RP) led to decreased relaxation or distensibility of corporal smooth muscle, and may lead to loss of length.

It is recognized that neural injury leads to end-organ structural alterations. Carrier et al. [19] in 1995 demonstrated that in a rat model of bilateral cavernous nerve transaction, there was a significant reduction in NO synthase (NOS)-staining nerves as early as 3 weeks post injury and that these reductions were sustained at the 6-month time point. Shortly thereafter, Klein et al. [20] demonstrated that following cavernous nerve injury, the corporal smooth muscle shows apoptotic changes; these findings were confirmed by User et al. [21]. Leungwattanakij et al. [22] further demonstrated that cavernous neurotomy leads to up-regulation of fibrogenic cytokines and collagenization of the corporal smooth muscle. It has also been postulated that the chronic absence of erectile activity leads to a state of cavernosal hypoxia (see Fig. 16-9) [23]. Finally, sympathetic hyperinnervation (termed *competitive sprouting* by some experts) refers to the concept that when autonomic nerves are injured, sympathetic fibers are biologically primed to recuperate from injury and regenerate more quickly, resulting in unantagonized sympathetic tone in the end organ [24]. Following cavernous nerve injury, this phenomenon results in a penile hypertonic state.

To synthesize these concepts into a working hypothesis, penile length changes can be divided into early and delayed changes. In response to the neural injury that occurs intraoperatively, the cavernous nerves undergo wallerian degeneration, and early on, when sympathetic nerve function is in the ascendancy, as stated above, the penis is a hypertonic organ—an organ exhibiting sympathetic overdrive. The clue that these changes are not the result of permanent structural sequelae is that on gentle penile stretch, the penis readily elongates from its "buried" position. It has been our clinical experience that this hypertonic state is most pronounced within the first 3 to 6 months after surgery. Of more concern are delayed structural changes, which result from true irreversible structural alterations in the corporal smooth muscle. These structural changes probably result from a combination of factors (as described above): neural injury–associated denervation apoptosis as well as cavernosal hypoxia-induced collagenization in men who experience delayed return of erectile function. The difference between these changes and early hypertonicity is evidenced by the reduced or absent penile stretch in the group with permanent smooth muscle alterations.

Post–Radical Prostatectomy Sexual Dysfunction and Quality of Life

Level of Sexual Function	Degree of Bother, % of Patients		
	None, Very Small, or Small	Moderate	Great
Good or very good	90	7	3
Very poor or poor	12	10	78

▶ **FIGURE 16-4.** Post–radical prostatectomy (RP) sexual dysfunction and quality of life. Litwin *et al.* [25,26] assessed the health-related quality-of-life outcomes of patients with clinically localized prostate cancer. This study demonstrated that patients with prostate cancer treated with surgery or radiation reported worse sexual function and bother than men of similar age without prostate cancer intervention. Globally, patients with a poor or very poor level of sexual functioning were greatly bothered. Those with a high level of sexual functioning cited low levels of bother. Fowler *et al.* [27] surveyed 1072 Medicare patients who underwent RP. Fifty-six percent of patients who had functional erections prior to surgery had postoperative erectile dysfunc-

tion (ED). When questioned about the degree of bother associated with their ED, 39% of the patients stated it was no problem, 29% stated it was a small problem, and only 32% stated it was a moderate/big problem. Stanford *et al.* [1] analyzed data from Surveillance, Epidemiology, and End Results (SEER) registries and reported on 1291 patients. Patients were followed prospectively for 2 years. After RP, 19% of the patients reported erections firm enough for intercourse and 44% reported no erections whatsoever. With regard to bother, of those with erectile function changes, 14% thought it no problem, 23% a small problem, and 42% a moderate/big problem. Despite these figures, 72% of the patients stated that they would choose surgery again.

Mechanisms of Post–Radical Prostatectomy Erectile Dysfunction

Neurogenic
  Neuropraxia is routine
  Stretch, traction, compression, cautery, transection injury
  Anatomic versus functional preservation
  Neural trauma leads to decrease in NOS staining
  Neural trauma leads to CCSM apoptosis
Arteriogenic
  Preoperative arterial insufficiency
  Accessory pudendal artery injury
  Defined postoperatively using vascular assessment
  Predictive of erectile function outcomes
Venogenic
  Denervation apoptosis
  Cavernosal hypoxia-induced fibrosis
  Structural alterations are time dependent
  Predictive of erectile function outcomes
Psychogenic
  Impact of cancer diagnosis on erectile function
  Impact of anxiety centered on reinitiation of intimacy

▶ **FIGURE 16-5.** Mechanisms of post–radical prostatectomy (RP) erectile dysfunction (ED). It is well established in the literature that the degree of nerve sparing is correlated with long-term erectile function outcomes [7]. Even in the hands of experienced high-volume surgeons who perform bilateral nerve-sparing RP, the maneuvers used to spare the nerves are potentially neuron threatening. Currently, for most surgeons, nerve sparing means that using their experience, the nerves appear anatomically intact and are not handled in a traumatic fashion. However, unless some functional assessment of the nerve is conducted after prostate removal (*eg*, intraoperative neurostimulation), how can an individual surgeon be certain that the nerves are functional? Supporting this issue is the fact that 15% of patients who have undergone documented non–nerve-sparing surgery will respond in some fashion to phosphodiesterase-5 inhibitors [28], a situation that can only exist when functioning nerve tissue remains. It is likely that stretching, compression, and traction injuries are more common than hitherto appreciated.

Numerous investigators have documented intraoperatively and by transrectal ultrasonography, angiography, and cadaveric dissection that there are arteries that do not travel with the internal pudendal system

(in Alcock's canal), course close to the prostate, and terminate in the corpora cavernosa (*see* Fig. 16-7) [29,30]. These arteries are called accessory pudendal arteries. Venous leakage may result post RP through two mechanisms, namely, denervation apoptosis and cavernosal hypoxia-induced fibrosis (*see* Fig. 16-8). There is a wealth of literature demonstrating that even temporary nerve injury may result in significant structural and cellular consequences in erectile tissue, including reduced nitric oxide synthase (NOS) staining, up-regulation of fibrogenic cytokines (especially transforming growth factor-β), and increased apoptotic indices eventuating in fibrosis.

Not frequently discussed by urologists is the concept of psychogenic ED in men post RP; however, it is well recognized that the diagnosis of prostate cancer may itself lead to erectile function changes. Furthermore, loss of confidence in erectile ability generates adrenaline because of anxiety about reestablishing intimacy [31], which is seen clinically in men who have a significant discrepancy in their erectile rigidity between nocturnal and sexual erections. Some of these men can improve their erectile function well past 2 years postoperatively, the generally accepted time limit for neural regeneration. CCSM—corpus cavernosum smooth muscle.

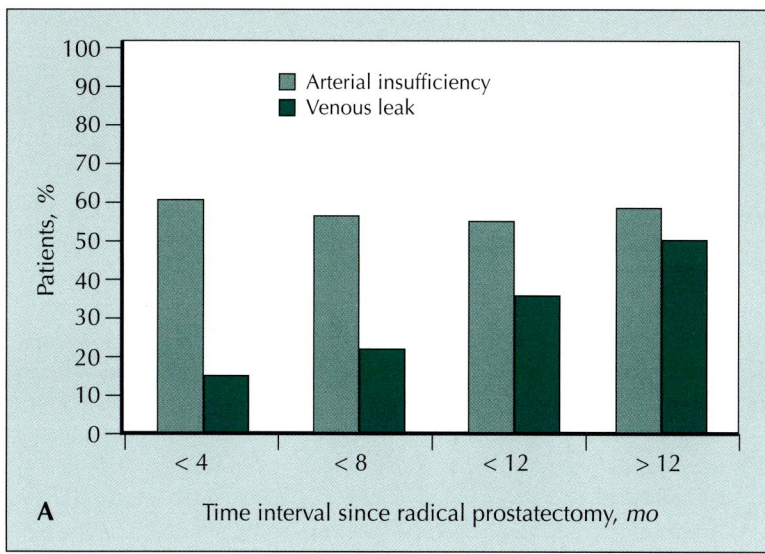

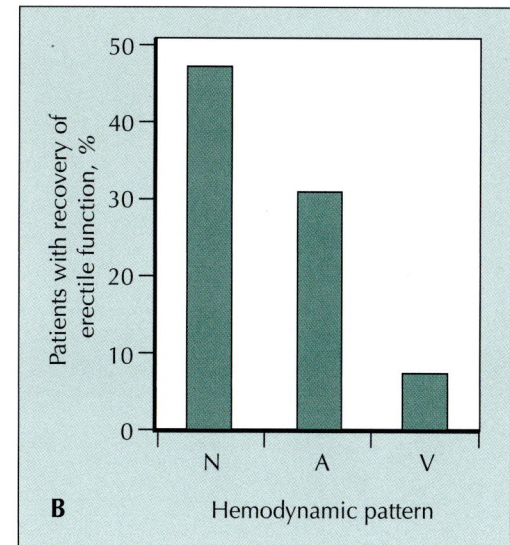

A Time interval since radical prostatectomy, *mo*

B Hemodynamic pattern

▶ FIGURE 16-6. Post–radical prostatectomy (RP) hemodynamics. There is good evidence that some men experience changes in vascular hemodynamics following RP [32,33]. It is postulated that this may result from intraoperative arterial injury. Mulhall and Graydon [32] published data on a group of patients who underwent both pre- and post-RP hemodynamic evaluation. In this small cohort (*n* = 16), 10 patients with post-RP erectile dysfunction (ED) underwent repeat dynamic infusion cavernosometry at 6 months and duplex ultrasonography at 24 months postoperatively. All the patients with ED demonstrated significant arteriogenic impotence and six of 10 patients had venous leakage documented. Only one patient (10%) recovered his erectile function between the sixth and the 24th postoperative month. In another analysis, Mulhall *et al.* [33] demonstrated a very strong correlation between the vascular diagnosis documented post RP and the return of spontaneous erectile function. **A,** Patients with normal (N) vascular status postoperatively had the highest chance of recovery of spontaneous erectile function (47%), followed by those with pure arterio-

genic (A) ED (31%); the lowest chance was seen in patients who had any degree of venous (V) leakage present post RP (8%). **B,** Of note, in this analysis, the incidence of venous leakage increased as the time after surgery increased, it being present in 14%, 21%, 35%, and 50% of patients at less than 4, 4 to 8, 8 to 12, and more than 12 months, respectively.

More recently, it has also been demonstrated that erectile homodynamic alterations are predictive of erectile function outcomes. Ohebshalom *et al.* (Unpublished data) studied 111 patients and found 29% to have normal postoperative penile hemodynamics, whereas 71% had abnormal hemodynamics. Fifteen percent were found to have a venous leakage component. Comparing normal with abnormal hemodynamic groups, there were differences in mean erectile function scores, percent erectile rigidity at 18 months, percent of patients with functional erections permitting sexual intercourse unassisted by pharmacologic agents, and percent of patients responding to sildenafil citrate as defined by vaginal penetration.

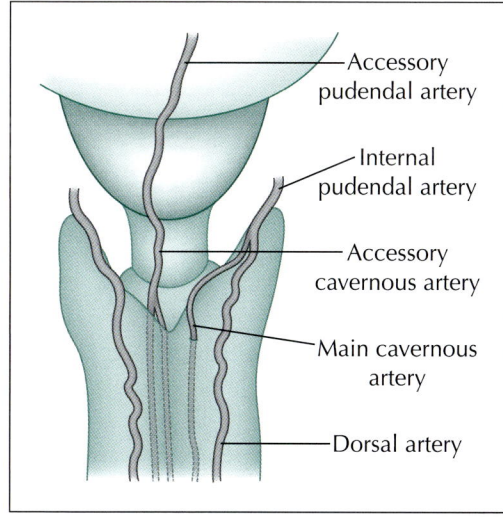

▶ FIGURE 16-7. Accessory pudendal arteries. It has been postulated that arteriogenic erectile dysfunction post radical prostatectomy (RP) results from injury to or transection of the accessory pudendal arteries. These arteries have been shown to course from various origins adjacent to the prostate and to travel caudally toward the corporal bodies [29]. Reports of accessory pudendal arteries range from 7% identified using angiography [34] to approximately 70% of men in cadaveric dissections; in some men, these vessels may represent the sole source of cavernous arterial inflow [29]. In 1999, Droupy *et al.* [30] assessed the functional role of accessory pudendal arteries in erection by transrectal color Doppler ultrasound following a pharmacologically induced erection. They found statistically significant increases in the diameter of the accessory arteries following intracavernosal medication administration. Spectral waveform analysis displayed significant increases in peak systolic velocity, demonstrating a functional role of these arteries in erection. Rogers *et al.* [35] examined the influence of accessory pudendal artery preservation on the recovery of sexual function after RP. Of the 2399 RP patients studied, 4% were identified as having accessory pudendal arteries. Fifty-two of 84 who underwent bilateral nerve-sparing surgery were compared with a control population without accessory pudendal arteries. Potency was defined as the ability to achieve unassisted intercourse with or without the use of sildenafil. In a Cox proportional hazards model, the effect of artery preservation increased the likelihood of potency more than twofold (RR, 2.65; 95% CI, 1.11, 6.32; *P* = 0.028).

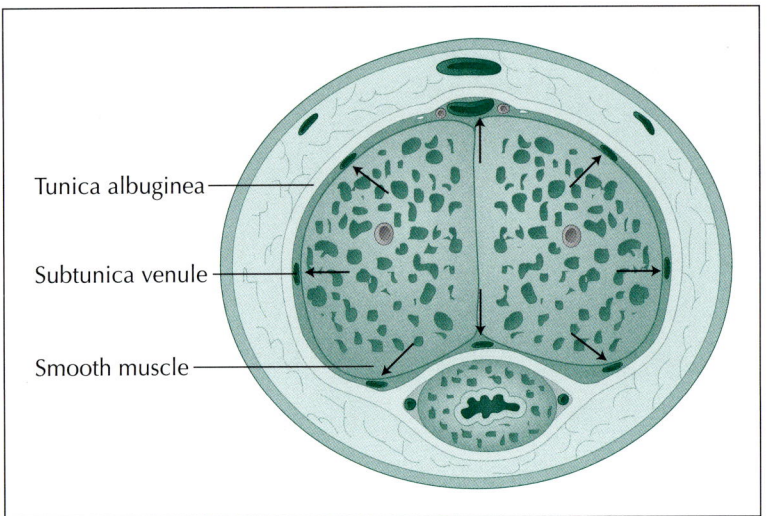

Tunica albuginea

Subtunica venule

Smooth muscle

FIGURE 16-8. Venocclusive mechanism. One of the ever-confusing concepts in sexual medicine is that of corporal vein occlusion. Such misunderstanding has led to the use of venous ligation surgery for venous leakage, without proven long-term benefits. Between the tunica albuginea and the corporal smooth muscle lies a plexus of venules known as the subtunical venous plexus [18]. Upon inflow of blood into the corpus cavernous sinusoids, the smooth muscle becomes engorged and expands in an outward direction (represented by the *fine arrows* in the figure). This expansion traps the subtunical venules between the muscle and the tunica. This is the veno-occlusive mechanism. Failure of the corporal smooth muscle to expand, diffusely or focally, results in persistent potency of some or all of the subtunical venules. This patency results in persistent outflow of blood form the corporal bodies, and this is venous leakage (synonymous with corporo-veno-occlusive dysfunction, veno-occlusive dysfunction, and venogenic erectile dysfunction) [36]. The most common etiology for venous leakage in all erectile dysfunction patients is adrenaline. This chemical will result in persistent contraction of the smooth muscle in the corporal bodies. However, in the post–radical prostatectomy patient, structural alterations that occur in the smooth muscle lead to its failure to expand and fully compress the subtunical venules.

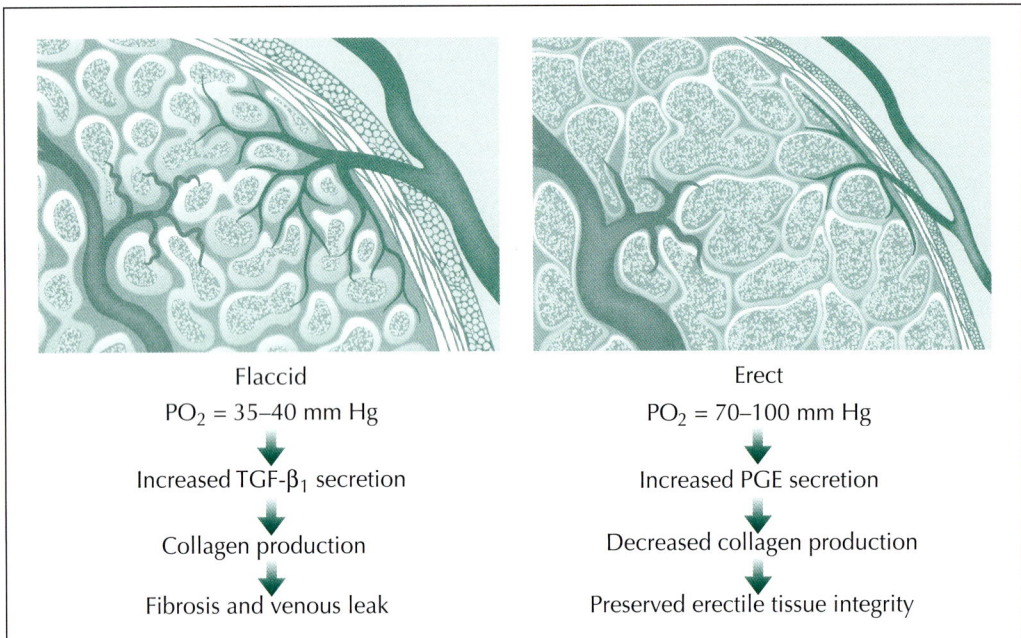

Flaccid
$PO_2 = 35\text{–}40$ mm Hg
⬇
Increased TGF-β_1 secretion
⬇
Collagen production
⬇
Fibrosis and venous leak

Erect
$PO_2 = 70\text{–}100$ mm Hg
⬇
Increased PGE secretion
⬇
Decreased collagen production
⬇
Preserved erectile tissue integrity

FIGURE 16-9. The concept of cavernosal oxygenation. It has been postulated that the chronic absence of erectile activity leads to a state of cavernosal hypoxia [23]. In the flaccid state, blood within the corporal bodies has a venous PO_2, which favors the secretion of fibrogenic cytokines such as transforming growth factor (TGF)-β. During erection, the corporal smooth muscle is oxygenated, resulting in the secretion of endogenous prostanoids (prostaglandin E_1 [PGE_1]), which in turn switch off fibrogenic cytokine production [37,38]. Thus, the health of erectile tissue relies to some extent on the balance between erection and flaccidity. In the patient who has no erectile activity, such as frequently occurs in the early phases post radical prostatectomy, the balance shifts in favor of hypoxia and collagen production. Sattar *et al.* [39] have postulated that there may be a correlation between corporal smooth muscle content and intracavernosal PO_2 level. Moreland *et al.* [38] demonstrated, in cell culture models at least, that corporal smooth muscle cells, when exposed to hypoxic conditions, preferentially secrete TGF-β, which is altered to PGE_1 once the cells are exposed to normoxic conditions [38].

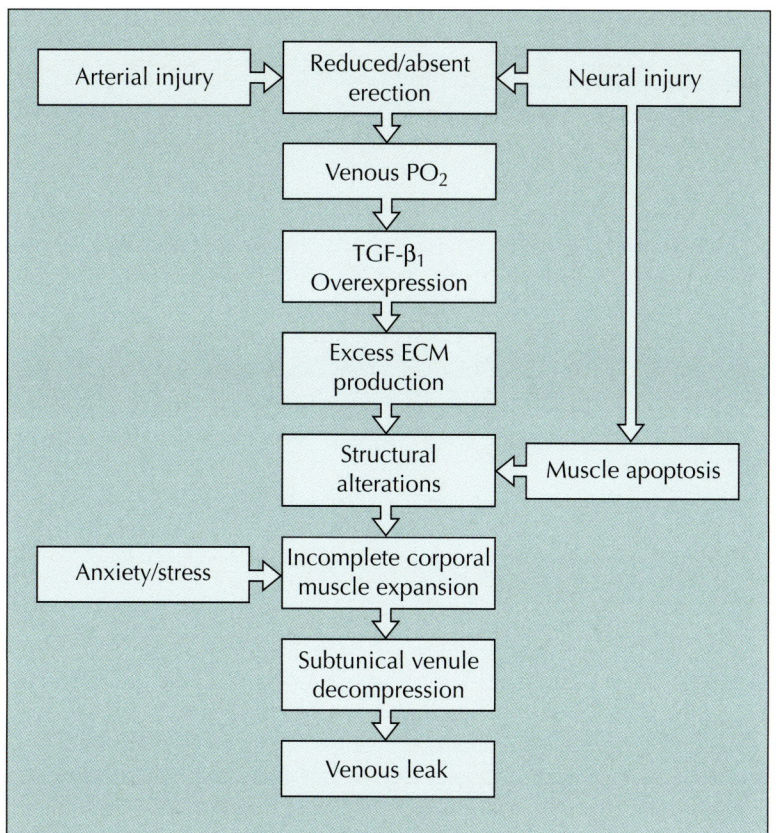

FIGURE 16-10. Pathogenesis of post–radical prostatectomy erectile dysfunction (ED). The previously outlined concepts can be synthesized into an algorithm for the genesis of permanent ED in men who have had nerve-sparing surgery. Neural injury can induce smooth muscle changes (apoptosis), even if the nerve injury is minor and transient. We have data from an animal model showing that cavernous nerve exposure in a rat without any overt dissection or manipulation leads to erectile function alterations [40]. The combination of nerve and arterial insults may lead to loss of erectile function, which in turn causes a state of chronic cavernosal hypoxia. This results in a change in the prostanoid–fibrogenic cytokine balance in favor of the latter, with resultant increased extracellular matrix (ECM; collagen) production and fibrosis of the smooth muscle in the corpora cavernosa. These changes cause the failure of subtunical venules to fully compress, a situation worsened by anxiety and stress-induced adrenaline secretion. All these factors lead to venous leakage. Thus, men who have had recovery from neuropraxia but whose erectile tissue has degenerated may suffer from long-term ED. TGF-β—transforming growth factor-β.

Determinants of Erectile Function Recovery

Definite predictors
  Degree of nerve sparing
  Preoperative erectile function
  Patient age
  Postoperative arterial insufficiency
  Postoperative venous leakage
Possible predictor
  Vascular comorbidities
Nonpredictors
  Tumor volume
  Preoperative PSA
  Surgical margin status

FIGURE 16-11. Determinants of erectile function recovery. It is irrefutable that the nerve-sparing status of a radical prostatectomy (RP) is predictive of the degree of recovery of erectile function, bilateral nerve sparing being associated with spontaneous and oral therapy–assisted erectile function results superior to those of unilateral nerve sparing, which in turn is more likely to lead to functional erections than is non–nerve-sparing surgery [41]. The term *nerve sparing* generally refers to the macroscopic preservation of the cavernous nerves. Although rarely reported in a quantitative fashion, at least to this point, there clearly are degrees of nerve sparing, depending on the amount of nerve handling, stretching, and electrocautery use during the RP, and preliminary reports suggest that such grading is predictive of erectile function outcomes [8]. Furthermore, the concept of bilateral, unilateral, and non–nerve-sparing surgery may be a historical one, as we should be moving toward the more meaningful idea of what percentage (proportion) of each cavernous nerve has been preserved.

Rabbani *et al.* [41] demonstrated that preoperative erectile function and patient age are predictive of erectile function outcomes. Mulhall *et al.* [32,33] showed in two separate studies that postoperative arterial insufficiency and venous leakage as defined by Doppler penile ultrasound correlate with post-RP erectile function outcomes. Although not proven at this point, it is likely that the presence of vascular risk factors such as hypertension, diabetes, and dyslipidemia is associated with poorer erectile function outcomes given their well-known association with erectile dysfunction in the general population. Not shown to be of predictive value for erectile function are pathologic stage, prostate-specific antigen (PSA) level, margin status, and tumor volume.

Prevalence of Post–Radical Prostatectomy Erectile Dysfunction

Study	Year	Patients, n	ED Rate, %
Parsons	2004	25	29
Hara	2003	54	73
Schover	2002	240	67
Abbou	2002	26	77
Theodorescu	2001	42	82
Costabile	2001	419	90
Stanford et al. [1]	2000	1291	60–72
Kao	2000	1069	88
Walsh et al.	2000	64	27
Catalona et al. [6]	1999	1870	32–53
Talcott	1998	125	69–75
Talcott et al. [47]	1997	94	70
Brasilis	1995	51	65–98
Lim	1995	89	96
Litwin et al. [25]	1995	98	52–71
Fowler	1995	1072	59

▶ **FIGURE 16-12.** Prevalence of post–radical prostatectomy (RP) erectile dysfunction (ED). On reviewing the literature, one finds a staggering discrepancy in the prevalence rates of ED following RP. What is the reason for this? Could it be that some centers are just far superior technically to others in nerve-sparing capabilities? It is extremely unlikely that this is the sole reason for the difference in ED rates after this operation. Since the initial description of the anatomic radical retropubic prostatectomy and the elucidation of the course of the cavernous nerves, many urologists have been trained to perform nerve-sparing surgery. The variability in anatomic location and distribution of these nerves combined with variations in nerve-sparing technique and nerve handling has resulted in variable erectile function outcomes after this operation. Reports from centers of high volume and excellence (generally single-institution and -surgeon series) have cited ED rates following RP of between 15% and 40% [6,41–43]. However, if studies of other multisurgeon and multi-institution experiences are included, post-RP ED rates as high as 91% have been reported [27,44–47]. The variability in these rates reflects the difficulty in studying erectile function after RP.

In an attempt to explain the variability in reported rates, there have been several problems. First, there has been variability in the definition of ED among the various studies. For example, the National Institutes of Health consensus conference definition used a definition that nowhere mentioned the use of erectogenic medications. Despite this, there is a contemporary trend to include men using and responding to oral erectogenic medications as being fully potent, which is inaccurate. Second, the means by which data regarding erectile function were collected was scientifically suspect. The modern approach to erectile function assessment includes the use of validated instruments, of which there are several, although the International Index of Erectile Function is the gold standard erectile function questionnaire [48]. With regard to this questionnaire, debate remains as to which score cutoff represents adequate postoperative function. Third, RP patients are among the most heterogeneous populations that exist with regard to erectile function assessment, and comparison among studies is fraught with problems. This heterogeneity is based on differences in mean patient age, mean duration post-RP, comorbidity profile, degree of nerve sparing, and level of nerve-sparing expertise. All these factors make comparison among series from different centers scientifically invalid.

◗ FIGURE 16-13. Maneuvers to minimize post–radical prostatectomy (RP) erectile dysfunction (ED). The nerve-sparing status of an RP is predictive of recovery of erectile function, bilateral nerve sparing being associated with spontaneous and oral therapy–assisted erectile function results superior to those of unilateral nerve sparing, which in turn is more likely to lead to functional erections than is non–nerve-sparing surgery. Identical degrees of nerve manipulation may be graded differently by different surgeons, and postoperative erectile function may be the only reliable surrogate of intraoperative nerve preservation that exists. In the final analysis, with good nerve-sparing technique, erectile function, both natural and medication-assisted, is more likely to be preserved than in cases in which the nerves cannot be spared. The question may be raised as to whether nerve-sparing surgery should ever be done in men with preoperative ED. We believe that the ability of these men to respond to oral therapy postoperatively depends to a large degree on cavernous nerve integrity. Therefore, we urge urologic oncologists to consider, when appropriate, nerve-sparing surgery in patients who are interested in postoperative sexual function, irrespective of their preoperative erectile function.

Nerve identification is sometimes difficult before and/or after the extirpation of the prostate because of patient anatomy and/or intraoperative bleeding [49]. The use of intraoperative cavernous nerve stimulation may aid in overcoming such difficulty and may translate into improved erectile function recovery postoperatively. This technique was initially described by Lue *et al.* [50] and was later formally developed as an intraoperative tool (CaverMap; Bluetorch Technologies, Ashland, MA) for nerve stimulation and tumescence monitoring [51]. The tip of the electrode is placed over the (suspected) cavernous nerve, and stimulation is conducted at multiple sites along the course of the nerves before and/or following prostatectomy. Tumescence is monitored by the presence of a penile strain gauge, which records changes in penile girth. Although data on neurostimulator-assisted prediction of erectile function outcomes have been somewhat mixed, there is good literature to suggest that failure to obtain a response on either side is predictive of no spontaneous erectile function post-RP. Furthermore, the presence of bilateral response is associated with reasonable erectile function outcomes, at least oral erectogenic drug response. Rates of erectile function recovery as high as 68% to 88% have been cited at 12 months postoperatively (Rabbani *et al.*, Unpublished data) [52,53]. The most damning study to date was from a group of highly experienced surgeons who found a high sensitivity of 88% but a low specificity of 54% when using intraoperative neurostimulation [54]. The authors suggested that this lack of specificity hampers the ability to judge what is safe to resect or to determine which tissue needs to be preserved intraoperatively. Despite this study, it likely that nerve function assessment using this technique will continue to be explored at select centers and that with further refinements in the technology, improved computer data generation, and a greater understanding of the implications of the data, intraoperative neurostimulation may in the near future assume a role in predicting at least return of oral therapy response following RP.

Resection of the neurovascular bundle (NVB) may be indicated in patients with advanced unilateral or bilateral disease (*ie*, multiple positive cores, length of positive core, high Gleason grade, and suggestion of extracapsular extension on imaging) to decrease the risk of positive surgical margins. Positive surgical margins increase the chance of treatment failure. Extracapsular extension increases the risk of a positive margin, and this occurs most frequently in the area of the NVB. Wide resection, which may include the NVB, decreases the risk of a positive surgical margin but increases the chance of postoperative ED

without intervention to restore continuity of the nerves [55]. The initial experience using nerve grafts was in rodents, more than a decade ago [56]. It is generally accepted that bilateral nerve resection translates to almost universal loss of spontaneous erectile function, although some men may still respond to oral erectogenic medication. Clinical studies indicate that bilateral nerve grafting may be associated with a 35% to 45% chance of being at least an oral erectogenic agent responder [57,58]. The data on unilateral nerve grafts are less convincing at this time. Cavernous nerve grafting is associated with minimal complications, which are limited to the morbidity associated with harvesting the sural nerves (genitofemoral nerve harvesting has no significant morbidity), such as incisional pain and hypoesthesia over the lateral aspect of the dorsum of the foot (a problem the majority of patients do not complain about) and increased operative time. Given the association between bilateral cavernous nerve resection and long-term failure to obtain spontaneous functional erections or a significant response to oral therapy, this technique appears to be a reasonable strategy to restore erectile function in men in whom bilateral nerve resection is either planned or is required intraoperatively. Larger randomized multi-institutional studies are required to definitively address the role of nerve grafting in the management of the RP patient.

Although the degree of neural trauma that occurs intraoperatively is a determinant of long-term neural function recovery, biologic factors that are involved in neural regeneration likely are important determinants of the completeness of neural recovery. Furthermore, these biologic factors likely are a major reason for the interindividual variation in erectile function recovery after this operation.

Immunophilins are molecules that are found in both immune and neural tissue, although they are found in far greater quantities in the neural tissues. The immunophilin ligand FK506 has been found to prevent axonal degeneration and to preserve electrically induced penile erections in the rat [59]. This agent is an immunosuppressant agent that has been used in transplant medicine for a number of years [60]. Other nonimmunosuppressant neuromodulators have also been explored in animal models [9]. In animal models of stroke and neurodegenerative disease, FK506 has been found to have potent neuroprotective effects. In the rat cavernous injury model, both FK506 and the nonimmunosuppressant agent GPI-1046 have been shown to preserve erectile function and cavernous nerve architecture.

In 1997, Montorsi *et al.* [61] introduced the concept of penile rehabilitation following RP in a randomized, controlled trial using early intracavernosal injections compared with no intervention in 30 men. This study demonstrated a threefold increase in the ability of men to obtain spontaneous erections at 6 months after surgery (67% vs 20%). This small study, which has never been repeated, has been put forth as the main supporting evidence in favor of the concept of penile rehabilitation. The mechanism by which penile injections promote erectile function recovery has been suggested to be the promotion of cavernosal oxygenation. Recently, a randomized, controlled study comparing daily sildenafil with placebo after RP demonstrated an improved ability for men in the treatment group to preserve their preoperative erectile function [62]. In this analysis, nightly use of sildenafil for 6 months after RP improved the ability to preserve preoperative erectile function level, with 27% of the men maintaining their preoperative function compared with 4% in the placebo group. It has been suggested that cavernosal oxygenation is the mechanism by which this regimen effected its improvement in erectile function. However, from clinical experience, few men in the early months after RP obtain any significant nocturnal response to sildenafil, so it is questionable whether oxygenation plays a major role in the improvement in erectile function outcomes. As an alternate hypothesis, preliminary but intriguing data exist demonstrating that sildenafil is an endothelial protectant and may also promote neurogenesis. Most recently, in a nonrandomized study by Mulhall *et al.* [63] comparing 48 men who committed to rehabilitation (in the form of three erections per week) with 74 men who did not, the rehabilitation patients experienced higher rates of recovery of spontaneous functional erections (52% vs 19%), a greater ability to respond to sildenafil (64% vs 24%), a shortened time course to respond to sildenafil, and an increased ability to respond to intracavernosal injections.

Management of Erectile Dysfunction Following Radical Prostatectomy

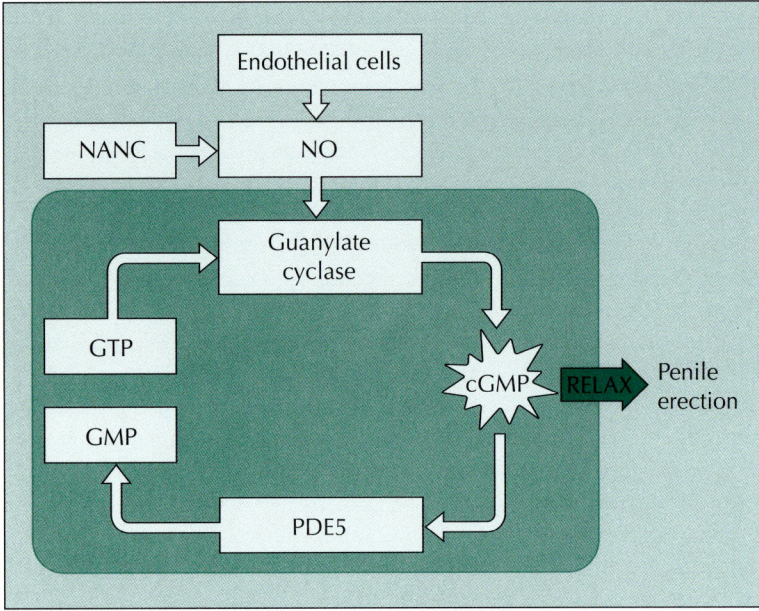

▶ **FIGURE 16-14.** Phosphodiesterase-5 (PDE5) inhibitors. PDE5 inhibitors (sildenafil, vardenafil, tadalafil) result in corporal smooth muscle relaxation through the accumulation of cGMP. cGMP is a second messenger that is formed as a result of the action of the cytoplasmic enzyme guanylate cyclase on guanosine triphosphate (GTP) [64]. Guanylate cyclase, in turn, is activated by the presence of nitric oxide (NO). NO arises from two sources in the corpus cavernosum. The

predominant source is the nerve endings that synapse directly on the corporal smooth muscle [18]. A secondary source is the endothelium that lines the cavernosal arteries and the sinusoids of the corporal bodies. Data support the fact that lower success rates with sildenafil are obtained in erectile dysfunction patients with dysfunction of their cavernous nerves. Such lower-motor neuropathies are seen most often in diabetic men with neuropathy and in patients in the early stages following radical prostatectomy (RP). Goldstein *et al.* [65] reported a 43% success rate in RP patients using a global assessment question (which generally overestimates the ability of men to have sexual intercourse).

In the RP patient population, it is well recognized that the success of these drugs depends on the time of the trial, the degree of nerve sparing, and the integrity of the corporal smooth muscle. Clinical experience demonstrates that men uncommonly respond to sildenafil with a penetration rigidity erection within the first 3 months after RP. It has been our experience that most men start to demonstrate reasonable efficacy at approximately 1 year after surgery. Raina *et al.* [28] demonstrated that duration after surgery of greater than 6 months was associated with an improved response to sildenafil. It has also been well documented that patients who have undergone bilateral nerve-sparing surgery do better than those who have undergone unilateral non–nerve-sparing surgery. Raina *et al.* [28] cited rates in their series of 76%, 53%, and 14%, respectively. In this series, other predictors of a positive outcome with sildenafil included age less than 65 years and better erectile function preoperatively. Company-sponsored data would suggest that all three drugs are approximately similar in their efficacy in this patient population. To date, there have been no head-to-head trials for these drugs in this population [66,67]. NANC—nonadrenergic-noncholinergic neurons.

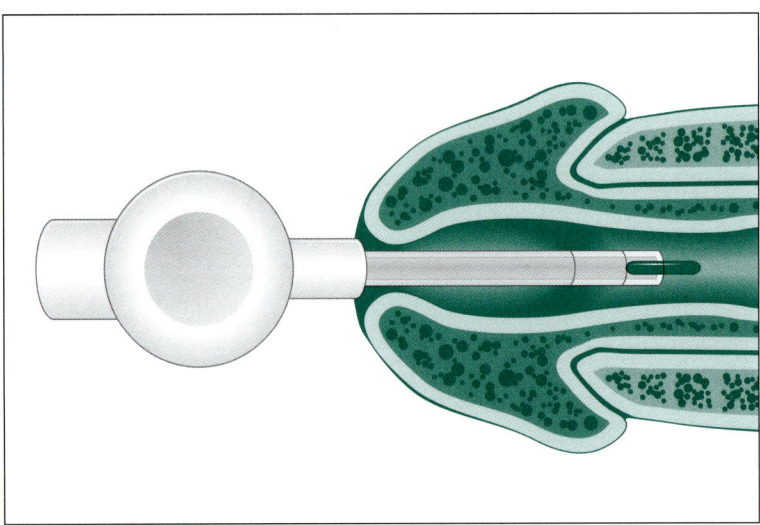

▶ **FIGURE 16-15.** Transurethral suppositories. Intraurethral administration of prostaglandin E_1 (MUSE; Vivus, Menlo Park, CA) elicits a marked cavernosal smooth muscle relaxation, which has been clearly demonstrated [68]. Tiny pellets are placed 2 to 3 cm into the distal urethra following urination. This is followed by massaging of the distal shaft. Approximately 20% of the medication is absorbed into the corpus cavernosum via inter-communicating veins. Eighty percent of the drug is absorbed into the systemic circulation, although it undergoes 99% metabolism on first pass through the lungs. The reported side effects include pain and hypotension. The only series that addresses MUSE in the radical prostatectomy (RP) patient population is that of Costabile *et al.* [69]. In this series of 384

men, of the patients who had an in-office success, 40% were capable of sexual intercourse at home. The most common side effect was pain, reported in 18% of patients in this series. Administration of intraurethral suppositories, although less intimidating than intracavernosal injection, is also somewhat complex. It is recommended that these medications initially be given in the office setting, with instruction and demonstration of competence as well as effectiveness before dispensing a prescription for at-home use. In our experience, lack of effectiveness and inconsistency of response are the main reasons for patient dropout. We use a starting dose of 1000 μg. The patient is instructed to void just prior to use of the medication. Voiding lubricates the urethra and makes the administration of the suppository easier. To minimize venous leakage and promote intra-cavernosal absorption, the patient is instructed to stand while the medication is absorbed. Gentle massage helps absorption. The effectiveness is assessed at 15 to 30 minutes. Detumescence is expected within 1 hour. The manufacturer supplies a variable-tension occlusive device (ACTIS) that is placed at the base of the penis just prior to medication administration, in an effort to increase success rates.

We have been disappointed with the efficacy of this device. The efficacy of this agent in the RP patient population in our hands is less than that reported by Costabile *et al.* [69], with approximately a 60% consistency rate [70] and more than a 50% incidence of pain at the 500- to 1000-μg doses. Nehra *et al.* [71] reported on the ability of a combined sildenafil-MUSE approach to salvage monotherapy failures. In 28 men who had failed either sildenafil or MUSE treatment, all 28 reported penetration rigidity erections with the combined approach (100 mg sildenafil and 500 μg MUSE). These data were confirmed by Mydlo *et al.* [72] in another series.

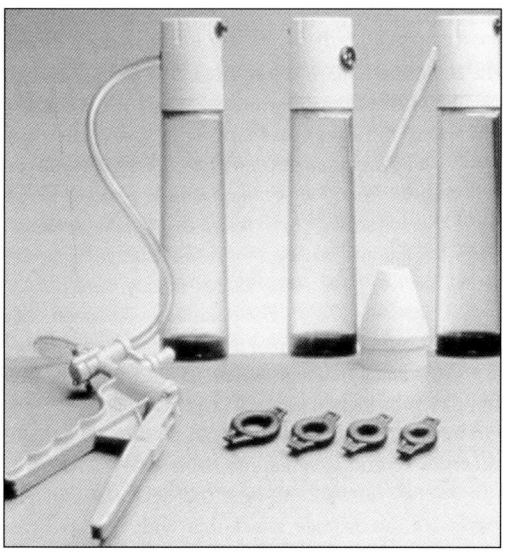

▶ **FIGURE 16-16.** Vacuum devices. At this time, to the best of our knowledge, there is no analysis of vacuum device therapy in the radical prostatectomy (RP) patient population. Of note, despite information to the contrary from vacuum device manufacturers, there are no data to support the use of vacuum device therapy as a rehabilitation strategy in this population. These devices have as advantages the fact that they are simple to use and do induce penile lengthening. They do not oxygenate the erectile tissue, as the majority of the inflow of blood is nonoxygenated blood, although there is a minimal increase in cavernosal artery flow without the use of a constriction ring. As a strategy, it is difficult to integrate into sexual relations because of the fact that the penis neither looks nor feels normal to patient or partner. Furthermore, the application of a constriction ring often results in significant discomfort for the patient. Only randomized studies to compare vacuum device therapy with no intervention or with regular oral or intracavernosal agents will answer the question regarding its role in post-RP sexual function rehabilitation. Soderdahl *et al.* [73] analyzed 44 patients who had been randomized to injection therapy or vacuum devices and after 15 uses, assessed patient satisfaction. Overall, superior erectile rigidity was obtained and patient and partner satisfaction was greater with injection therapy. Overall determinants of injection preference included age less than 60 years, erectile dysfunction duration of less than 12 months, and a history of RP.

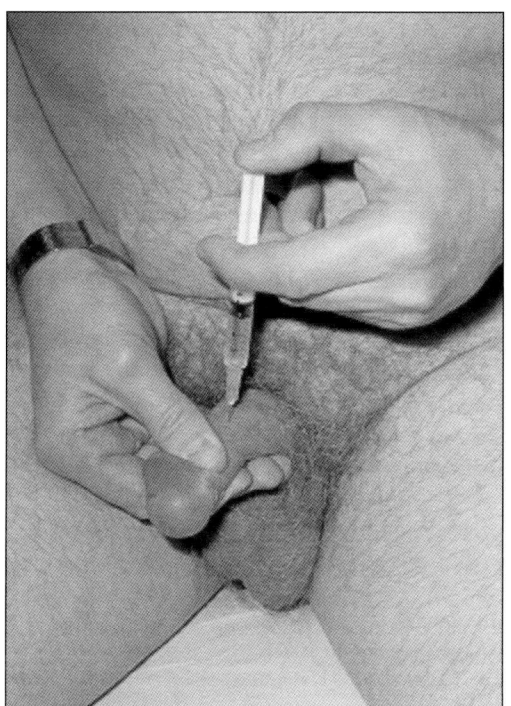

▶ **FIGURE 16-17.** Intracavernosal injection therapy. In the radical prostatectomy (RP) patient population using combination agents, 95% success rates can be achieved with injection therapy [63]. The advantages of injection therapy are the efficacy, consistency, and rigidity profiles. The disadvantages include the need for the use of a needle, pain (with prostaglandin E_1 [PGE_1]-containing medications), priapism, and cost. The use of combination agents is preferred over single agents to minimize side effects and maximize effectiveness [74]. For example, the combination of papaverine, phentolamine, and PGE_1 (known as trimix) has been shown to be more effective than high-dose alprostadil alone and, especially in this population, has a lower incidence of painful erections (because of the lower concentration of alprostadil). The advantage of intracavernosal agents compared with oral agents is that the injection medications bypass the need for nitric oxide. Thus, patients with a largely neurogenic form of erectile dysfunction (ED; post-RP, for example) who fail oral therapy are routinely successfully treated with low-dose intracavernosal injection if they commence injection therapy within a year of RP. The one major prerequisite for injection therapy response is a responsive corporal smooth muscle.

As the erectile undergoes structural damage in the absence of erectile activity, the longer after surgery a patient starts injections, the less likely he is to respond. Although sildenafil has become the most prescribed medication for the treatment of ED, intracavernosal therapy still represents a cornerstone of therapy. In a series by Brannigan *et al.* [75], 74 patients were asked to compare trimix to sildenafil with regard to rigidity of erection, overall sexual satisfaction, and preference for future use. All patients, regardless of etiology of ED, reported a more rigid erection using trimix versus sildenafil. The majority of patients (60%) who had undergone a prostatectomy chose to continue using trimix as their preferred treatment. The potential side effects—fibrosis, priapism, bleeding, and bruising—can be thus minimized by using combination medications, carefully titrating to the correct dose in the clinic, and thoroughly educating the patient on injection technique [74]. Fibrosis may occur as a nodule, plaque, or penile curvature. Pastorini *et al.* [76] found the incidence is 1% with alprostadil, 12% with papaverine, and 9% with papaverine and phentolamine (bimix), although these incidences are far in excess to those experienced in our population of injection patients. Linet and Neff calculated that priapism occurred in 1.3% of 8090 patients in 48 studies with alprostadil. Patients in our clinic are instructed that prolonged erections constitute a medical emergency. If the patient has an erection that lasts longer than 2 hours and is not relieved by ejaculation, he is instructed to call the office for advice and should be in the emergency department by the fourth hour. Patients who still have an erection are treated with intracavernosal α-adrenergic agonists (phenylephrine).

In a retrospective analysis of 102 RP patients who had used injection therapy at the Cleveland Clinic, Raina *et al.* [77] cited a 68% efficacy rate. In this study, there was no difference in response between patients who had nerve-sparing and those who had non–nerve-sparing surgery. The overall dropout rate was 52%; however, if patients who had return of spontaneous or pill-assisted erectile function are excluded, the dropout rate was only 29%.

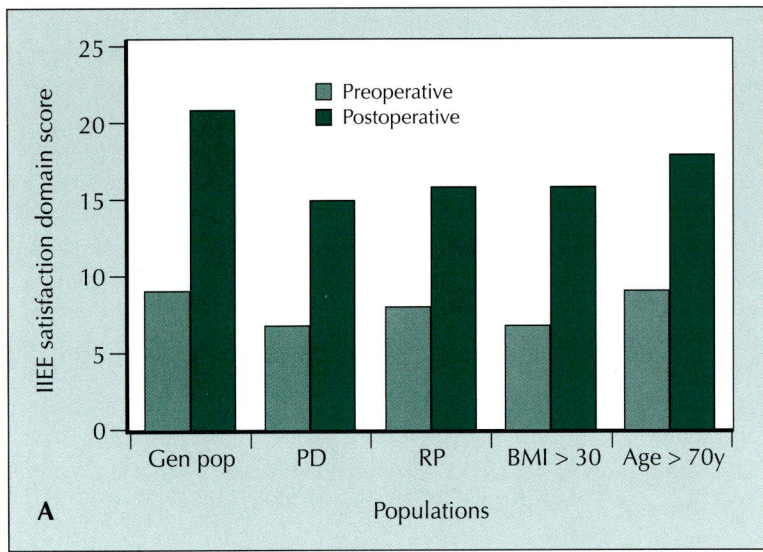

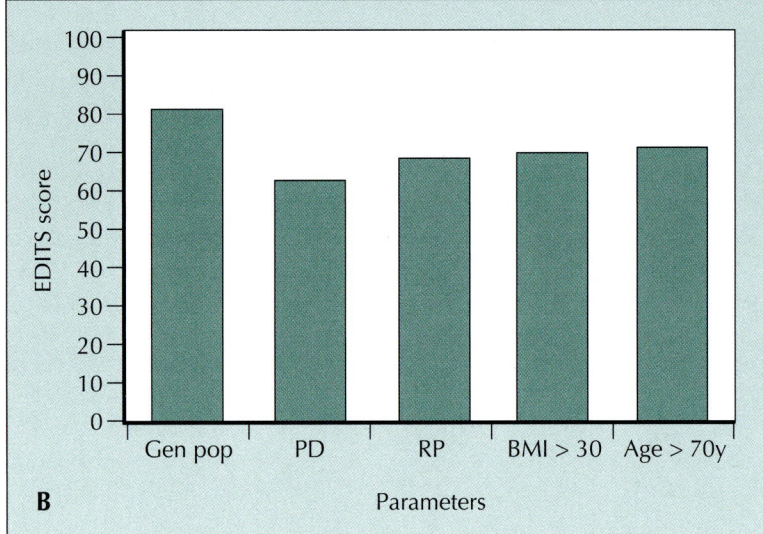

▶ **FIGURE 16-18.** Penile prosthesis surgery. Penile implants remain a key strategy in the management of patients with erectile dysfunction (ED). The majority of patients for which it is a treatment option have found other options ineffective; have structural damage to the corpora, as occurs after radical prostatectomy (RP); or are unwilling to consider alternative treatments or find such options unpalatable [78]. Overall satisfaction rates with penile prosthetic surgery are high, with more than 80% of patients and their partners happy with the result of the implant [79,80]. It is likely that the satisfaction level with implants is high largely because of excellent penile rigidity and rapidity of response, resulting in an associated improvement in sexual relations [81]. On the other hand, a number of studies have highlighted implant complications and disadvantages such as pain, postoperative appearance of the penis, insufficient firmness, altered erectile sensation, reduced penile length compared with recalled preoperative dimensions, decreased sensation during ejaculation, and difficulty with using the prosthetic devices as major reasons for dissatisfaction with penile implants [79,82].

Khoudary *et al.* [83] reported on 50 men who underwent a combination procedure of non–nerve-sparing radical retropubic prostatectomy and placement of a penile prosthesis. A retrospective chart review was conducted. The group was compared with a group of 72 men undergoing RP alone during the same time interval. The mean time to sexual intercourse was 12.7 weeks. No prosthesis infections had occurred at a mean last follow-up of 1.7 years. Eight percent of the men required revision of their inflatable penile prosthesis. **A** and **B**, Akin-Olugbade *et al.* [84] reported on determinant of satisfaction following penile implant surgery and demonstrated that RP was associated with significantly lower scores on a global sexual satisfaction question, International Index of Erectile Function (IIEF) satisfaction domain, and ED inventory of treatment satisfaction (EDITS) compared with those of the general implant population. On multivariable analysis, RP remained a significant factor associated with lower satisfaction (RR, 2.2).

For the patient who has preoperative ED, and has explored oral and injection agents, and has failed these options or finds them unsatisfactory, simultaneous implant placement with RP is a reasonable option. We advocate placement of only the implant (three-piece) reservoir at the time of the RP, with delayed placement of the cylinders/pump. For patients with functional erections prior to RP, we advocate implant surgery only for those who have developed postoperative ED and who have explored oral and injection therapies and have either failed them or find them unsatisfactory. We advocate a conservative approach until at least 12 to 18 months after surgery. BMI—body mass index; PD—Peyronie's disease.

Penile Rehabilitation Program

Comprehensive preoperative counseling
Immediate oral agent trial (at time of catheter removal)
Early evaluation (4–8 wk)
Move directly to ICI if oral therapy fails early
Regular erectile activity
Regular follow-up
Rechallenge with oral agent regularly if patient failed therapy early
Follow-up to 24 mo
All patients presenting within 12 mo of surgery are offered nightly PDE5 inhibitor therapy
  as an adjunct

▶ **FIGURE 16-19.** Penile rehabilitation program. Based on the concepts that are outlined in this chapter, at Memorial Sloan-Kettering Cancer Center, we have in place a structured rehabilitation program for the prostatectomy patient. For the highly motivated and concerned patient, preoperative counseling is encouraged to give the patient realistic expectations as well as information on rehabilitation strategies for the earliest phases following the operation. At the time of urinary catheter removal, the patient is given a prescription for a phosphodiesterase-5 (PDE5) inhibitor and asked to define if he is a responder to this agent using the maximum dose with sexual stimulation over the ensuing 2 to 4 weeks. Many men are not interested in sexual relations at this early stage, so they are instructed to assess PDE5 inhibitor response through self-stimulation. After the patient has tried maximum-dose PDE5 inhibitors, he presents to the sexual medicine urologist to discuss the results. This appointment will have been made either preoperatively, at the time of hospital discharge, or at the time of catheter removal. At this visit, the next stage of penile rehabilitation is discussed. If the patient has responded with a penetration-hardness erection to oral agents, he is assigned to oral agent–based rehabilitation; if he has not responded, he is asked to consider injection therapy. The vast majority of patients are not PDE5 inhibitor responders in the first 3 months after surgery, and for some who respond early postoperatively, this response may diminish over the course of the first 3 months following the operation.

Patients are encouraged to get three penetration rigidity erections per week (with oral agents or injections). They are informed that this does not mandate sexual relations three times per week, as it is the physical process of the erection that is of benefit to the corporal smooth muscle and endothelium, so sexual relations and orgasm are of no added benefit. On the other four (nonerection) nights, patients are encouraged to use a low-dose PDE5 inhibitor at bedtime. In our practice, we predominantly use sildenafil at 25 to 50 mg mhs (100-mg pill split into halves or quarters), depending on cost to the patient. The purpose of this latter strategy is not to induce erection in the early stages after surgery but rather to protect endothelium and corporal smooth muscle. Of note, patients who are using injection therapy regularly are not prescribed tadalafil because of the long half-life (17.5 hours), which may lead to circulating tadalafil when a man uses his next injection and to priapism.

Patients are followed on a 4-month basis until 24 months after surgery. Those who fail PDE5 inhibitors in the early stages after surgery are encouraged to rechallenge themselves on a regular basis, at least every 2 months in the first year and every month in the second year. In our practice, the time to peak sildenafil response is greater than 20 months after radical prostatectomy. ICI—intracavernosal injection.

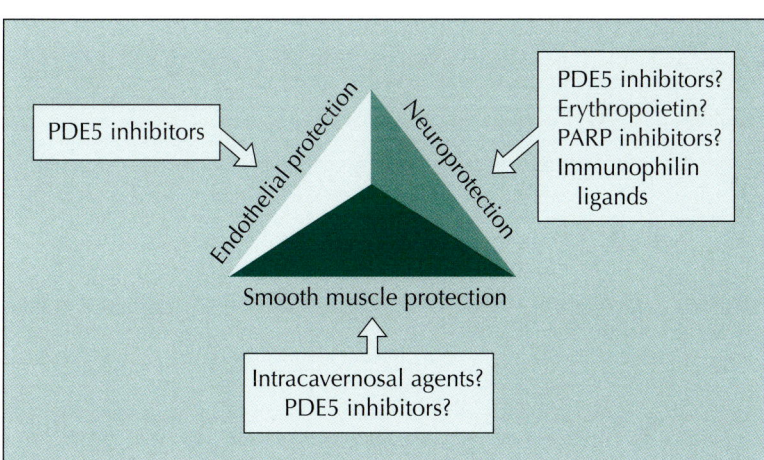

▶ **FIGURE 16-20.** The future of post–radical prostatectomy (RP) sexual function preservation. It is probable that the future of sexual rehabilitation after RP will see a greater level of proactivity on the part of urologists in an effort to optimize outcomes. The optimal approach will likely be a trimodal strategy that makes efforts to protect the cavernous nerves, the endothelium of the cavernosal sinusoids, and the corporal smooth muscle. Ongoing investigation is being conducted into immunophilin ligands such as tacrolimus and the GPI compounds as neuromodulatory agents; however, there is interest in other agents, such as poly(adenosylribose) polymerase (PARP) inhibitors, erythropoietin, and phosphodiesterase-5 (PDE5) inhibitors, for the same reason. It is believed that the best way to protect corporal smooth muscle is to generate erections with oxygenated blood. At this time, the only two strategies that do this with efficacy are intracavernosal injection agents and, in certain cases, PDE5 inhibitors. The only endothelial protectants that we have identified to date are PDE5 inhibitors. More basic research is being conducted in this area than ever before.

1. Stanford JL, Feng Z, Hamilton AS, *et al.*: Urinary and sexual function after radical prostatectomy for clinically localized prostate cancer. The Prostate Cancer Outcomes Study. *JAMA* 2000, 283:354–360.

2. Harlan LC, Potosky A, Gilliland FD, *et al.*: Factors associated with initial therapy for clinically localized prostate cancer: Prostate Cancer Outcomes Study. *J Natl Cancer Inst* 2001, 93:1864–1871.

3. Bokhour BG, Clark JA, Inui TS, *et al.*: Sexuality after treatment for early prostate cancer: exploring the meanings of 'erectile dysfunction.' *J Gen Int Med* 2001, 16:649–655.

4. Guest JF, Das Gupta R: Health-related quality of life in a UK-based population of men with erectile dysfucntion. *Pharmacoeconomics* 2002, 20:109–117.

5. Walsh PC, Donker PJ: Impotence following radical prostatectomy: insight into etiology and prevention. *J Urol* 1982, 128:492–497.

6. Catalona WJ, Carvalhal GF, Mager DE, Smith DS: Potency, continence and complication rates in 1870 consecutive radical retropubic prostatectomies. *J Urol* 1999, 162:433–438.

7. Quinlan DM, Epstein JI, Carter BS, Walsh PC: Sexual function following radical prostatectomy: influence of preservation of neurovascular bundles. *J Urol* 1991, 145:998–1002.

8. Touijer AK, Trabulsi E, Hassen W, *et al.*: Evaluation of erectile function at 3 months in a contemporary series of laparoscopic radical prostatectomy. *J Sex Med* 2004, 151:108–109.

9. Burnett AL, Becker RE: Immunophilin ligands promote penile neurogenesis and erection recovery after cavernous nerve injury. *J Urol* 2004, 171:495–500.

10. Barnas J, Pierpaoli S, Ladd P, *et al.*: The prevalence and nature of orgasmic dysfunction following radical prostatectomy. *BJU Int* 2005, 94:603–605.

11. Goriunov VG, Davidov MI: Sexual readaptation after the surgical treatment of benign prostatic hyperplasia [in Russian]. *Urol Nefrol (Mosk)* 1997, Sep-Oct:20–24.

12. Koeman M, van Driel MF, Schultz WC, Mensink HJ: Orgasm after radical prostatectomy. *Br J Urol* 1996, 77:861–864.

13. Bergman B, Nilsson S, Petersen I: The effect on erection and orgasm of cystectomy, prostatectomy and vesiculectomy for cancer of the bladder: a clinical and electro-myographic study. *Br J Urol* 1979, 51:114–120.

14. Steg A, Zerbib M, Conquy S: Sexual disorders after an operation for benign prostatic hypertrophy [in French]. *Ann Urol (Paris)*, 1988, 22:129–133.

15. Fraiman MC, Lepor H, McCullough AR: Changes in penile morphometrics in men with erectile dysfunction after nerve-sparing radical retropubic prostate-ctomy. *Mol Urol* 1999, 3:109–115.

16. Munding MD, Wessells HB, Dalkin BL: Pilot study of changes in stretched penile length 3 months after radical retropubic prostatectomy. *Urology* 2001, 58:567–569.

17. Savoie M, Kim SS, Soloway MS: A prospective study measuring penile length in men treated with radical prostatectomy for prostate cancer. *J Urol* 2003, 169:1462–1464.

18. Lue TF: Erectile dysfunction. *N Engl J Med* 2000, 342:1802–1813.

19. Carrier S, Zvara P, Nunes L, *et al.*: Regeneration of nitric oxide synthase–containing nerves after cavernous nerve neurotomy in the rat. *J Urol* 1995, 153:1722–1727.

20. Klein LT, Miller MI, Buttyan R, *et al.*: Apoptosis in the rat penis after penile dener-vation. *J Urol* 1997, 158:626–630.

21. User HM, Hairston JH, Zelner DJ, *et al.*: Penile weight and cell subtype specific changes in a post–radical prostatectomy model of erectile dysfunction. *J Urol* 2003, 169:1175–1179.

22. Leungwattanakij S, Bivalacqua TJ, Usta MF, *et al.*: Cavernous neurotomy causes hypoxia and fibrosis in rat corpus cavernosum. *J Androl* 2003, 24:239–245.

23. Moreland RB: Is there a role of hypoxemia in penile fibrosis: a viewpoint presented to the Society for the Study of Impotence. *Int J Impot Res* 1998, 10:113–120.

24. Zhou S, Chen LS, Miyauchi Y, *et al.*: Mechanisms of cardiac nerve sprouting after myocardial infarction in dogs. *Circ Res* 2004, 95:76–83.

25. Litwin MS, Hays RD, Fink A, *et al.*: Quality-of-life outcomes in men treated for localized prostate cancer. *JAMA* 1995, 273:129–135.

26. Litwin MS, Flanders SC, Pasta DJ, *et al.*: Sexual function and bother after radical prostatectomy or radiation for prostate cancer: multivariate quality-of-life analysis from CaPSURE. Cancer of the Prostate Strategic Urologic Research Endeavor. *Urology* 1999, 54:503–508.

27. Fowler FJ, Barry MJ, Lu-Yao G, *et al.*: Patient-reported complications and follow-up treatment after radical prostatectomy. The National Medicare Experience: 1988–1990 (updated June 1993). *Urology* 1993, 42:622–629.

28. Raina R, Lakin MM, Agarwal A, *et al.*: Long-term effect of sildenafil citrate on erectile dysfunction after radical prostatectomy: 3-year follow-up. *Urology* 2003, 62:110–115.

29. Aboseif SR, Breza J, Orvis BR, *et al.*: Erectile response to acute and chronic occlusion of the internal pudendal and penile arteries. *J Urol* 1989, 141:398–402.

30. Droupy S, Hessel A, Benoit G, *et al.*: Assessment of the functional role of accessory pudendal arteries in erection by transrectal color Doppler ultrasound. *J Urol* 1999, 162:1987–1991.

31. Schover LR: Sexual rehabilitation after treatment for prostate cancer. *Cancer* 1993, 71:1024–1030.

32. Mulhall JP, Graydon RJ: The hemodynamics of erectile dysfunction following nerve-sparing radical retropubic prostatectomy. *Int J Impot Res* 1996, 8:91–94.

33. Mulhall JP, Slovick R, Hotaling J, *et al.*: Erectile dysfunction after radical prostate-ctomy: hemodynamic profiles and their correlation with the recovery of erectile function. *J Urol* 2002, 167:1371–1375.

34. Rosen MP, Greenfield AJ, Walker TG, *et al.*: Arteriogenic impotence: findings in 195 impotent men examined with selective internal pudendal angiography. Young Investigator's Award. *Radiology* 1990, 174:1043–1048.

35. Rogers CG, Trock BP, Walsh PC: Preservation of accessory pudendal arteries during radical retropubic prostatectomy: surgical technique and results. *Urology* 2004, 64:148–151.

36. Mulhall JP, Damaser MS: Development of a mathematical model for the pre-diction of the area of venous leak. *Int J Impot Res* 2001, 13:236–239.

37. Moreland RB, Traish A, McMillin MA, *et al.*: PGE$_1$ suppresses the induction of collagen synthesis by transforming growth factor-beta 1 in human corpus caver-nosum smooth muscle. *J Urol* 153:826–834.

38. Moreland RB, Gupta S, Goldstein I, Traish A: Cyclic AMP modulates TGF-beta 1–induced fibrillar collagen synthesis in cultured human corpus cavernosum smooth muscle cells. *Int J Impot Res* 1998, 10:159–163.

39. Sattar AA, Salpigides G, Vanderhaeghen JJ, *et al.*: Cavernous oxygen tension and smooth muscle fibers: relation and function. *J Urol* 1995, 154:1736–1739.

40. Mullerad M, Donohue JF, Li PS, *et al.*: Functional sequelae of cavernous nerve injury in the rat: model dependency. *J Sex Med* 2004, 1:39.

41. Rabbani F, Stapleton AMF, Kattan MW, *et al.*: Factors predicting recovery of erections after radical prostatectomy. *J Urol* 2000, 164:1929.

42. Walsh PC, Marschke P, Ricker D, Burnett AL: Patient-reported urinary continence and sexual function after anatomic radical prostatectomy. *Urology* 2000, 55:58–61.

43. Walsh PC: Sexual function and bother after radical prostatectomy or radiation for prostate cancer: multivariate quality-of-life analysis from CaPSURE. *J Urol* 2000, 163:370.

44. Jonler M, Messing EM, Rhodes PR, Bruskewitz RC: Sequelae of radical pro-statectomy. *Br J Urol* 1994, 74:352–358.

45. Leandri P, Rossignol G, Gautier JR, Ramon J: Radical retropubic prostatectomy: morbidity and quality of life. Experience with 620 consecutive cases. *J Urol* 1992, 147:883–887.

46. Siegel T, Moul JW, Spevak M, *et al.*: The development of erectile dysfunction in men treated for prostate cancer. *J Urol* 2001, 165:430–435.

47. Talcott JA, Rieker P, Propert KJ, *et al.*: Patient-reported impotence and incon-tinence after nerve-sparing radical prostatectomy. *J Natl Cancer Inst* 1997, 89:1117–1123.

48. Rosen RC, Riley A, Wagner G, *et al.*: The international index of erectile function (IIEF): a multidimensional scale for assessment of erectile dysfunction. *Urology* 1997, 49:822–830.

49. Myers RP: Radical prostatectomy: pertinent surgical anatomy. *Urol Clin North Am* 1994, 21:

50. Lue TF, Gleason CA, Brock GB, *et al.*: Intraoperative electrostimulation of the cavernous nerve: technique, results and limitations. *J Urol* 1995, 154:1426–1428.

51. Klotz L, Herschorn S: Early experience with intraoperative cavernous nerve stimu-lation with penile tumescence monitoring to improve nerve sparing during radical prostatectomy. *Urology* 1998, 52:537–542.

52. Klotz L, Heaton J, Jewett M, *et al.*: A randomized phase 3 study of intraoperative cavernous nerve stimulation with penile tumescence monitoring to improve nerve sparing during radical prostatectomy. *J Urol* 2000, 164:1573–1578.

53. Chang SS, Peterson M, Smith JA Jr: Intraoperative nerve stimulation predicts postoperative potency. *Urology* 2001, 58:594–597.

54. Walsh PC, Marschke P, Catalona WJ, *et al.*: Efficacy of first-generation Cavermap to verify location and function of cavernous nerves during radical prostatectomy: a multi-institutional evaluation by experienced surgeons. *Urology* 2001, 57:491–494.

55. Scardino PT, Kim ED: Rationale for and results of nerve grafting during radical prostatectomy. *Urology* 2001, 57:1016–1019.

56. Quinlan DM, Nelson RJ, Walsh PC: Cavernous nerve grafts restore erectile function in denervated rats. *J Urol* 1991, 145:380–383.

57. Kim ED, Nath R, Kadmon D, *et al.*: Bilateral nerve grafts during radical retropubic prostatectomy: 1-year follow-up. *J Urol* 2001, 165:1950–1956.

58. Kim ED, Scardino PT, Kadmon D, *et al.*: Interposition sural nerve grafting during radical prostatectomy. *Urology* 2001, 57:211–216.

59. Burnett AL: Rationale for cavernous nerve restorative therapy to preserve erectile function after radical prostatectomy. *Urology* 2003, 61:491–497.

60. Starzl TE, Todo S, Fung J, *et al.*: FK 506 for liver, kidney, and pancreas transplantation. *Lancet* 1989, 2:1000–1004.

61. Montorsi F, Guazzoni G, Strambi LF, *et al.*: Recovery of spontaneous erectile function after nerve-sparing radical retropubic prostatectomy with and without early intracavernous injections of alprostadil: results of a prospective, randomized trial. *J Urol* 1997, 158:1408–1410.

62. Padma-Nathan H, McCullough A, Giuliano F, *et al.*: Nightly post-operative sildenafil dramatically improves the return of spontaneous erections following a bilateral nerve-sparing radical prostatectomy [abstract]. *J Urol* 2003, 169:Abstract 1402.

63. Mulhall JP, Land S, Parker M, *et al.*: The use of an erectogenic pharmacotherapy regimen following radical prostatectomy improves recovery of spontaneous erectile function. *J Sex Med* 2005, 2:532–539.

64. Boolell M, Allen MJ, Ballard SA: Sildenafil: an orally active type 5 cyclic GMP–specific phosphodiesterase inhibitor for the treatment of penile erectile dysfunction. *Int J Impot Res* 1996, 8:47–52.

65. Goldstein I, Lue TF, Padma-Nathan H, *et al.*: Oral sildenafil in the treatment of erectile dysfunction. Sildenafil Study Group. *N Engl J Med* 1998, 338:1397–1404.

66. Brock G, Nehra A, Lipshultz LI, *et al.*: Safety and efficacy of vardenafil for the treatment of men with erectile dysfunction after radical retropubic prostatectomy. *J Urol* 2003, 170:1278–1283.

67. Montorsi F, Nathan HP, McCullough A, *et al.*: Tadalafil in the treatment of erectile dysfunction following bilateral nerve sparing radical retropubic prostatectomy: a randomized, double-blind, placebo controlled trial. *J Urol* 2004, 172:1036–1041.

68. Padma-Nathan H, Hellstrom WJ, Kaiser FE, *et al.*: Treatment of men with erectile dysfunction with transurethral alprostadil. Medicated Urethral System for Erection (MUSE) Study Group. *N Engl J Med* 1997, 336:1–7.

69. Costabile RA, Spevak M, Fishman IJ, *et al.*: Efficacy and safety of transurethral alprostadil in patients with erectile dysfunction following radical prostatectomy. *J Urol* 1998, 160:1325–1328.

70. Mulhall JP, Jahoda AE, Ahmed A, *et al.*: Analysis of the consistency of intraurethral prostaglandin E(1) (MUSE) during at-home use. *Urology* 2001, 58:262–266.

71. Nehra A, Blute ML, Barrett DM, Moreland RB: Rationale for combination therapy of intraurethral prostaglandin E(1) and sildenafil in the salvage of erectile dysfunction patients desiring noninvasive therapy. *Int J Impot Res* 2002, 14(Suppl 1):S38–S42.

72. Mydlo JH, Volpe MA, Macchia RJ: Initial results utilizing combination therapy for patients with a suboptimal response to either alprostadil or sildenafil monotherapy. *Eur Urol* 2000, 38:30–34.

73. Soderdahl DW, Thrasher JB, Hansberry KL: Intracavernosal drug-induced erection therapy versus external vacuum devices in the treatment of erectile dysfunction. *Br J Urol* 1997, 79:952–957.

74. Mulhall JP: Intracavernosal injection therapy: a practical guide. *Tech Urol* 1997, 3:129–134.

75. Brannigan RE, Spitz A, Schatte EC: Comparison of sildenafil citrate (Viagra) versus trimix intracavernosal injection (ICI) as treatment for erectile dysfunction (ED) [abstract]. *J Urol* 1999, 161:214.

76. Pastorini S, Marino G, Cocimano V, *et al.*: Complications of intracavernous pharmacologic infusion in impotence. Long-term results [in Italian]. *Minerva Urol Nefrol* 1993, 45:109–112.

77. Raina R, Lakin MM, Thukral M, *et al.*: Long-term efficacy and compliance of intracorporeal (IC) injection for erectile dysfunction following radical prostatectomy: SHIM (IIEF-5) analysis. *Int J Impot Res* 2003, 15:318–322.

78. Eardley I, Sethia K: Surgery for erectile dysfunction. In *Erectile Dysfunction: Current Investigation and Management*, edn 2. Philadelphia: Mosby; 2003:

79. Garber BB: Mentor Alpha 1 inflatable penile prosthesis: patient satisfaction and device reliability. *Urology* 1994, 43:214–217.

80. Montorsi F, Guazzoni G, Bergamaschi F, Rigatti P: Patient-partner satisfaction with semirigid penile prostheses for Peyronie's disease: a 5-year followup study. *J Urol* 1993, 150:1819–1821.

81. Tefilli MV, Dubocq F, Rajpurkar A, *et al.*: Assessment of psychosexual adjustment after insertion of inflatable penile prosthesis. *Urology*, 1998, 52:1106–1112.

82. Whalen RK, Merrill DC: Patient satisfaction with Mentor inflatable penile prosthesis. *Urology* 1991, 37:531–539.

83. Khoudary KP, DeWolf WC, Bruning CO, Morgentaler A: Immediate sexual rehabilitation by simultaneous placement of penile prosthesis in patients undergoing radical prostatectomy: initial results in 50 patients. *Urology* 1997, 50:395–399.

84. Akin-Olugbade Y, Ahmed A, Parker M, *et al.*: Determinants of patient satisfaction following penile prosthesis surgery. *J Sex Med* 2005, in press.

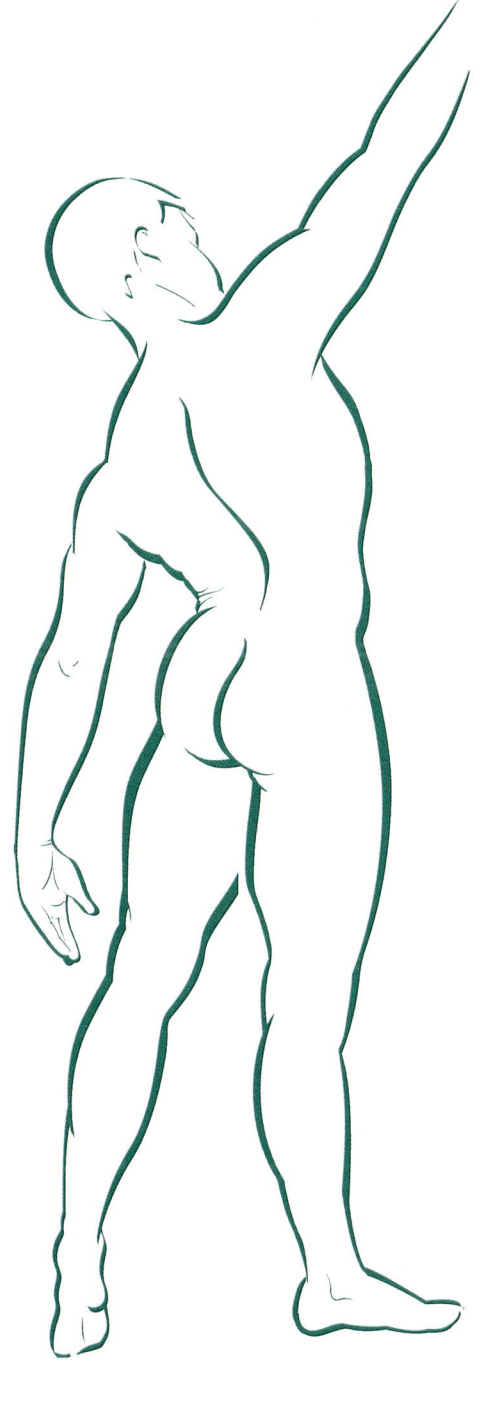

Management of Metastatic Prostate Cancer

17

Kenneth J. Pienta

Prostate cancer is curable if detected when confined to the gland, but treatment remains palliative once the disease has metastasized. The propensity of prostate cancer to metastasize to bone has been documented through several autopsy programs and a systematic protocol performed by Roudier *et al.* [1], which evaluated the prevalence of osseous involvement in patients who have died from prostate cancer. They found that 100% of patients had histologic evidence of bone involvement [1–5]. This propensity to metastasize to bone is accompanied by an osteoblastic reaction in the bone that is unmatched by any other type of cancer. The interaction of the osteoclasts and osteoblasts of the bone stroma and the prostate cancer cells that lead to this osteoblastic response is largely undefined, however endothelin-1, transforming growth factor-β, bone morphogenetic proteins, and several other cytokines have been implicated [6–8].

Less well recognized is the prevalence of metastases to other organs in the late stages of the disease. In addition to the bone, common sites of involvement include the lymph nodes, lung, adrenal glands, and liver. Although the pattern of prostate cancer metastasis remains unexplained, it appears that prostate cancer cells metastasize, in part, to organs with high levels of the chemokine stromal-derived factor-1 (SDF-1, CXCL12) [9–13]. The stromal cell components of different organs and tissues secrete chemokines that act as local chemoattractants for normal and cancer cells in the circulation [14]. Prostate cancer cells up-regulate the receptor for SDF-1, CXCR4, when they are exposed to the hypoxic environment of the primary tumor [15,16]. The continued definition of the factors involved in prostate cancer tumorigenesis and metastasis is an area of active investigation and will allow for the development of novel therapeutic strategies in high-risk patients as well as those with advanced disease.

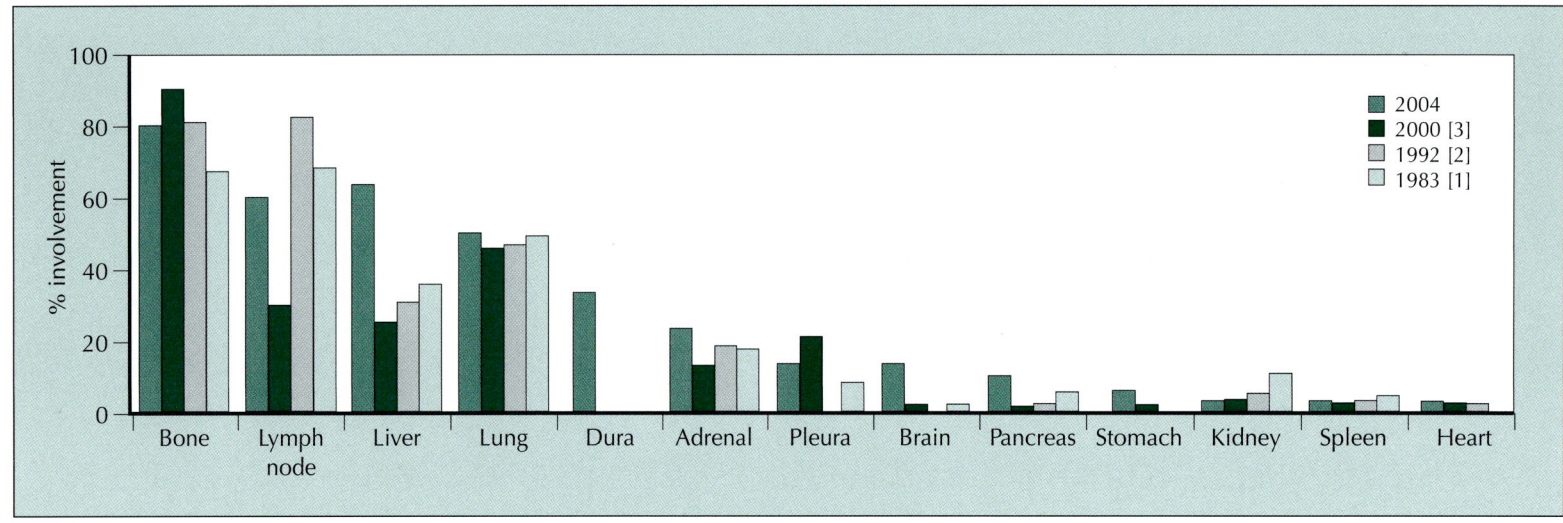

▶ **FIGURE 17-1.** Prevalence of metastases in various organs in patients dying of prostate cancer. Bone, lymph nodes, liver, and lung are the most common sites of disease. The involvement of these sites may reflect a tropism secondary to high levels of the chemokine stromal derived factor-1.

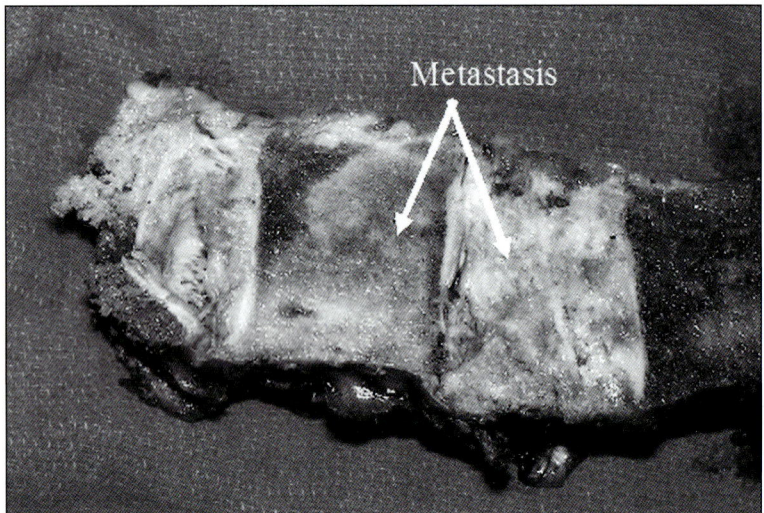

▶ **FIGURE 17-2.** Osteoblastic metastases in bone. The osteoblastic reaction common to prostate cancer is seen here in the vertebral column of a patient with late-stage prostate cancer.

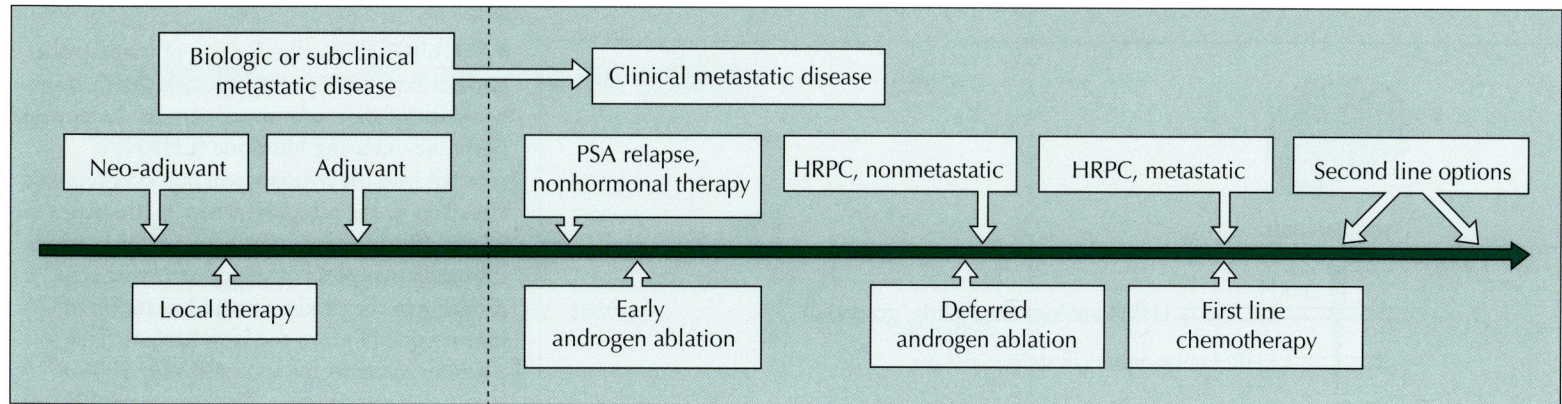

▶ **FIGURE 17-3.** The timeline of metastatic disease in a patient treated for prostate cancer. Note that metastasis occurs in a patient subclinically long before it is recognized clinically, generally by an increase in serum prostate-specific antigen (PSA). Treatment type depends on where in the disease course a patient lies.

Biologically, metastatic prostate cancer is defined by the point at which prostate cancer cells successfully leave the prostate gland and establish themselves at a distant site. Clinically, metastatic prostate cancer is first defined by the presence of a rising PSA level in the blood after local treatment or salvage local therapy. When a patient is identified with metastatic prostate cancer, the immediate questions become when to treat them and how to treat them.

No study has evaluated in a rigorous manner whether there is a survival benefit in treating a patient with metastatic disease, as evidenced by a rising PSA, early or waiting until the disease has progressed further [17]. A few studies were done addressing the question of early versus delayed therapy in the pre-PSA era. The concept of watchful waiting, *ie*, waiting to treat until the development of symptoms, was first piloted in the 1970s after the results of trials in patients within the Veterans Administration suggested that delaying therapy until the onset of symptoms did not increase prostate cancer–specific mortality in patients with locally advanced or metastatic disease [18,19]. In a reanalysis of the these studies, early medical castration with the estrogen diethylstilbestrol was found to improve actuarial survival rates for patients with locally advanced and metastatic disease when compared with placebo. Early treatment appeared to be most beneficial for younger patients [18,19]. From 1985 until 1993, a Medical Research Council (MRC) trial randomized 938 men with locally advanced or asymptomatic metastatic prostate cancer to either immediate (at the time of diagnosis) or deferred (on development of symptoms) treatment with monotherapy [20]. Although this study has been criticized because of the lack of uniform staging in the patients, it demonstrated an increase in disease-specific and overall survival in patients treated with immediate androgen deprivation. Patients treated with deferred therapy suffered significantly more comorbid events associated with their disease. Additionally, men with metastatic disease at presentation developed an indication for treatment at a median of 9 months of observation, and few remained untreated at the time of death. A recent abstract regarding longer-term data from the MRC trial, however, reported that although immediate therapy continued to improve disease-specific survival, overall survival differences were becoming considerably smaller [21]. Interestingly, more patients in the immediate-therapy arm died of nonprostate cancer. It is unclear whether the hormonal therapy conferred adverse events leading to morbidity and mortality or the hormonal treat-

ment controlled the prostate cancer, allowing other comorbid conditions to run their natural course.

Most recently, the question of when to treat patients with early metastatic prostate cancer has been discussed in terms of PSA kinetics. Serum PSA levels are known to increase with tumor growth and disease progression of metastatic disease after relapse and correlate with the pathologic state of the disease [22,23]. Therefore, a rapid change in PSA doubling time (PSADT; also described as PSA velocity) would potentially indicate increased tumor growth and/or a change in tumor aggressiveness. Pound *et al.* [24] evaluated PSADT from PSA levels during follow-up evaluation after radical prostatectomy in men who did not receive hormone therapy. A PSADT of less than 10 months was associated with the development of subsequent clinical metastasis. Similarly, D'Amico *et al.* [25] reported PSADT in 94 patients with localized prostate cancer treated with external-beam radiation who presented with PSA failure. They found that a PSADT of 12 months or less correlated with high-risk disease and increased prostate cancer–related deaths.

These studies of hormonal therapy in patients with metastatic disease have been complemented by studies in the primary treatment adjuvant setting demonstrating a survival advantage for men treated with primary therapy plus hormonal therapy versus primary therapy alone. The European Organization for Research and Treatment of Cancer randomized 415 men with locally advanced prostate cancer at presentation to radiation alone versus radiation with concurrent goserelin therapy [26]. The Kaplan-Meier estimate of overall survival at 5 years was 79% for the combined treatment group, compared with 62% for the group receiving radiation alone (*P* = 0.001). From 1988 to 1993, the Eastern Cooperative Oncology Group evaluated the impact of immediate hormonal therapy on 98 men who underwent radical prostatectomy and pelvic lymphadenectomy who were found to have nodal metastases [27]. Patients were randomized to androgen deprivation or to routine follow-up. After a median follow-up of 7.1 years, the group who received immediate hormonal therapy had a statistically significant improvement in overall survival (*P* = 0.02), progression-free survival (*P* < 0.001), and prostate cancer–specific survival (*P* = 0.001). After 10 years, the actuarial survival of patients treated with immediate therapy was approximately 80%, compared with only 55% in patients treated with deferred androgen deprivation (*P* = 0.02). Although such data cannot be extrapolated to patients with metastatic prostate cancer as manifested by a rising PSA, the conclusions of these studies provide additional evidence in support of early androgen deprivation. The current clinical trend is to treat patients with aggressive disease (initial high Gleason score, fast PSADT) with early hormonal therapy [28]. HRPC—hormone-refractory prostate cancer.

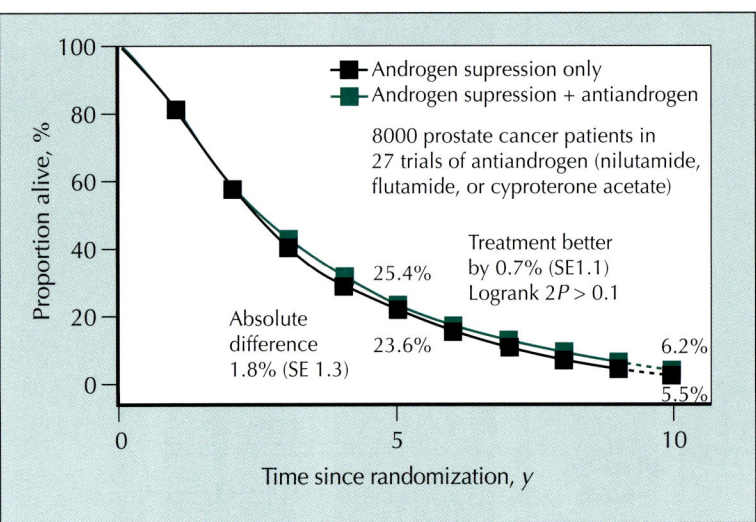

▶ **FIGURE 17-6.** Ten-year survival in the 27 randomized trials of complete androgen blockade versus monotherapy. Survival differences between patients treated with complete androgen blockade versus monotherapy with surgical or medical castration are generally considered minor.

Hormonal therapy in the most traditional sense consists of inducing castration levels of testosterone in the patient (*see* Fig. 17-4) [17]. More than 60 years ago, Huggins and Hodges [33] achieved these levels with estrogen administration and then with surgical castration. The estrogenic compound diethylstilbestrol, no longer manufactured in the United States, acts as a potent inhibitor of luteinizing hormone (LH) secretion, thereby indirectly lowering testosterone secretion [34]. The gold standard for eliminating gonadal androgen secretion remains bilateral orchiectomy. Within hours of surgical castration, 95% reduction in serum testosterone level is achieved. The luteinizing hormone–releasing hormone (LHRH) analogues currently approved by the US Food and Drug Administration potently bind and stimulate the pituitary LHRH receptors. This sustained agonist activity initially results in a marked increase in LH and testosterone secretion ("testosterone flare") but is followed by a decline to castra-

tion testosterone levels after 2 to 4 weeks. Current LHRH agonists, such as leuprolide and goserelin acetate, are available in depot formulations capable of suppressing testosterone secretion for 3, 4, or 12 months per subcutaneous injection [35]. Abarelix is a pure LHRH antagonist that does not induce an initial increase in LH [36].

Antiandrogens block the effects of androgens by competitively binding the androgen receptor. The nonsteroidal antiandrogens flutamide, bicalutamide, and nilutamide are used in the initial month of hormonal therapy to block the potential effects of the testosterone flare or are used in combination with the LHRH agonists. The combination of testicular androgen suppression and adrenal androgen blockade (termed maximal androgen blockade, total androgen blockade, or total androgen suppression) was initially thought to improve outcomes in patients with metastatic disease [37]. However, benefits of combined androgen blockade, such as time to progression and overall survival, are minimal at best [38]. Current standard of care leaves the decision of monotherapy versus combined androgen blockade with the physician and patient. (*Adapted from* Prostate Cancer Trialists' Collaborative Group [38]; with permission.)

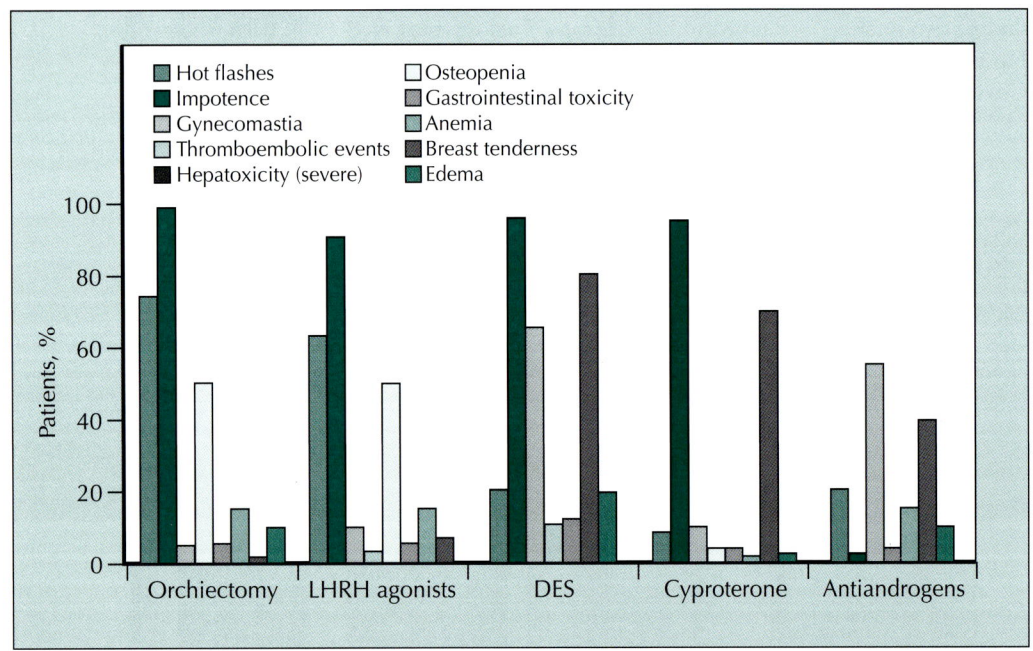

▶ **FIGURE 17-7.** Side effects of hormone therapy. Castration levels of testosterone lead to several side effects. Individual side effects vary widely between patients. For many years, androgen deprivation therapy (hormonal therapy that lowers testosterone to castrate levels) was considered to be well tolerated. Loss of libido and hot flashes were often the only side effects told to patients. Several other toxicities have now been described, including fatigue, weight gain, depression, osteopenia, anemia, muscle atrophy, gyne-

comastia, loss of cognitive function, and decrease in high-density lipoprotein [39–44]. Symptoms may be relieved partially by a variety of agents. The addition of an estrogen for patients treated by medical or surgical castration may lessen the frequency or severity of hot flashes as well as loss of bone density. Other agents, such as venlafaxine, may also reduce the severity of hot flashes [45]. The antiandrogens and cyproterone (a steroidal antiandrogen not used in the United States) are associated with a rare but potentially fatal hepatotoxicity, and should be used with caution in patients with preexisting liver disease. Patients on therapy should have liver enzyme measurements monitored. Gynecomastia can be lessened with a very short course of radiation therapy to the breasts, but only if initiated prior to treatment.

Long-term treatment with androgen deprivation may lead to osteopenia and osteoporosis [44,46–48]. Many patients initiating hormonal therapy are elderly and have a component of osteopenia before therapy begins, and this is exacerbated by castration. Several studies have demonstrated that the rate of fractures increases with time as men remain on hormonal therapy for extended periods.

(*Continued on next page*)

▶ **FIGURE 17-7.** (*continued*) One study found that 50% of men on androgen blockade for at least 12 months had asymptomatic vertebral fractures; however, the clinical relevance of these fractures remains undefined [49]. As has been observed in breast cancer, prevention of osteopenia/osteoporosis in these patients may be useful in prevention of fractures and other skeletal events [50]. A study of 47 men with hormone-sensitive prostate cancer compared bone mineral density (BMD) in men receiving leuprolide alone with that in men receiving a combination of pamidronate and leuprolide [51]. Pamidronate showed significant protection of BMD in the lumbar spine, greater trochanter, and total hip. Although the study lasted only 48 weeks, it underscored the startling amount of bone loss in patients on leuprolide alone for this period: 3.3% in the lumbar spine, 2.1% in the trochanter, and 1.8% in the total hip. The bisphosphonate zoledronic acid has been demonstrated to decrease fractures in men with hormone-refractory prostate cancer when given as an adjunctive treatment [52]. Zoledronic acid is approved in the United States for use in men with metastatic hormone-refractory prostate cancer and in the European Union for any patient with bone metastases, including prostate cancer patients. Currently, there is no validated method to determine which patients might benefit most from bisphosphonate therapy in the setting of hormone therapy. At present, no data suggest that bisphosphonates should be used routinely to prevent BMD loss in men with normal BMD at the start of therapy. Osteopenia that is present at the start of therapy or that develops during hormonal therapy may be treated with calcium and vitamin D supplements as well as approved bisphosphonates.

Because of the side effects associated with androgen deprivation, several strategies are being tested to lessen the toxicity of therapy whereas still depriving the prostate cancer cells of androgen stimulation. These include intermittent androgen blockade, treatment with high-dose nonsteroidal antiandrogen, and treatment with combinations of nonsteroidal antiandrogen and a 5α-reductase inhibitor.

The concept of intermittent androgen blockade developed out of laboratory studies that suggested tumors could be controlled equally well by intermittent castration as well as continuous castration and early phase II studies that demonstrated that taking patients off therapy and allowing their testosterone to rise improved quality of life [53–57]. In general, patients are placed on androgen blockade for a period of 6 to 9 months and after nadir of prostate-specific antigen (PSA) is established, treatment with luteinizing hormone–releasing hormone (LHRH) analogues is withheld. Over the course of the next several months, testosterone rises. Subsequent to the testosterone rise and improvement in quality of life, however, the androgen-dependent cancer cells begin to proliferate, producing PSA. At some point, generally when the PSA rises to between 4 and 10 ng/mL, androgen deprivation is reinstituted. This cycling continues until the patient develops androgen-independent cancer. The Southwest Oncology Group, the National Cancer Institute of Canada, the South European Uro-Oncological Group, and the German Cancer Society are studying the effects of intermittent androgen blockade on progression-free survival, overall survival, and quality of life via large multicenter, randomized phase III clinical trials. Until the results of these ongoing phase III studies are available, this approach has to be regarded as experimental.

Combining a nonsteroidal antiandrogen (flutamide, bicalutamide, nilutamide) with finasteride blocks the conversion of testosterone to its active metabolite dihydrotestosterone, and also prevents testosterone and dihydrotestosterone from binding to the androgen receptor (*see* Fig. 17-4). This approach, often termed sequential androgen blockade, results in androgen deprivation at the cellular level but leaves circulating testosterone levels intact. In phase II trials, this therapy has resulted in a decrease in serum PSA in the majority of men while maintaining sexual potency [58–61]. This form of treatment has not been tested against traditional androgen deprivation in the phase III setting, and its impact on survival remains unknown. Although initially used mainly in men with advanced disease who wished to maintain potency, it is now being used in the nonprotocol setting to treat men with biochemical failure after primary therapy (PSA-only disease). This type of treatment remains unproven, and its impact is uncertain. At least one study, however, has demonstrated that approximately 80% of men treated with sequential androgen blockade respond to androgen deprivation therapy when their PSA starts to rise [62].

The traditional dose of bicalutamide to achieve its effect as a nonsteroidal antiandrogen is 50 mg/d. Studies have reported that a dose of 150 mg/d is as effective as castration or combined androgen blockade in patients with advanced prostate cancer. Use of a high-dose antiandrogen monotherapy approach has sometimes been referred to as peripheral androgen blockade (PAB) [63–66]. PAB has been compared with classic androgen deprivation in two open-label, randomized trials. Data were collected from 805 patients with demonstrable metastatic (M1) prostate cancer and 480 patients with biochemically advanced (M0) disease. Analysis at a median follow-up period of 6.3 years in M0 patients demonstrated no statistically significant difference in overall survival or time to progression between bicalutamide 150 mg monotherapy and medical or surgical castration. There was an overall survival advantage of 6 weeks in favor of castration in patients with M1 disease. PAB with high-dose bicalutamide was generally well tolerated as compared with androgen deprivation treatment. There was a high rate (approximately 50%) of gynecomastia. These data suggest that PAB may become a viable alternative for patients requiring androgen blockade and has led to approval in many countries outside the United States as a standard of care.

To investigate the role of antiandrogen monotherapy in earlier disease settings, the bicalutamide Early Prostate Cancer program undertook three randomized, double-blind, placebo-controlled trials prospectively designed for combined analysis [66]. A total of 8113 men with T1b to T4, M0, any N (N0 in one trial) prostate cancer were randomized to bicalutamide 150 mg/d (4052) or placebo (4061) in addition to standard care (radical prostatectomy, radiotherapy, or watchful waiting). At a median 5.4 years of follow-up, bicalutamide significantly improved progression-free survival in the overall population. Patients with locally advanced disease gained most benefit from bicalutamide in terms of progression-free survival, irrespective of underlying therapy. Overall survival was similar in the bicalutamide and placebo groups, across the program and in each trial, although the follow-up time period is too early to determine overall survival. The data suggest that bicalutamide provides benefit in patients with locally advanced disease. Further analysis of the data suggests that bicalutamide monotherapy is not appropriate for patients at low risk of disease progression. (*Adapted from* Hellerstedt and Pienta [17].)

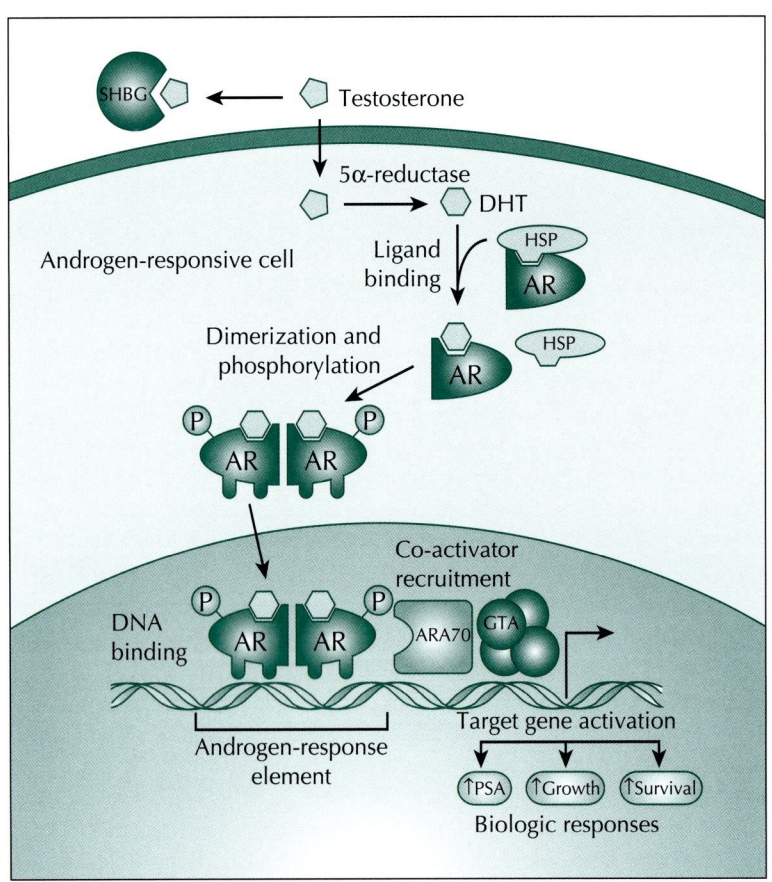

▶ **FIGURE 17-8.** The androgen pathway. Testosterone circulates in the blood bound to albumin and sex hormone–binding globulin (SHBG) and exchanges with free testosterone. Free testosterone enters prostate cells and is converted to dihydrotestosterone (DHT) by the enzyme 5α-reductase. Binding of DHT to the androgen receptor (AR) induces dissociation from heat-shock proteins (HSPs) and receptor phosphorylation. The AR dimerizes and may bind to androgen-response elements in the promoter regions of target genes. Coactivators (such as ARA70) and corepressors also bind the AR complex, facilitating or preventing, respectively, transcription. Activation or repression of target genes leads to biological responses including growth, survival, and the production of prostate-specific antigen (PSA).

During androgen-dependent progression, prostate cancer cells depend primarily on the androgen receptor for growth and survival [67–69]. When the androgen receptor is inactive, it is bound to heat-shock proteins in the cytoplasm of prostate cells. The androgen dihydrotestosterone binds to the androgen receptor, dissociating it from heat-shock proteins. The dihydrotestosterone-bound androgen receptor translocates into the nucleus, dimerizes, and binds to the androgen-response elements, thereby activating genes involved in cell growth [67]. GTA—gene transfer agent. (*Adapted from* Feldman and Feldman [67]; with permission).

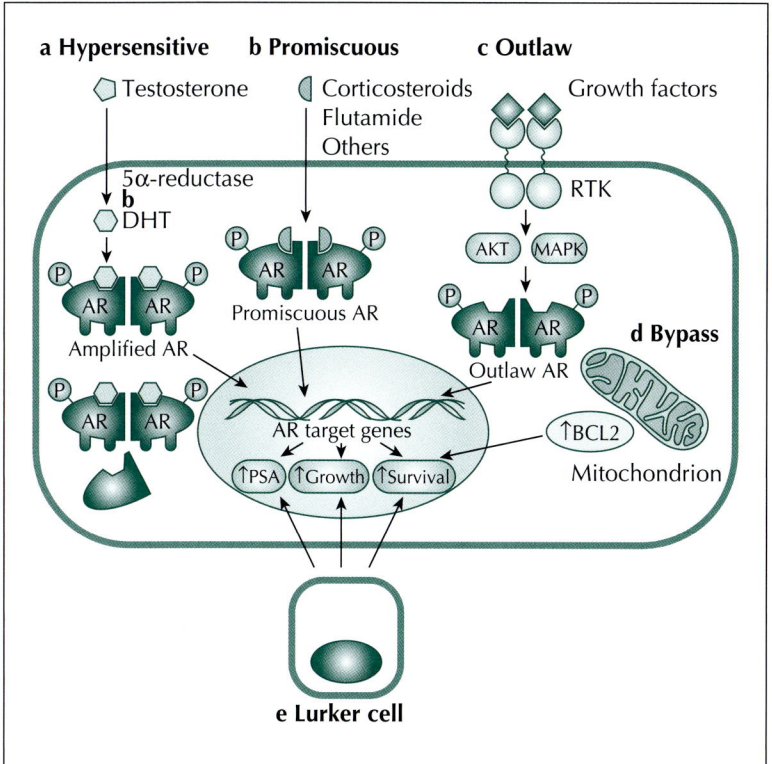

◗ **FIGURE 17-9.** Possible pathways to androgen independence. During androgen-independent progression, prostate cancer relies on various cellular pathways, some involving the androgen receptor (AR) and others bypassing it [67–69]. The AR may be amplified and therefore may be activated by reduced levels of dihydrotestosterone (DHT). In the hypersensitive pathway (*a*), more androgen receptor (AR) is produced (usually by gene amplification), or AR has enhanced sensitivity to compensate for low levels of androgen, or more testosterone is converted to the more potent androgen, DHT, by 5α-reductase. In the promiscuous pathway (*b*), the specificity of the AR is broadened so that it can be activated by nonandrogenic molecules normally present in the circulation. In the outlaw pathway (*c*), receptor tyrosine kinases (RTKs) are activated, and the AR is phosphorylated by either the AKT (protein kinase B) or the mitogen-activated protein kinase (MAPK) pathway, producing a ligand-independent AR. In the bypass pathway (*d*), parallel survival pathways, such as that involving the antiapoptotic protein BCL2 (B-cell lymphoma 2), obviate the need for AR or its ligand. In the lurker cell pathway (*e*), androgen-independent cancer cells that are present all the time in the prostate—possibly epithelial stem cells—might be selected for by therapy. Multiple studies have now demonstrated that AR is amplified in androgen-independent cancers [70–72]. These studies suggest that hormone-refractory prostate cancer is not "androgen independent" in the classic sense but rather is "castration independent," and that the cancer is now able to use very low levels of androgen to grow.

The specificity of the AR can also be broadened so that it can be activated by nonandrogenic molecules normally present in the circulation, creating a "promiscuous receptor." It has also been demonstrated that a mutated androgen receptor may be activated by various other ligands. Deregulated growth factors and cytokines can activate the AR, usually with the help of androgen-receptor coactivators. These "outlaw" pathways may lead to direct phosphorylation and subsequent activation of the AR, or may "bypass" the AR completely. For example, the loss of PTEN

reverses the inhibition of the phosphatidylinositol 3-kinase (PI3-K)–AKT pathway, permitting activated AKT to phosphorylate BAD. This activation results in the release of BCL2, which eventually leads to cell survival [69]. Other postulated mechanisms of androgen independence include the involvement of other cells that support the growth of the cancer cells. Neuroendocrine cells may secrete neuropeptides that induce the growth of adjacent cells or androgen-independent cancer cells may be present all the time in the prostate (possibly stem cells), supporting the growth of androgen-independent cells as the androgen-dependent cells die as a result of hormone therapy.

Some patients treated with combined androgen blockade develop a promiscuous AR, and the antiandrogen that was previously inhibiting prostate cancer growth starts to fuel it. Withdrawal of the antiandrogen may lead to a regression in disease as measured by a decrease in prostate-specific antigen (PSA) or in tumor size [73–75]. Withdrawal responses have been seen with the antiandrogens flutamide, bicalutamide, and nilutamide, as well as with estrogens, megestrol acetate, estramustine, and the antiangiogenic agent TNP-470 [75–78]. Withdrawal responses generally occur in 10% to 20% of patients who have been on combined androgen blockade and last approximately 4 to 6 months.

There is no standard second-line therapy for patients failing first-line hormonal treatment. The addition of antiandrogens, single-agent steroids, estrogens, and the adrenal-suppressive agent ketoconazole are the most common agents used [79–85]. These agents have demonstrated response rates of 10% to 50%, with activity generally measured in months. These agents have gained in popularity in recent years as more and more patients present with "PSA-only" hormone-refractory prostate cancer (*see* Fig. 17-3). These patients have a rising PSA on first-line hormonal therapy, and their only evidence of disease is an increase in PSA. The impact of survival of second-line hormonal therapy, especially in this PSA-only hormone-refractory setting is unclear. (*Adapted from* Feldman and Feldman [67]; with permission.)

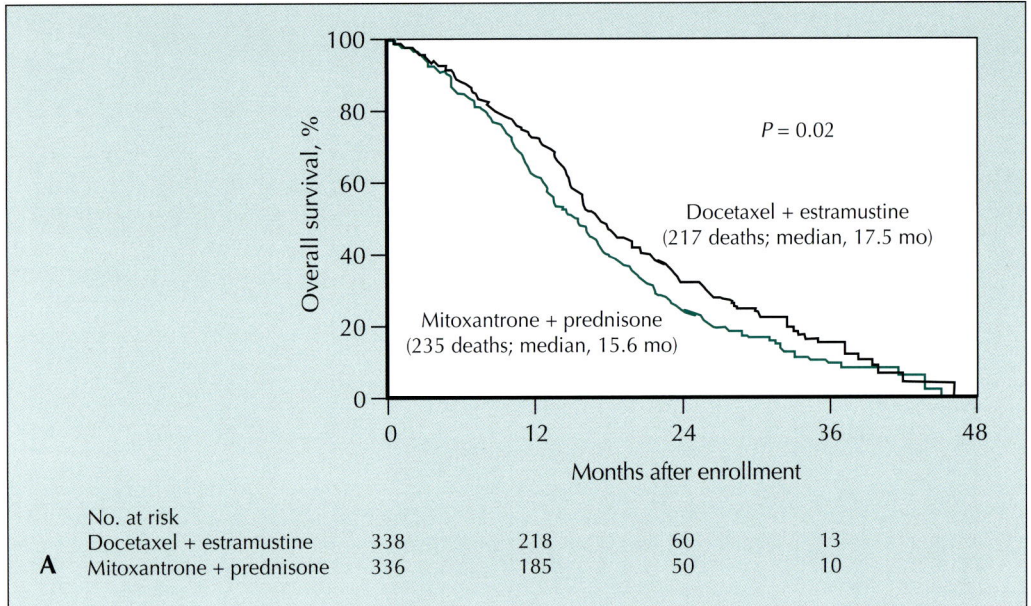

▶ FIGURE 17-10. First-line chemotherapy. **A,** Kaplan-Meier estimates of overall survival among men with androgen-independent prostate cancer treated with mitoxantrone and prednisone or docetaxel and estramustine. **B,** Kaplan–Meier estimates of the probability of overall survival in the patients treated with docetaxel plus prednisone in two different schedules versus mitoxantrone and prednisone.

Docetaxel is a semisynthetic taxane analogue from the European yew (*Taxus baccata*) that acts by altering microtubule dynamics, causing cell cycle arrest during mitosis. It has also been demonstrated to promote apoptosis via BCL2 phosphorylation. In hormone-refractory prostate cancer, docetaxel has been studied as a single agent or in combination with estramustine and in different schedules with demonstrated efficacy. With the recent publication of two large phase III trials demonstrating a survival advantage in hormone-refractory prostate cancer, docetaxel has become the new standard of care for first-line treatment in this setting.

Both trials randomized docetaxel verses mitoxantrone, an agent that has been shown to improve quality of life but has failed to demonstrate any survival benefit [86]. A Southwest Oncology Group/Intergroup trial studied 770 patients randomized to mitoxantrone (12 mg/m^2) and prednisone (5 mg twice daily) (M/P) versus docetaxel 60 mg/m^2 on day 2 and estramustine 280 mg/m^2 three times daily on days 1 to 5 (D/E), each on a 21-day cycle. The primary end point was overall survival, and secondary end points included progression-free survival, objective response rate, and prostate-specific antigen (PSA) decline rate. Patient stratification was to type of progression (PSA-only vs evaluable disease), pain, and performance status. Overall survival was significantly higher in the D/E arm, 18 months versus 16 months for the M/P arm (*P* = 0.01). Also statistically significant were PSA response rate, 50% in the D/E group versus 27% in the M/P, and objective response rate 17% versus 11%. Neutropenia (grades 3 to 5) was similar for both groups (D/E, 16.1%; M/P, 12.5%), but the D/E group did have higher rates of neutropenic fevers, cardiovascular events, nausea and vomiting, metabolic disturbances, and neurologic events. Two clotting events were noted in the D/E group and none in the M/P group, but this difference was not statistically significant. The authors' conclusion was that D/E should be considered a standard of care secondary to a 20% increase in overall survival, progression-free survival, and in both PSA and objective response rates [86].

Another multicenter phase III study was TAX-327. This was a three-arm trial comparing mitoxantrone 12 mg/m^2 every 3 weeks with prednisone 5 mg twice daily to either docetaxel 30 mg/m^2 weekly 5 of 6 weeks or docetaxel 75 mg/m^2 every 3 weeks and prednisone 5 mg twice daily [87]. In this study, 1006 patients were enrolled and were stratified by pain level or performance status. A median survival advantage was found for the every-3-week schedule of docetaxel compared with mitoxantrone (18.9 vs 16.4 months, *P* = 0.009). Weekly docetaxel demonstrated a trend toward improved survival but failed to reach statistical significance (median survival, 17.3 months; *P* = 0.3). Furthermore, the every-3-week docetaxel regimen had a significant improvement in pain rate, PSA response rate, tumor response rate, and quality of life. Toxicity in the every-3-week docetaxel schedule was a 32% rate of grade 3 to 4 neutropenia, and patients in this group suffered more adverse events than those in the mitoxantrone group (26% vs 20%). Interestingly the weekly docetaxel group experienced an adverse event rate of 29%, higher than the group on the 3-week schedule. Phase II data had suggested a similar efficacy with a reduction in neutropenia [26]. The Food and Drug Administration (FDA)-approved regimen for treating advanced prostate cancer is docetaxel 75 mg/m^2 every 3 weeks in combination with prednisone 5 mg orally twice a day.

Although docetaxel has become the standard first-line therapy for hormone-refractory prostate cancer, mitoxantrone plus prednisone has been demonstrated to have significant palliative activity in patients experiencing pain from advanced prostate cancer. Tannock *et al.* [80] demonstrated that the percentage of patients achieving pain relief or having declines in analgesic consumption was substantially higher in those receiving mitoxantrone. These data were confirmed by another phase III trial conducted by Kantoff *et al.* [88] of the Cancer and Leukemia Group B [88]. These studies demonstrated that approximately one third of patients receiving mitoxantrone chemotherapy demonstrated significant pain relief for an average of 8 months. Mitoxantrone is FDA approved and is given in a dosage of 12 to 14 mg/m^2 intravenously every 3 weeks with 10 mg prednisone, or the equivalent of hydrocortisone is given orally daily.

Radiation therapy has long been known to provide effective palliation for patients with advanced prostate cancer.

(*Continued on next page*)

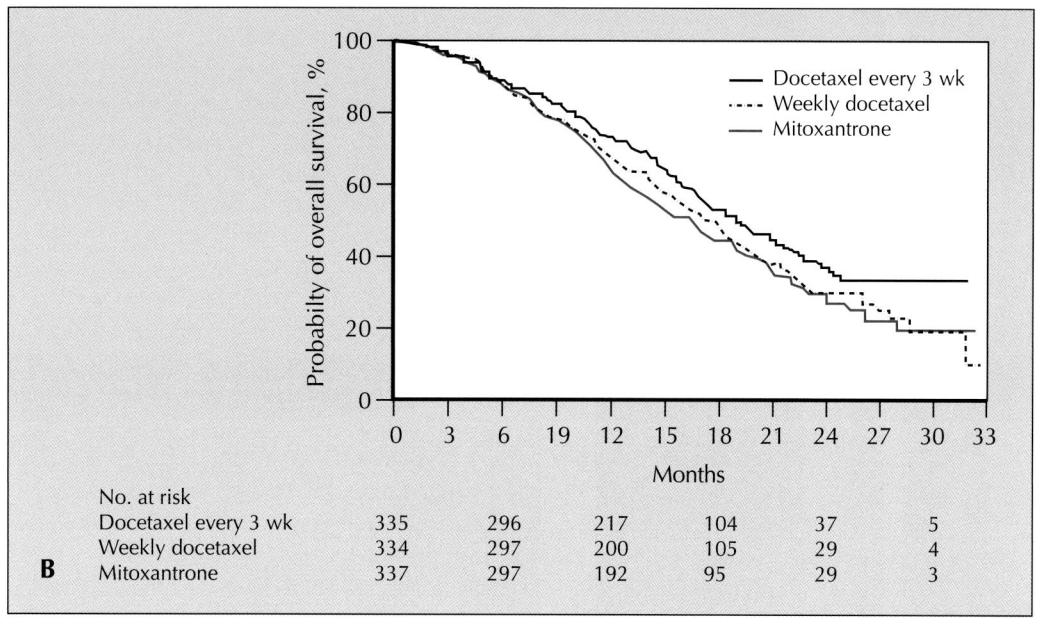

No. at risk						
Docetaxel every 3 wk	335	296	217	104	37	5
Weekly docetaxel	334	297	200	105	29	4
B Mitoxantrone	337	297	192	95	29	3

▶ **FIGURE 17-10.** (*Continued*) For patients with single sites of osseous pain or with limited obstructing masses or lymph nodes, external beam radiation has been demonstrated to be very effective in controlling progressive disease. For patients with multiple sites of bone involvement and pain, systemic radioisotopes administered intravenously have significant therapeutic effects. The two most commonly used radioisotopes are strontium and samarium. These isotopes demonstrate significant differences in physical half-life and particle energy. Porter *et al.* [89] demonstrated in a phase III trial that strontium was more effective than placebo in the control of painful metastases when given as an adjunct to local radiation. Patients with hormone-refractory metastatic prostate cancer received local field radiotherapy and either strontium-89 as a single injection of 10.8 millicuries (mCi) or placebo. Although no significant differences in survival or relief of pain at the index site were noted, intake of analgesics over time demonstrated a significant reduction in the arm treated with strontium-89. Progression of pain as measured by sites of new pain or the requirement for radiotherapy showed statistically significant differences between the arms in favor of strontium-89. Quality-of-life analysis demonstrated the overall superiority of strontium-89, with alleviation of pain and improvement in physical activity being statistically significant. These data demonstrate the effectiveness of strontium; however, strontium has a very long half-life of almost 60 days in bone and may lead to decreased blood element counts, especially of platelets. This makes strontium difficult to give in a setting in which patients are also eligible for chemotherapy.

Sartor *et al.* [90] demonstrated in a phase III trial that 1 mCi/kg samarium was more effective than placebo in controlling pain secondary to bone metastases. Mild transient bone marrow suppression was the only adverse event associated with samarium administration. The mean nadir white blood cell and platelet count at 3 to 4 weeks after treatment was 3800/μL and 127,000/μL, respectively. Counts recovered to baseline after approximately 8 weeks. No grade 4 decreases in either platelets or white bloods cells were documented. These findings demonstrate that samarium

is both safe and effective for the palliation of painful bone metastases in patients with hormone-refractory prostate cancer and suggest that the agent can be successfully integrated with chemotherapy regimens.

It is well known that prostate cancer produces predominantly osteoblastic metastases (*see* Fig. 17-2). The production of an osteoblastic metastasis is the result of a complex interaction between prostate tumor cells, osteoclasts, and osteoblasts. Before the osteoblasts are activated, osteoclasts first break down the bone and initiate bone remodeling. Bisphosphonates are analogues of pyrophosphate, a normal constituent of the bone matrix, and bind to bone surfaces (hydroxyapatite crystals), making them less available to osteoclast resorption. Additionally, bisphosphonates inhibit recruitment of osteoclast precursors, prevent the migration of osteoclasts toward bone, and inhibit the production of prostaglandin-E_2, interleukin-1, and other proteolytic enzymes. In a placebo-controlled, randomized clinical trial, zoledronic acid (4 mg via a 15-minute infusion every 3 weeks for 15 months) reduced the incidence of skeletal-related events (SREs) in men with hormone-refractory metastatic prostate cancer [52]. Among 122 patients who completed a total of 24 months of study, fewer patients in the 4-mg zoledronic acid group than in the placebo group had at least one SRE (38% vs 49%, $P = 0.028$). The annual incidence of SREs was 0.77 for the 4-mg zoledronic acid group versus 1.47 for the placebo group ($P = 0.005$). The median time to the first SRE was 488 days for the 4-mg zoledronic acid group versus 321 days for the placebo group ($P = 0.009$). Compared with placebo, 4 mg of zoledronic acid reduced the ongoing risk of SREs by 36% (risk ratio, 0.64; 95% CI, 0.485–0.845; $P = 0.002$). The authors concluded that long-term treatment with 4 mg of zoledronic acid is safe and provides sustained clinical benefits for men with metastatic hormone-refractory prostate cancer, and this agent has been approved for the treatment of men with bone metastases who have failed hormonal therapy. (*Part A adapted from* Petrylak *et al.* [86]; with permission; *part B adapted from* Tannock *et al.* [87]; with permission.)

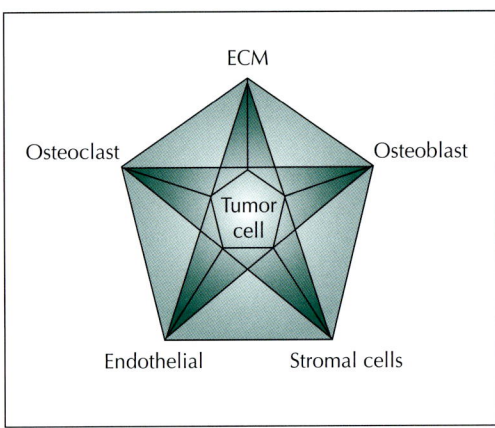

FIGURE 17-11. The vicious pentagon of prostate tumor cell–bone microenvironment interactions. The relationship between the tumor cell and the surrounding tissue is a complex environment. Tumor cells in the bone interact with the extracellular matrix (ECM), stromal cells, osteoblasts, osteoclasts, and endothelial cells to coordinate a sophisticated series of interactions to promote tumor cell survival and proliferation, leading to a "pentagon of pain" for patients with advanced prostate cancer. These interrelationships identify a paradigm shift in understanding prostate cancer growth in bone and lead to the ability to design targeted therapies to interrupt the vicious cycle of the tumor cell with its microenvironment.

The traditional paradigm for prostate cancer treatment, as well as all cancer treatment, has been to target the tumor cell directly. For the first time, it has been demonstrated that chemotherapy with docetaxel increases survival in patients with hormone-refractory prostate cancer. These current chemotherapy regimens debulk the tumor but cannot eradicate late-stage disease. The paradigm of targeting the tumor cell is now being expanded beyond classic chemotherapy, not only with the identification of new chemotherapy agents and new targeted signal transduction agents, but with the recognition that cancer cells exist in complex microenvironments that offer therapeutic targets.

Cancer chemotherapy that directly targets the tumor cells can now be divided into two general categories, classic chemotherapy and "targeted" therapy. Several new chemotherapeutic agents are under active investigation, and the list continues to evolve rapidly. These agents include the epothilones, which target microtubules, and satraplatin, which inhibits DNA replication. Targeted therapy now generally refers to inhibiting specific signal transduction molecules important in cell growth. These agents include inhibitors of the epidermal growth factor receptor, HER2/neu, and mammalian target of rapamycin (mTOR) [91–94]. Combining these new agents with inhibitors of the greater tumor microenvironment is already being accomplished. Several strategies have been developed to inhibit osteoclast activity. Bisphosphonates inhibit recruitment of osteoclast precursors, prevent the migration of osteoclasts toward bone, and inhibit the production of prostaglandin-E_2, interleukin-1, and other proteolytic enzymes [95]. An osteoclast differentiation factor has been identified as having significant homology to the receptor activator of nuclear factor-κB ligand (RANK-L, also known as osteoprotegerin and osteoclast differentiation factor). RANK-L binding to RANK stimulates bone resorption, is required for osteoclastogenesis, and is important in tumor cell interactions with the bone microenvironment [96]. The RANK–RANK-L axis may be disrupted by an osteoprotegerin decoy receptor (AMGN-0007) [97].

As previously noted, the most common histology of prostate cancer bone metastases is a disorganized osteoblastic response. The osteoblast plays a key role in the bone metastasis microenvironment as several growth factors (eg, insulin-like growth factor-1, transforming growth factor-β, endothelin-1, fractalkine) produced by osteoblasts and osseous stromal cells act as chemoattractants for prostate cancer cells, as well as promote tumor growth and proliferation [98]. Targeting the osteoblast and the osteoblast axis is an underdeveloped area; however, one promising example of osteoblast targeted therapy appears to be the endothelin-1A (ETA) receptor. Endothelin-1 has been shown to be an important mediator of tumor growth and tumor cell survival in prostate cancer [99]. Several compounds are under investigation as a novel class of chemotherapeutic compounds that target the ETA receptor [100]. Currently, one of the most promising ETA receptor antagonist is atrasentan, an orally bioavailable compound that has a 1800-fold higher affinity for the ETA receptor compared than for the endothelin-1B receptor, with an ETA receptor–binding constant of 34 picomoles [101]. Phase III studies in prostate cancer utilizing atrasentan have been performed, and currently atrasentan is being targeted to slow prostate tumor growth in patients without overt metastases (Zonnenberg, Unpublished data).

The other stromal elements that have been shown to participate in cancer metastasis include fibroblasts, smooth muscle cells, endothelial cells, and inflammatory cells [102–104]. It appears that targeting these stromal components of the microenvironment may be effective in reducing the development of metastases. The new blood vessel growth associated with tumors, ie, neoangiogenesis, remains a therapeutic target of major interest [94]. Clinical trials are now studying several new compounds that inhibit the vascular endothelial growth factor receptor as well as the integrins necessary for blood vessel growth [105,106]. A more general approach is to target the whole microenvironment compartment with systemic radioisotopes. Radioisotopes are effective therapeutic agents for the management and palliation of bone-specific disease because of the high levels of retention by bone metastases (highest in damaged bone, less in normal bone tissue, and none outside of bone). Adding systemic radioisotopes to chemotherapy regimens for patients with advanced prostate cancer appears to increase response rates and survival [107,108]. The radioisotopes have the potential to interrupt the axes of interaction among the cancer cells, the osteoclasts, and the osteoblasts, as well as the stromal cells. All of these data suggest that systemic or local radiation may play a role in controlling metastasis by a variety of mechanisms. Further exploration of how this could be applied to the human disease setting needs to be done in the preclinical and clinical settings.

Cancer should be considered a multicellular organ involving both heterogenous cancer cells and multiple normal cell types interacting with the tumor cells and, therefore, must be treated as such. Treating the tumor cell represents only one avenue for attacking the disease of advanced prostate cancer. It is imperative that we expand the therapeutic target options to include the cancer as "organ" and not just the cancer as "tumor cell." At the level of the tumor cell, cancer has developed multiple methods centering on genetic mutation to promote self-survival and perpetuation. The pliability of cancer cells to mutate into several different phenotypes in an attempt to find one that will survive and colonize at the metastatic site is a tremendous hurdle to overcome in the pursuit of better cancer therapies. The future of cancer therapy resides in combining classic chemotherapy with the ability of new agents to focus on targeted signal transduction pathways and to exploit relationships of the cancer cell with the host environment.

1. Roudier MP, True LD, Higano CS, *et al.*: Phenotypic heterogeneity of end-stage prostate carcinoma metastatic to bone. *Hum Pathol* 2003, 34:646–653.

2. Saitoh H, Hida M, Shimbo T, *et al.*: Metastatic patterns of prostatic cancer. Correlation between sites and number of organs involved. *Cancer* 1984, 54:3078–3084.

3. Harada M, Iida M, Yamaguchi M, *et al.*: In *Prostate Cancer and Bone Metastasis.* Edited by Karr JP and Yamanaka H. New York: Plenum Press; 1992:173–182.

4. Bubendorf L: Metastatic patterns of prostate cancer: an autopsy study of 1589 patients. *Hum Pathol* 2000, 31:578–583.

5. Shah RB, Mehra R, Chinnaiyan AM, *et al.*: Androgen-independent prostate cancer is a heterogeneous group of diseases: lessons from a rapid autopsy program. *Cancer Res* 2004, 64:9209–9216.

6. Guise TA, Mohammad KS: Endothelins in bone cancer metastases. *Cancer Treat Res* 2004, 118:197–212.

7. Brown JM, Zhang J, Keller ET: Opg, RANKl, and RANK in cancer metastasis: expression and regulation. *Cancer Treat Res* 2004, 118:149–172.

8. Tantivejkul K, Kalikin LM, Pienta KJ: Dynamic process of prostate cancer metastasis to bone. *J Cell Biochem* 2004, 91:706–717.

9. Kucia M, Jankowski K, Reca R, *et al.*: CXCR4-SDF-1 signalling, locomotion, chemotaxis and adhesion. *J Mol Histol* 2004, 35:233–245.

10. Rubin MA, Putzi M, Mucci N, *et al.*: Rapid ("warm") autopsy study for procurement of metastatic prostate cancer. *Clin Cancer Res* 2000, 6:1038–1045.

11. Howard OM, Galligan CL: An expanding appreciation of the role chemokine receptors play in cancer progression. *Curr Pharm Des* 2004, 10:2377–2389.

12. Liang Z, Wu T, Lou H, *et al.*: Inhibition of breast cancer metastasis by selective synthetic polypeptide against CXCR4. *Cancer Res* 2004, 64:4302–4308.

13. Sun YX, Wang J, Shelburne CE, *et al.*: Expression of CXCR4 and CXCL12 (SDF-1) in human prostate cancers (PCa) in vivo. *J Cell Biochem* 2003, 89:462–473.

14. Zlotnik A, Yoshie O: Chemokines: a new classification system and their role in immunity. *Immunity* 2000, 12:121–127.

15. Ceradini DJ, Kulkarni AR, Callaghan MJ, *et al.*: Progenitor cell trafficking is regulated by hypoxic gradients through HIF-1 induction of SDF-1. *Nat Med* 2004, 10:858–864.

16. Staller P, Sulitkova J, Lisztwan J, *et al.*: Chemokine receptor CXCR4 downregulated by von Hippel-Lindau tumour suppressor pVHL. *Nature* 2003, 425:307–311.

17. Hellerstedt BA, Pienta KJ: The current state of hormonal therapy for prostate cancer. *CA Cancer J Clin* 2002, 52:154–179.

18. Byar DP, Corle DK: Hormone therapy for prostate cancer: results of the Veterans Administration Cooperative Urological Research Group studies. *NCI Monogr* 1988, 7:165–170.

19. Cox RL, Crawford ED: Estrogens in the treatment of prostate cancer. *J Urol* 1995,154:1991–1998.

20. Medical Research Council Prostate Cancer Working Party Investigators Group: Immediate versus deferred treatment for advanced prostatic cancer: initial results of the Medical Research Council trial. *Br J Urol* 1997, 79:235–246.

21. Medical Research Council Prostate Cancer Working Party Investigators Group: Immediate versus deferred hormone therapy for prostate cancer: how safe is androgen deprivation? *BJU Int* 2000, 86:220.

22. Stamey TA, Yang N, Hay AR, *et al.*: Prostate-specific antigen as a serum marker for adenocarcinoma of the prostate. *N Engl J Med* 1987, 317:909–916.

23. Partin AW, Carter HB, Chan DW, *et al.*: Prostate specific antigen in the staging of localized prostate cancer: influence of tumor differentiation, tumor volume and benign hyperplasia. *J Urol* 1990, 143:747–752.

24. Pound CR, Partin AW, Eisenberger MA, *et al.*: Natural history of progression after PSA elevation following radical prostatectomy. *JAMA* 1999, 281:1591–1597.

25. D'Amico AV, Cote K, Loffredo M, *et al.*: Determinants of prostate cancer-specific survival after radiation therapy for patients with clinically localized prostate cancer. *J Clin Oncol* 2002, 20:4567–4573.

26. Bolla M, Gonzalez D, Warde P, *et al.*: Improved survival in patients with locally advanced prostate cancer treated with radiotherapy and goserelin. *N Engl J Med* 1997,337:295–300.

27. Messing EM, Manola J, Sarosdy M, *et al.*: Immediate hormonal therapy compared with observation after radical prostatectomy and pelvic lymphadenectomy in men with node-positive prostate cancer. *N Engl J Med* 1999, 341:1781–1788.

28. Loblaw DA, Mendelson DS, Talcott JA, *et al.*: American Society of Clinical Oncology recommendations for the initial hormonal management of androgen-sensitive metastatic, recurrent, or progressive prostate cancer. *J Clin Oncol* 2004, 22:2927–2941.

29. Chang C, Kokontis J, Liao S: Molecular cloning of the human and rat complementary DNA encoding androgen receptors. *Science* 1988, 240:324–326.

30. Litvinov IV, De Marzo AM, Isaacs JT: Is the Achilles' heel for prostate cancer therapy a gain of function in androgen receptor signaling? *J Clin Endocrinol Metab* 2003, 88:2972–2982.

31. Beato M: Gene regulation by steroid hormones. *Cell* 1989, 56:335–344.

32. Onate S, Tsai S, Tsai M, *et al.*: Sequence and characterization of a coactivator for the steroid hormone receptor superfamily. *Science* 1995, 270:1354–1357.

33. Huggins C, Hodges CV: Studies on prostate cancer: I. The effect of castration of estrogen and of androgen injection on serum phosphatases in metastatic carcinoma of the prostate. *Cancer Res* 1941, 1:293–297.

34. Shupnik MA, Schreihofer DA: Molecular aspects of steroid hormone action in the male reproductive axis. *J Androl* 1997, 18:341–344.

35. Sharifi R, Knoll LD, Smith J, *et al.*: Leuprolide acetate (30 mg depot every 4 months) in the treatment of advanced prostate cancer. *Urology* 1998, 51:271–276.

36. Wong SL, Lau DT, Baughman SA, *et al.*: Pharmacokinetics and pharmacodynamics of a novel depot formulation of abarelix, a gonadotropin-releasing hormone (GnRH) antagonist, in healthy men ages 50 to 75. *J Clin Pharmacol* 2004, 44:495–502.

37. Labrie F, Dupont A, Belanger A, *et al.*: New approach in the treatment of prostate cancer: complete instead of partial withdrawal of androgens. *Prostate* 1983, 4:579–594.

38. Prostate Cancer Trialists' Collaborative Group: Maximum androgen blockade in advanced prostate cancer: an overview of the randomised trials. *Lancet* 2000, 355:1491–1498.

39. Stone P, Hardy J, Huddart R, *et al.*: Fatigue in patients with prostate cancer receiving hormone therapy. *Eur J Cancer* 2000, 36:1134–1141.

40. Tayek JA, Heber D, Byerley LO, *et al.*: Nutritional and metabolic effects of gonadotropin-releasing hormone agonist treatment for prostate cancer. *Metabolism* 1990, 39:1314–1319.

41. Diamond T, Campbell J, Bryant C, *et al.*: The effect of combined androgen blockade on bone turnover and bone mineral densities in men treated for prostate carcinoma: longitudinal evaluation and response to intermittent cyclic etidronate therapy. *Cancer* 1998, 83:1561–1566.

42. Hedlund PO: Side effects of endocrine treatment and their mechanisms: castration, antiandrogens, and estrogens. *Prostate Suppl* 2000, 10:32–37.

43. Atala A, Amin M, Harty JI: Diethylstilbestrol in treatment of post orchiectomy vasomotor symptoms and its relationship with serum follicle-stimulating hormone, luteinizing hormone, and testosterone. *Urology* 1992, 39:108–110.

44. Higano CS: Understanding treatments for bone loss and bone metastases in patients with prostate cancer: a practical review and guide for the clinician. *Urol Clin North Am* 2004, 31:331–352.

45. Quella SK, Loprinzi CL, Sloan J, *et al.*: Pilot evaluation of venlafaxine for the treatment of hot flashes in men undergoing androgen ablation therapy for prostate cancer. *J Urol* 1999, 162:98–102.

46. Diamond TH, Higano CS, Smith MR, *et al.*: Osteoporosis in men with prostate carcinoma receiving androgen-deprivation therapy: recommendations for diagnosis and therapies. *Cancer* 2004, 100:892–899.

47. Krupski TL, Smith MR, Chan Lee W, *et al.*: Natural history of bone complications in men with prostate carcinoma initiating androgen deprivation therapy. *Cancer* 2004, 101:541–549.

48. Smith MR: Management of treatment-related osteoporosis in men with prostate cancer. *Cancer Treat Rev* 2003, 29:211–218.

49. Modi S, Wood L, Siminoski K, *et al.*: A comparison of the prevalence of osteoporosis and vertebral fractures in men with prostate cancer on various androgen deprivation therapies: preliminary report. *Proc Am Soc Clin Oncol* 2001, 20:2420.

50. Theriault RL, Lipton A, Hortobagyi GN, *et al.*: Pamidronate reduces skeletal morbidity in women with advanced breast cancer and lytic bone lesions: a randomized, placebo-controlled trial. Protocol 18 Aredia Breast Cancer Study Group. *J Clin Oncol* 1999, 17:846–854.

51. Smith MR, McGovern FJ, Zietman AL, *et al.*: Pamidronate to prevent bone loss during androgen-deprivation therapy for prostate cancer. *N Engl J Med* 2001, 345:948–955.

52. Saad F, Gleason DM, Murray R, *et al.*: Long-term efficacy of zoledronic acid for the prevention of skeletal complications in patients with metastatic hormone-refractory prostate cancer. Zoledronic Acid Prostate Cancer Study Group. *J Natl Cancer Inst* 2004, 96:1480; author reply 1480–1481.

53. Sato N, Gleave ME, Bruchovsky N, *et al.*: Intermittent androgen suppression delays progression to androgen independent regulation of prostate specific antigen gene in the LNCaP prostate tumor model. *J Steroid Biochem Mol Biol* 1996, 58:139–146.

54. de Leval J, Boca P, Yousef E, *et al.*: Intermittent versus continuous total androgen blockade in the treatment of patients with advanced hormone-naive prostate cancer: results of a prospective randomized multicenter trial. *Clin Prostate Cancer* 2002, 1:163–171.

55. Moul JW, Fowler JE Jr: Evolution of therapeutic approaches with luteinizing hormone–releasing hormone agonists in 2003. *Urology* 2003, 62:20–28.

56. Pether M, Goldenberg SL, Bhagirath K, *et al.*: Intermittent androgen suppression in prostate cancer: an update of the Vancouver experience. *Can J Urol* 2003, 10:1809–1814.

57. Goldenberg SL, Gleave ME, Taylor D, *et al.*: Clinical experience with intermittent androgen suppression in prostate cancer: minimum of 3 years' follow-up. *Mol Urol* 1999, 3:287–292.

58. Fleshner NE, Trachtenberg J: Combination finasteride and flutamide in advanced carcinoma of the prostate: effective therapy with minimal side effects. *J Urol* 1995, 154:1642–1645.

59. Ornstein DK, Rao GS, Johnson B, *et al.*: Combined finasteride and flutamide therapy in men with advanced prostate cancer. *Urology* 1996, 48:901–905.

60. Kirby R, Robertson C, Turkes A, *et al.*: Finasteride in association with either flutamide or goserelin as combination hormonal therapy in patients with stage M1 carcinoma of the prostate gland. International Prostate Health Council (IPHC) Trial Study Group. *Prostate* 1999, 40:105–114.

61. Brufsky A, Fontaine-Rothe P, Berlane K, *et al.*: Finasteride and flutamide as potency-sparing androgen-ablative therapy for advanced adenocarcinoma of the prostate. *Urology* 1997, 49:913–920.

62. Ornstein DK, Smith DS, Andriole GL: Biochemical response to testicular androgen ablation among patients with prostate cancer for whom flutamide and/or finasteride therapy failed. *Urology* 1998, 52:1094–1097.

63. Baltogiannis D, Giannakopoulos X, Charalabopoulos K, *et al.*: Monotherapy in advanced prostate cancer: an overview. *Exp Oncol* 2004, 26:185–191.

64. Sieber PR, Keiller DL, Kahnoski RJ, *et al.*: Bicalutamide 150 mg maintains bone mineral density during monotherapy for localized or locally advanced prostate cancer. *J Urol* 2004, 171:2272–2276.

65. Schellhammer PF, Davis JW: An evaluation of bicalutamide in the treatment of prostate cancer. *Clin Prostate Cancer* 2004, 2:213–219.

66. Wirth MP, See WA, McLeod DG, *et al.*: Casodex Early Prostate Cancer Trialists' Group. Bicalutamide 150 mg in addition to standard care in patients with localized or locally advanced prostate cancer: results from the second analysis of the early prostate cancer program at median followup of 5.4 years. *J Urol* 2004, 172:1865–1870.

67. Feldman BJ, Feldman D: The development of androgen-independent prostate cancer. *Nat Rev Cancer* 2001, 1:34–45.

68. Nelson WG, De Marzo AM, Isaacs WB: Prostate cancer. *N Engl J Med* 2003, 349:366–381.

69. Debes JD, Tindall DJ: Mechanisms of androgen-refractory prostate cancer. *N Engl J Med* 2004, 351:1488–1490.

70. Tindall D, Horne FM, Hruszkewycz A, *et al.*: Symposium on androgen action in prostate cancer. *Cancer Res* 2004, 64:7178–7180.

71. Chen CD, Welsbie DS, Tran C, *et al.*: Molecular determinants of resistance to antiandrogen therapy. *Nat Med* 2004, 10:33–39.

72. Shah RB, Mehra R, Chinnaiyan AM, *et al.*: Androgen-independent prostate cancer is a heterogeneous group of diseases: lessons from a rapid autopsy program. *Cancer Res* 2004, 64:9209–9216.

73. Scher HI, Kelly WK: The flutamide withdrawal syndrome: its impact on clinical trials in hormone-refractory prostate cancer. *J Clin Oncol* 1993, 11:1566–1572.

74. Figg WD, Sartor O, Cooper MR, *et al.*: Prostate specific antigen decline following the discontinuation of flutamide in patients with stage D2 prostate cancer. *Am J Med* 1995, 98:412–414.

75. Bissada NK, Kaczmarek AT: Complete remission of hormone refractory adenocarcinoma of the prostate in response to withdrawal of diethylstilbestrol. *J Urol* 1995, 153:1944–1945.

76. Dawson NA, McLeod DG: Dramatic prostate specific antigen decrease in response to discontinuation of megestrol acetate in advanced prostate cancer: expansion of the antiandrogen withdrawal syndrome. *J Urol* 1995, 153:1946–1947.

77. Nishiyama T, Terunuma M: Prostate specific antigen and prostate acid phosphatase declines after estramustine phosphate withdrawal: a case report. *Int J Urol* 1994, 1:355–356.

78. Sartor O: Prostate-specific antigen changes before and after administration of an angiogenesis inhibitor. *Oncol Rep* 1995, 2:1101–1102.

79. Fowler JE Jr: Endocrine therapy for localized prostate cancer. *Urol Ann* 1996, 10:57–77.

80. Tannock IF, Osoba D, Stockler MR, *et al.*: Chemotherapy with mitoxantrone plus prednisone or prednisone alone for symptomatic hormone-resistant prostate cancer: a Canadian randomized trial with palliative end points. *J Clin Oncol* 1996, 14:1756–1764.

81. Small EJ, Baron AD, Fippin L, Apodaca D: Ketoconazole retains activity in advanced prostate cancer patients with progression despite flutamide withdrawal. *J Urol* 1997, 157:1204–1207.

82. Osbom JL, Smith DC, Trump DL: Megestrol acetate in the treatment of hormone refractory prostate cancer. *Am J Clin Oncol* 1997, 20:308–310.

83. Smith DC, Redman BG, Flaherty LE, *et al.*: A phase II trial of oral diethylstilbestrol as a second-line hormonal agent in advanced prostate cancer. *Urology* 1998, 52:257–260.

84. Ryan CJ, Small EJ: Role of secondary hormonal therapy in the management of recurrent prostate cancer. *Urology* 2003, 62:87–94.

85. Harris KA, Weinberg V, Bok RA, *et al.*: Low dose ketoconazole with replacement doses of hydrocortisone in patients with progressive androgen independent prostate cancer. *J Urol* 2002, 168:542–545.

86. Petrylak DP, Tangen CM, Huaain MH, *et al.*: Docetaxel and estramustine compared with mitoxantrone and prednisone for advanced refractory prostate cancer. *N Engl J Med* 2004, 351:1513–1520

87. Tannock IF, de Wit R, Berry WR, *et al.*: Docetaxel plus prednisone or mitoxantrone plus prednisone for advanced prostate cancer. *N Engl J Med* 2004, 351:1502–1512.

88. Kantoff PW, Halabi S, Conaway M, *et al.*: Hydrocortisone with or without mitoxantrone in men with hormone-refractory prostate cancer: results of the cancer and leukemia group B 9182 study. *J Clin Oncol* 1999, 17:2506–2513.

89. Porter AT, McEwan AJ, Powe JE, *et al.*: Results of a randomized phase-III trial to evaluate the efficacy of strontium-89 adjuvant to local field external beam irradiation in the management of endocrine resistant metastatic prostate cancer. *Int J Radiat Oncol Biol Phys* 1993, 25:805–813.

90. Sartor O, Reid RH, Hoskin PJ, *et al.*: Quadramet 424Sm10/11 Study Group. Samarium-153-lexidronam complex for treatment of painful bone metastases in hormone-refractory prostate cancer. *Urology* 2004, 63:940–945.

91. Thompson JE, Thompson CB: Putting the rap on Akt. *J Clin Oncol* 2004, 22:4217–4226.

92. van der Poel HG: Smart drugs in prostate cancer. *Eur Urol* 2004, 45:1–17.

93. Semenza GL: Targeting HIF-1 for cancer therapy. *Nat Rev Cancer* 2003, 3:721.

94. Uehara H: Angiogenesis of prostate cancer and antiangiogenic therapy. *J Med Invest* 2003, 50:146–153.

95. Winquist E, Berry S: A randomized, placebo-controlled trial of zoledronic acid in patients with hormone-refractory metastatic prostate carcinoma. *J Natl Cancer Inst* 2004, 96:1183–1184.

96. Kitazawa S, Kitazawa R: RANK ligand is a prerequisite for cancer-associated osteolytic lesions. *J Pathol* 2002, 198:228–236.

97. Body JJ, Greipp P, Coleman RE, *et al.*: A phase I study of AMGN-0007, a recombinant osteoprotegerin construct, in patients with multiple myeloma or breast carcinoma related bone metastases. *Cancer* 2003, 97:887–892.

98. Shulby SA, Dolloff NG, Stearns ME, *et al.*: CX3CR1-fractalkine expression regulates cellular mechanisms involved in adhesion, migration, and survival of human prostate cancer cells. *Cancer Res* 2004, 64:4693–4698.

99. Mohammad KS, Guise TA: Mechanisms of osteoblastic metastases: role of endothelin-1. *Clin Orthop* 2003, 415:S67–S74.

100. Nelson JB, Nabulsi AA, Vogelzang NJ, *et al.*: Suppression of prostate cancer induced bone remodeling by the endothelin receptor A antagonist atrasentan. *J Urol* 2003, 169:1143–1149.

101. Lee D: Clinical trials of atrasentan in hormone-refractory prostate cancer. *Clin Prostate Cancer* 2003, 2:84–86.

102. Chung LW, Baseman A, Assikis V, *et al.*: Molecular insights into prostate cancer progression: the missing link of tumor microenvironment. *J Urol* 2005, 173:10–20.

103. Edlund M, Sung SY, Chung LW: Modulation of prostate cancer growth in bone microenvironments. *J Cell Biochem* 2004, 91:686–705.

104. Cooper CR, Chay CH, Gendernalik JD, *et al.*: Stromal factors involved in prostate carcinoma metastasis to bone. *Cancer* 2003, 97:739–747.

105. Figg WD, Kruger EA, Price DK, *et al.*: Inhibition of angiogenesis: treatment options for patients with metastatic prostate cancer. *Invest New Drugs* 2002, 20:183–194.

106. Veronese ML, O'Dwyer PJ: Monoclonal antibodies in the treatment of colorectal cancer. *Eur J Cancer* 2004, 40:1292–1301.

107. Tu SM, Millikan RE, Mengistu B, *et al.*: Bone-targeted therapy for advanced androgen-independent carcinoma of the prostate: a randomised phase II trial. *Lancet* 2001, 357:336–41. [Published erratum in *Lancet* 2001, 357:1210.]

108. Akerley W, Butera J, Wehbe T, *et al.*: A multiinstitutional, concurrent chemoradiation trial of strontium-89, estramustine, and vinblastine for hormone refractory prostate carcinoma involving bone. *Cancer* 2002, 94:1654–1660.

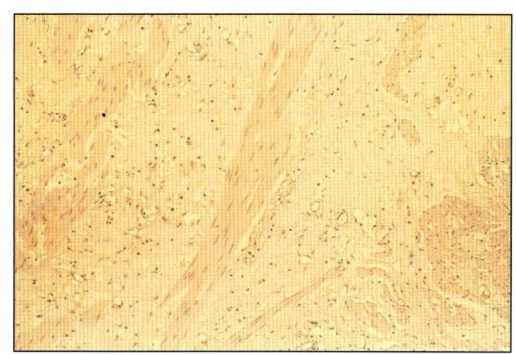

▶ **FIGURE 1-24.**

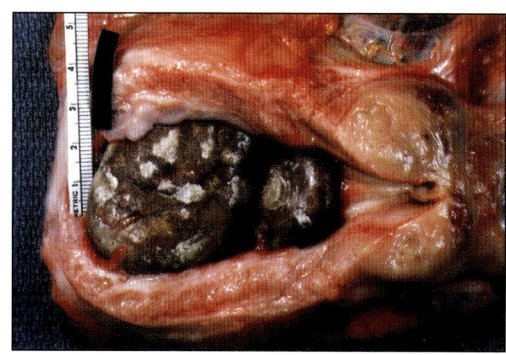

▶ **FIGURE 1-26.**

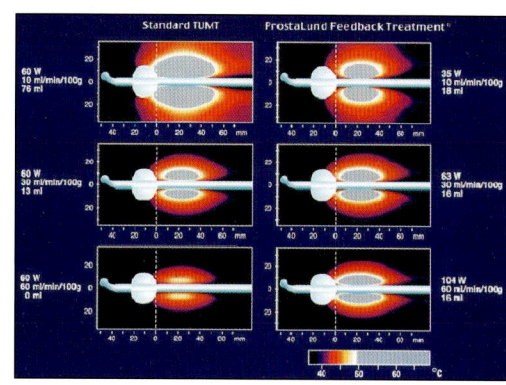

▶ **FIGURE 4-4.**

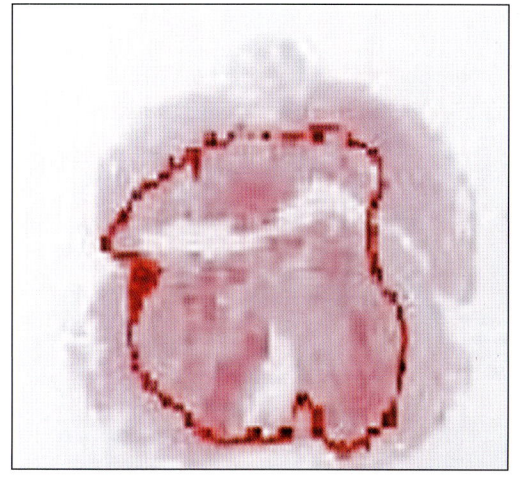

▶ **FIGURE 4-6.**

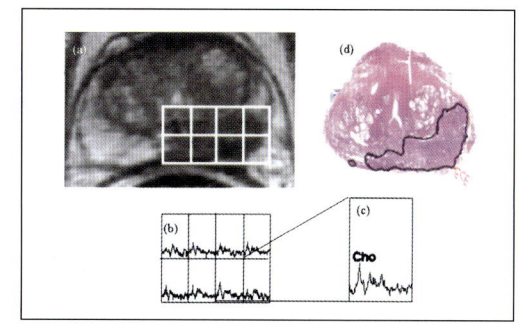

▶ **FIGURE 9-9C.**

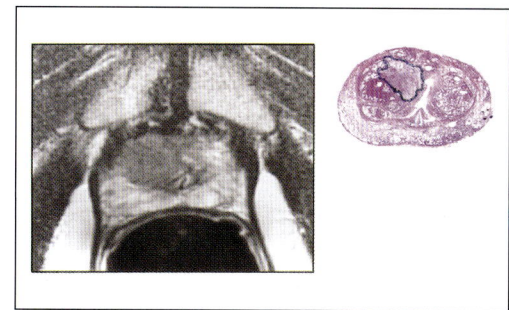

▶ **FIGURE 9-9D.**

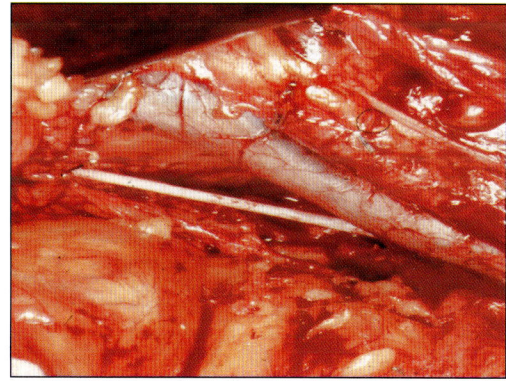

▶ **FIGURE 11-5B.**

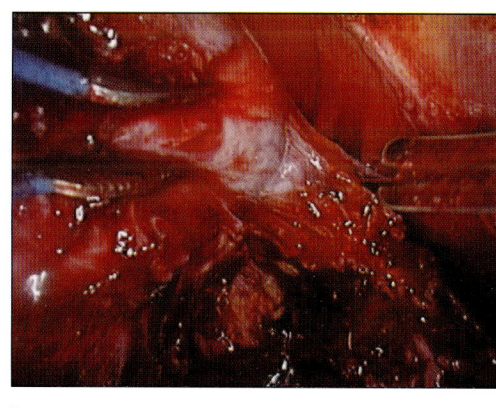

▶ **FIGURE 12-10.**

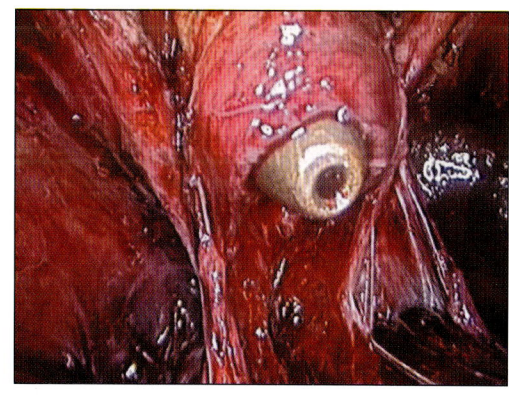

▶ **FIGURE 12-13.**

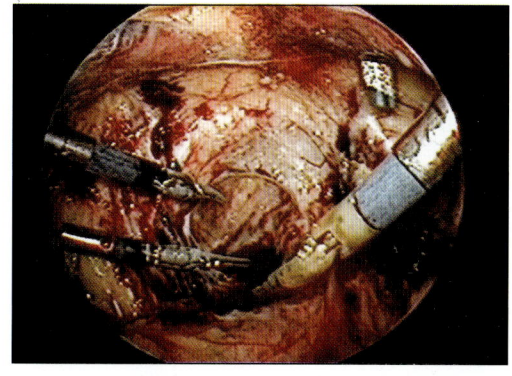

▶ **FIGURE 13-6.**

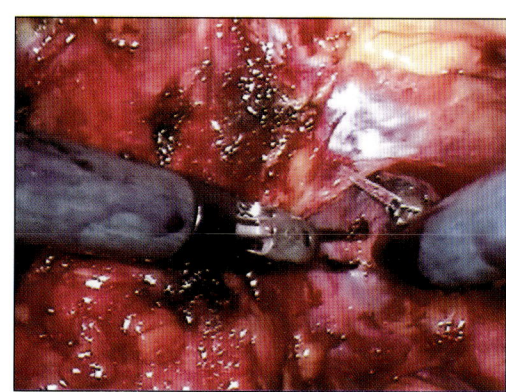

▶ **FIGURE 13-8A.**

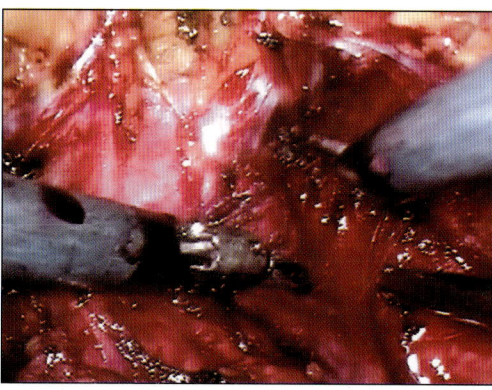

▶ **FIGURE 13-8B.**

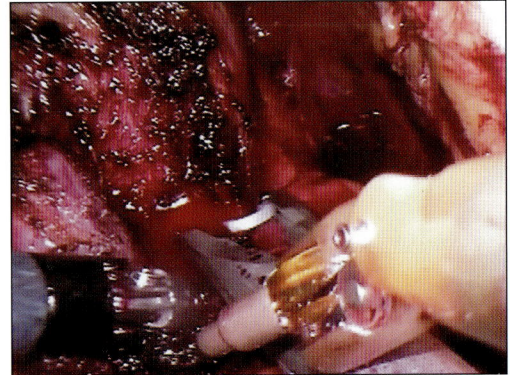

▶ FIGURE 13-15A.

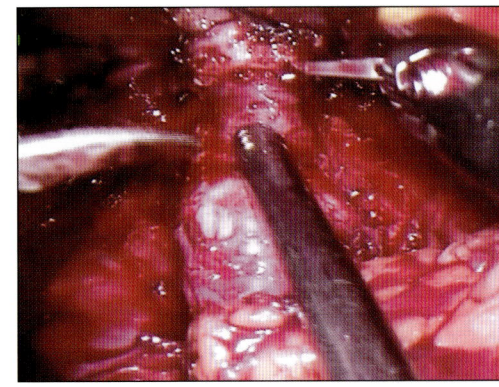

▶ FIGURE 13-16.

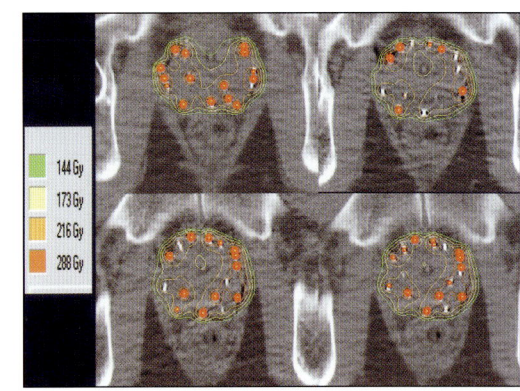

▶ FIGURE 14-10.

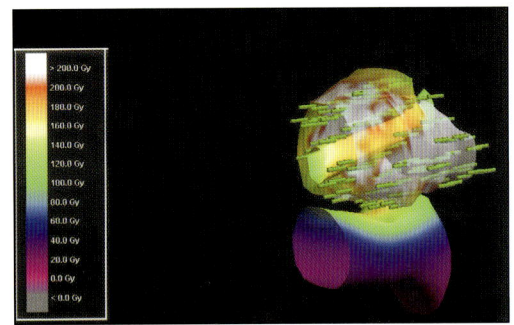

▶ FIGURE 14-12.

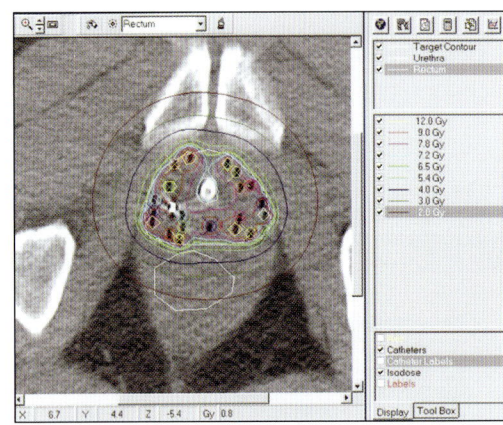

▶ FIGURE 14-17B.

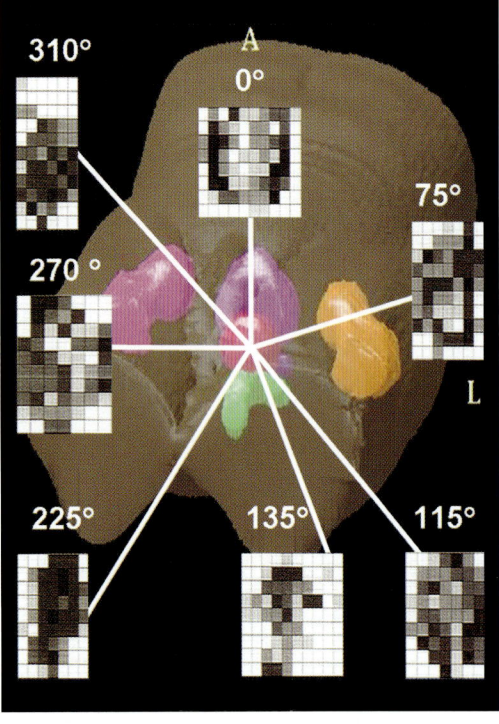

▶ FIGURE 15-13.

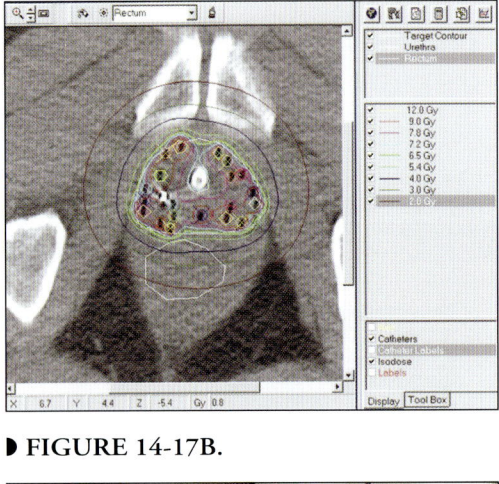

▶ FIGURE 15-11.

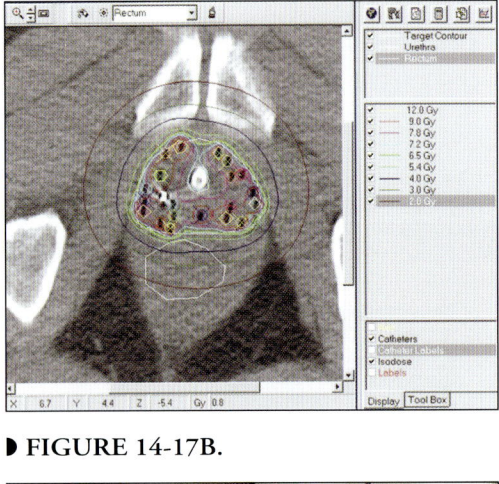

▶ FIGURE 15-12.

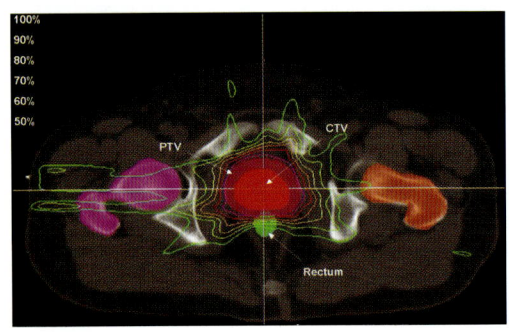

▶ FIGURE 15-14.

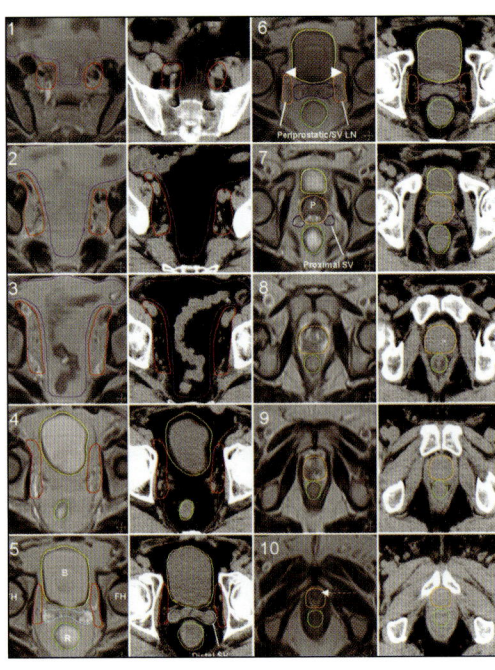

▶ FIGURE 15-16.

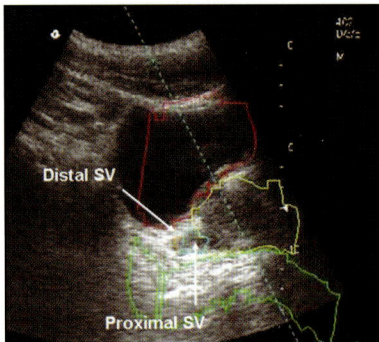

▶ FIGURE 15-18B.

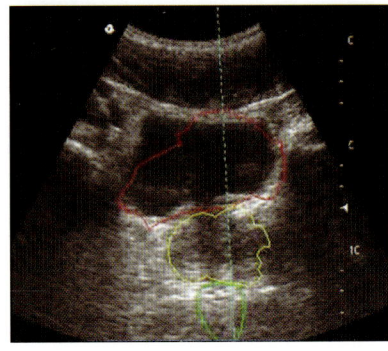

▶ FIGURE 15-18A.